W0080123

Lecture Notes of the Institute
for Computer Sciences, Social Informatics
and Telecommunications Engineering 61

Balwant Godara
Konstantina S. Nikita (Eds.)

Wireless Mobile Communication and Healthcare

Third International Conference
MobiHealth 2012
Paris, France, November 21-23, 2012
Revised Selected Papers

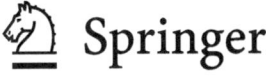 Springer

Volume Editors

Balwant Godara
Institut Supérieur d' Électronique de Paris
Minarc research team
75006 Paris, France
E-mail: bgodara@isep.fr

Konstantina S. Nikita
National Technical University of Athens
School of Electrical and Computer Engineering
15780 Athens, Greece
E-mail: knikita@ece.ntua.gr

ISSN 1867-8211   e-ISSN 1867-822X
ISBN 978-3-642-37892-8   e-ISBN 978-3-642-37893-5
DOI 10.1007/978-3-642-37893-5
Springer Heidelberg Dordrecht London New York

Library of Congress Control Number: 2013935555

CR Subject Classification (1998): K.4, J.3, C.2, H.2.8, C.5.3

Typesetting: Camera-ready by author, data conversion by Scientific Publishing Services, Chennai, India

Printed on acid-free paper

Springer is part of Springer Science+Business Media (www.springer.com)

Preface

The present volume includes the articles presented during the Third International Conference on Wireless Mobile Communication and Healthcare, Mobihealth, that took place in Paris (France) during November 21–23, 2012.

We received a total of 66 proposals. After a rigorous review process involving about 40 reviewers, members of the Technical Programme Committee, and (external experts invited to review with an average of 2.23 reviews per paper), 34 papers were accepted for the final program, yielding an acceptance rate of 59%. Moreover, three experts were invited to present their recent work in a special session on "implantable systems," in order to complete the main conference.

These papers were divided into nine sessions (corresponding to the tracks of the conference):

- Track 1: Wearable, Outdoor and Home-Based Applications
- Track 2: Remote Diagnosis and Patient Management
- Track 3: Data Processing
- Invited Session: Implants
- Track 4: Sensor Devices and Systems
- Track 5: Biomedical Monitoring in Relation to Society and the Environment
- Track 6: Body Area Networks
- Track 7: Telemedicine Systems for Disease-Specific Applications
- Track 8: Data collection and Management

In keeping with the scope of the conference, three keynotes were invited, to speak on the *"Personal Health Record Project in France"* (Anne Monnier of the ASIP Santé Agency of the French Ministry of Health); *"Implantable Active Medical Devices"* (Alain Ripart, chief scientific advisor of the Sorin Group); and *"Standardization Issues in Body-Area Networks"* (Jean Schwoerer of France Telecom and member of the IEEE 802.15.6 group).

The special scope of the conference was the use of ICT for healthcare in developing nations, and this was highlighted by an invited talk on 'Computerization of the Medical Consult for Children Under Five Years of Age in Rural Areas of Burkina Faso', given by Guillaume Deflaux, of the Swiss-based NGO Terre des Hommes. The tutorial entitled "ICT-Enabled Healthcare in Developing Countries" was a major event in this special scope.

The conference also included two side-event workshops. The first, entitled "Wireless Physical Layer Communications for Emerging Healthcare Applications" (*IWAWPLC*) attracted eight presentations. The second, "Personalized Healthcare Services, Wearable Monitoring and Social Media Pervasive Technologies" (*APHS*), included ten presentations.

Technically co-sponsored like its predecessors by the IEEE EMBS Society, this third edition of MobiHealth took place over three days, and included a total of 90 participants from 29 countries. The three days followed the same format. The tone of each day was set by the keynote that started the day. Following this, there were three sessions of four to five papers each, related to the same overall theme as the keynote of the day. The day ended with a "special event": the tutorial on day 1, a panel discussion on the "Concerto" FP7 project on day 2, and the invited talk by Terre des Hommes on day 3. The third day included the two workshops in parallel to the main conference, *IWAWLPLC* in the morning and *APHS* in the afternoon.

First and foremost, we would like to thank the 40-odd reviewers who helped ensure that the selected papers were relevant and of high quality. A special thanks to Asimina Kiourti who was in-charge of the special session, the tutorials, and workshops.

Our gratitude also goes to the participants who responded favorably to our invitations:

- The three keynotes: Monnier, Ripart, and Schwoerer
- The four invited speakers: Garda (Paris VI University, France), Marinkovic (ABB Company, Switzerland), Tanner (EPFL University, Switzerland), and Deflaux (Terre des Hommes).
- The participants of the panel on "Concerto": Dr. Martini (Kingston University, UK), Mr. Iacobelli (Thales Communications and Security, France), Mr. Lecroart (Nec Technologies, France), Mr. Moretti (CNIT Reseach Centre, Italy), and Mr. Takács (Budapest University of Technology and Economics, Hungary).
- The organizers of the two workshops: Prof. Scanlon (Queen's University, UK) and Prof. Nepa (University of Pisa, Italy) for IWAWPLC and Prof. Spanakis (Forth, Greece) for APHS.

We also thank our two student volunteers, Paul de Laforcade and Coumba Cissé, for their presence and their charm. To conclude, we would stress that without the support of the efficient and close-knit team, and our school, the Institut Supérieur d'Electronique de Paris (ISEP), the organization of MobiHealth would have been a much more daunting task.

November 2012   Konstantina Nikita
                                                                 Balwant Godara

Organization

Steering Committee Members

Founding Chair

James C. Lin	University of Illinois at Chicago, USA
Dimitrios Koutsouris	National Technical University of Athens, Greece
Janet Lin	University of Illinois at Chicago, USA
Arye Nehorai	Washington University, St. Louis, USA
Konstantina S. Nikita	National Technical University of Athens, Greece
George Papadopoulos	University of Cyprus

General Co-chairs

Balwant Godara	ISEP Paris, France
Konstantina Nikita	NTUA Athens, Greece

Technical Program Co-chairs

Laura M. Roa	IEEE Fellow, University of Seville, Spain
Nikolaos Bourbakis	IEEE Fellow, Wright State University, USA

Publication Chair

Thomas Ea	ISEP, France

Workshops and Tutorials Chairs

Asimenia Kiourti	NTUA Athens, Greece
Emmanouil Spanakis	Computational Medicine Laboratory, Institute of Computer Science, FORTH
William Scanlon	Queen's University, Belfast, UK and University of Twente, The Netherlands
Paolo Nepa	University of Pisa, Pisa, Italy

Technical Program Committee

Balwant Godara	ISEP Paris, France
Konstantina S. Nikita	NTUA Athens, Greece
Nizamettin Aydin	Yildiz Technical University, Turkey
Paolo Bernardi	La Sapienza University of Rome, Italy
Maria Christopoulou	NTUA Athens, Greece
Dimitrios I. Fotiadis	University of Ioannina, Greece
Thomas Falck	Philips Research Europe, Eindhoven, The Netherlands
Irene Karanasiou	NTUA Athens, Greece
Alexandros Karargyris	National Institute of Health, Bethesda, USA
Mohan Karunanithi	Australian e-Health Research Center, Australia
Ilkka Korhonen	VTT Information Technology, Finland
Luis Kun	National Defense University, DC, USA
Niels Kuster	ITIS Foundation/ETH, Switzerland
Efthyvoulos Kyriakou	Frederick University, Cyprus
Norbert Leitgeb	Graz University of Technology, Austria
Dimitris Lymberopoulos	University of Patras, Greece
James Lin	University of Illinois at Chicago, USA
Janet Lin	University of Illinois at Chicago, USA
Ilias Maglogiannis	University of Central Greece, Greece
Tom Martin	Virginia Tech, VA, USA
Paolo Nepa	University of Pisa, Italy
Alexandros Pantelopoulos	West Wearable Health Institute, CA, USA
Andriana Prentza	University of Piraeus, Greece
Javier Reina-Tosina	University of Seville, Spain
Dan Schonfeld	University of Illinois at Chicago, USA
Koichi Shimizu	Hokkaido University, Japan
Toshiyo Tamura	Chiba University, Japan
Manolis Tsiknakis	ICS-FORTH, Crete, Greece
Kamya-Yekeh Yazdandoost	University of Oulu, FInland
Konstantia Zarkogianni	NTUA Athens, Greece
Mi Zhang	University of Southern California, CA, USA
Yuan-Ting Zhang	Chinese University of Hong Kong, Hong Kong

Table of Contents

Session 3: Data Processing

Session 4: Sensor Devices and Systems

Session 5: Biomedical Monitoring in Relation to Society and the Environment

Session 6: Body Area Networks

Session 7: Telemedicine Systems for Disease-Specific Applications

Session 8: Data Collection and Management

Invited Session "Implants"

Workshop on "Advances in Wireless Physical Layer Communications for Emerging Healthcare Applications" (IWAWPLC 2012)

Workshop on "Advances in Personalized Healthcare Services,Wearable Mobile Monitoring, and Social Media Pervasive Technologies" (APHS 2012)

CareBox: A Complete TV-Based Solution for Remote Patient Monitoring and Care

António Santos, Rui Castro, and João Sousa

Fraunhofer Portugal AICOS, Rua Alfredo Allen 455, 4200-135 Porto, Portugal
{antonio.santos,rui.castro,joao.sousa}@fraunhofer.pt
http://www.fraunhofer.pt

Abstract. Influent voices from different areas like government and insurance companies already realized the savings that could be done with remote health monitoring and assistance systems. The TV is still the technology that older adults feel more comfortable with, and therefore we present *CareBox*, a new prototype that perfectly integrates with TV viewing experience and uses this almost ubiquitous mean to provide some features that they really feel the need in their daily lives: health agenda, medication intake and vital sign measurement scheduling and alerts, vital sign monitoring, videoconference with doctors and other features that may be also useful for doctors like support for medical questionnaires and health videos.

Keywords: Ambient Assisted Living, Telemedicine, Homecare, eHealth, Remote monitoring, TV, Set-top box.

1 Introduction

The majority of older adults are affected with chronic conditions and acute illnesses. Isolation (either physical or social) has been a social weapon that is covertly lowering the results of any care service.

Remote patient monitoring systems have been around for many years and are seen as a solution to reduce the costs for health care, which are still raising due to the increasing of life expectancy [1], but only few had been effectively working in the real world. Lack of interoperability is one of the main reasons for this. The creation of health information standards like ASTM-CCR or HL7 came to promote the interoperability and the adoption of this kind of technology.

CareBox is one of the main results from the EU-funded research projects eCAALYX [2] and CAALYX-MV [3] and was thought-out and designed with all these issues in mind. It aims at using well-known and standard technology to provide a full-featured and easy-to-use remote patient monitoring service, focusing on interoperability standards to allow its adoption by many stakeholders. Apart from the aforementioned features, it was completely designed to be adaptable to any environment and electronic medical record. This will certainly open many doors for the development and integration of new and innovative features.

B. Godara and K.S. Nikita (Eds.): MobiHealth 2012, LNICST 61, pp. 1–10, 2013.

2   State of the art

Fortunately, there are a lot of projects under the telemonitoring and homecare topics but few provide TV-based interfaces for the patient. There are essentially two main alternatives to provide them to the final user: either through an expansion (widget, plugin, etc.) to the official STB firmware of a DTV service provider or through a dedicated STB. Both have benefits and drawbacks. The former alternative allows the software to be easily distributed and maintained, being the costs significantly reduced due to the fact of not needing a dedicated hardware for the service. However, there are major drawbacks like the fact of having rather limited hardware support and little to no control over the operating system. Also, the homecare service can only reach population that holds a subscription to the DTV service. There are several examples of projects that use this approach like KeepInTouch [4], HERA [5], DIGA [6] and Panaceia-ITV [7].

The other alternative to provide TV-based patient monitoring and care services is through a dedicated STB. This approach allows having full control over the system and better hardware support, therefore not depending on any DTV service provider. On the other hand, the costs can be significantly higher. IN-HOME [8], OLDES [9], Avicena [10] and the work in [11] are example of projects that followed this approach.

CareBox fits in this latest category of care services using a dedicated STB. However, it stands out for its open and modular design, adjustable to any needs and focusing on interoperability, the integrated support for several vital sign sensors, the special care on the user interface and the drive for a smooth and intuitive integration with the TV viewing experience.

3   System Design

Providing a modular architecture to *CareBox* means not only there was the care to decouple the presentation layer from the logical layer, but also to decouple the communications layer from the logical layer. Also, there was the focus on using free, open and standardized technologies and protocols to promote the use of the system in every use case. *CareBox* was developed to be running on a *Nvidia ION*-based Mini-PC (Intel Atom 1.6GHz CPU, 2GB RAM) (Fig. 1). The operating system runs on an internal USB pen and is a modified version of the *OpenELEC* distribution, which targets at providing a complete XBMC media center with minimum software requirements, complemented by a *Firefox* web browser for generic use. Having complete control over the *Linux* operating system allows us to provide support for several hardware components, namely peripherals used in the system: dongles for vital-sign sensors, webcams, remote controls, etc.

Most of the implementation was done using the scripting and skinning capabilities that XBMC media center provides to develop plugins using the *Python* programming language.

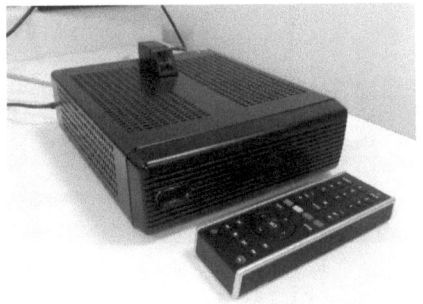

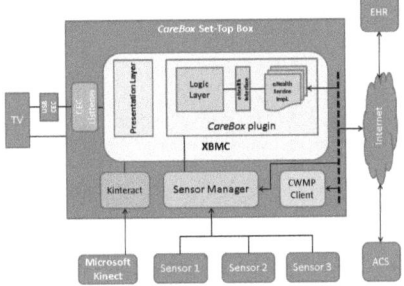

Fig. 1. *CareBox*   **Fig. 2.** *CareBox* architecture

One of the strongest points in *CareBox* is its focus on interoperability. The modular design regarding the communications layer allows the system to support different protocols and communication schemas and technologies, being quite easy to switch from one module to another and to implement new ones. Currently, and since the system was developed under the support of the eCAA-LYX project, only the implementation for the protocol used by the care server developed in the project is available, as well as an early, but quite usable, implementation for the *eHealthCom* [12] server. Nevertheless, implementations for subsets of the ASTM-CCR and HL7-CCD specifications are underway. These implementations will explore all the possibilities of using the standards for every feature available. In case that is not possible, extensions to the standards will be used.

The management of the system can be done remotely since *CareBox* provides an expandable CWMP (TR-069) client that allows not only remote configuration but also remote firmware upgrade through the use of an Auto-Configuration Server (ACS).

4   Technical Details

4.1   General Considerations

CareBox firmware image features a small footprint (slightly more than 120 MB, plus 100 MB if compiled with support for Microsoft *Kinect*) and a quite short cold boot time (nearly 20-30 seconds on a USB pen), although it supports a standby mode.

The system was properly set up in order to include several libraries and frameworks needed for some *CareBox* features. It can use either Ethernet or Wi-Fi to access the Internet and comes with an RF remote control that allows a simple operation of the set-top box. This remote is also programmable so that it can also control the TV set through InfraRed.

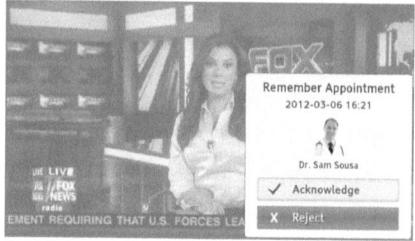

Fig. 3. *Reminders interface (Google TV)*

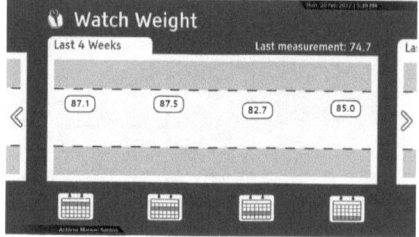

Fig. 4. *Weight graphics*

4.2   Multi-User Support

CareBox was also designed to have multi-user support. Depending on the protocol and caretaker server, the configuration can hold data for more than one user, to be used in scenarios where *CareBox* is shared by multiple users in the same location.

Two login mechanisms are available: one is having a simple user selection interface, without any authentication method. This is the simpler to deploy, although it may raise privacy issues. The second mechanism came to address these issues and uses a fingerprint sensor connected to the STB (via USB) (Fig. 1). Right after validating a fingerprint, the user is automatically logged in and may be logged out manually or by idle timeout.

4.3   User Interface

Regarding the graphical user interface, a lot of care was taken in this matter. It must be emphasized that the system was primarily designed to be used by elderly people, as it was a main requirement of the eCAALYX project, and the current minimalist design is based on the work made by [13] and [14]. The output of this work came from some tests made with real people using low-fidelity prototypes and mock-ups.

4.4   Agenda and Reminders

In order to help the patients in their schedules, a useful medical agenda was developed to ease the tracking of their medication, vital sign measurements and appointments. To raise the usefulness of the system, a reminders system was developed and uses the TV to warn the patient for upcoming events (Fig. 3). It uses time frames based on patient's daily routine: *Wake-up time, Breakfast, Lunch, Dinner* and *Bed time*. This information, alongside last intake time, allows for a quite effective reminders system, alerting the patient for medication at the right time. *CareBox* holds medication information based on common parameters used in standards like ASTM-CCR or HL7. Specifically, medication frequency is based on what SNOMED CT defines.

4.5   Vital Sign Monitoring

Another main feature of *CareBox* is the ability to read vital sign measurements from some sensors (using Bluetooth) and provide the patient with easy reading graphics that represent their evolution. The TV acts as a wizard providing all the guided steps for taking measurements. There is no local storage, although a retry system may be triggered in case of a sporadic network failure. The patient also has the ability to select from within different time frames for each vital sign when viewing the graphics. All the measurements are grouped in time blocks and all the measurements taken within that time block are processed in order to have a mean value that will be shown on the graphic (Fig. 4). While this is straightforward regarding weight, things are a bit trickier in what it takes to blood pressure, since there's no explicit separation of systolic and diastolic graphics. In this case, the mean arterial pressure calculation (MAP) is used, based on the values of the diastolic pressure (DP) and systolic pressure (SP) (1).

$$MAP \simeq \frac{2}{3}(DP) + \frac{1}{3}(SP) \tag{1}$$

CareBox also supports vital sign thresholds per patient, represented as red areas at the top and at the bottom of the graphics.

4.6   Questionnaires

Medical questionnaires are a useful tool for the doctors to retrieve medical data from the patients. Functional Impairment (Barthel Index) or Geriatric Depression Scale questionnaires are common examples in the context of treatments of elderly people with chronic conditions. Although most of them are designed in order to have questions of dichotomous nature, the system supports any number of questions with any number of possible answers.

4.7   Health Videos

Another topic that isn't being vastly explored by this kind of systems is the possibility of using them also for pedagogic purposes. Allowing the patient to watch videos related to their condition, or just providing generic health-related videos (daily exercises, how to use a sensor, etc.) is of utmost importance. Therefore, and exploring the fact of having the system developed on top of a media center framework, *CareBox* easily provides this feature, supporting almost every video and audio format (Fig. 5).

4.8   Videoconference and Emergency Call

A patient will feel much more safe and confident if he knows that he can establish a visual communication with his doctor (or even with his own family) in a quite easy way, anywhere, anytime. As for the doctor, he will certainly be pleased to be able to video-call his patients anywhere, using common technology like, for

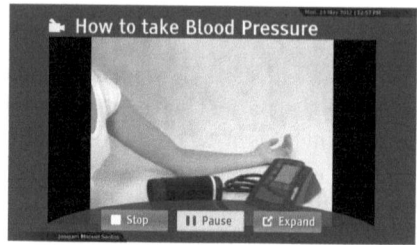
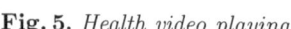

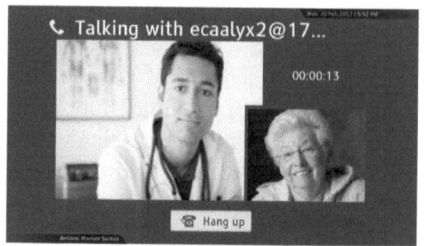

Fig. 5. *Health video playing*   **Fig. 6.** *A running video call*

instance, his own smartphone. Therefore, *CareBox* provides an integrated VoIP client that can be used to start or receive audio/video calls with/from doctors, as long as the needed configuration parameters are provided (Fig. 6). Following the care of using standard technology, this client uses the SIP standard (used by most of existing VoIP services) and currently supports H.263, H.263+ and H264 video codecs (MP4 and VP8 are currently being worked on) and PCMU, PCMA, Speex and Siren audio codecs (GSM and G.726 are also currently being worked on).

The whole client is developed on top of a stack of open-source libraries and frameworks, namely *GStreamer*, *Telepathy*, *Farstream* and *Sofia-SIP*. *CareBox* is provided with a webcam (it includes the microphone) but it should support any webcam compliant with the UVC specification and supported by the *Video4Linux* 2 drivers. *CareBox* also offers an Emergency Call service, which basically uses the VoIP client to make an audio call to a pre-defined contact.

4.9 TV Integration

CareBox is provided as a set-top box that simply connects to an available input on the TV. Although it supports analog connection through VGA output (it provides an adapter for SCART/S-Video connection), *CareBox* also provides a digital HDMI output (for both video and audio) and explores some unused capabilities of this type of connection.

The HDMI-CEC standard allows a device to be able to control others through an HDMI connection. The standard defines several messages and commands that can be used by a device to achieve optimal integration and ease some common operations by the users. *CareBox* supports the HDMI-CEC standard, at least a subset that allows it to be perfectly integrated within the patient's TV viewing experience. Most of the times, the patient will of course be watching his favourite TV shows so if, for instance, a medication reminder is fired or *CareBox* is receiving a call from a doctor, there should be a way for the patient to be instantly notified. *CareBox* can do it through the use of an USB-CEC adapter [15] and a carefully designed and developed daemon for this purpose. When such a scenario happens, *CareBox* will immediately switch the TV input to the one used by itself and the user is asked to follow up the event. When it finishes, *CareBox* will do the reverse and will switch the TV back to the previous input.

Another interesting thing is that the support for the HDMI-CEC standard allows the user to use the TV remote to control the *CareBox*. So there's no need to be always switching the remotes to control either the TV or the *CareBox*. This is a really important feature given the usual resistance by the elderly people to learn to use new input devices.

Currently, most TV manufacturers do support this standard (or at least a subset), although sometimes published under commercial sounding names like *Simplink* (LG), *Anynet+* (Samsung), *Bravia Link* (Sony), *EasyLink* (Philips), etc.

4.10   Google TV Port

With the recent developments on *Google TV*, a clear window of opportunity has opened in what it takes to developing applications for the TV. The video overlaying ability is clearly an added value in this system, allowing notifications on top of the TV image (Fig. 3). Therefore, *CareBox* also has a port for *Google TV*, which can be later distributed as an application through *Google Play*. This port is almost fully functional, when compared with the current features of the standalone version, only missing the support for taking measurements and a VoIP client due to limitations on the support to USB peripherals, including webcams.

4.11   Microsoft Kinect support

Foreseeing the need to promote body activity, *CareBox* has provided the support for Microsoft *Kinect* (support for other similar devices like Asus *Xtion Pro* can be easily added) through the integration of the OpenNI/NITE middleware stack and the development of a natural interaction driver, *Kinteract* [16], that detects some common hand movements (directions, wave, push, backward, etc.) and maps them into pre-configured standard keyboard events, which are then sent into the Linux user level input subsystem (*uinput*). XBMC will then react normally like being controlled by the remote control, allowing the user to easily navigate through the *CareBox* user interface. Taking into account that *CareBox* is primarily designed to be used by older people, some subjects with ages between 60 and 75 were asked to do some movements they feel as appropriate to control the user interface in what it relates to the common actions (up, down, left, right, select, back, etc.). The idea is to improve *Kinteract* so that it can accurately detect some common gesture patterns applied by these users, thus reducing the learn curve, improving the results and therefore motivating the user to select this interaction method more often.

5   Results

Up until now, the only trustful results are the ones that are coming out from the field trials that took place in Germany with 10 patients. All the features were tested except for the *Videoconference/Emergency Call*. The field trials were divided in two phases. The first phase took place in January 2012 and focused more on the usability and stability of the system, with a limited set of features being tested. In what it takes to the home system, namely the STB, it was tested with just the *Health Status* (vital signs) and *Health Agenda* (and *Reminders*) features enabled. Also, the user interface was still in a draft mode and not as stylish as the one presented in this document. The results were not as positive as expected [17]. The patients found the navigation confusing, mainly due to the fact of having the main menu showing all the options, even if some of them were still not available for testing. To worsen things up, the remote control was not working properly due to a manufacturing error and the patients also found the keys too small. Also, the long waiting periods on every request to the Caretaker server (which were due to major issues on the implementation of the server) lowered the rating of the system. Nevertheless, the patients were able to work with the STB after minor training and all the implementation, including all under the hood and system-level applications, was found to be working properly, without major issues being detected. The second phase of the field trials took place in March and April 2012 and already included a larger set of features, except again for the *Videoconference/Emergency Call*. The patients immediately noticed an increase on the usability and the overall results were more positive, even taking into account the learning effect inherent to these second trials. Apart from some minor issues, the overall impression included some considerations and recommendations like: the remote control should be more tailored for this scenario, with only the necessary buttons; long loading times (due to severe connection issues to the Caretaker Server); no immediate visualization of the measurement value on the TV after using a sensor (not an issue anymore since the STB can now act as sensor gateway); learning curve still too steep. Massive field trials will be taken in different countries in the already running CAALYX-MV project, which basically runs a market validation of all the prototypes that came out from the eCAALYX project. These field trials will comprise about 80-100 patients over three different countries.

Also, Fraunhofer Portugal AICOS has recently made another round of internal tests with ten older adults in order to validate the implementation of the user interface and collect feedback in order to improve it. The results of the tests [18] showed that the overall user interface layout is now appropriate, although some interesting findings and recommendations were provided and are already implemented.

6   Conclusions and Future Work

CareBox tries to gather all import features into a single product that can be easily distributed and managed. Currently, and despite still being under heavy development, there are already some foreseen features being implemented like expanding the support to medical information standards (HL7 and ASTM-CCR) and extending the support to sensors using technologies like *ANT+*, *Zigbee* or

Z-Wave. New features are also in the pipeline: promote user mobility with movement games using Kinect, support for the visualization of more vital signs, including physical activity data, and adding new services like, for instance, home automation using recent standards like *OpenURC.* Last but not least, the development of a simplified interface for smartphones could also be of major importance, allowing the user to interact with the system (for instance, acknowledging medication reminders, making/receiving calls, etc.).

Acknowledgements. The authors wish to thank their work colleagues Pedro Saleiro, António Rodrigues, Luis Carvalho, Carlos Resende, Paula Silva, Francisco Nunes, Cláudia Peixoto and Bernardo Pina for all their time and support to this project.

References

1. Continua Health Alliance, Industry Statistics (2012)
2. Enhanced Complete Ambient Assisted Living Experiment, http://www.ecaalyx.org
3. Complete Ambient Assisted Living Experiment-Market Validation, http://www.caalyx-mv.eu
4. Angius, G., Pani, D., Raffo, L., Randaccio, P.: KeepInTouch: A Telehealth System to Improve the Follow-up of Chronic Patients. In: International Conference on Collaboration Technologies and Systems, CTS (2011)
5. Spanoudakis, N., Grabner, B., Kotsiopoulou, C., Lymperopoulou, O., Moser-Siegmeth, V., Pantelopoulos, S., Sakka, P., Moraitis, P.: A Novel Architecture and Process for Ambient Assisted Living - The HERA approach. In: 10th IEEE International Conference on Information Technology and Applications in Biomedicine, ITAB (2010)
6. Oliveira, M., Santos, M., Cunha, P., Bezerra, J.: Implementing Home Care Application in Brazilian Digital TV. In: Information Infrastructure Symposium (2009)
7. Maglaveras, N., Lekka, I., Chouvarda, I., Koutkias, V., Gatzoulis, M., Kotis, T., Tsakali, M., Maglavera, S., Danelli, V., Zeevi, B., Balas, E.: Congenital Heart Disease Patient Home Care Services Using the Interactive TV: The PANACEIA-ITV Approach. Computers in Cardiology (2003)
8. Vergados, D.: Service personalization for assistive living in a mobile ambient healthcare-networked environment. Personal and Ubiquitous Computing 14 (September 2010)
9. Novák, D., Uller, M., Rousseaux, S., Mráz, M., Smrz, J., Stepanková, O., Haluzík, M., Busuoli, M.: Diabetes management in OLDES project. In: Annual International Conference of the IEEE Engineering in Medicine and Biology Society (2009)
10. Guillén, S., Arredondo, M.T., Traver, V., García, J.M., Fernández, C.: Multimedia Telehomecare System Using Standard TV Set. IEEE Transactions on Biomedical Engineering (2002)
11. Faro, A., Giordano, D., Kavasidis, I., Spampinato, C.: A Web 2.0 Telemedicine System integrating TV-centric Services and Personal Health Records. In: 10th IEEE International Conference on Information Technology and Applications in Biomedicine, ITAB (2010)

12. Ferreira, L., Ambrósio, P.: Towards an Interoperable Health-Assistive Environment: the eHealthCom Platform. In: IEEE-EMBS International Conference on Biomedical and Health Informatics (2012)
13. Nunes, F.: Healthcare TV Based User Interfaces for Older Adults. Master's thesis, Faculdade de Engenharia da Universidade do Porto (2010)
14. Santos, J.: Personal Health Channel. Master's thesis, Faculdade de Engenharia da Universidade do Porto (2010)
15. USB-CEC Adapter,
    `http://www.pulse-eight.com/store/products/104-usb-hdmi-cec-adapter.aspx`
16. Melo, T.: Gesture Recognition for Natural Interaction with Applications. Master's thesis, Faculdade de Ciências da Universidade do Porto (2012)
17. Prescher, S., Bourke, A.K., Koehler, F., Martins, A., Ferreira, H.S., Sousa, T.B., Castro, R.N., Santos, A., Torrent, M., Gomis, S., Hospedales, M., Nelson, J.: A Ubiquitous Ambient Assisted Living Solution to Promote Safer Independent Living in Older Adults Suffering from Co-morbidity. In: 34th Annual International Conference of the IEEE Engineering in Medicine & Biology Society, EMBC (2012)
18. Nunes, F.: Usability Testing eCAALYX TV UI. Fraunhofer Portugal AICOS (2012)

Biomedical Monitoring
of Non-hospitalized Subjects
Using Disruption-Tolerant Wireless Sensors

Frédéric Guidec[1], Djamel Benferhat[1], and Patrice Quinton[2]

[1] IRISA, Université de Bretagne-Sud, France
{Frederic.Guidec,Djamel.Benferhat}@univ-ubs.fr
[2] IRISA, ENS Cachan Bretagne, France
Patrice.Quinton@bretagne.ens-cachan.fr

Abstract. The proliferation of private, corporate and community Wi-Fi hotspots in city centers and residential areas opens up new opportunities for the collection of biomedical data produced by sensors carried by mobile non-hospitalized subjects.

In this paper we investigate the possibility of using these many hotspots as gateways for biomedical data transmission. A disruption-tolerant application is presented, that can record biomedical data while the subject is not in the range of a Wi-Fi hotspot, and upload recorded data to a remote monitoring center whenever a hotspot is located nearby. Results of a field trial are presented, with a scenario involving a subject wearing an ECG-enabled sensor, walking in the streets of a residential area.

Keywords: wireless networking, delay/disruption-tolerant networking, sensor networking, biomedical monitoring.

1   Introduction

Wireless sensors open up interesting opportunities for biomedical monitoring, such as the long-term, continuous monitoring of subjects in a clinical environment or at home [1,2]. In a typical deployment scenario, one or several wireless sensors are attached to a subject, and a wireless base station is installed in this subject's surroundings. This base station can either record the data received from the sensors, or it can forward these data directly to a remote site, such as a physician's desktop computer or a hospital's monitoring center. In any case, since the sensors are wireless the subject can move freely around the base station, while an endless stream of data flows from the sensors he is carrying to the base station. This freedom of movement is however hampered by the short transmission range of current off-the-shelf wireless sensors. Indeed, most of these sensors include low-power radio transceivers, with which actual transmission ranges usually do not exceed a few meters. For this reason most research projects targeting health monitoring on mobile subjects rely either on dedicated base stations that

B. Godara and K.S. Nikita (Eds.): MobiHealth 2012, LNICST 61, pp. 11–19, 2013.

must be deployed specifically for that purpose [3], or assume ubiquitous connectivity to 2.5/3G infrastructure [4].

The concept of *Disruption-Tolerant Networking*[1] *(DTN)* is a means to cope with challenging situations where continuous transmissions cannot be guaranteed. When considering a scenario involving mobile wireless devices, the general idea is to apply the *store, carry, and forward* principle: a device that is temporarily disconnected from the network can *store* data for a while in a local cache, carry these data while moving towards a location where network connectivity can be restored, and ultimately *forward* the data when circumstances permit.

Applying the store, carry and forward principle in wireless biomedical sensors is an appealing prospect. Indeed, a clinician monitoring a subject remotely does not necessarily need to receive data concerning this subject in real time. In most cases a time lag of a few minutes is perfectly tolerable. Using the store, carry and forward principle therefore makes sense in order to give greater mobility to the monitored subject. To the best of our knowledge this approach has not been investigated much so far, although disruption-tolerant solutions for *non-biomedical* sensor-based applications have already been proposed in the literature [5,6,7].

The solution we consider specifically in this paper consists in using any accessible Wi-Fi hotspot as a gateway for data uploading. Nowadays, Wi-Fi hotspots can be counted in millions. Besides corporate hotspots, most DSL providers distribute residential gateways that include a builtin Wi-Fi access point, which can operate a private and public Wi-Fi hotspot simultaneously. When a DSL subscriber accepts to enable the public hotspot service on his own residential gateway, he can in return access any other public hotspot deployed by the same DSL provider in the country. The millions of public hotspots managed by a single provider therefore constitute a wide community network that covers a significant part of urban areas. A subject should thus be able to attend to his daily business, while the sensing system he's wearing relies on nearby hotspots to upload data to a monitoring center.

The remainder of this paper is organized as follows. The SHIMMER platform we use in this project for data acquisition on mobile subjects is described in Section 2. Section 3 presents the main features of the transmission chain we designed in order to support the disruption-tolerant transmission of data between subjects and a monitoring center. In Section 4 we present the results of one of the field trials we conducted in order to validate this approach. Section 5 concludes this paper.

2   Overview of SHIMMER Sensors

In this project we use SHIMMER platforms in order to acquire biomedical data on non-hospitalized subjects (see Fig. 1). The SHIMMER platform is a programmable lighweight wireless sensing system that can record and transmit physiological and kinematic data in real-time [8]. Data acquisition is performed on up to 8 channels through a 12-bit AD converter. Several kinds of expansion

---

[1] The term Delay-Tolerant Networking is also used in the literature.

modules are available, including physiological sensors such as ECG (electrocardiography), EMG (electromyography) and GSR (galvanic skin response) sensors, as well as kinematic sensors for 3-axis angular rate sensing and 3-axis low field magnetic sensing.

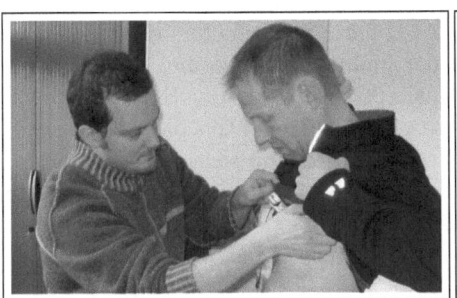 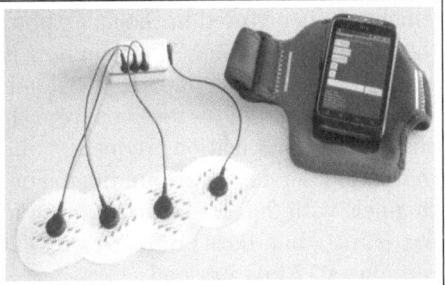

Fig. 1. A volunteer is equipped with an ECG-enabled SHIMMER sensor and a smartphone (which can be worn in an armband or in a pocket)

Two low-power radio transceivers operating in the 2.4 GHz ISM band are included in the platform: an IEEE 802.15.4/ZigBee compliant CC2420 transceiver, and a WML-C46A class 2 Bluetooth transceiver. Since none of these standards can be used to connect directly to a Wi-Fi (IEEE 802.11) access point, an additional wearable device is required to serve as a relay between a SHIMMER sensor and a Wi-Fi access point. In the solution we propose this relaying device is an Android smartphone, which can receive data continuously from the sensor through a Bluetooth RFCOMM link, and forward these data whenever possible to nearby Wi-Fi access points, while tolerating the transient connectivity to such access points.

3   Protocol for Data Acquisition and Transmission

We developed specific code in nesC (a dialect of C) for the SHIMMER sensors, and a Java application for Android smartphones. The main features of this code are detailed below.

Data Acquisition on a SHIMMER Sensor. This acquisition is performed on two 12-bit channels, with a sampling frequency that can be adjusted as needed. The nature of the data depends on the kind of expansion module that is associated with the main unit. In any case the data stream produced by the sensor is transmitted on-the-fly to the smartphone through a Bluetooth RFCOMM link.

Transmission between Sensor and Smartphone. Each sensor must be paired with a specific smartphone, and two paired devices must of course be carried by the same subject. Once a smartphone is paired with a sensor, an RFCOMM link is established between them. Through this link, the smartphone can control the sensor, and send simple commands in order to adjust the sampling frequency or resolution, to start or stop data acquisition, etc. When data acquisition is enabled on a sensor, a continuous data stream is sent to the smartphone through the RFCOMM link.

The data stream received by the smartphone is packetized in small bundles, which are then stored in the smartphone's SD-card, awaiting for transmission to the monitoring center. The bundle's header includes an identifier of the source sensor and a timestamp. Its payload is simply a byte array that contains a sequence of data bytes received from the sensor. The size of this payload depends on the data acquisition frequency and resolution on the sensor, as well as on the period set for data bundling. For example, data acquisition on two 12-bit channels with 200 Hz sampling produces a continuous data stream at 4.8 kbps. Assuming a bundle is produced every 20 seconds on the smartphone, each bundle contains a 12 kiB payload.

Hotspot Discovery, Selection, and Authentication. When a subject enters a hotspot, the smartphone he is carrying must detect the Wi-Fi access point that serves this hotspot and attempt to associate with it. If the association succeeds, the smartphone must send a DHCP request in order to obtain IP parameters from a DHCP server. Finally, some form of authentication may be required before access to the Internet is granted.

In order to ensure hotspot discovery, selection, and authentication in our project we rely on Wi2Me, an Android-based application that has been designed specifically to support fast handover between hotspots in corporate and community networks [9].

Wi2Me notably uses active probe requests (rather than the standard's default passive scan) in order to locate nearby hotspots, and Kalman filters to characterize signal attenuation tendencies and select interesting hotspots accordingly. When connecting to a selected hotspot Wi2Me can authenticate with this hotspot using the standard WPA (Wi-Fi Protected Access) procedure, or through an HTTPS captive portal.

Transmission between Smartphone and Remote Server. Once the Wi2Me application has managed to establish a connection and to authenticate with a nearby hotspot, the disruption-tolerant Android application we designed can start uploading data bundles to a server that is the entry point of the monitoring center. This application basically behaves like a client thread with respect to the server. Whenever a "Connected" notification is issued by the Wi2Me program, this thread attempts to open a TCP session with the server. If this attempt fails, the thread waits for a few seconds before initiating another attempt. Once a TCP session is established, bundles stored in the local cache are sent to the server sequentially, and each bundle received by the server is acknowledged explicitly at application level. This approach allows the client thread to detect and react to transmission failures, which typically occur when the subject carrying the smartphone moves out of the radio range of the current hotspot.

The Wi-Fi connection is then broken unexpectedly, and the TCP session must be closed unilaterally on the client side while TCP segments (containing fragments of data bundles) are still pending in the client socket's send buffer. The client thread then waits for the next "Connected" notification from the Wi2Me program, and as soon as this notification is received it tries to open a new TCP session with the server. If a bundle sent during the previous TCP session has not been acknowledged yet, then this bundle is sent again. Afterwards, the client thread resumes its normal routine activity, which consists in sending available data bundles one after another, and waiting for an acknowledgement after each bundle.

Several strategies can be devised in order to determine which data bundles should be sent first when a smartphone establishes a connection with a new hotspot. An option is for example to preserve the chronological ordering of data bundles, uploading the oldest bundles first. In the current implementation we decided to favor the transmission of "fresh" data first, and to fill the gaps by uploading older bundles whenever possible. The application's client thread was therefore implemented in such a way that "real-time" bundles (i.e. those produced during a radio contact between the sensor and the base station) get uploaded to the monitoring center first, and the time remaining during a contact window is used to upload "older" bundles, that is, bundles that are stored on the smartphone's micro-SD card and that have not been uploaded to the monitoring center yet. A graphical application running in the monitoring center can thus display the latest data concerning a subject, while allowing an operator to rewind the data stream in order to display past data if necessary.

4   Experimental Results

In order to validate our approach, we conducted several field trials involving volunteers carrying SHIMMER sensors and HTC Wildfire S smartphones.

Several scenarios were considered, with subjects staying at home, going to work, shopping, etc. In this section we present the results observed with a subject wearing an ECG-enabled SHIMMER sensor, walking along the streets and footpaths of a residential area. During this trial the smartphone was configured so as to split the ECG data stream received from the sensor in 16 kiB bundles, each bundle containing 20 seconds of recorded data. Additionally, the Wi2Me application running on the smartphone was configured so as to seek and connect to any community hotspot administered by either of the French network operators Free and SFR.

The subject was first equipped at home with an ECG-enabled sensor and a smartphone (Fig. 1). After a few minutes he went for a 4.6 km walk, and came back home about an hour later. Figure 2 shows the route followed by the subject during his walk, as well as the community hotspots his smarphone managed to connect to along that route. Figure 3 shows the timeline of data bundles storage and transmissions during this experiment, as well as the connectivity status of the smartphone.

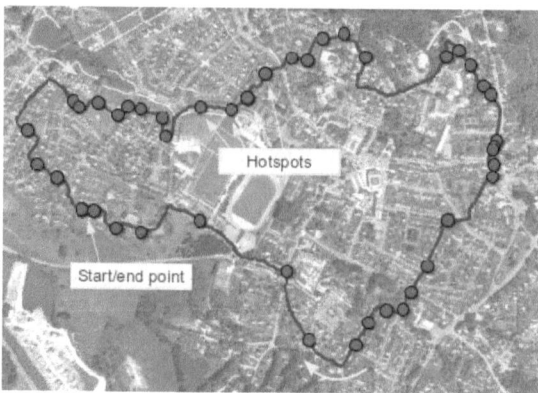

Fig. 2. Route followed by the volunteer subject during the experiment. The green circles represent community hotspots used by his smartphone to upload ECG data while he walked along streets and footpaths.

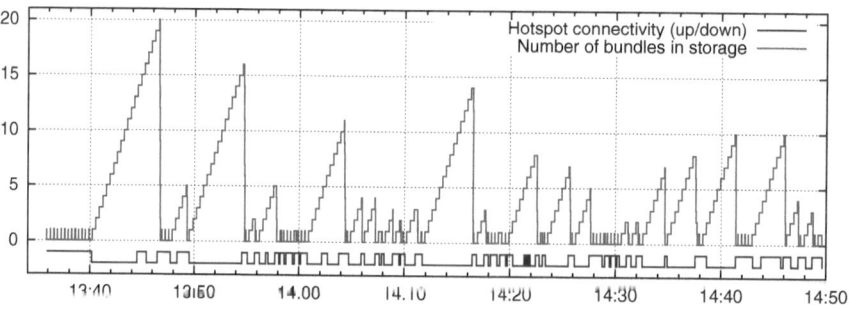

Fig. 3. Timeline of data storage and transmissions during the experiment

At 13:35 both devices were switched on. The sensor immediately started monitoring the cardiac activity of the subject, while the smartphone connected to the subject's own Wi-Fi access point (the most accessible hotspot at that time). The bundles of ECG data produced were therefore transmitted in real time to the remote server. At 13:40 the subject went out. The smartphone then disconnected from the access point, and started storing data bundles. At 13:44 the smartphone connected to a second hotspot, but did not manage to upload bundles through that hotspot. At 13:46 it connected to a third hotspot, and this time it managed to upload through that hotspot the 20 bundles stored in its cache. Since the connection with that hotspot was maintained for almost one minute, the smartphone additionally managed to upload a couple of "fresh" bundles before the connection was broken. As the subject continued walking in the streets further connections were established with community hotspots, until the subject came back home around 14:47.

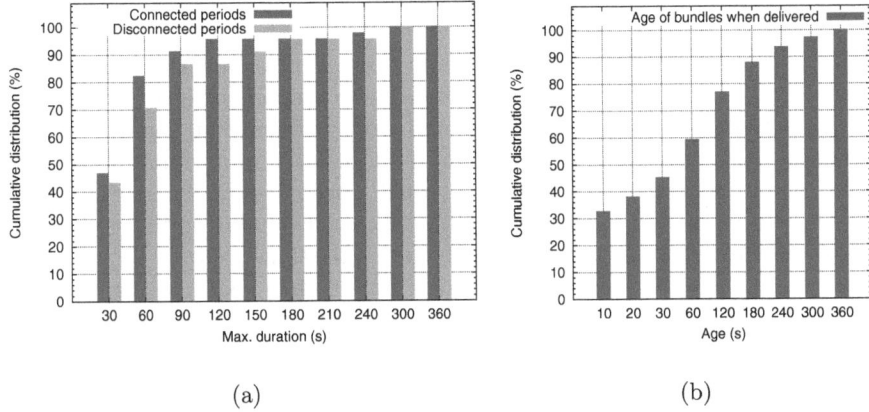

Fig. 4. Cumulative distribution (a) of hotspot connectivity periods, and (b) of the age of bundles at delivery time

This trial lasted 74 minutes, and 45 hotspots were used for data uploading in the meantime. Figure 4.a shows the cumulative distribution of connected and disconnected periods. It can be observed that about 80% of the connections to hotspots lasted less than one minute, which is consistent with the fact that the subject was mobile –and walking at a steady pace– most of the time during the period considered. Similarly, it can be observed that more than 90% of the disconnected periods lasted less than 2.5 minutes. This observation confirms that the density of community hotspots in a residential area is such that a disruption-tolerant application like ours can find many opportunities to upload data to a remote server. The delay before data bundles can reach the server of course depends on the frequency of connections with hotspots. As shown in Figure 4.b, during this trial most bundles reached the server in less than one minute, and no bundle was more than 6 minutes old when it reached the server.

During this trial the battery level on the smartphone dropped by 40%. Since the GPS receiver was enabled in order to record the route followed by the subject, this figure is not a good indication of the autonomy of the system. According to measurements we performed in our laboratory, a SHIMMER sensor with an ECG expansion module can run for almost 10 hours on its built-in battery, while sending data continuously on a Bluetooth RFCOMM link. A HTC Wildfire S smartphone maintaining a Bluetooth connection with a SHIMMER sensor and establishing episodic connections with nearby Wi-Fi hotspots depletes its battery in 5 to 7 hours, depending on the frequency of radio contacts with these hotspots. In contrast, it is worth mentioning that if the smartphone uses 3G transmissions instead of Wi-Fi transmissions its battery is depleted in less than 3 hours.

These figures confirm that with a combination of Bluetooth and Wi-Fi transmissions (with disruption tolerance on the Wi-Fi segment) a subject can be monitored during his daily activity, provided the smartphone's battery can be recharged at least once or twice during the meantime.

5   Conclusion

In this paper we investigated the possibility to collect biomedical data on non-hospitalized mobile subjects. The approach we propose involves off-the-shelf wireless sensors for data acquisition, and smartphones that can record data continuously and upload these data whenever possible to a remote monitoring center. Transient connectivity with personal, corporate, or community Wi-Fi hotspots is used by a disruption-tolerant application running on the smartphone to perform data uploading transparently and opportunistically.

Results of a field trial involving a subject walking in a residential area confirm that the density of community hotspots in such an environment is sufficient to ensure regular updates of the data collected by the monitoring center. Other trials conducted in different conditions (subject at work, shopping, practising sports, etc) have led to similar conclusions.

There are of course circumstances when the smartphone carried by a subject may be unable to connect to a Wi-Fi hotspot for long periods of time. In such circumstances it may be useful to resort to 3G transmissions, if only to upload a minimal set of data while waiting for the next hotspot connection. With this approach the major bottlenecks are the lower transmission rate (for upload) and the power-greedy nature of 3G transmissions. In future papers we shall propose a combination of these solutions, balancing transmission delays with cost and longevity.

References

1. Alemdar, H., Ersoy, C.: Wireless Sensor Networks for Healthcare: a Survey. Computer Networks 54(15), 2688–2710 (2010)
2. Konstantas, D., Herzog, R.: Continuous Monitoring of Vital Constants for Mobile Users: the MobiHealth Approach. In: 25th Annual International Conference of the IEEE EMBS, pp. 3728–3731 (2003)
3. Babovic, Z., Crnjin, A., Racocevic, G., Stankovic, M., Peric, Z., Cirkovic, I., Damjanovic, I., Milutinovic, V.: Prosense Reaseach Activities in Belgrad (2009)
4. Konstantas, D., Jones, V., Herzog, R.: MobiHealth Innovative 2.5-3G Mobile Services and Applications for Healthcare. In: Proceedings of the Eleventh Information Society Technologies (IST) Mobile and Wireless Telecommunications, pp. 43–52 (2002)
5. Pisztor, B., Musolesi, M., Mascolo, C.: Opportunistic Mobile Sensor Data Collection with SCAR. In: Proc. IEEE Int'l Conf. on Mobile Adhoc and Sensor Systems (MASS 2007), pp. 1–22. IEEE Press (2007)
6. Jain, S., Shah, R., Brunette, W., Borriello, G., Roy, S.: Exploiting Mobility for Energy Efficient Data Collection in Wireless Sensor Networks. MONET 11(3), 327–339 (2006)
7. Nayebi, A., Sarbazi-Azad, H., Karlsson, G.: Routing, Data Gathering, and Neighbor Discovery in Delay-Tolerant Wireless Sensor Networks. In: 23rd IEEE International Symposium on Parallel and Distributed Processing, IPDPS 2009, Rome, Italy, May 23-29, pp. 1–6. IEEE CS (2009)

8. Burns, A., Greene, B., McGrath, M., O'Shea, T., Kuris, B., Ayer, S., Stroiescu, F., Cionca, V.: SHIMMER: A Wireless Sensor Platform for Noninvasive Biomedical Research. IEEE Sensors Journal (9), 1527–1534 (2010)
9. Castignani, G., Lampropulos, A.M., Blanc, A., Montavont, N.: Wi2Me: A Mobile Sensing Platform for Wireless Heterogeneous Networks. In: IEEE International Workshop on Sensing, Networking, and Computing with Smartphones (ICDCS 2012), Macau, China (June 2012)

ANT+ Medical Health Kit for Older Adults

Ricardo Belchior[1], Diogo Júnior[1], and António Monteiro[2]

[1] Associação Fraunhofer Portugal Research, Rua Alfredo Allen 455, 4200-135 Porto, Portugal
[2] Faculdade de Engenharia da Universidade do Porto, Rua Dr. Roberto Frias, s/n 4200-465 Porto, Portugal

Abstract. This paper describes the research made on current mobile health monitoring systems targeting the elderly and the development of an elderly-oriented solution, serving as a proof-of-concept of the research done. It provides a scientific contribution by specifying a system with characteristics never combined before, when applied to the health monitoring of older adults. Also, a prototype for that system was developed and evaluated with its end users – the elderly.

The proof of concept solution allows the patient to measure his weight and blood pressure with ANT+ sensors connected to his Android smartphone. The measured data is stored on the mobile device for later reading and sent through the network, to a medical entity. This entity can, whenever desired, analyse that information and give an appropriate feedback to the patient through a web application.

Keywords: health monitoring, mobile health system, wireless sensors, ANT+, Android.

1 Introduction

Rising life expectancy and declining birth rates are ageing the population of most developed countries all over the world and in a few years there will be a large portion of senior citizens in our society [12]. Therefore, it is very important to figure out ways to improve their well-being and quality of life.

Unfortunately, the elderly are more likely to suffer from certain types of diseases when compared to younger people and if a problem is not detected in time, serious problems can arise, resulting in a longer and more difficult treatment. Which means they need to be monitored more often in order to detect changes in their condition as early as possible [13]. Long trips to the hospital, expensive medical appointments or the lack of specialized doctors in remote areas, are all motives that constantly lead an older person not to have proper health cares [3].

In addition, if the patient eventually gets worse, he will probably have to pay for several medications and different treatments. Treatments that usually also have costs for the hospital; several studies have shown that the health care expenditures increase significantly for the elderly [7]. Eventually if the patient needs to be hospitalized, these numbers will obviously rise and the simple fact of being in the hospital can bring more problems to his health condition [9].

B. Godara and K.S. Nikita (Eds.): MobiHealth 2012, LNICST 61, pp. 20–29, 2013.
© Institute for Computer Sciences, Social Informatics and Telecommunications Engineering 2013

Summing up, the lack of proper monitoring might end up bringing costs to both patient and health system.

Recent improvements in sensor technology have allowed the creation of small, light weight and wireless devices that are practical and easy to use by almost everyone. The result is that much of the process of clinical examination, once done in uncomfortable and harsh environments, can now be done at the patient's place of comfort. Combining this technology with the computing power of a smart-phone and its connectivity to the Internet, there is a large number of possibilities to try to reduce some of the problems regarding the elderly. Renowned entities are already embracing these trends, as the Medical Technology Policy Committee of the IEEE USA refers: "Appropriate adoption of existing and emerging technology can improve the efficiency and quality of health care delivery, restrain cost increases and, perhaps most importantly, improve the quality of life for our ageing population" [2].

1.1   Motivation

The motivation of this work was to apply the growing use of communication technologies, namely the smart-phones and the Internet, in order to:

- **Prevent health problems** — Frequent monitoring of the elderly can avoid severe health problems [13,3]. This monitoring often consists of checking a few parameters, like the heart rate, the blood pressure, among others. Most of these values can be read with wireless sensors and then sent to a common smart-phone. A possible scenario is one in which a patient has a blood pressure monitor at home, does a couple readings and those values are sent to the patient's smart-phone. The mobile device is then able to store those values and send them to the patient's doctor that can, at a later moment, give a more accurate feedback to the patient;
- **Enhance the doctor-patient communication** — Nowadays with the Internet, it is very easy to send big amounts of information in a fast and cheap way. As a result, information that was once only available through direct contact with the patient, can now be easily sent with a smart-phone;
- **Reduce costs** — Both smart-phones and the Internet are becoming more and more accessible to the population in terms of costs and availability. This fact makes the solution being here presented, a feasible and useful product to the patients and also to the health system. A study states that with mobile healthcare, costs related to data collection can be reduced by 24% and costs in elderly care can be reduced by 25% [17,7,9].

1.2   Goals

The goal of this study was to research on mobile health systems for the elderly, using the ANT+ wireless technology and create a system as proof of concept with the interactions presented on Figure 1.

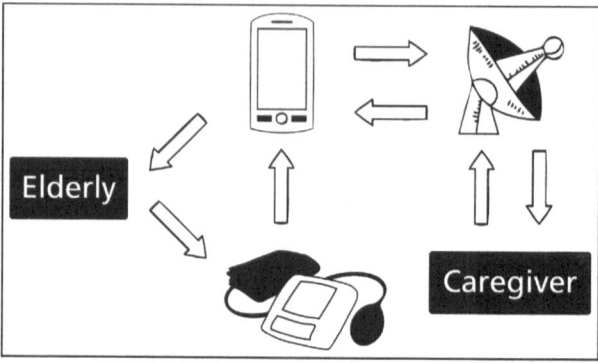

Fig. 1. System architecture

A certain patient would have his sensor that would capture one of several values, including heart rate, blood pressure, weight, body fat, among others. The sensor would then receive the data from the patient and send it to the smart-phone, allowing him to immediately read the collected data. At the same time, that data would be sent through the network to a medical entity, who could analyse it thoroughly and contact the patient again, if necessary. The same information could be registered in a remote server, in charge of the medical entity, so that the doctor would be able to review the historical data from any patient, at any time.

1.3   ANT+

ANT+ is a wireless sensor network technology, designed to enable communications between self powered devices in an extensible network environment, easing the collection, automatic transfer and tracking of sensor data for monitoring of all personal wellness information. This ability to transfer data between sensors is a feature built on top of the base ANT protocol, a proprietary technology. Rod Morris, director of ANT Wireless states at the ANT+ website [18], that ANT is the lightest protocol available that still has the ability to scale into complex network topologies and communication methods, achieving lower costs and power. It is capable of being powered by a coin cell battery, operating on it for up to several years. ANT+ is said to be compact, with a small stack size; scalable, supporting complex network topologies; flexible, supporting ad hoc network reconfiguration; focused, by not being a standard development organization; and proven, because of the millions of nodes delivered around the world.

Ant+ has several device profiles defining the network parameters and the structure of data, so that different products are able to communicate seamlessly. Current ANT+ profiles are currently available for the following devices: Heart Rate Monitor, footpod, Bicycle Speed and Cadence, Bicycle Power, Weight Scale, Multi-Sport Speed and Distance (Radar, GPS).

It is a quite recent technology and not much research has been done using it. Besides, most of the products available on the market focus on sports and fitness, instead of health and well being. One of the innovative points of this study was to take advantage of this technology and apply it to health services.

2   Work Description

The following subsections describe the work done during this study, starting with a review on the state of the art research, followed by a description on the system requirements specification and architecture, both usability tests that were conducted and the implementation of the working prototype.

The prototype consisted on a mobile application developed under the Android operating system, to be used by the patient and to connect with the ANT+ sensor devices; and a web application developed in Ruby On Rails, targeted for the physicians and in charge of receiving and transmitting data to each patient's mobile application.

2.1   State of the Art

Research was made on all areas whose domain intersects this study, going from similar mobile health systems, to designing applications for the elderly, to the technologies being used.

Although related projects have already been developed, some do not use the technologies in this study, others are seeking the detection of health problems in real-time and others are simply not targeted to the elderly [10,5,3,1]. Seto et al. [16] conducted a comprehensive study on mobile health monitoring, providing insights on the main features contributing to a successful heart failure telemonitoring system, claiming it should provide immediate self-care and clinical feedback, it should be easy to use and the perceived benefits of using the system should be clear to everyone involved

Holzinger et al. [6] review the major problems of the elderly using mobile phones, as a way to understand what developers can change to create applications capable of reaching their needs; categorizing their problems into cognitive, motivational, physical and perceptive. Regarding the patient's attitudes and perceptions, it should also be noticed that not all the elderly will be willing to adopt such a monitoring system. A study from Marzegalli et al. [8], showed that some patients embraced the use of mobile applications for remote monitoring, although they were not willing to replace the personal contact with their health workers and older patients with disabilities will find it difficult to adapt to such systems.

The researcher Sarasohn-Kahn [15], is concerned that too much application development is carried out by specialists without the involvement of patients. She believes that the challenges to the smart phone growth include finding the right business model and privacy issues. A report by Fox and Purcell [4] presents the same opinion by stating that despite already existing hundreds of health oriented applications, few of them are designed thinking about the patient in the first place.

At the moment of writing this paper, no project was found that combined the ANT+ technology with the Android platform, together with a web application, for health monitoring of the elderly. Also, this research reinforced the importance of usability when aiming for the elderly. At last, it was noticed that no evaluation metrics were found on the prototypes developed within these studies, leaving little room for a proper comparison with the prototype built for the current study.

2.2   Requirements Elicitation

For a better requirements specification, interviews were conducted with a few medical specialists, bringing a better knowledge on general health care and on the clinicians opinions regarding this project. As expected, some of these thoughts confirmed what other studies have already stated. The main opinions that resulted from the interviews are presented next:

- Hypertension and diabetes would be the most easily detected diseases, within the monitoring system here envisioned, using a blood pressure monitor and glucose meter, respectively[1].
- A better knowledge of the disease by the patient himself is always beneficial and integrating some kind of hint advisor before and/or after each measurements, would be interesting, thereby confirming the study from Seto et al. [16].
- Regarding the user interface, they thought to be very important to keep things simple and not complicate processes and operations for both patients and physicians.
- Giving constant feedback from the clinician to his patient is an important feature, although it may be hard for him to handle extra workload and a proper delegation of work between doctors and nurses should be made.
- Similar systems currently being used are focused on real-time monitoring, with the patient having to walk with a device at all time. The flexibility and mobility provided by the system being developed here would be a big advantage.
- All interviewed clinicians referred the importance of separating the information presented to patients and physicians. For instance, if an anomaly is detected perhaps it is not wise to show it to the patient right away, or even show it at all. This type of information may worry the patient in a way that is not beneficial for either patient and physician.

Given all the insights and after weighting the pros and cons, important decisions were made on the features to be developed on the working prototype.

2.3   System Architecture

A description of how physical components interact between each other is presented on Figure 2. This diagram was grouped by: devices which solely interact

---

[1] During this study, the only available devices were a weight scale and a blood pressure monitor.

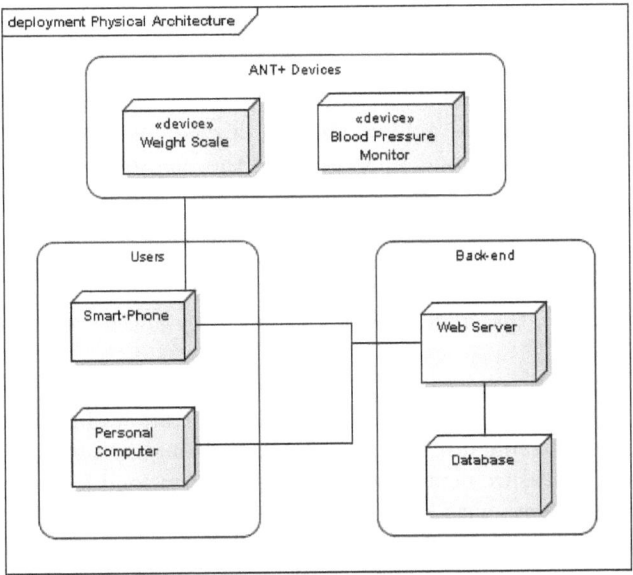

Fig. 2. Physical Model

with ANT+ technology, devices which remain on the back-end and devices used by patients and physicians.

On the users devices there is the smart-phone, which is used by the elderly and interacts with all available ANT+ devices – weight scale and blood pressure monitor. The other device on this group is the personal computer, used by either patients or physicians. Both users devices interact with the web server on the back end group, serving as the connection point between the system users. At last, the web server connects with its database in order to store and retrieve the system's persistence data.

2.4   Low-Fidelity Usability Tests

Once the system was thoroughly planned, low-fidelity usability tests were conducted with 9 elderly between 62 and 81 years old and in average, 71.6 years old, willing to help the project. The tests followed instructions advised by human-computer interaction experts, such as the think aloud protocol [14] or how to properly introduce the test to the participant [11].

This phase resulted in user-interface prototypes and its advantages were significant: a much better understanding of the users by the developer and the output provided – user interface prototypes – which ended up saving much of the development time, thereby accomplishing a better quality in the proof-of-concept solution.

2.5   Implementation

The mobile application development, started by implementing the ANT+ communication with the available devices – a weight scale and a blood pressure monitor. Then the Android application was developed, allowing the elderly to measure his weight and blood pressure with the help of the smart-phone and if desired, send those values to his clinician — the values are stored on a local database for later reading. He is also able to communicate with his clinician by sending and receiving messages through the application interface. Furthermore, if a physician schedules a measurement with one of the sensor devices, within the web application, the smart-phone appropriately notifies the elderly of such measurement.

The web application was targeted for the clinicians, although patients also have access to it. From a clinician point-of-view, it allows him to choose what patients he wants to monitor. Once a patient is being monitored by him, he is able to: view his measurements and messages history; send him a new message; schedule measurements with a custom frequency; and specify threshold values for each sensor, so that he is warned whenever a measurement value is too high or too low. From the patient's point-of-view, he can access the web application in order to view his measurements and messages history and also send the physician a new message.

2.6   Prototype Usability Tests

Once both mobile and web applications were done, it was time to test the prototype with its end users, the elderly. Similarly to the usability tests previously conducted, 9 elderly were involved in the tests, this time between 59 and 74 years old and in average, 67.8 years old. These tests were conducted within an apartment, so the elderly could feel more confortable, relaxed and the tasks they would do could be simulated with the maximum possibly realism.

The goal was to simulate the entire process of the system's usage: the patient goes to an appointment in the hospital or clinic, then goes home with both smart-phone and ANT+ devices, and when a scheduled alarm appears on the phone he measures himself with the corresponding device and sends the values to his physician. Then on the web application side, a clinician analyses the patient's measurements and sends a feedback message to the patient. Now back to the patient, he receives that message, reads it and gives an answer to his physician. To finish the process, the patient uses the smart-phone to review his latest measurements. In each session the smart-phone was given to the participant and the entire session was recorded from three angles: one camera on the living room, another on the bedroom and the last one on the smart-phone itself, recording everything the elderly was doing.

All testes were made in average, in 29 minutes, with a standard deviation of 5 minutes. The graph presented on Figure 3, shows how much time each measurement took, from the moment a participant received an alarm in the smart-phone, to the moment he sent the values to his physician. Each blood

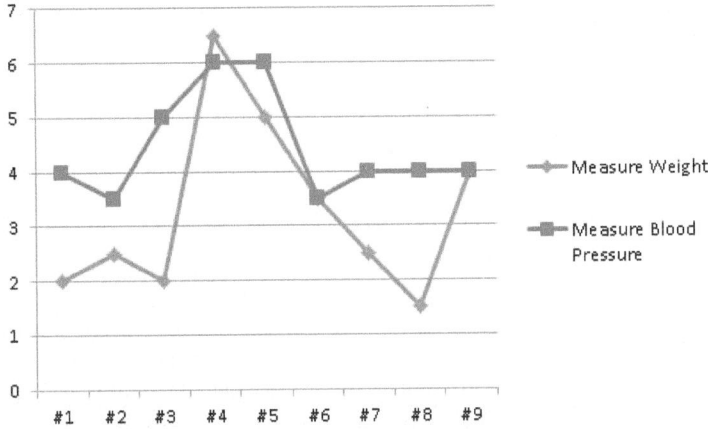

Fig. 3. Duration of Measure on Prototype Tests

pressure measurement took in average 4 minutes and 30 seconds, while the weight measurement took in average, 3 minutes and 20 seconds. Comparing these times with the ones taken on the low fidelity usability tests, a decrease in the duration of each measure was visible. This proves that not only the mobile application matched the success of the usability prototypes, but it also made both operations quicker. The peak on participants number 4 and 5 can be explained by those participants clearly difficulties, when comparing to the remaining participants. One of them, was the oldest participant, while the other had a chronic injury in his fingers.

All of them told that any difficulties found in each task would only occur on first usage and if they were to make the test again, it would be much easier and much quicker.

On the remaining tests – reading the feedback message, writing it back to the physician and viewing the latest measurements – several difficulties were found and the times taken on each of them are not conclusive. The user-interface used on these tests, was not subject to prior usability tests and although it followed a few guidelines taken from the first usability tests (font type, size, background and text colors, etc.), participants still found some obstacles. These difficulties only prove the importance of conducting usability tests with the end-users of a system.

3   Conclusion and Future Work

One of the innovating points of this study was to apply ANT+ devices to health care services and its usage was proved to be as effective as any other wireless technology, with the advantage of achieving very low costs and power, by today standards. During development, the ANT+ chip was used quite often and still, no significant changes in the battery life of the smart-phone were noticed. Its current competitor, Bluetooth 4.0, is still integrating with current devices and it is still early to tell which of them is a better choice.

The advantages that may arise from this project were visible through the developed working prototype. The results on Figure 3 show us that on average, an elderly would take less then ten minutes to measure important health values and send them to his physician. As a monitoring operation, we believe it is a non-intrusive and acceptable duration for the elderly to do on a regular basis.

The tests participants were all clearly motivated on the work being made and several even asked where they could buy such a product. In the country where this study was made, Portugal, no similar mobile health system has ever been implemented. Their only concern was the cost of buying such devices, which is understandable given the current economic crisis. Although with the right partnerships and a sensible business model it may actually become a reality in the near future.

Future work should start by refining the working prototype. The approach on getting the data from the blood pressure device could be enhanced, as well as implementing the HTTP-Secure protocol for transferring data from the mobile device to the web server. Also, conducting prototype tests for the web application on the physicians point-of-view, would be very important in order to evaluate the developed prototype. Conducting more usability tests would also be valuable, especially on the user interfaces that were not tested during this work. At last, efforts could be made together with health specialists, in order to look for other devices to be integrated with the prototype here developed.

References

1. Boulos, M.K., Wheeler, S., Tavares, C., Jones, R.: How smartphones are changing the face of mobile and participatory healthcare: an overview, with example from ecaalyx. BioMedical Engineering OnLine (2011)
2. IEEE-USA Medical Technology Policy Committee. Technologies for addressing the health care needs of our aging population (November 2009)
3. Chan, V., Ray, P., Parameswaran, N.: Mobile e-health monitoring: an agent-based approach. IET Communications 2(2), 223–230 (2008)
4. Fox, S., Purcell, K.: Chronic disease and the internet. Technical report, Pew Research Center's Internet & American Life Project (2010)
5. Gay, V., Leijdekkers, P.: A health monitoring system using smart phones and wearable sensors. International Journal of ARM 8(2) (2007)
6. Holzinger, A., Searle, G., Nischelwitzer, A.K.: On some aspects of improving mobile applications for the elderly. In: Stephanidis, C. (ed.) Universal Acess in HCI, Part I. LNCS, vol. 4554, pp. 923–932. Springer, Heidelberg (2007)
7. Mayhew, L.: Health and elderly care expenditure in an aging world. Research report (International Institute for Applied Systems Analysis) (2000)
8. Marzegalli, M., Lunati, M., Landolina, M., Perego, G.B., Ricci, R.P., Guenzati, G., Schirru, M., Belvito, C., Brambilla, R., Masella, C., Stasi, F.D., Valsecchi, S., Santini, M.: Remote monitoring of crt-icd: The multicenter italian carelink evaluation – ease of use, acceptance, and organizational implications. Pacing Clin. Electrophysiol. (2008)

9. Creditor, M.C.: Hazards of hospitalization of the elderly. Annals of Internal Medicine 118(3), 219–223 (1993)
10. Milosevic, M., Shrove, M.T., Jovanov, E.: Applications of smartphones for ubiquitous health monitoring and wellbeing management. Journal of Information Technology and Application (2011)
11. Nielsen, J.: Usability Engineering. Morgan Kaufmann Publishers Inc., San Francisco (1993)
12. Population Division of the Department of Economic and Social Affairs of the United Nations Secretariat. World population prospects: The 2010 revision. Technical report, United Nations (2011)
13. Scanaill, C.N., Ahearne, B., Lyons, G.M.: Long-term telemonitoring of mobility trends of elderly people using sms messaging. IEEE Transactions on Information Technology in Biomedicine 10(2), 412–413 (2006)
14. Senger, C.J.: Thinking Aloud Protocols: A Tool for Teaching (1992)
15. Sarasohn-Kahn, J.: How smartphones are changing health care for consumers and providers. Technical report, California HealthCare Foundation (2010)
16. Seto, E., Kevin Leonard, J., Joseph Cafazzo, A., Barnsley, J., Masino, C., Heather Ross, J.: Perceptions and experiences of heart failure patients and clinicians on the use of mobile phone-based telemonitoring. J. Med. Internet Res. 14(1), 25 (2012)
17. The Socio-Economic Impact of Mobile Health. Technical report, The Boston Consulting Group and Telenor Group (2012)
18. Morris, R.: Why ant?, http://www.thisisant.com/why-ant

Smart Media Services through TV Sets
for Elderly and Dependent Persons

Tayeb Lemlouma and Mohamed Aymen Chalouf

IRISA Laboratory, University of Rennes I,
IUT of Lannion, BP 30219, Rue Edouard Branly, 22302 Lannion Cedex, France
{tayeb.lemlouma,mohamed-aymen.chalouf}@irisa.fr

Abstract. This paper deals with providing adapted media content and services for elderly and dependent persons living alone. In our approach, providing solutions and technologies for elderly requires to consider the simplification of architectures and the acceptance of the user. We propose to provide content and services using familiar TV sets and to consider medical advices and recommendations in using media and TV programs. As the user control is a key criterion in adopting context-aware systems, we consider the user actions and preferences. The proposed media selection scheme considers the evolution of the user preferences based on the recent user behavior patterns.

Keywords: Healthcare, TV program recommendation, recommendation systems, user behavior, pervasive computing, home automation, smart home.

1   Introduction

Smart homes represent an application of pervasive environments that involves the integration of different services by using a common communication system. Smart home technology promises tremendous benefits for an elderly and dependent persons living alone. The environment provides user context-aware services like comfort, healthcare, safety and energy conservation. Many smart home projects and architectures have been conducted over the last decades [1]. However, proposed systems are always faced to the problem of their adoption and real use by the general public. For elderly, this situation is explained by the system complexity and the acceptance of new technologies. For example, DLNA digital home systems [2] are already integrated in about 74 % of existing home consumer electronics but with only 6 % of real users [3]. This fact is due mainly to the complexity of the technology and the lack of intelligent services/components that help users to find content, configure and connect their terminals.

Robles and Kim [4] concluded in their review that a main challenge of installing a smart home system is balancing the complexity of the system against its usability. Based on the work of [5], half of all computer-based information systems related to health care fail due to user resistance and staff interference. The main reason is that users were asked to significantly alter traditional workflow patterns to accommodate the system, rather than the system accommodating the users. According to a study done

B. Godara and K.S. Nikita (Eds.): MobiHealth 2012, LNICST 61, pp. 30–40, 2013.
© Institute for Computer Sciences, Social Informatics and Telecommunications Engineering 2013

within 300 people of 65-85 years old [6], elderly are constantly faced to the ever-evolving technology and need appropriate support in order to satisfactorily meet with the difficulties of everyday living. The study shows that elderly are able to handle the TV sets (99.4%) while only 67.7% of them are able to use a simple wireless phone. Old people are using television more than other media and devices for many reasons. Mainly, because of the easy combined availability of verbal and visual information and sometimes to replaces lost social contacts, maintain a sense of participation in society and combat feelings of loneliness. Decreases in the ability to read and lower attendance at religious services and organizations both lead to increased TV viewing [7].

Providing smart media services through TV sets allow elderly and disabled to have personalized content adapted to their needs without leaving their homes and without complex home architectures. Furthermore, enabling smart services using familiar TV sets simplifies the use of advanced technologies and makes their integration in home easily accepted by elderly. The trends in smart homes research indicate an increasing popularity of using middleware. The use of middleware is efficient to integrate heterogeneous multivendor devices that coexist in the same system [1].

UNIVERSALLY [8], [9] is a middleware based architecture that provides media services in digital homes. The goal of UNIVERSALLY is to simplify and optimize digital home architectures and make their use intuitive. The system used an optimized way to deliver media services for heterogeneous renderers connected through different access technologies [8], [9]. In this work, we extend UNIVERSALLY in order to offer personalized media content and smart services though TV sets. Provided content are dynamically selected from TV programs and other media items (stored in the proposed system or coming from the Internet). Provided services depend on the elderly situation and could be notifications to take medicine or to go to sleep, incoming calls from family or assistance organisms, etc.

The new system components are designed to be easily used in both advanced digital homes (e.g. a DLNA compatible home [2]) and in simple homes where a simple TV set is used by the elderly. The idea behind the use of TV sets is to take advantage of the observed increased TV viewing by elderly living alone to personalize the watched media content. This automatic personalization, called also *media selection*, is made according to the elderly situation, preferences over the time, needs of contact and assistance. Moreover, at any moment, the user has the choice to control or change automatic selected media content and services. This aspect aims to further facilitate the user adoption of the system as it was pointed in many previous works regarding the satisfaction of the user in using context-aware applications [10].

Our cost-effective approach tuned towards preferences and needs of the users and the use of the familiar TV set (already existed in the elderly home) would accelerate the rapid adoption of the system and increases the acceptance of advanced technologies and services by elderly. The reminder of this paper is organized as follows. Principles of the context aware media selection are presented in Section 2. In Section 3, our proposed media selection scheme is discussed. The system rules required in providing our smart services are described in Section 4. Rules concern the system behavior in handling events and the user actions. The system implementation and experimentations are presented in Section 5. Conclusions are given in Section 6.

2   Context-Aware Media Selection

In order to provide smart services through the elderly TV set, the system must be able, at any moment, to display the most appropriate media content or service. This is the primary scope of the *context-aware media selection* problem. For TV programs, previous works have addressed the problem in the form of TV recommendation techniques. These techniques aim to avoid the blindly zapping of channels and help users to find their favorite TV programs. In [11], a recommendation system is presented for Web-TV content based of the user preferences and users rating. Recommendation techniques can be classified mainly into two common categories: *Content-based* recommendations and *Collaborative filtering* recommendation [12], [13]. In the first category, the similarities between the watched content and new content are considered. The second category is based on the content recommendations of other TV viewers having similar preferences as the user. Collaborative rating and filtering are not considered in our work because we believe that rating the viewed content does not simplify the system for the elderly. Our objective is to leave the elderly using the TV set as usual with its own remote controller.

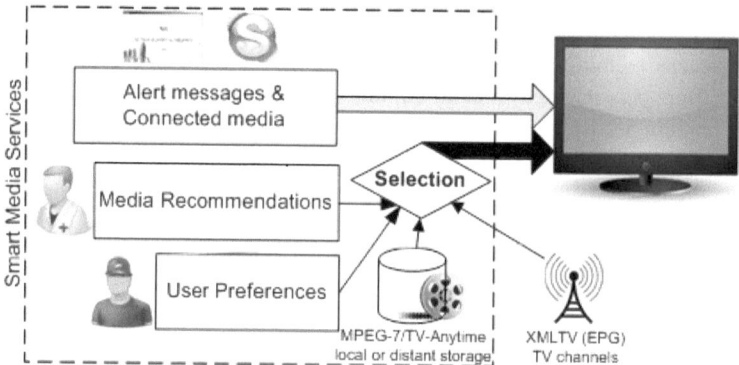

Fig. 1. Media selection based on the *Media Recommendations, User Preferences* and the description of TV channel content and available external media

Bearing in mind that the focus is on comfort and healthcare for elderly and dependent persons, our model considers the following aspects (Fig. 1):

- *Media Recommendations* for the user considered as elderly or a dependent person. These recommendations are intended to be advised by the referring doctor, a caregiver or a healthcare assistant that follows the elderly. For example, these recommendations aim to find what external media[1] content is considered adapted to the user situation (age, health situation and culture). In other words, what content can be better for the user than any arbitrary TV channel content. Moreover, media

---

[1] We define an external media as a media content (video or audio) that does not come from a current TV channel but from a local or distant storage used by our system.

recommendations include the maximal recommended time to spend in watching TV, times to take medicine for the elderly and recommended time to sleep.

- *User preferences*. The content the user likes to watch as expressed by him. The content can come from a TV channel or an external media. The user preferences are expressed once. However, our system may change the preferences over the time according to the user behavior.
- *Alert messages*. Alert content for health and safety such as the notification when it is time to take medicine.
- *Connected media*. The received calls from family, friends or assistance organisms.

Table 1. An example of a *Media Recommendations* profile

Media Recommendations	
Content Category	**Percentage per Week**
Relaxation Atmosphere: Laid back (Calm, relaxed, easy-going)	50%
Daily news, regular program carrying breaking and current news stories	20%
Leisure/Hobby/Lifestyle, Personal/Lifestyle/Family, Fitness/Keep-fit and House Keeping	15%
Humanities, Culture/Tradition/Anthropology/Ethnic studies	10%
Sports, Winter sports, Ice-skating	5%
Other Variables	**Value(s)**
Maximal Recommended TV Time per Day	5h per day
Medicines Times	10:00 AM, 04:00 PM
Level of Hearing	medium
Time to Sleep	10:00PM

Table 2. An example of a *User Preferences* profile (a French viewer)

User Preferences	
Content Category	**Percentage per Week**
Similar structure as the Media Recommendations profile but with the user favorite categories	
Favorite presenters/actors	**Value(s)**
Presenter/actor	Louis de Funès
Presenter/actor	Tex
Other Variables	**Value(s)**
Preferred Sport	Ice-skating
Preferred General Channel	M6
Preferred News Channel	iTélé
Preferred programs	**Value(s)**
Title / Channel	Les feux de l'amour / TF1
Title / Channel	Un dinner presque parfait / M6
Title / Channel	Les Z'amours / France 2

Recommendations and user preferences are stored in the form of two separate profiles that include the needs and preferences regarding the content. In Tables 1 and 2, we give an overview extracted from a *Media Recommendations* and *User Preferences* profile. Recommendations and preferences profiles are stored in RDF [16]; the media content categorization uses the schema defined in the ETSI TV-Anytime specification (version 1.7.1) [14]. Media content analysis is done on the metadata provided by the used media formats MPEG-7 and TV-Anytime. The content analysis of TV channels is applied on an XMLTV format [17] based on EPG data received using a TV card.

3   Media Selection Scheme

As shown in Fig. 1, we consider alert messages and connected media a priority. This means that when it is time to display an alert message or when a call is received, it will be displayed on the TV set. Hence, the media selection problem will be limited to the media recommendations, the user preferences and the available media items (external media and current TV channel content). The media diversity of the selected content is also considered to avoid boring the TV viewer with the same category of content.

3.1   Proposed Scheme

The media selection is applied on available media sources: external media items and current TV channel programs. The result of the media selection is the decision to either play an external media item or select a TV channel program. The selection is based on the metadata of the content: MPEG-7 or TV-Anytime for external items and XMLTV for TV channel content. Each media item viewed by the elderly is logged. A log entry includes mainly the fields represented in Table 3.

Table 3. A log entry of the elderly TV viewing activities

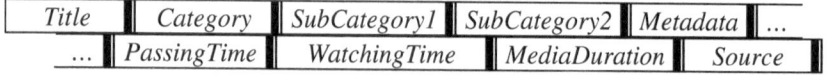

Title	Category	SubCategory1	SubCategory2	Metadata	...
...	PassingTime	WatchingTime	MediaDuration	Source	

The media selection scheme performs the following phases:

- **Phase 1:** Based on the user behavior patterns in the seven last days, find the set of media items S_1 that fulfills the requirements of the *Media Recommendation* profile. This means to do the best effort to reach the given percentage per category and to keep the given proportion between the different percentages.
- **Phase 2:** Order the S_1 set according the score function *MediaScore* that takes into account the recent behavior patterns of the user. The *MediaScore* function will be discussed later. We denote S_2 the set returned at the end of this phase.
- **Phase 3:** Order the S_2 set according to the current *User Preferences* profile. Items of S_2 are evaluated according to the user preferences dimensions in the following order: does the item belong to the preferred programs list? Is there any favorite presenter/actor in the media item? Does the item fulfill the preferred

content categories percentage and proportions between percentages? Finally, evaluate the item according to the other variables of the *User Preferences* profile. We denote S_3 the set returned at the end of this phase.

- **Phase 4:** Select the top media item of S_3.
- **Phase 5:** Update the log of the user behavior patterns with the selected item in Phase 4.

If the user performs a selection action (example turning off the TV set or zapping a selected program), the system will apply the ***UpdateUponAction*** procedure as follows:

- Updates the log of the user behavior patterns,
- Updates the current preferences according to the passing time, watching duration and media duration of the last viewed item using the *MediaScore* function.
- Updates the current elderly status regarding to the requirements of the Media Recommendations profile. This means to update the different percentages of viewed content categories and subcategories, the daily time spent in watching TV and initializing the energy saving timer (if the TV set still on). The energy saving timer serves to turn off the TV set if no action from the user is captured within a fixed time value (*EnerySavingValue* constant). The default value of *EnerySavingValue* in our system is four hours.

At a given moment, the number of available TV programs and external media items is important. Performing the previous phases requires a non-negligible computing time that can affect negatively the elderly experience. Indeed, the computing time required for the media selection implies that the elderly will have no displayed content before the result of the selection. Our approach is to perform the different phases of the media selection scheme offline, i.e. when the TV set is off or when the user is already watching a media item. The result of the selection is stored temporarily. When the user performs a new action, the temporarily result is updated in order take into account only the time spent to watch the last item (*WatchingTime* value). If the user zaps quickly a media item, updating the temporarily result of the media selection will be fast because the last zapped item will not affect significantly neither the media selection result nor the user behavior patterns. Indeed, as we will see later, if the user spent a short time to watch a media item, this implies that the score of this item will not be significant. This is due to the recent passing time of the media item and its short watching time value.

3.2   Evaluating the Media Score

Our scheme aims to further facilitate the elderly adoption of the system. As stated earlier, previous works have pointed the user's need of control in order to satisfy him in using context-aware applications [10]. Our system gives the user the choice to control and change selected media content at any moment. Our scheme includes this user control patterns to adjust the user preferences and so the scores associated to media content items. If the user selects and spends more time on watching a given media item, the item's score will be increased. If the user spends less time or simply ignores an automatic selected item, the item's score will be decreased. The tacit assumption is that the elderly selection of media is a reflection of his preferences that can be learned. However, as the elderly preferences may change over time, we focus on the recent behavior patterns of the user.

The following equations are used to evaluate the score of a media item I according to the viewing patterns of the user (using logs). We consider the watching time and the passing time of similar media items j. WatchingTime (j) returns the time that user spent to watch the item j divided by the total duration of j. In (1), we consider that an item I will have a better score if the viewer found an interest to stay for a long time watching similar content. Content similarities consider the same category and subcategories with similar metadata. However, in order to avoid boring the user with repeated selections of the same content and the same categories, we will consider the passing time importance factor δ. PassingTime$_j$ returns the most recent week in which the item j was watched. In order to avoid repeated selections that return the same result, the δ factor will be positive if the item was watched recently but at least one week ago. As the elderly preferences may change over time, items watched before the last four weeks will have a negative importance factor (Equation 2). In (2), α is a constant that adjusts the importance factor δ to be in the range of 0 to 100 (for a passing time from one to four weeks). The value of α is 44,44.

$$MediaScor\,(I) = \sum_{j} \delta_j \cdot WatchingTime(j) \tag{1}$$

$$\delta_j = -\alpha \cdot \left(Pas\sin gTime_j - 1\right) \cdot \left(Pas\sin gTime_j - 4\right) \tag{2}$$

4   Rules Implementation

In this section, we present the different rules required to implement smart media services through the TV set of the user. The system takes into account the *Media Recommendations* and the *User Preferences* profile discussed previously. Services include displaying available TV programs, external media items, incoming calls and different alerts. The implementation of incoming calls detection and termination is done based on the network capture of the traffic. The user actions are capture using an infrared sensor (see Section 5). Rules implementation follows the condition/action model i.e. when a given condition is satisfied the smart system performs a given action. In our system, conditions are related to the user control or particular events.

User control (**rules: R1, R2, R3**)
R1 (condition): *the user turns on the TV Set*
R1 (actions):

- Apply the Media Selection Scheme;
- Display the selected Item on the TV Set;
- Initialize the energy saving timer;
- **If** (*time to sleep* OR *the maximal recommended TV time per day* is exceeded) **Then** Display an alert message every thirty minutes;

R2 (condition): *the user turns off the TV Set*
R2 (actions):
- Apply the *UpdateUponAction* procedure (Section 3.1); (except the initialization of the energy saving timer)
- Stop playing any external media if it was displayed on the TV set;

R3 (condition): *the user zaps the current media item*
R3 (actions):
- Perform the user's action; (this means that the system will accept the user control. The media selection process will not be called. The system lets the TV set displays the desired TV channel)
- Apply the *UpdateUponAction* procedure (Section 3.1)

Events (rules: R4, R5, R6, R7, R8)

R4 (condition): *a media item is completely watched*
R4 (actions):
- Updates the *WatchingTime* value of the last watched item; (this field is updated in the user's log with the value of: current time minus the *PassingTime* value)
- Apply the Media Selection Scheme;
- Display the selected Item on the TV Set;

R5 (condition): *it is time to sleep* OR *the maximal recommended TV time is exceeded*
R5 (actions): Display an alert message every thirty minutes;
R6 (condition): *it is time to take medicine*
R6 (actions):
- Display an alert message;
- Perform a pause on the current media item if it is an external media;

R7 (condition): *no user action is received within the value of EnerySavingValue*
R7 (actions):
- Turn off the TV set;
- Apply the *UpdateUponAction* procedure (Section 3.1); (except the initialization of the energy saving timer)

R8 (condition): *a call is received*
R8 (actions):
- Display the call on the TV set;
- Perform a pause on the current media item if it is an external media;
- Exclude the call interruption in the *WatchingTime* value calculation;

In addition to the previous rules, the system performs a volume adjustment each time the TV set is turned on or when an external media item or a new TV program is displayed. Volume adjustment is based on the *Level of Hearing* value (*normal, medium, hard, very hard*) expressed in the *Media Recommendations* profile. Volume adjustment is based on the real volume as sensed by the system using an embedded microphone (Section 5). This choice is due to the difference of the real output TV volume between: a TV channel and another one; a TV program and an external media; different models of TV sets and finally between the volume of a TV program and its included commercial advertisements.

5   System Implementation and Experimentation

In order to validate our approach, we have enriched the UNIVERSALLY system [8], [9] by the implementation of the context-aware media selection scheme, the user control management and rules of the user control and events (Fig. 2).

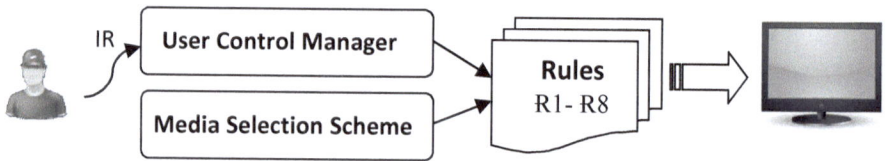

Fig. 2. The system components

In order to implement the *User Control Manager*, we use a USB infrared receiver and transmitter (*USB-UIRT* [15]). The device allows learning and receiving the infrared signals that the user transmits using his remotes. The device allows performing different actions on the TV set according to the specified rules. The implemented basic actions are: turning on/off the TV set, adjusting the volume, selecting the TV video/audio source (channels or PC) and the selection of TV channels. Actions are implemented using the *USB-UIRT trydrv* and *uutx* commands [15]. The infrared receiver/transmitter is connected to a personal computer (*DELL Precision M6300*) where the system components are implemented. The TV set (*Sony KDL-46Z5500*) is connected to the PC through a scart and audio cables. For incoming calls, we use a web camera (*Logitech HD Webcam C310*) with a built-in microphone used also in volume sensing and adjustment discussed in section 4. Figure 3 shows three tested scenarios in the house of *Marie* a 60 years old elderly person. In (A), the system selected automatically a preferred program ("*almost perfect dinner*", in French "*un dinner presque parfait*", from the French *M6* channel). In (B), *Marie* received a skype call from her daughter *Lydie*. The system switches automatically the TV set to the computer call. *Marie* was able to perform the call using the camera with built-in microphone used by the platform. In (C), *Marie* was watching a selected media item; the system notifies her to take her medicine.

6   Conclusion

In this paper we have described how smart media services can be provided to elderly and dependent persons using their TV sets. We have proposed a media selection scheme base on the *Media Recommendations* and *User preferences* profile. The system considers the media recommendations to provide content and services adapted to the user situation and health. Selected media are closer to the user needs and preferences than any arbitrary TV content obtained after a blindly zapping. Our proposed scheme considers the change and evolution over time of the user preferences and makes selected media items dynamically adapted to current preferences. The proposed approach made the system tuned towards preferences and needs of the elderly. The use of TV sets increases the acceptance of advanced technologies and services by elderly. The user's acceptance of the proposed system was a key criterion in our approach. Unfortunately this aspect is generally ignored in previous context aware approaches. The next step of our work will concern the evaluation of the user acceptance and quality of experience in using our system. Concretely, one of the identified metric is to measure, over time, the number of media items returned as a result of our selection scheme and zapped by the user. This number should decrease if the user is satisfied. Also, we will consider the time spent to watch selected items and enabling the dynamic change of the proposed *Media Recommendations* profile.

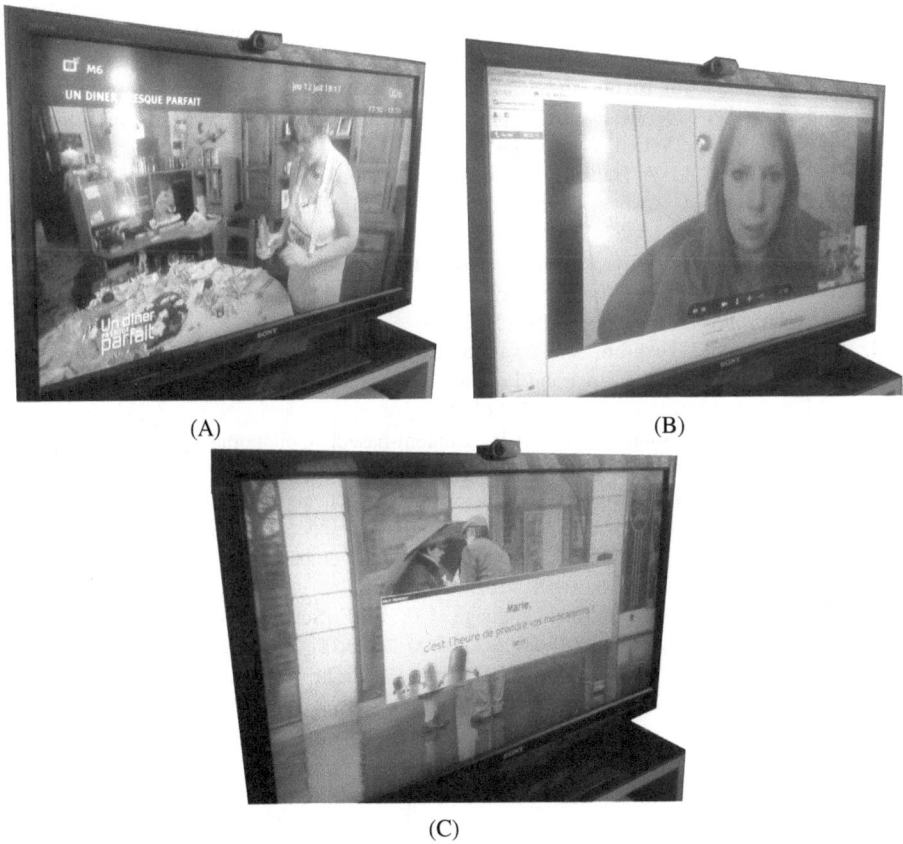

Fig. 3. Three tested scenarios: preferred program (A), incoming call (B) and medicine notification (C)

References

1. Alam, M.R., Reaz, M.B.I., Ali, M.A.M.: A Review of Smart Homes-Past, Present, and Future. IEEE Transactions on Systems, Man, and Cybernetics, Part C: Applications and Reviews PP(99), 1–14 (2012)
2. Digital Living Network Alliances: DLNA Overview and Vision Whitepaper (2007), http://www.dlna.org/
3. In-Stat: UPnP and DLNA—Standardizing the Networked Home. Research Information (2010)
4. Robles, R.J., Kim, T.-H.: Review: Context Aware Tools for Smart Home Development. International Journal of Smart Home 4(1), 1–12 (2010)
5. Anderston, J., Aydin, C.: Evaluating the Impact of Health Care Information Systems. International Journal of Technology Assessment in Health Care 13(2), 380–393 (1997)
6. Roupa, Z., Nikas, M., Gerasimou, E., Zafeiri, V., Giasyrani, L., Kazitori, E., Sotiropoulou, P.: The Use of Technology by the Elderly. Health Science Journal 4(2), 118–126 (2010)
7. Media and Values. Studies Analyze Elderly Use of Television, Media and Values, Issue 45, Center for Media Literacy (2010)
8. Lemlouma, T.: UNIVERSALLY: A Context-Aware Architecture for Multimedia Access in Digital Homes. In: IEEE International Conference on Advanced Infocomm Technology (ICAIT 2012), Paris, France (2012)
9. Lemlouma, T.: Improving the User Experience by Web Technologies for Complex Multimedia Services. In: Proc. 8th International Conference on Web Information Systems and Technologies (WEBIST), Porto, Portugal, pp. 444–451 (2012)
10. Criel, J., Claeys, L.: A Transdisciplinary Study Design on Context-aware Applications and Environments. A Critical View on User Participation within Calm Computing. Observatorio Journal 5, 57–77 (2008)
11. Chen, K.-C., Teng, W.-G.: Adopting User Profiles and Behavior Patterns in a Web-TV Recommendation System. In: IEEE 13th International Symposium on Consumer Electronics, Kyoto, Japan, pp. 320–324 (2009)
12. Adomavicius, G., Tuzhilin, A.: Toward the Next Generation of Recommender Systems: A Survey of the State-of-the-Art and Possible Extensions. IEEE Transactions on Knowledge and Data Engineering 17(6), 734–749 (2005)
13. Balabanovi, M., Shoham, Y.: Fab: Content-based, Collaborative Recommendation. Communications of the ACM 40(3), 66–72 (1997)
14. ETSI, Broadcast and On-line Services, Search, Select, and Rightful Use of Content on Personal Storage Systems ("TV-Anytime"); Part 3: Metadata; Sub-part 1: Phase 1 - Metadata Schemas, ETSI TS 102 822-3-1 V1.7.1 (November 7, 2011)
15. USB-UIRT (2012), http://www.usbuirt.com/
16. RDF Vocabulary Description Language 1.0: RDF Schema, W3C Recommendation (February 10, 2004), http://www.w3.org/TR/rdf-schema/
17. XMLTV Project: XMLTV DTD (2012), http://xmltv.cvs.sourceforge.net/viewvc/xmltv/xmltv/xmltv.dtd

User Centered Design of an Interactive Mobile Assistance and Supervision System for Rehabilitation Purposes

Florian Klompmaker[1], Anke Workowski[2], Wolfgang Thronicke[3],
Florian Ostermair[3], Detlev Willemsen[2], and Jan-Dirk Hoffmann[2]

[1] University of Paderborn, C-LAB,
Fürstenallee 11, 33102 Paderborn, Germany
florian.klompmaker@c-lab.de
[2] Schüchterman-Schiller'sche Kliniken Bad Rothenfelde GmbH & Co.KG
Ulmenallee 5 – 11, 49214 Bad Rothenfelde, Germany
{AWorkowski,DWillemsen,JHoffmann}@schuechtermann-klinik.de
[3] Atos IT Solutions and Services GmbH, C-LAB,
Fürstenallee 11, 33102 Paderborn, Germany
{wolfgang.thronicke,florian.ostermair}@c-lab.de

Abstract. This paper describes the user centered development of a mobile assistance and supervision system for cardiac disease patients. Smartphones are used to collect data from wireless sensors like ECG, blood pressure or oxygen saturation sensors while a patient is exercising outdoors. All data from the wireless sensors as well as GPS information is sent to a supervision center where doctors and sport therapists analyze the data in a collaborative and interactive setting. We here present the User Centered Design process, the technical realization as well as the interaction modalities of our system.

Keywords: Mobile rehabilitation, cardiac diseases, telemedicine, mobile assistance, interactive visualization, supervision, user centered design.

1 Introduction

Cardiorespiratory fitness is a health protective factor. "Fit people", persons with a high fitness level, have a longer life expectancy [1] since physical activity reduces the risk of a cardiac event by the positive adaptation of the musculoskeletal and cardiovascular system [2]. Therefore, in Germany health initiatives have been established to increase the motivation for physical activity. Such initiatives are not set up for specific diseases but address the average population.

Cardiovascular diseases (CVD) remain the number-one cause of deaths worldwide, with more than 80% of deaths from CVD in low- and middle-income countries [3]. The reduction of mortality is associated with the activity level. People with CVD need an adapted and monitored training to avoid over exertions and prevent further cardiac events. Cardiac rehabilitation is established after a cardiac event in order to minimize the cardiovascular risk factors in the long term. However, existing studies indicate that the success of this kind of rehabilitation only persist for about one year [4] since

B. Godara and K.S. Nikita (Eds.): MobiHealth 2012, LNICST 61, pp. 41–50, 2013.
© Institute for Computer Sciences, Social Informatics and Telecommunications Engineering 2013

follow-up offers don't exist and patients tend to abort continuous exercises and a healthy lifestyle.

In Germany outpatient heart groups are the only offer of cardiology secondary prevention. However, these groups are not nationwide represented and temporally inflexible, so that only about 13-40% of CVD patients participate [5]. Therefore, health initiatives that are geared specifically to elderly and persons with CVD are extremely necessary. For that reason within the ITEA2 research project "OSAmI - Open Source Ambient Intelligence Commons", funded by the Federal Ministry of Education and Research in Germany, an indoor bicycle ergometer with an integrated telemonitoring system was developed. In collaboration with computer-, information- and sports scientists as well as medical technicians an intelligent bicycle ergometer for patients with CVD was built. The ergometer bike can be controlled by a patient via a 15" touch screen that is mounted to the handlebar. The vital data of a patient is measured using a 3-lead-ECG, an oxygen saturation sensor and a blood pressure sensor. All sensors use Bluetooth for sending the vital data wirelessly to a nearby receiver station. This station is connected to the Internet and sends all vital data and all bike data in real-time to a medical center, where supervisors observe the data. A supervisor can adapt the training and remotely change the bike settings. Further on, the system has an integrated alarm system to prevent over- and under-loads [6].

Since heart patients need different types of training regarding different histories of CVD and because of the different cardiorespiratory level, the OSAmI system offers three different exercise types: heart rate controlled training, constant load training and interval training. To gather personal feelings about the current wellbeing of the patient, they need to answer questionnaires before and after every training in order to get information about medication intake, the deterioration of the disease, the perceived difficulty of the training etc. The OSAmI system has a huge potential to motivate and support elderly people and patients with CVD to physical activity [7]. A training can be absolved flexible in time and under safe conditions, because the vital data is live monitored and the supervisor is able to adapt the load and duration of the training immediately. The attractiveness of this form of training was rated very high in a first user study [8].

However, an indoor ergometer training can be very monotonous. Therefore, we developed an outdoor scenario that is introduced in this paper. Patients participating in the OSAmI program can take their wearable equipment outside. A mobile gateway like a smartphone is needed to collect the data from the wireless sensors and send it to the medical center for supervision. Further on, GPS information is collected and also transmitted. The vital data can be monitored while patients are hiking or cycling outdoors producing a save feeling for them. Further on, the mobile gateway is able to locate the trained person. If an acute cardiac event happens, the emergency doctor can locate the patient rapidly.

The structure of this paper is as follows: We will first address some related work in the area of mobile supervision and observation systems as well as our work on User Centered Design (UCD) within the OSAmI project. Next we will describe the technical realization of the mobile scenario. We will further on introduce an interactive setup that allows a team of medical experts to supervise the mobile data on a tabletop device. The paper ends with a conclusion and some ideas for future work.

2   Related and Previous Work

Since smartphones are wide spread these days and millions of mobile Apps have been programmed and published, there are also many of them that address sportsmen or people who need extra care. Many so-called sport tracker applications are available, e.g. Endomondo[1] or Sports Tracker[2]. These Apps are available for various kinds of smartphones and besides GPS data they are also able to measure the heart rate of the user via chest straps. As long as a mobile data connection is available the data is transmitted to a portal where the community can see the current location and heart rate of a user. However, supervising cardiac disease patients is much more critical since a huge amount of data like ECG has to be transmitted in real-time. Therefore, until now these applications are only suitable for sportsmen, not for cardiac disease patients to control exercise.

In the area of medical assistance many mobile application scenarios have been developed and realized. Also applications that analyze ECG data have been created, e.g. for ECG monitoring at night-time [9]. Other systems collect data that is not that dynamic and critical, like the weight of a patient, her nutrition during a day or general activity analysis [10] using acceleration or GPS sensors. The home-based cardiac rehabilitation care model "TuneWalk" [11] is a measurement system and software tool for a mobile phone platform. This mobile application gives guidance to the patients during home exercises using heart rate and physical activity analysis and also stores long-term information about their progress during the weeks of the rehabilitation program. The measured data is sent to a server for remote exercise performance analysis and consultation by the patient's personal mentor. However, most approaches are quite simple and do not consider real-time transmission of vital data or live supervision. Further on, they do not address the special use case of rehabilitation and sport exercises.

Cardiac disease patients require individual training plans and often also live supervision and adaptation of these plans. For every critical patient medical supervisors need to know the vital data like ECG, blood pressure and oxygen saturation in real-time. The OSAmI system offers all the technical components that are needed to turn this scenario into reality.

However, in order to create a medical product also the usability is an important factor. User Centered Design (UCD) is an established methodology in the software-industry that focuses on the users of a future system and aims to create solutions that fits the users needs, their requirements and supports their tasks and goals. The usability of products gains in importance not only for the users of a system but also for manufacturing organizations. According to Jokela [12], the advantages for users are far-reaching and include increased productivity, improved quality of work, and

---

[1] http://www.endomondo.com/

[2] http://www.sports-tracker.com/

increased user satisfaction. Manufacturers also profit significantly through a reduction of support and training costs [12]. In order to create usable solutions it is necessary to involve potential users in early stages and during the process of development. UCD adds to this by providing methods applicable at different stages in the process of development.

To sum up, technical approaches exist that address sportsmen or elderly people who need special care. However, to the knowledge of the authors no system exists that offers the mobile collection of vital data like ECG, transmits this data in real-time to a supervision center and offers supervisors the possibility to observe multiple patients at the same time in a collaborative setting. Therefore, we will describe the technical realization within a UCD process that included patients, doctors, sports therapists and sport scientists in the next sections.

3   The Mobile Client

This section describes the technical realization of the mobile rehabilitation client that runs on a smartphone. It's main task is to manage the communication to the supervision center and transmit the sensor data. Further on it must provide an easy to use user interface and assist a patient especially in critical situations.

On technical level the system is message-based. All clients as well as the server application share a common XML-based message format and connect transparently using the XMPP protocol. With XMPP an arbitrary number of devices can be used platform-independently. The protocol supports presence detection and various communication schemes like publish-subscribe, notifications, etc. The architecture distinguishes between three categories: mobile trainee clients, mobile coach clients and stationary clients. The mobile trainee client (realized with Android™) connects to the vital data sensors using Bluetooth but also other communication technologies like ANT+ have been implemented. The monitored data is processed using the C-LAB context store[3] component, which is an open-source framework for designing arbitrary context processing solutions. Whenever communication is available monitored data is send to the central server. On this server the coach clients are registered as recipients of the data. The combined data is then transferred to these clients. The architecture allows simultaneous use of a mobile coaching client and the stationary solution (see next chapter).

On the client side the information from the sensors and the user portal is processed. The trainee can see her training schedule and her position on the map including the tracks (see figure 2). In one of our first interview sessions with patients we found out that patients want to be able to see their own vital data on a display [8] (which isn't the case during an on-site ergometer training in the clinic). Therefore, the vital data is displayed and if predefined limits are violated automated warnings are given. The warnings are presented using multimodal feedback via audio, vibration feedback and

---

[3] http://www.c-lab.de/en/publications/services_downloads/
c_lab_open_source/contextstore/

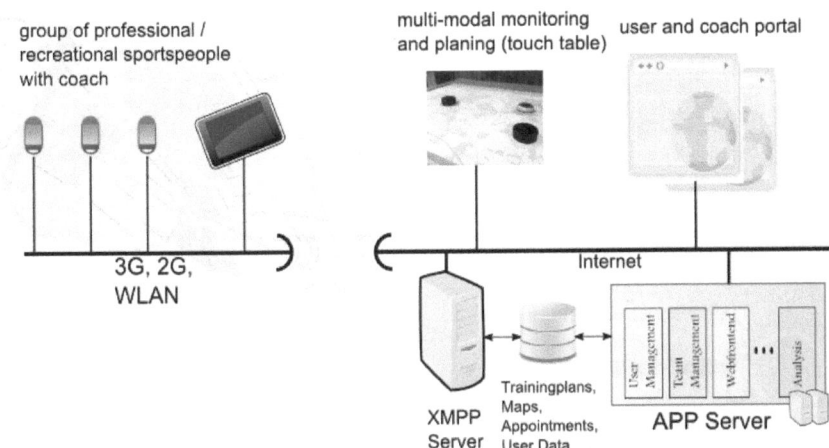

Fig. 1. OSAmI architecture

visually on the smartphone screen. This ensures that she is informed about important information even though she's currently exercising without having the device in front of her (e.g. wearing it in a pocket). An online supervisor receives the same data and alerts. Additionally she can directly modify the training parameters, or contact the trainee. In a medical scenario the recorded data can be discussed with the trainees and the training plans can be adapted. The screenshots in figure 2 demonstrate the mobile trainee application in action.

On the server (see figure 1) the training data is managed and the training plans are provided for the trainee. Training plans can contain different activities of various sport types with specific constraints on the vital data. They are based on one of the OSAmI-Trainings presented in the beginning (heart rate controlled, constant load or interval). Connection loss is handled transparently. If the connection is restored all buffered data is transmitted automatically so there is no "gap" in the final training report.

The entire system has been realized by COTS (Samsung Galaxy Tab, Samsung Galaxy I9000) and standard open-source server implementations. The results from our earlier studies for designing the user interfaces and icons [8] were used during the development. In the next section we will described how the vital and GPS data of the mobile clients is supervised by medical experts in a collaborative setting.

4   Collaborative Supervision

During one of our on-site studies [13] we have observed that the supervision of cardiac disease patients during rehabilitation exercises can ideally be performed in teams. In the cardiology clinic *Schüchtermann Schiller'sche Kliniken* in Bad Rothenfelde, Germany, we observed that often teams of two or three sport therapists or doctors supervise a group of about 16 patients exercising on ergometer bicycles.

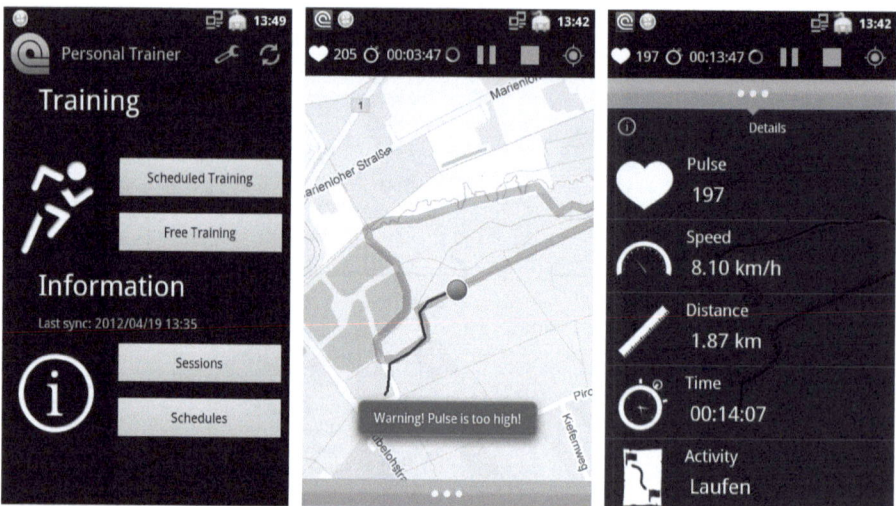

Fig. 2. Screenshot of the mobile client

Since outdoor exercises are much more dynamic they require a more concentrated observation. Therefore, we think that a supervision team of four or five sport therapists, doctors or other medical experts might be suitable to observe a group of up to 20 patients. This is because there might be several patients at the same time that need detailed supervision, the risk of missing a critical situation is lower but also because the supervision can be best performed within a collaborative decision process, so discussions between supervisors are very important. The challenge is to create a working environment that supports group work, enables the visualization of huge amount of data and supports collaborative decision processes at the same time. Further on, everyone from the group must be able to interact with the system at any time and the usability of the system has to taken into account because critical decisions have to be made within seconds frequently.

Therefore, we extracted the requirements for a collaborative supervision system within a UCD process that included interviews and observations. During a first visit we observed an on-site training in the clinic in order to get familiar with the current training setup and procedure. We recognized that supervising sport therapists not that much focus on the two large-scale monitors where all the vital data of the patients is presented but often walk around in order to visually observe the patients and talk to them. During a second where visit we held interviews with four sport therapists we got the feedback that the overall well-being of a patient can best be analyzed by observing their behavior, movements, skin color or sweating condition. Since such kind of observation is not possible in remote situations it is very important that:

- More than one supervisor is present in order to reduce the risk for overseeing a critical event. We therefore designed the supervision application in such a way that about five supervisors can use it coactively.
- All information about the patients is available to every supervisor. Since displaying all information at the same time would end up in a confusing user

interface only the most important things (alerts and GPS positions) are presented while all other data is callable on demand. The presented information must be visible from different position and adjustable by every supervisor easily.

- Algorithms for the automatic detection of events like over- or under exceeding a limit previously assigned to a vital data value are used and alarms occur.
- Supervisors can send feedback like audio or text messages to the patients.
- Routines for handling malfunctions in the data transmissions exist (e.g. informing the patients about connection errors and giving hints on how to proceed or pause the training).

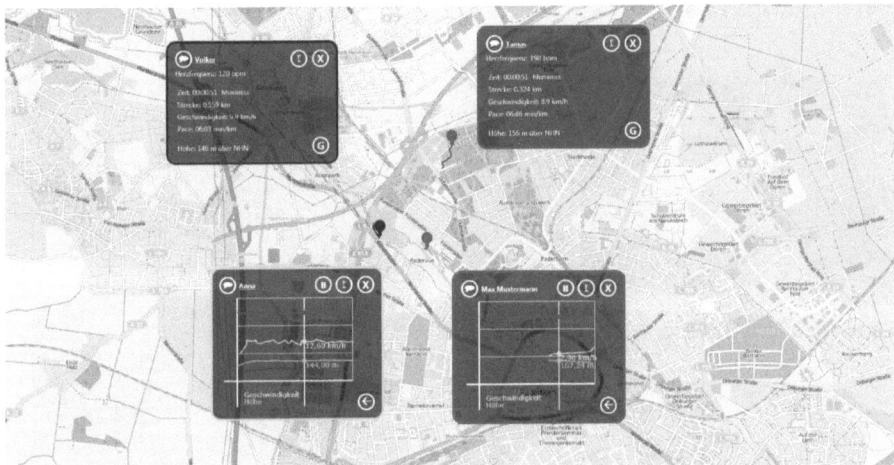

Fig. 3. Screenshot of the tabletop application showing details of four simultaneously exercising patients

Using this requirements we created a prototype application on our multitouch table useTable[4] (see figures 3 and 4). The useTable offers a 72" horizontal multitouch screen with full HD image projection. Past research has proven interactive tables to be especially beneficial for collaborative decision support systems [14,15]. The size of the useTable is perfect for groups of five or six people distributed on all sides of the table. Besides multitouch the useTable is also able to detect physical objects (*tangibles*) that are placed on the screen. We used these tangibles for map manipulation. After a tangible is placed on the table zooming can be performed by rotating the tangible and moving the map is performed by moving the tangible. Since only one map-tangible exists everyone in the group can see and understand what is happening and which person is currently interacting with the map. This realization perfectly addresses the interaction awareness [16] of the group. Further on, multitouch gestures for map interaction would end up in chaos because often multiple persons are touching the table at the same time. Figure 3 shows a screenshot of the application. It can be seen that four patients are exercising at

---

[4] http://www.usetable.de

this time. The windows with detailed information about vital data can be popped up or minimized by touching the patient's icon on the map. Users can switch between textual and graphical representation by clicking a button in the window. If an alarm occurs (e.g. the vital data has exceeded a predefined limit or a patient's smartphone lost it's connection), the information window pops up automatically. All windows on the screen can be moved, rotated and scaled using multitouch gestures allowing everyone on every side of the useTable to see the data and interact with it. In order to change the limits for heart rates etc. a user has to identify herself by placing a so-called chief-tangible on the table. Doing so creates a popup window that allows for such kind of manipulations (see figure 4, right). This addresses the required rights and role-management since not every supervisor is allowed to change these values for every patient.

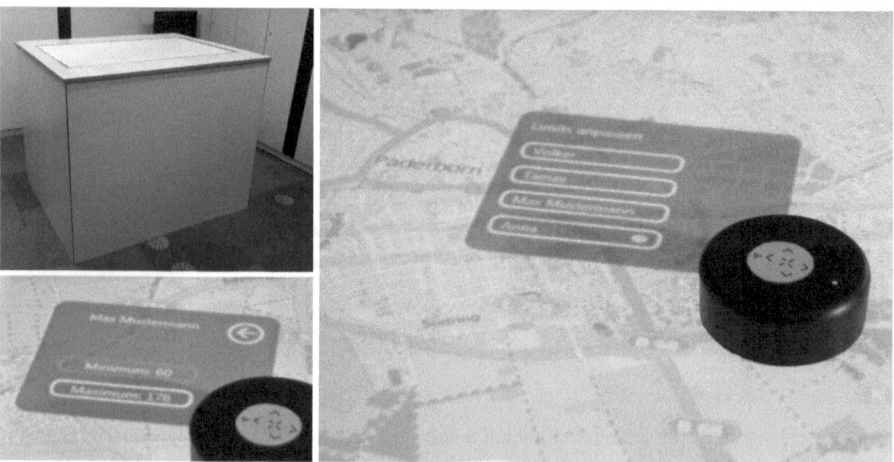

Fig. 4. Picture of the useTable (top left) and a tangible object allowing an authenticated changing of heart rate limits (right: select patient, bottom left: change limits)

In the third step of the UCD process we invited qualified clinic staff (doctors, sport therapists and sport scientists) to review this prototype and got positive but also critical feedback. In general the system was evaluated as highly interactive and very useful. However, there is still some work to do to address the specific use case of collaborative supervision of heart disease patients. Therefore, the next version of the system will include a third party ECG renderer. Further on the authentication through the tangible objects has to be improved. At the moment the recognition is done by a simple black and white pattern that can be easily reproduced. We are currently working on an RFID based authentication [17]. Last, we are planning to implement algorithms that address the loss of connection of a smartphone during exercises. For a limited period of time the system could forecast this situations and also forecast future positions and vital data based on available routes and altitude profiles.

5   Conclusion

In this paper we introduced the mobile OSAmI system that we developed within a User Centered Design process. Cardiac disease patients can use their smartphone for collecting vital data like ECG, blood pressure or oxygen saturation from wireless sensors. This data, as well as the GPS position, is sent to an observation center where a team of medical experts can supervise the training of multiple trainees in a collaborative setting including an interactive tabletop device.

Even though the User Centered Design process is still ongoing and the system still a prototype we think that this approach has a huge potential. In the next iteration of the process step we plan to solve the problem of loosing network connectivity by predicting positions and vital data developments. After doing some refinements on the visualization and interaction the next review by experts from the clinic is planned. Further on, the developed technology is also suitable for other use case scenarios.

References

1. Sattelmair, J., Pertman, J., Ding, E.L., Kohl, H.W., Haskell, W., Lee, I.-M.: Dose response between physical activity and risk of coronary heart disease. Circulation 124, 789–795 (2011)
2. Lee, C.D., Folsom, A.R., Blair, S.N.: Physical activity and stroke risk. A meta-analysis. Stroke 34, 2475–2482 (2003)
3. Mendis, S., Puska, P., Norrving, B. (eds.): Global Atlas on Cardiovascular Disease Prevention and Control. World Health Organization, Geneva (2011)
4. EUROASPIRE II Study Group: Lifestyle and risk factor management and use of drug therapies in coronary patients from 15 countries: principal results from EUROASPIRE II Euro Heart Survey Programme. Eur. Heart J., 554–572 (2001)
5. Bjarnason-Wehrens, B., Held, K., Karoff, M.: Herzgruppen in Deutschland – Status quo und Perspektiven. Herz 31, 559–565 (2006)
6. Busch, C., Baumbach, C., Willemsen, D., Nee, O., Gorath, T., Hein, A., Scheffold, T.: Supervised training with wireless monitoring of ECG, blood pressure and oxygen-saturation in cardiac patients. J. Telemed. Telecare 15(3), 112–114 (2009)
7. Workowski, A., Busch, J.-C., Hoffmann, J.-D., Müller, F., Dohndorf, O., Willemsen, D., Stewing, F.J., Eichelberg, M., Krumm, H.: Acceptance of telemonitoring in cardiology secondary prevention – evaluation results of the research project OSAmI Commons. In: Congress of The Royal Society of Medicine: eHealth & Telemedicine 2012 - 3 million and Rising: Integrating Care, Mainstreaming Technology, London (2012) (in press)
8. Klompmaker, F., Nebe, K., Busch, C., Willemsen, D.: User Centered Design Process of Osami-D - Developing User Interfaces for a Remote Ergometer Training Application. In: Proceedings of HEALTHINF (2011)
9. Vehkaoja, A., Verho, J., Comert, A., Honkala, M., Lekkala, J.: Wearable System for EKG Monitoring - Evaluation of Night-Time Performance. Wireless Mobile Communication and Healthcare 83, 119–126 (2012)
10. Salminen, J., Koskinen, E., Kirkeby, O., Korhonen, I., Walters, D.: A home-based care model for outpatient cardiac rehabilitation based on mobile technologies. In: 3rd International Conference on Pervasive Computing Technologies for Healthcare (2009)

11. Mattila, J., Ding, H., Mattila, E., Särelä, A.: Mobile tools for home-based cardiac rehabilitation based on heart rate and movement activity analysis. In: Conf. Proc. IEEE Eng. Med. Biol. Soc. 2009, pp. 6448–6452 (2009)
12. Jokela, T.: An assessment approach for user-centred design processes. In: Proceedings of EuroSPI (2001)
13. Klompmaker, F., Nebe, K., Busch, C., Willemsen, D.: Designing context aware user interfaces for online exercise training supervision. In: 2nd Conference on Human System Interactions (2009)
14. Ha, V., Inkpen, K.M., Mandryk, R.L.: Direct intentions: the effects of input devices on collaboration around a tabletop display. In: TableTop 2006, pp. 177–184 (2006)
15. Scott, S.D., Carpendale, M.S.T., Inkpen, K.M.: Territoriality in collaborative tabletop workspaces. In: Proceedings of the 2004 ACM Conference on Computer Supported Cooperative Work, pp. 294–303 (2004)
16. Gutwin, C., Greenberg, S.: A descriptive framework of workspace awareness for real-time groupware. In: Computer Supported Cooperative Work (CSCW), vol. 11(3), pp. 411–446 (2002)
17. Klompmaker, F., Fischer, H., Jung, H.: Authenticated Tangible Interaction using RFID and Depth-Sensing Cameras Supporting Collaboration on Interactive Tabletops. In: The Fifth International Conference on Advances in Computer-Human Interactions, pp. 141–144 (2012)

One IMU Is Sufficient:
A Study Evaluating Effects of Dual-Tasks on Gait in Elderly People

Rolf Adelsberger[1], Nathan Theill[2], Vera Schumacher[2],
Bert Arnrich[1], and Gerhard Tröster[1]

[1] Federal Institute of Technology Zurich, ETHZ, Switzerland
[2] University of Zurich, Zurich, Switzerland
{rolf.adelsberger,bert.arnrich,gerhard.troester}@ife.ee.ethz.ch,
n.theill@inapic.uzh.ch,v.schumacher@psychologie.uzh.ch

Abstract. In industrialized countries the share of elderly subjects is increasing. Hence, diseases or symptoms associated with aging are more common than they were in the past. As a consequence, more effort is invested into research analyzing the effects of aging on the motion and cognition. However, economical and flexible methods to measure motion and its cross-effects with cognition are still missing. Therefore, we developed a new approach which neither requires a specific location, large infrastructural requirements, nor does it require large investments. We base our setting on match-box sized inertial measurement units (IMUs) attached to the participants' legs. 47 elderly subjects participated in our study where we analyzed the interplay between cognitive load and gait features. We show that it is feasible to automatically detect episodes of interest, e.g. straight path, during walking periods of a subject only using IMU data. Our approach detects the steps autonomously and calculates gait features without supervision. The results demonstrate that cognitive load induces a significant increase ($p = 0.007$) in step-duration variability from $16ms$ (baseline) to $21ms$ (load). Our findings demonstrate that IMUs are a proved alternative to static setups that usually require a non-trivial infrastructure, e.g. optical movement tracking.

Keywords: wearable computing, gait analysis, elderly people, risk of falling, imu, sensors.

1 Introduction

Increasing age might affect people in motoric skills as well as in cognitive performance. In general, the ability to sit, stand, walk and to perform activities of daily living (ADL) can be condensed in the term *mobility*. Mobility contributes the lion's share to an elderly persons' independence and as such is a combination of mental resources and their physical expressions. Limited motoric or mental capabilities result in a lowered mobility and with reduced mobility the risk of falling (RoF) increases [1]. If we can objectively measure mobility of a person,

B. Godara and K.S. Nikita (Eds.): MobiHealth 2012, LNICST 61, pp. 51–60, 2013.
© Institute for Computer Sciences, Social Informatics and Telecommunications Engineering 2013

there might be a model to predict her RoF. This is our main motivation: To estimate automatically the mobility of elderly people with future applications for safety in mind (e.g. reducing RoF).

In this paper we focus on gait features as they are by nature closely linked to RoF. It is known that gait features are affected by cognitive load levels of a subject. Especially for elderly people the *threshold level* where gait-feature-changes are noticeable is low [2] (compared to younger individuals' levels), sometimes as low as a task of subtracting numbers.

We demonstrate that a sensor-based automatic acquisition and analysis setup is a efficient alternative to the currently used methods. To this purpose we are looking at the step duration and its dynamics in situations with and without cognitive load. We present the analysis and results of a study with elderly people (aged 65+) and analyze the changes of gait features between a baseline setting (i.e. common walk) and a setting where the subjects were under elevated cognitive load while walking. We compare state-of-the-art (SoA) to our approach and show that we can detect the differences between situations with elevated cognitive load and situations without.

Furthermore, our longer-term goal is it to contribute to a transparent estimation system - not requiring any special action by the subjects - to make statements about a human's relative mental load level and the consequences for her motoric performance. We position our work as an initial contribution to that goal.

2   Related Work

2.1   Tests Not Using Electronic Devices

In general, in geriatrics the term mobility refers to a person's aptitude of performing a physical task in her everyday life. The definition of mobility is usually tailored to a specific target group, e.g. hospitalized patients or subjects at home and to a specific environment, e.g. medical care facility, home etc. [3, 4].

One of the most often used mobility indices (MI) is the timed-up-and-go test (TUG) first introduced by Podsialdo et al. [5] which is analyzed in more detail by Thrane et al. in [6]. TUG is often used as an indicator for RoF of a person. It measures the time a person needs to rise from a chair and walk a given distance. The *Short Physical Performance Battery* (SPPB) [7] focuses on the lower extremities and their functionality. SPPB can be divided into three sections: Balance Tests, Gait Speed Test and Chair Stand Tests (similar to TUG). The *Motor Assessment Scale* (MAS) [8] analyzes 8 motor functions. In particular, it also assesses transition movements (standing up), static tasks (standing still) and dynamic tasks (walking).

2.2   Tests with Electronic Devices

Webster et al. [9] introduced the GAITRite sensor system used for the evaluation of walking performance[1]. This sensor system consists of a pressure sensitive mat

---

[1] GAITRite Gold, CIR Systems, Easton, PA.

in various sizes. The largest model is about $1m$ wide and $7.5m$ long, allowing for the analysis of step length, step width and frequency. Webster et al. compared the system's performance to a state-of-the-art optical 3D motion tracking system, e.g. VICON. Van Iersel et al. [10] investigated the effect of cognitive dual tasking on balance of older adults. They used the GAITRite system for data acquisition and extracted spatial features of gait (e.g. stride length) and temporal gait features (time variability). Hollman et al. [11] performed a study incorporating older and younger subjects. In that study they analyzed the differences of dual-task walking between the two age groups. Kuys et al. [12] used a system to evaluate spatio-temporal gait features of stroke patients: the researchers used the data from the system to compute the MAS gait score of the patients. In [13] Bamberg et al. present a sensor system that provides three pressure measuring points as well as orientation data of the feet using intertial measurement units (IMU). All system components were integrated in a shoe. The authors used that system to analyze heel-strike and toe-off events during gait periods as well as the feet orientation. Within a sport focused setting Strohrmann et al. [14] used IMUs attached to the legs to analyze the running behavior of healthy younger people.

2.3 Evaluating Cognitive Features

Theill et al. [15] suggest that performing simple mathematical calculations[2] suffices to generate sufficient cognitive load to induce a measurable physical response of a subject. In their paper they present a precise method for measuring situations with cognitive loads of varying degree. Schaefer et al. [16] demonstrate that elderly subjects, when put under cognitive load, express an increased variance in step frequency and might even show difficulties maintaining balance. They used a variant of the N-Back test [17] to induce elevated cognitive load levels in their subjects. Schaefer et al. contributed to the motivation of evaluation training impact on cognitive performance and motoric fitness.

Cinaz et al. developed in [18] a system to estimate mental workload using the heart rate variability. They were able to train a classifier separating the instances of low mental workload from samples with higher mental workload. Cinaz et al. showed that the links between cognitive load and physical expression are abundant and feasible to measure.

3 Experiment

3.1 Hypotheses and Approach

We aimed at demonstrating the feasibility of using sensor data from IMUs to automatically detect periods of regular walk. During those intervals distinguished between situations without and situations with cognitive load. For this purpose we have setup a study where elderly people were asked to perform a simple

---

[2] e.g. starting from 50 subtract consecutively 2.

walking task once with, and once without a cognitive task in parallel. In the following sections we are going to provide the details.

3.2   Participants

Elderly people at the age 65 or older were recruited for the study. The inclusion criteria for participants was an age within the range $[\geq 65, 85 \leq]$. The applicants for participation had to pass a cognitive screening test [19] in order to be included in the study. To assess their overall motor activity we asked them to perform TUG. We were interested in healthy subjects with no evident disabilities. Subjects included in our study tested normal in the cognitive test and in the motoric evaluation, TUG. Out of 63 participants 47 individuals (32 female and 16 male) successfully completed the study and we could use their data for our evaluation[3]. The subjects' demographics are listed in Table 1 .

Table 1. Age distribution of the 47 subjects

	Min	Max	Mean	Std.Dev.
overall	65	84	71.77	4.89
female	65	81	71.71	4.70
male	65	84	71.88	5.33

3.3   Measurement Setup

For the testings we equipped the subjects with sensor devices. In order to track gait features of our subjects we used four IMUs by XSens [20]. With Velcro straps we attached on each shin and each thigh a sensor having the x-axis pointing towards ground (cf. Figure 1a). Four sensors at these locations allowed us to track more features than just step durations: angles between shin and thigh, leg orientation etc. The devices were tethered; the data was sent to and power comes from a gateway device (transmit station) that was worn by a belt around the subjects' waist. We configured the devices to report raw acceleration, rotation rate values, but also Euler angles which reflect the orientation in space relative to the earth.

At 50Hz motion data was streamed via Bluetooth to a standard notebook where we stored it for later analysis. Higher sampling was not possible due to bandwidth limitation of the Bluetooth system.

The subjects were additionally recorded on video for a validity check of our automatic feature calculations. Data analysis was performed offline using MATLAB®.

---

[3] For the first 15 subjects our measurement setup suffered a technical problem and the recordings failed. One subject did not perform a testing at all. Our set therefore contains data from 47 subjects.

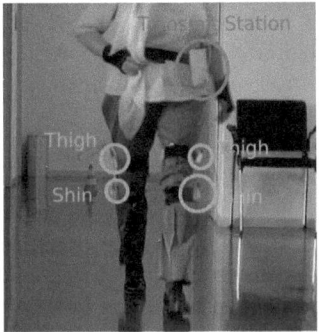 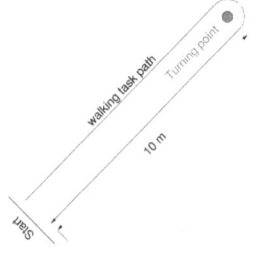

(a) Subject with four sensors and one gateway.

(b) The path for tasks 1 and 2.

Fig. 1. Test procedure illustrations

3.4 Test Procedure

At the beginning of the test session the mental test [19] (Mini Mental State Evaluation, MMSE) was presented to the subjects in direct interaction with an expert. This study controller (a psychologist) asked the questions and noted the answers of the subjects on the evaluation sheets. We required the subjects to score above 26 to be included in our study.

Motoric testing was performed with an instance of TUG: subjects were asked to sit on a regular chair. The controller then asked the subjects to stand up. Time until completion was measured starting from the issue of the command until the subject was in an upright position. TUG scores above 10 seconds are considered as noticeable [7].

During testings, subjects were two times required to walk down a aisle of length 10m, turn around and walk back again (baseline testing, task 1). In the second part of the testing we asked them to do the walk as before but now while subtracting from a random number provided by us (arbitrarily chosen from the set [501, 502, 503]) at each step a specific number, i.e. 7 (task 2).

4 Methods

We primarily wanted to compare statistics of the data from the baseline task to data from the cognitive-load task. To this purpose we firstly needed to detect the intervals in our data that were of interest, e.g. periods of straight walking, segmented by turning points. These intervals were detectable using the magnetometer data. In Figure 2a an axis of a magnetometer is plotted in blue. In the high frequency spectrum the steps are visible, the four changes of the mean value correlate with the walking direction of the subject. We calculated the turning points by first applying a smoothing, e.g. low-pass, filter to the data (red curve). Then, we used the sign of the slope (magenta) of this curve as the limits for the intervals. Finally, we declared the turning point as the mid-point of a decreasing interval. To maintain comparability to related work we analyzed the walking interval for the first $20m$, $(2 \times 10m)$. Therefore, only data until the second turning point (start position) was used. The turning points were detected by our algorithm without false positives. At each turning point we disregarded two steps before and one step afterward since we were only interested in statistics from straight walk.

Next we detected the steps using SoA [14] on the accelerometer signals. The steps manifest themselves as peaks in the accelerometer signal. In Figure 2b a fragment of a data set is shown: the accelerometer signal is in blue, the step locations are marked with red circles. Our focus lied on the variances of step

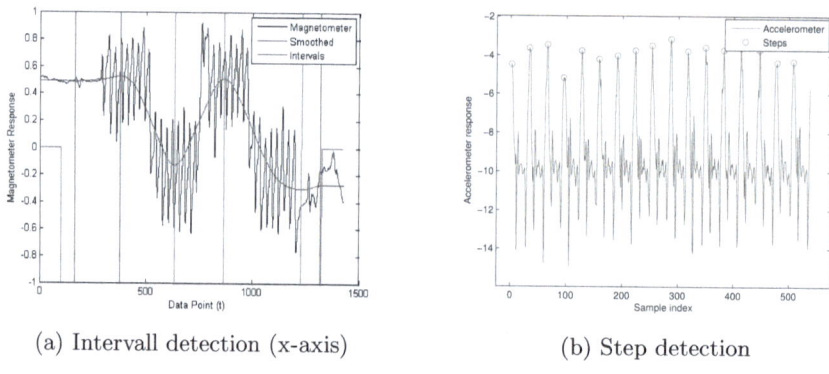

(a) Intervall detection (x-axis)   (b) Step detection

Fig. 2. Analyzing gait data

duration for task 1 and task 2. Hence, the time delays between individual steps served as input for our further analysis: For each subject we calculated the step durations for the baseline task (task 1) and for the cognitively loaded task (task 2) in milliseconds. Next, we calculated for each task $t = \{1, 2\}$ for each subject i the mean μ_t^i, the median m_t^i and standard deviation σ_t^i (or variance, resp.) of the step durations. We denote the collection of all μ_k^j of all subjects for task k as the vector $\bar{\mu}_k$. The definitions for $\bar{\sigma}_k$ and $\bar{m}_k$ are analogous. Since we are interested in individual changes we calculated the difference of μ^i and σ^i between the two tasks for each subject i: $\tilde{\mu}^i$ and $\tilde{\sigma}^i$, resp. $\tilde{\mu}^i := \mu_2^i - \mu_1^i$, $\tilde{\sigma}^i := \sigma_2^i - \sigma_1^i$. So, $\tilde{\mu}^3$ is the positive or negative change of the mean value of the step durations for subject 3.

In our analysis we looked at the set of means for both tasks, $\bar{\mu}_1$, and $\bar{\mu}_2$, resp. We also considered the sets of standard deviation for both tasks, $\bar{\sigma}_1$ and $\bar{\sigma}_2$. Finally, we also analyzed the set of individual progresses, $\bar{\tilde{\mu}}$ and $\bar{\tilde{\sigma}}$.

In order to make a statement about the development of gait features between task 1 and task 2 we needed to compare the variances of step duration of the first task to those variances from the second task. A requirement for a valid comparison is the two sets originate from the same distribution, e.g. a Normal distribution. The distribution parameters for each of the sets might be different.

We used the Lilliefors test [21] based on the Kolmogorov-Smirnov test [22] to verify task-1 data and task-2 data are from the same distribution family. Lilliefors' test performs better for smaller sample sizes than the Kolmogorov-Smirnov test.

For visualization the QQ-Plot [23] allows for graphical comparison of two distributions: it draws the quantiles of two empirical distributions against each other.

Finally, the variances of the two data sets were analyzed with a person-independent analysis of variance (ANOVA[4]).

5   Results

The validation of equality of distribution between the two sets yielded a positive result: in Figure 3a we show that the baseline data set and the cognitive load set originate from the same distribution family. The blue points represent the quantiles of the distributions. The abscissa represents the distribution for task 1 the ordinate is for task 2. Indicated in red is the linear interpolation line for the two sets. As can be seen the two sets relate in a linear manner to each other.

The evaluation of the Lilliefors test [21] for either set accepted the null hypothesis of the data originating from a normally distributed population with a confidence level $\alpha = 0.05$.

During evaluation we noticed that the sensor at the shin positions produced the best signal-to-noise (SNR) ratio. The shin sensors were less susceptible to *motion noise* that may be introduced by low-friction clothing (like synthetic trousers) and the sensor devices moving uncontrolled relatively to the leg or textile. We believe this result is caused by a looser attachment of the thigh sensors as a consequence of the thigh being by nature more sensitive to pressure than the shin. A tight Velcro was considered uncomfortable at that position. Too tight strappings might even have had an impact on the gait pattern. The shin, however, is not that sensitive and the muscular tissue does not perform large movements. Due to this reasons we decided to evaluate for each subject data solely from one (e.g. the left) shin sensor. A manual verification of the peak positions proved that the step detection algorithm worked with 100% accuracy.

Cognitive load had a significant impact on the gait features. This effect on the variance of step duration can be seen in Figure 3b where we draw probability plots for the two sets. In the plot data points (e.g. step durations) are plotted against their probability. The blue points mark the data points from the first task, the data of the second task is in green.

We performed a person-independent ANOVA test: In Table 2a we list the results of our analysis. In each line we report the mean value for the features $\bar{\mu}_k$, $\bar{\sigma}_k$ and the median, m_k resp., introduced in Section 4 . Additional to the mean values of the features we provide also the standard deviation. All values are in milliseconds. The F column are the F-numbers from ANOVA[5]. The $p-$values in

---

[4] Using a one-tailed significance level of p = .05.

[5] F-statistics from the ANOVA test: $F = \dfrac{\text{between-group variability}}{\text{within-group variability}}$.

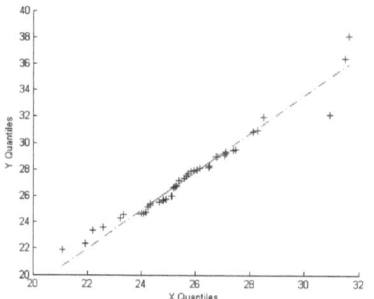

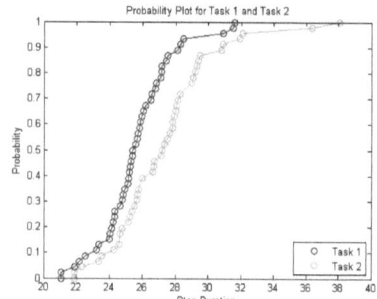

(a) QQ-Plot of mean values for baseline task and cognitive load task

(b) Cumulative Probability plot for baseline task and cognitive load label

Fig. 3. Comparing tasks

Table 2. Results of analysis

(a) ANOVA

Feature	Task 1 (ms)	Task 2 (ms)	F	p
$\bar{\sigma}_k$	16.84 ± 5.17	21.64 ± 10.62	6.62	0.007
$\bar{m}_k$	513.04 ± 45.41	547.39 ± 63.82	8.85	0.0038
$\bar{\mu}_k$	514.93 ± 44.24	549.01 ± 62.88	9.04	0.0034

(b) Mean changes.

Feature	Value (ms)
$\bar{\bar{\sigma}}$	4.8065
$\bar{\bar{\mu}}$	34.0807

the last column in Table 2a indicate that all three features differ significantly between the two testings.

Table 2b depicts the mean changes on gait features induced by the cognitive task. The standard deviation between the baseline task (task 1) and the cognitive load task has increased by $4.8ms$ (mean). The mean of the mean values increased by $34.1ms$. The variability of the step duration changes from baseline to cognitive loaded situations and the mean step duration increases. Our findings are comparable to previous findings of related work [10, 11].

6   Conclusion and Future Work

In this paper we have taken the first step towards an autonomous mobility assessment system by automatically analyzing the correlations of gait features and cognitive load with an IMU setup. We have shown that by using step duration it is possible to distinguish between situations of cognitive load and those without. We have also provided a proof-of-concept for the feasibility of performing the analysis automatically. In our paper we successfully demonstrated that with a minimal setup of one single inertial measurement sensor it is feasible to conduct studies equivalent to SoA, but requiring substantially less infrastructure, e.g. no cameras, no human resources etc. at arbitrary locations.

We are going to base our future work on the results and findings of this study. We further believe that for future gait analysis it is possible to reduce the hardware requirements even more. We envision a single-sensor setup - untethered - providing us with gait features like the ones used here but also with additional ones. We believe that there are training effects over longer periods of time: redoing task 2 several times over a longer time span might reduce the effect of the cognitive load. We want to measure this progression in the future. Also, generalizing our setup even more in order to allow for many more movement features is planned for the future.

We envision a automatic system to assess mobility: an unobtrusive self-contained sensor system that constantly monitors the movement of its wearer. This paper represents a part of the whole, but for the future we want to add additional modalities and more importantly at some point leave the lab setting and go into real life environments.

References

1. Scott, V., Votova, K., Scanlan, A., Close, J.: Multifactorial and functional mobility assessment tools for fall risk among older adults in community, home-support, long-term and acute care settings. Age and Ageing 36(2), 130–139 (2007)
2. Hausdorff, J.M., Schweiger, A., Herman, T., Yogev-Seligmann, G., Giladi, N.: Dual-task decrements in gait: contributing factors among healthy older adults. J. Gerontol. A Biol. Sci. Med. Sci. 63(12), 1335–1343 (2008)
3. de Morton, N.A., Davidson, M., Keating, J.L.: Reliability of the de morton mobility index (demmi) in an older acute medical population. Physiotherapy Research International: the Journal for Researchers and Clinicians in Physical Therapy (October 2010)
4. Kuys, S.S., Brauer, S.G.: Validation and reliability of the modified elderly mobility scale. Australasian Journal on Ageing 25(3), 140–144 (2006)
5. Richardson, S., Podsiadlo, D.: The timed 'up and go': A test of basic functional mobility for frail elderly persons. Journal of the American Geriatrics Society 39(2), 142–148 (1991)
6. Thrane, G., Joakimsen, R.M., Thornquist, E.: The association between timed up and go test and history of falls: the tromso study. BMC Geriatr. 7, 1+ (2007)
7. Guralnik, J.M., Simonsick, E.M., Ferrucci, L., Glynn, R.J., Berkman, L.F., Blazer, D.G., Scherr, P.A., Wallace, R.B.: A short physical performance battery assessing lower extremity function: Association with self-reported disability and prediction of mortality and nursing home admission. Journal of Gerontology 49(2), M85–M94 (1994)
8. Carr, J.H., Shepherd, R.B., Nordholm, L., Lynne, D.: Investigation of a new motor assessment scale for stroke patients. Physical Therapy 65(2), 175–180 (1985)
9. Webster, K.E., Wittwer, J.E., Feller, J.A.: Validity of the gaitrite walkway system for the measurement of averaged and individual step parameters of gait. Gait & Posture 22(4), 317–321 (2005)
10. van Iersel, M.B., Ribbers, H., Munneke, M., Borm, G.F., Rikkert, M.G.O.: The effect of cognitive dual tasks on balance during walking in physically fit elderly people. Archives of Physical Medicine and Rehabilitation 88(2), 187–191 (2007)

11. Hollman, J.H., Kovash, F.M., Kubik, J.J., Linbo, R.A.: Age-related differences in spatiotemporal markers of gait stability during dual task walking. Gait & Posture 26(1), 113–119 (2007)
12. Kuys, S.S., Brauer, S.G., Ada, L.: Test-retest reliability of the GAITRite system in people with stroke undergoing rehabilitation.. Disabil. Rehabil. 33(19-20), 1848–1853 (2011)
13. Bamberg, S., Benbasat, A., Scarborough, D., Krebs, D., Paradiso, J.: Gait analysis using a shoe-integrated wireless sensor system. IEEE Transactions on Information Technology in Biomedicine 12, 413–423 (2008)
14. Strohrmann, C., Harms, H., Tröster, G., Hensler, S., Müller, R.: Out of the lab and into the woods: kinematic analysis in running using wearable sensors. In: Ubicomp, pp. 119–122 (2011)
15. Theill, N., Martin, M., Schumacher, V., Bridenbaugh, S.A., Kressig, R.W.: Simultaneously measuring gait and cognitive performance in cognitively healthy vs. cognitively impaired older adults: The basel motor-cognition dual task paradigm. Journal of the American Geriatrics Society 59, 1012–1018 (2011)
16. Schaefer, S., Schumacher, V.: The interplay between cognitive and motor functioning in healthy older adults: Findings from dual-task studies and suggestions for intervention. In: Gerontology, pp. 1–8 (2010)
17. Kirchner, W.K.: Age differences in short-term retention of rapidly changing information. Journal of Experimental Psychology 55(4), 352–358 (1958)
18. Cinaz, B., La Marca, R., Arnrich, B., Tröster, G.: Monitoring of mental workload levels. In: Proceedings of IADIS eHealth Conference, pp. 189–193 (2010)
19. Folstein, M.F., Folstein, S.E., McHugh, P.R.: "Mini-mental state". a practical method for grading the cognitive state of patients for the clinician. Journal of Psychiatric Research 12, 189–198 (1975)
20. XSens, http://www.xsens.com/
21. Lilliefors, H.W.: On the kolmogorov-smirnov test for normality with mean and variance unknown. Journal of the American Statistical Association 62, 399–402 (1967)
22. Kolmogorov, A.N.: Sulla determinazione empirica di una legge di distribuzione. Giornale dell'Istituto Italiano degli Attuari 4, 83–91 (1933)
23. Wilk, M.B., Gnanadesikan, R.: Probability plotting methods for the analysis of data. Biometrika 55, 1–17 (1968)

On the Use of Nomadic Relaying for Emergency Telemedicine Services in Indoor Environments

Inam Ullah, Zhong Zheng, Edward Mutafungwa, and Jyri Hämäläinen

Aalto University, School of Electrical Engineering,
Department of Communication and Networking,
P.O. Box 13000, 00076 Aalto, Espoo, Finland
{firstname.lastname}@aalto.fi

Abstract. The need for high-quality on-the-spot emergency care necessitates access to reliable broadband connectivity for emergency telemedicine services used by paramedics in the field. In a significant proportion of recorded cases, these medical emergencies would tend to occur in indoor locations. However,broadband wireless connectivity may be of low quality due to poor indoor coverage of macro-cellular public mobile networks, or may be unreliable and/or inaccessible in the case of private Wi-Fi networks. To that end, relaying is emerging as one of promising radio access network techniques that provide coverage gain with improved quality of service. This paper analyzes the use of nomadic relays that could be temporarily deployed close to a building as part of the medical emergency response. The objective is to provide improved indoor coverage for paramedics located within the building for enhanced downlink performance (throughput gain, lower outage probability). For that scenario, we propose a resource sharing algorithm based on static relay link with exclusive assigned subframes at the macro base station (MBS) coupled with access link prioritization for paramedic's terminals to achieve max-min fairness. Via comprehensive system-level simulations, incorporating standard urban propagation models, the results indicate that paramedics are always able to obtain improved performance when connected via the relay enhanced cell (REC) networks rather than the MBS only.

Keywords: Emergency Telemedicine, Relay Node, Relay Enhanced Cell, Indoor Coverage, Long-Term Evolution, Outage Probability.

1 Introduction

Emergency telemedicine is the usage of telecommunication technologies by Emergency Medical Services (EMS) providers (hospitals,paramedics,etc) so as to ensure a rapid and coordinated medical care to patients at emergency sites [1, 2]. This typically enables emergency use cases, such as, setting up a communications link to provide field paramedics with expert opinion from physicians at a hospital or trauma center, thus enabling better-informed diagnosis or medical interventions by the EMS responder. Or then, a high-speed link may enabling sharing of large amounts of patient measurements or images prior to transfer to relevant trauma center.

B. Godara and K.S. Nikita (Eds.): MobiHealth 2012, LNICST 61, pp. 61–68, 2013.

Contemporary modern communication technologies, especially the wireless tech-nologies (e.g modern wireless,Wireless Local Area Network or WLAN,satellite,etc) improves the intra- and inter-organization (hospitals,fire brigade,police station,etc) collaborations in emergency or disaster management [2,3]. Furthermore, the continued developments in mobile broadband networks are now opening new possibilities in emergency telemedicine for exchange of diagnostic-quality digital medical images (e.g. ultrasound scans) and high-resolution interactive or streaming video from emergency sites [3]. Nevertheless, these broadband mobile network technologies also inherit some network limitations(resources scarcity,link throughput,etc), particularly in indoor environments, where the distant outdoor MBS yields poor radio links with low SINR levels (Signal-to-Interference-and-Noise-Ratio) due to in-building penetration loss and distant-dependent path losses [4,5]. This will in-turn leads to less than optimum quality of service (e.g. reduced link throughput) which may prove to be unreliable for emergency telemedicine applications, particularly for indoor environments where most medical emergencies have been noted to frequently occur [6].

Relaying is emerging as one of the promising radio access techniques for provid-ing coverage gain and improved quality of service in cell edge and/or indoor environ-ments [4,11–17]. This paper aims to show the relaying benefits (one being the improved throughput in indoor environment) in a REC network from the perspective of the indoor emergency telemedicine use case. To that end, we perform a comparative study of the REC network performance (in terms of throughput and outage probability) against that of the conventional macrocellular connectivity used in existing mobile networks. In the remaining part of the paper, Section 2 presents the comparative analysis of com-munication technologies and potential benefits in indoor emergency telemedicine use case scenarios, while Section 3 outlines the system model considered for this study. Simulation methodology and results with conclusive remarks are provided in Sections 4 & 5 respectively.

2 Nomadic Relaying for Emergency Telemedicine Services

A number of wireless networking technologies are considered for use to support indoor emergency telemedicine services [3]. Private WLANs are one of the most common means for subscribers to provide broadband wireless extensions to their residential fixed access lines. However, these WLANs may expose patient data on poorly secured open networks or may be inaccessible to EMS responders due to access controls settings by the WLAN access point (AP) owner. Moreover, lack of centralized management of private APs means that guarantee of services (through admission control, traffic flow prioritization etc.) cannot be provided for emergency telemedicine users [6].

The shortcomings when sharing the commercial networks has prompted the deployment of dedicated *Professional Mobile Radio* (PMR) systems launched, in order to enable a reliable network coverage for the emergency responders (e.g, Terrestrial Trunked Radio (TETRA), Association of Public Safety Communications Officials International Project(APCO-25)) [7]. However, these PMR networks are typically narrowband systems which lack capabilities to support the advanced multimedia emergency telemedicine applications. Broadband satellite communications provides

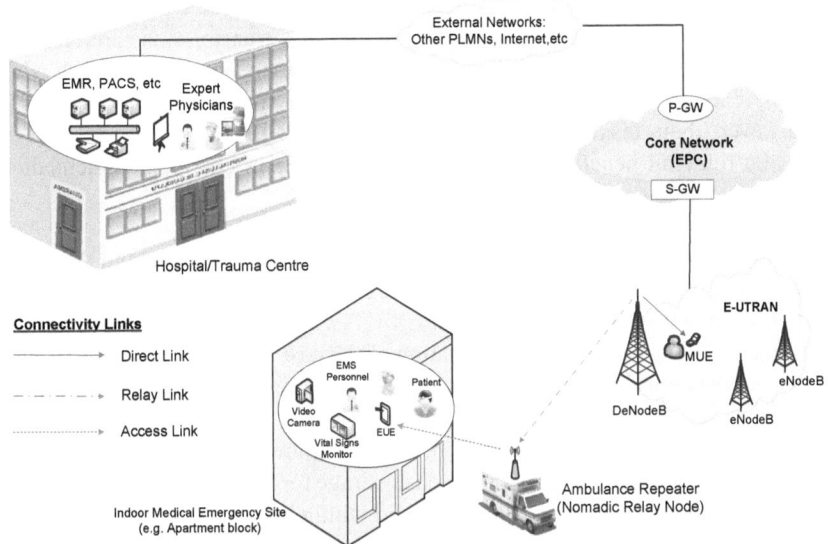

DeNodeB = Donor Enhanced Node-B, EMR = Electronic Medical Records, EMS = Emergency Medical Service, EUE = Emergency User Equipment, E-UTRAN = Evolved UMTS Radio Access Network, EPC = Evolved Packet Core, MUE = Macrocellular User Equipment (Common UE), REC = Relay Enhanced Cell, PACS = Picture Archiving and Communications System, P-GW = Packet Data Network Gateway, S-GW = Serving Gateway.

Fig. 1. Usage of a nomadic relay node to provide improved coverage in indoor emergency areas

another alternative. However, the satellite terminals cannot be used for high data rate indoor service provision due to bulky terminals, stringent line-of-sight requirements and high latency [3, 6, 8]. As a result mobile broadband networks (and evolutions beyond 3G) provide arguably the most attractive option for emergency telemedicine use cases [3, 8]. This is also previously noted in various experimental telemedicine studies or practical implementations in third generation (3G) mobile networking environments [9, 10]. However, these networks employ conventional macrocell deployment for providing coverage in a wide-area. Yet, in many cases they also admit some difficulties for enabling improved services with guaranteed QoS in indoor environments [4].

To that end, multi-hop relaying emerges as a promising deployment scenario, pro-vides an improved network performance gains in the existing macro-overlaid networks. Relay node (RN) being a low-power base station, can be considered as an intermediate access point between User Equipment (UE) and 3GPP Long Term Evolution Advanced (LTE) compliant macro base station, known as Donor Evolved Node B (DeNB) [11]. Likewise, nomadic relaying being semi-static in nature, allows temporary RN deploy-ment in emergency areas, even providing additional indoor coverage [12].

Figure 1 presents a schematic end-to-end overview of relay enhanced cellular (REC) network for emergency telemedicine scenario, comprises a two-hop nomadic RN (N-RN) deployed within the macro-overlaid network. From the network operator perspective, all the emergency telemedicine devices (tablet PC,Smartphone,etc.) would be consider as a UE providing broadband access to the mobile network. The mobile core network can be accessed by EMS responders, either via the DeNB direct link or alternatively, via the two-hop relaying where the UE-RN transmissions are facilitated by the Access link while the RN-DeNB transmission is done via a wireless Relay link.

Yet the relaying benefits being explored from the mobile operator-subscriber aspect,however, their feasibility for public safety need to be examine. Below are few two-hop relaying benefits justifying the relay usage in emergency telemedicine scenarios.

- Enabling high spectral efficiency with improved network coverage and throughput at dead spot (due to shadowing) or at cell edge (poor eNB coverage) [13, 14].
- With low capital/operational cost (CAPEX/OPEX) and low power constraints, the benefits might probably be the elimination of the cost barrier in making RNs available in large volumes and ease of operation (e.g. in terms of powering requirements) [15].
- Wireless relay link with no line of sight (LOS) requirements, enabling flexible RN deployment options to provide improved coverage for EMS responders from relay-deployed-ambulance near to patients located within indoor environments [15].
- Decode-and-forward (DF) relaying though increases the system complexity, intended to provide a noiseless signal transmission via a two-hop link in urban environments (where the signals certainly experience multipath fadings) [16].
- A multimode relaying directly route the user data to mobile operator core network via internet via wired and/or wireless link. Thus, incorporates a diversity to emergency telemedicine, in case of macrocellular network being unavailable or destroyed [17].

3   System Model

A LTE-Advanced compliant RN has been proposed to use for the considered emergency communication scenario. The adopted relay operates with the type 1 inband configuration, where the relay and access link transmissions are time-division multiplexed and operate at the same carrier frequency. Moreover, the relay link can coexist with direct link, sharing the same frequency spectrum with DeNB users, enabling a full frequency reuse [11]. Consequently, the REC network performance depends on a resource partitioning strategy between the relay and direct links, along with an effective scheduling technique to allocate relay resources on the access link. Orthogonal Frequency Division Multiple Access (OFDMA) is employed as a radio interface for LTE-Advanced DL transmission, splitting the system bandwidth into narrow orthogonal subcarriers each with 15 kHz spectrum bandwidth. Furthermore, in 3GPP LTE-Advanced, a physical layer radio frame composed of 10 subframes, has a total duration of 10 msec. Each subframe comprises two consecutive 0.5 msec time slot. Hence, twelve consecutive orthogonal subcarriers are aggregated into physical resource block (PRB), which comprises a total bandwidth of 180 kHz and 0.5 msec duration. The PRB is used as a basic resource element for assigning the network resources to UE by a 3GPP eNB scheduler.

In the downlink, an inband RN quits transmission towards UEs on access link, while during the reception from DeNB via relay link, however, an RN needs to enable a backward compatibility towards Rel-8 UEs by sending cell-specific reference and control signals in all DL subframes. Hence, it facilitates the configuration of Multi-Media Broadcast over Single Frequency Network (MBSFN) subframes in DL, allowing the RN to inform the Rel-8 UEs, not to expect transmission from RN, by sending control signals in the first OFDM symbols of a blank subframe [18]. In this study, three subframes has been reserved as the MBSFN subframes for DL relay link transmissions at the DeNB side. In remaining seven subframes, a simultaneous transmission of eNB and RN enabled on direct and access link respectively, creates an interference to neighbouring cells. Moreover, all the eNB interference towards RN, are avoided, as all the cells use the same frame format. To that end, a Max-Min Fairness (MMF) scheduling technique is used to distribute the network resources at eNB on direct link as well as at RN with relay link constraint. From cellular system perspective, this algorithm aims to maximize the minimum user throughput by allocating more network resources to UEs with low Signal-to-Interference-and-Noise-Ratio (SINR), with a condition that all UEs obtain same throughput level. The UE throughput is calculated for given SINR level as follows [19];

$$TP_{user} = BW_{PRB}.BW_{eff}.\log_2\left(1 + \left(\frac{SINR}{SINR_{eff}}\right)\right) \quad (1)$$

where (1) represents a modified version of Shannon's capacity formula with parameters known as the bandwidth efficiency (BW_{eff}) and SINR efficiency $(SINR_{eff})$ with values of 0.88 and 1.25 respectively. They presents the performance loss to the network implementation and signal processing losses, while (BW_{PRB}) is bandwidth of one PRB (valued 180 kHz). The COST231-Walfisch-Ikegami (WI), path loss model is adopted in the simulations, which models both indoor and outdoor radio propagations [5]. The selected channel model accounts for distance-dependent path loss, shadowing as well as indoor penetration loss. To estimate the indoor losses, external and internal walls penetration losses has been explicitly modelled in line with COST 231 report [5].

4   Methodology and Results

The simulated network consists of seven hexagonal cellular eNB sites each possess three sectorized RF antennas to provide coverage to three sectors. Furthermore, it is assumed that there are 10 UEs randomly located in each sector. A $5 * 5$ grid layout residential building is assumed in central sector at two locations,i.e. cell center and cell edge. The building includes eight EMS responders (each with one emergency UE or EUE) scattered in random locations within the building. A vehicular nomadic RN is located 50 meter away from the building and provides indoor coverage. In simulations, we assumed downlink scenario with 3GPP use case 1 (Urban)and Inter-Site Distance (ISD) of 500m. It represents the typical case, where indoor emergency incident could occur. The baseline scenario with eNB only deployment is used as a reference.

Table 1 enlists the system parameters used in simulation. Via comprehensive system level simulations, a comparative study of eNB only and REC networks performance is carried out, in terms of cumulative distribution function (CDF) of indoor EUE data rates. Moreover, we also examine the impact of RN transmission on the performance

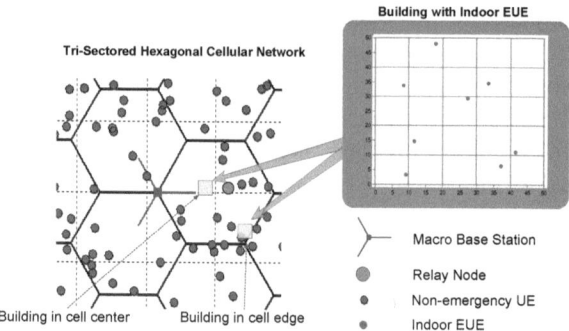

Fig. 2. Relay enhanced cellular (REC) network

Table 1. Simulation parameters

Parameters	Value
DeNB Parameters	
Carrier Frequency	$800\ MHz$
Transmission Bandwidth	$10\ MHz$,48 PRBs for data & 2 PRB for signalling
eNB Transmit Power	$46\ dBm$
eNB Elevation Gain	$14\ dBi$
eNB Antenna Pattern	$A(\theta) = -\min\left[12\left(\dfrac{\theta}{\theta_{3dB}}\right)^2, A_m\right]$ $\theta_{3dB} = 70°$ and $A_m = 25\ dB$
RN Parameters	
RN Transmit Power	$30\ dBm$
RN Antenna Pattern	Omni-directional
RN-eNB Elevation Gain	$7\ dBi$
UE Parameters	
UE Transmit Power (Maximum)	$23\ dBm$
UE Received Diversity Gain	$3\ dBi$

of non-emergency UEs of only those eNBs, which are serving the indoor EUE. Figure 3 indicates the simulations carried out for cell center and cell edge with UE performance constraint of 2 Mbps. Figure 3 (left) shows that the REC network outperforms the eNB only deployment, with almost 70% indoor EUEs in cell center case and 77% indoor EUEs in cell edge case, achieve a data rate of higher then 6 Mbps (i.e. from mid to high data rate levels). This gain is due to the fact that indoor EUE receive good enhanced signal quality from RN as well as experience less competition for radio resources. However, in addition to performance constraint of 2 Mbps, the high power eNB creates interference towards the indoor EUEs, resulting a 2% outage in the cell center scenario, which is negligible for the cell edge scenario where the eNB interference decays over the long distance. Similarly, figure 3 (right) shows the CDF plots for outdoor non-emergency UE data rates. The results demonstrate the deterioration impact of RN deployment on the performance of outdoor non-emergency UEs, due to the RN

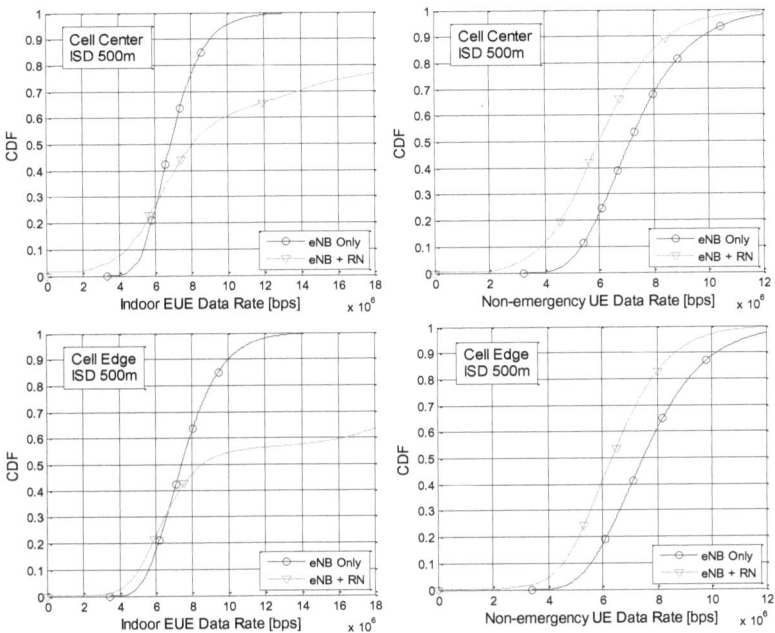

Fig. 3. CDFs of indoor EUE (left) and non-emergency UE (right) data rates

interference power. However, this degradation is insignificant as compared to the indoor coverage provided in emergency events.

5   Conclusion and Future Work

This paper investigated the benefits of improved indoor coverages enabled by REC network deployments in emergency telemedicine scenarios. Moreover, this paper outlined the architectural implementation of REC network as well as yields a comparative analysis of RN deployment to legacy eNB only networks in 3GPP downlink urban scenario. Simulation results show that indoor coverage has been significantly improved in relay-based system , with only insignificant performance degradation for outdoor non-emergency UEs.

In future work, we will investigate the performance of multiple un-coordinated REC used by various PMR organizations. These RNs coexist and operate in the same frequency band , compete for the available radio resources at eNB. Hence, a scheduling mechanism with pre-defined requirement will be needed for optimal RN operations.

Acknowledgement. This work was prepared in HEWINETS project framework, and was supported in part by the Finnish Funding Agency for Technology and Innovation (TEKES), Cassidian and Ericsson Finland.

References

1. Sluyter, A.J.: The role of Communication Systems in Emergency Medical Services. IEEE Transactions on Vehicular Technology 25(4), 175–186 (1976)
2. Ziadlou, D., Eslami, A., Hassani, H.R.: Telecommunication methods for implementation of telemedicine systems in crisis. In: Broadband Communications, Information Technology and Biomedical Applications, Gauteng, pp. 268–273 (2008)
3. Pattichis, C.S., Kyriacou, E., Voskaride, S., Pattichis, M.S., Lstepanian, R., Schizas, C.N.: Wireless Telemedicine Systems An Overview. IEEE Antennas and Propagation Magazine 44(2), 143–153 (2002)
4. Holma, H., Toskala, A.: WCDMA for UMTS: HSPA Evolution and LTE, 5th edn. Wiley and Sons Ltd., Chichester (2010)
5. COST 231, COST Action 231 Digital mobile radio towards future generation systems Final report. Luxembourg: Office for Official Publications of the European Communities (1999)
6. Mutafungwa, E., Zheng, Z., Hämäläinen, J., Husso, M., Korhonen, T.: On the use of Home Node Bs for Emergency Telemedicine Applications in Various Indoor Environments. Special Issue of the International Journal on E-Health and Medical Communications 2(1), 91–109 (2011)
7. Ketterling, H.: Introduction to Digital Professional Mobile Radio. Artech House, Boston (2004)
8. Shimizu, K.: Telemedicine by mobile communication. IEEE Journal of Engineering in Medicine and Biology Magazine 18, 32–44 (1999)
9. Banitsas, K., Konnis, G., Koutsouris, D.: 3G Networks in Emergency Telemedicine - An In-Depth Evaluation and amp; Analysis. In: 27th Annual International Conference of the Engineering in Medicine and Biology Society, IEEE-EMBS 2005, pp. 2163–2166 (2006)
10. Gállego, J.R., Hernández-Solana, A., Canales, M., Lafuente, J., Valdovinos, A., Fernández-Navajas, J.: Performance analysis of multiplexed medical data transmission for mobile emergency care over the UMTS channel. IEEE Transactions on Information Technology in Biomedicine 9(1), 13–22 (2005)
11. 3GPP TR 36.814.: Requirements for further advancements for Evolved UTRA (E-UTRA Release 9), physical layer aspects version 9.0.0 (March 2010)
12. Sydir, J.: Harmonized Contribution on 802.16j (Mobile Multihop Relay) Usage Models. IEEE 802.16 Broadband Wireless Access Working Group (July 2006)
13. Beniero, T., Redana, S., Raaf, B., Hämäläinen, J.: Effect of Relaying on Coverage in 3GPP LTE-Advanced. In: Vehicular Technology Conference, pp. 1–5 (2009)
14. Bou Saleh, A., Redana, S., Raaf, B., Hämäläinen, J.: On the coverage extension and capacity enhancement of inband relay deployments in LTE-Advanced networks. Journal of Electrical and Computer Engineering, 1–12 (2010)
15. Bulakci, Ö., Redana, S., Raaf, B., Hämäläinen, J.: Performance Enhancement in LTE-Advanced Relay Networks via Relay Site Planning. In: VTC, pp. 1–5 (2010)
16. Bou Saleh, A., Redana, S., Riihonen, T., Raaf, B., Hämäläinen, J.: Performance of Amplify-and-Forward and Decode-and-Forward Relays in LTE-Advanced. In: VTC IEEE 70th, pp. 1–5 (2009)
17. Teyeb, O., Phan, V.V., Raaf, B., Redana, S.: Dynamic Relaying in 3GPP LTE-Advanced Networks. EURASIP Journal on Wireless Communication and Networking (2009)
18. R1-091294, On the design of relay node for LTE-advanced, Texas instruments, 3GPP TSG RAN WG1 (March 2009)
19. Mogensen, P., Na, W., Kovacs, I.Z., Frederiksen, F., Pokhariyal, A., Pedersen, K.I., Kolding, T., Hugl, K., Kuusela, M.: LTE Capacity Compared to the Shannon Bound. IEEE VTC (2007)

A Mobile Healthcare System for Sub-saharan Africa

Bakia Bisong[1], Etienne Asonganyi[2], Andrii Gontarenko[1],
Alexander Semenov[1], and Jari Veijalainen[1]

[1] University of Jyvaskyla
Mattilanniemi 2, FI-40014, Jyväskylä, Finland
[2] Kumba District Hospital, Station Road
Kumba, Cameroon
{holmes.b.j.bisong,alexander.v.semenov,
jari.a.veijalainen}@jyu.fi,
{etienne.asonganyi,velotelo}@gmail.com

Abstract. The disparity between healthcare systems in developed countries and underdeveloped countries is huge, particularly due to the fact that the healthcare infrastructure of former is based on a sophisticated technological infrastructure. Efforts are being made worldwide to bridge this disparity and make healthcare services affordable even to the most remote areas of undeveloped countries. Recent growth of mobile networks in underdeveloped countries argues for building mHealth systems and applications on their basis. However, peculiarities of the area introduce difficulties into potential use cases of mobile devices, thus making the copying of mHealth services from developed countries inapplicable. In this paper, we present the functional requirements for a patient medical record system running partially on mobile devices and architectural choices for this system. Requirements are based on the circumstances of the Republic of Cameroon. In addition we discuss the country-level benefits that may appear after deployment of such a system.

Keywords: mHealth, Functional Requirements, Cameroon.

1 Introduction

Cameroon is a sub-Saharan African state with a population of about 20 million, according to a 2012 estimate [1]. As of 2007 about 70% of the population aged 15 and above were literate. Despite the fact that the country (and Africa in general) has a very low Internet penetration rate, the country is experiencing a mobile boom that is going through the developing and least-developed countries nowadays. As of 2011, there were close to 10 million mobile subscribers in Cameroon [1]. There are three mobile operators in Cameroon, and the coverage rate is about 80% population-wise.

The handset base consists of cheap Chinese phones, secondhand phones imported from Europe, and some new smartphones. Inflow of these phones into the market is uncontrolled. In the smartphone category, BlackBerry phones recently have shown a greater influx, as operators such as MTN have made them available to clients, along

B. Godara and K.S. Nikita (Eds.): MobiHealth 2012, LNICST 61, pp. 69–78, 2013.

with the normal uncontrolled inflow. The operator offers unlimited Internet access for 15/38 €/mth if the subscription includes BlackBerry/GALAXYtab [2].

The healthcare system is very inefficient. Lack of infrastructure and competent staff makes it very difficult to provide adequate healthcare. The government allocates about 5.6% of the GDP to the healthcare sector [3]. In Cameroon, patients' medical records are stored in so-called hospital books, which are solely kept by the patients. They are small booklets issued by hospitals. Besides that, hospitals compile and keep patients' partial medical history in paper files. The hospital books are quite vulnerable to destruction and are easily lost. So a patient may not have a complete or even a partial written medical record available for future use.

Currently, a large volume of data is moved from the paper to the digital form, and digital docflow systems are widespread in developed counties. A similar system or simply camera phones might be used to move the information in the hospital books and manual cards into a digital format. One can also ponder whether the information from the hospital books could be manually typed into a new digital system in character format in a country where the labor is cheap.

In this paper we propose a system through which patients would have their medical data stored on their mobile phones, thereby eradicating the problem of vulnerability of hospital books and paper-based storage.

The paper is structured as follows. In section 2 we consider related work in this area. In section 3 we analyze the business requirements of the proposed systems, taking into consideration the existing constraints. In section 4 we propose possible variants mHealth systems and discuss shortly the deployment of our current prototype. Section 5 concludes.

2   Related Work

There is a large body of literature about mHealth in developed countries, but a general assumption is that mHealth systems augment heavily networked medical record and medical image systems, rather than act as a backbone system. Therefore, we do not handle them in this context. In [4] the authors describe a phone based mHealth system. The authors discuss problems that arose during the deployment and arrive at six core findings that should guide mobile health system designs. The results are preliminary, though.

The District Health Information System (DHIS2) project was run at the University of Oslo, Norway [5]. It aimed at the collection and analysis of health information in Vietnam. The main causes of failure were that DHIS2 was not fully implemented prior to deployment in Vietnam, and the system could not provide vital reports when needed. Besides that, problems such as lack of computers, insufficient skills of the staff, and bad management also contributed to the failure of the project.

Paper [6] examines the use of mobile devices, particularly Android-based tablets, in rural healthcare. Paper [7] discusses mWash mobile phone applications, which aim at helping the people who do not have access to safe water and sanitation by mainly using mobile phones for the collection and dissemination of information regarding water sources. Though the application domain differs from the one proposed in this paper, the environments are similar (cf. below).

FrontlineSMS and RapidSMS are frameworks that allow two-way data exchange between a computer and a mobile device. FrontlineSMS [8] is an appropriate solution for some remote areas with GSM network coverage for the transfer of data directly between residents of those areas and service providers. These frameworks are considered here since most of Sub-Saharan Africa, and Cameroon in particular, relies solely on two GSM networks, although 3G license competition is ongoing [9].

Berg et al. [10] implemented an application that allows the storage of outgoing data on a mobile device if there is no network connection and sends those data when the connection is reestablished. Similar functionality might be desirable for the system proposed in this paper for the same reasons.

Paper [11] describes a project carried out at the University of Botswana to improve learning facilities and bring healthcare provision closer to the rural population. Relevant material about projects under resource-poor settings in low-and middle-income countries was traced referring to various mHealth projects at different stages of implementation in several countries in [12]. Some of these projects are reviewed here, but others, such as [13], Expedited Results System to Improve Early Infant Diagnosis [14], and Fitun Warmline AIDS Hotline [15] are also relevant. Paper [21] describes a mobile system aimed at collecting the data from a sensor measuring blood glucose. Software is installed on a cellphone, and the sensor is sending the information via Bluetooth. Paper [22] describes the progress of telehealth projects in Sub-Saharan Africa and concludes that many projects are up and running. Some of them are in a pilot phase, and the future of mHealth is hard to predict in general. Paper [23] discusses applications of mHealth systems in Botswana and concludes that the success of mHealth projects demonstrates the potential of the technology. Paper [24] discusses mHealth in resource-limited settings, and describes an mHealth project in Kenya: patients would get SMS messages reminding about the need to take their medicine and enquiring about their health status. Paper [25] discusses the TRACnet system in Rwanda. Its architecture and use experiences are of high relevance for our work, although the goal of the system is different. Its success shows that mHealth is possible in Africa. Paper [26] discusses general barriers for mHealth in Africa.

3   Requirements for a Patient-Centered System

3.1   Stakeholder Identification

In this section we discuss the requirements for the proposed mHealth system, taking into consideration the peculiarities of the Sub-Saharan region. According to [16], getting stakeholders involved in the requirements-elicitation process of a system eliminates the need for two of the most ineffective requirements-elicitation techniques: clairvoyance and telepathy. When identifying the stakeholders of the proposed system, we referred to stakeholder-identification models presented in [17, 18]. From these works the following stakeholders were identified: patients who are the users of the system, doctors, nurses, developers of the system, and maintenance personnel of the system. Apart from these basic stakeholders, other stakeholders such as the government of Cameroon represented by the Ministry of Public Health, the Medical Council, local hospitals, clinics, and health centers are relevant. Some individual stakeholders were included in the elicitation process of the requirements, but not all categories had their say.

3.2   Business Requirements and Constraints

Medical records of patients are not only very important for medical staff and the patients, but to a greater extent can be useful to the government as a whole. Although a paper-based version of the storage is simple and reliable, many of the developing countries or at least some private hospitals are moving to the usage of special information systems aimed at the storage of the medical data. An example of a special-purpose system is TRACnet in Rwanda [25].

In general, information system architecture always spans certain power relations between the stakeholders. The developed countries started to develop their medical information systems during 1960s, first based on the available mainframes. This was typically a top-down endeavor, where government and public and private hospitals were controlling the development. Patients were not at all included as stakeholders, or they had a minor role. Hospitals and governments controlled the structure the information systems and the information stored into the medical record systems. In Finland, healthcare districts and municipal health centers were allowed to decide for themselves during 1990s what kind of systems they would use. This led to large interoperability problems between different healthcare units. One argument was the privacy legislation that imposes strict rules upon the transfer and use of the patient's data that are at the same time owned by the government or private enterprises, not by the patient.

Only in the recent years governments have begun to change their policies and open access for patients to their own data. In Finland this will happen by 2014, when KanTA [19] will be taken into full use. The e-prescription service is now almost fully functional, and by 2014 complete copies of citizens' electronic medical records will be stored into the central repository. They can be accessed by the patients and healthcare personnel over the Web using PCs or smartphones. Usage of such an IS as KanTA provides obvious benefits such as access to a rather complete medical record of a patient that is currently lacking, soon a rather complete picture of the current medication of the patient, enabling easy searching of the data, simple data transfer, and so on. However, deployment and maintenance costs of such systems might be rather high, since they require a number of computers, large data storage, expensive software support, and skilled personal for maintaining the system. KanTA is maintained by KELA—The Social Insurance Institution of Finland, which has a long record of massive population-wide insurance and social benefit systems.

Deployment of the massive country-wide health information systems in underdeveloped countries might become almost completely insuperable. The first problem is the lack of funding and skilled personnel. The second problem is the almost complete lack of the ICT infrastructure, so the hospitals can only provide basic facilities and it would be difficult to equip computer and server rooms. This would also require a lot of electricity that should be constantly supplied. The third problem is a frequent occurrence of electricity shortages, and the lack of Internet connections. Thus, an important business requirement and a constraint is the usage of very cheap infrastructure, e.g., mobile phones, since currently they are very widespread and the government would not need to pay for them. A further requirement is making the architecture of the system reliable, taking into account all the realities of Cameroon, including harsh conditions for the ICT equipment that has to operate under constant high temperatures of about 30–35 degrees Celsius during the dry season, high humidity during the rainy season, and dust from the roads that in rural areas are not paved.

3.3 Central Functional and Non-functional Requirements

The system consists of a number of mobile handsets and a central component that can communicate over mobile telecom networks (2G–4G) or fixed Internet using SMS, MMS, or data services. The central component can further be implemented as one entity running on one site (one or several server computers), or it can be implemented as a distributed system consisting of several components running on fixed servers at various sites, communicating over wireless or wireline data connections with each other. "The system" consists of mobile handsets controlled by the patients, and the central component is controlled by the hospital(s) and possibly by the central government.

- F1 The system shall facilitate storage and manipulation of patient medical records on mobile phones. Rationale: Patients can carry digital medical records with them all the time, and presumably phones are less often lost than hospital books.
- F2 Medical records of a certain person are stored into a mobile phone controlled by him or her. Children's medical records can be stored into mobile phones under the control of their parents. Rationale: In this way the privacy is maintained
- F3 Medical records of a certain person can be stored and manipulated at the central component. Rationale: This component is hosted by the hospitals (and government) and storage and manipulation are dictated by their needs. The central component also acts as a backup point for the medical data.
- F4 The system shall provide the capability for medical personnel to access the Internet and transfer the data using a wireless data connection. Rationale: The transfer of medical data can easily be done via the Internet.
- F5 The system shall provide the possibility to transfer medical data using SMS as a bearer, in addition to GPRS, HSPA, and WLAN. Rationale: In the absence of an Internet connection medical data can still be transferred—at least important extracts such as blood type and diseases (cf. TRACnet).
- F6 The system shall be equipped with the capability of handling images. Rationale: Doctors could improve diagnosis with image files, and patient records can be images.
- F6.1 The system shall support the transfer of images from a mobile phone to the central component. Rationale: The doctor could improve diagnosis if he is supported with images from past treatments.
- F6.2 The system shall support the transfer of images from a computer to a mobile phone. Rationale: The patient would be able to take home images such as X-rays or ECG-plots needed for future diagnosis and treatments.

- F6.3 The system shall support the transfer of images from mobile phone to mobile phone. Rational: This is helpful for clinics equipped only with mobile devices.
- F6.4 The system shall support transfer of image files from a computer to a computer. Rationale: This is helpful for the interaction between hospitals equipped with computers.
- F7 The system shall enforce authentication through PIN codes and passwords at least. Rationale: This is useful for security and privacy reasons, for both doctors and patients.
- F8 Patients shall have access to their own medical data residing at the central component. Rationale: The patient might not have complete medical data on her mobile phone or she might have lost the mobile phone and needs to access medical data remotely or locally from the central component.
- F9 Patients and healthcare personnel must have a unique identity inside the system. Rationale: This is necessary for enforcing access control and protecting the privacy of the data.
- F10 Special infrastructure and interfaces shall exist that would allow the transfer of currently existing medical data (in form of paper-based hospital books) to a digital format into the mobile handsets and central component. Rationale: This is useful for patients who still have hospital books during the transition period.
- F11 The system interfaces should be designed so that illiterate people can also use the system.

In addition, we describe the following *non-functional requirements* (NF):

- NF1 The system must not lose data when electricity shortage takes place in the hospital or the handset runs out of power.
- NF2 Core functions of the system should still run even without Internet connection
- NF3 The system must provide high enough performance for hospitals and patients.
- NF4 The system design must minimize software and communication costs.

4   Architectural Solutions

In this section we present two architectural solutions that correspond to the described requirements. The "system" that is required is inherently distributed, because we want the mobile phones be part of "the system."

4.1   Decentralized Solutions

In theory, we might base the entire distributed system on the portable terminals, without any central components. The data would be carried in the terminals of the patients, doctors, and nurses, and replicated for safety and availability reasons into other terminals. Obviously, the smartphones/tablets/laptops of the doctors and nurses should contain their patients' data, but data could be further replicated. This kind of architecture would have many unsolved challenges, though. Evident ones are data privacy issues (e.g., a patient's data could be copied to other patients' phones), synchronization costs (e.g., who pays the network transmission costs?), and reliability and availability issues (e.g., in spite of copying, the data might be lost and unreachable when needed by the doctor for various reasons).

The individual patient's data is placed on his or her own mobile terminal in any case (Fig. 1.). Data storage and its user interface are implemented as an application on top of the mobile operating systems. Data can be uploaded to the terminal from another fixed or mobile terminal over various network bearers (SMS, GPRS, HSPA, etc.) and short-range links (USB, IR, BT, ZigBee, WLAN). The terminal can be handed over to a doctor or nurse, and he/she can find out the data him/herself and update it. The application on the terminal should provide the necessary interfaces.

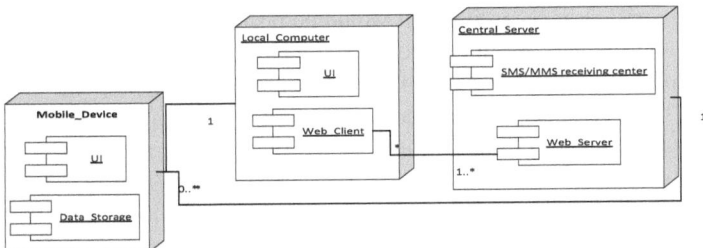

Fig. 1. Decentralized system

For the processing of SMS and MMS messages on patients' and doctors' terminals, it is necessary to have special software (possibly deployed at the mobile operator's central location), which would handle the received SMS or MMS messages. The mobile phone would send an encoded message to a defined number, and later this message would be received and processed. This is similar to TRACnet functionality.

The main benefit of this kind of system is perhaps that it does not cost anything or almost anything for the government, because it does not need to invest in the infrastructure. The patients would pay for the infrastructure. A challenge is the communication of the patient data from the handset to the doctor and vice versa. Another issue is that the data on the cell phone might be lost. This can be remedied by copying the data to a memory card, for example. This might be necessary also when the phone is changed and the medical data need to be moved to a new phone.

For better reliability it would be possible to make a hybrid system, which would contain central backup storage, in addition to the data on cell phones. Thus, if data from phone were lost, it would be possible to recover the data from the central backup system. This could be maintained even by a telecomm operator.

We can also consider that there is a central component that can be hosted by one hospital or by the government (centralized central component) or by many hospitals and government agencies (decentralized central component).

4.2   Single Central Component Solution

First, we discuss a centralized system, i.e., one in which medical data are stored on a central server (cf. Fig. 1). Central storage on the server would contain a copy of the medical data of all the patients in the country. This would be a massive centralized solution with all relevant data up- and downloadable from/to the mobile phones and other networked computers and mobile terminals. This kind of solution is now emerging in Finland in the form of KanTA. Only a government could host such a component due to the high costs. In a country with 20 million people, this could require a datacenter, placed where the power supply in the country is most stable. This kind of architecture would mean a single point of failure. Access to the server farm should be possible from fixed and mobile terminals. TRACnet [25] seems to have this kind of architecture.

4.3   Multitude of Central Components

The above can be modified so that the country is divided into regions and each region has a central component, as in Fig 1. It would be hosted by a suitable hospital. In this basic setting, not all the central components would be interoperable. The patient data would be stored into the handsets of the patients and into the local hospital data repositories. Each component would contain data of the patients registered to the area of the hospital in question. Such a component would be one server-level installation with a suitable data management and Web access software (e.g., LAMP stack). In each hospital there could be several computers or mobile devices used by the doctors for downloading patients' data from the server storage and uploading the data there. This kind of central component architecture would require a LAN or WLAN in the hospital. The architecture would correspond to the current situation as concerns the healthcare organization. A strong point is that patients could carry their medical records in their phones and if treated outside the region still have the data with them. The data could also be fetched to another hospital, if the patient allows it or accesses the data him or herself with his or her phone. This scheme works better in cases where fewer people need treatment outside of their region.

The main part of a central component is a DBS, e.g., a PostgreSQL database.

4.4   Loosely Coupled Central Components

The above architecture can be developed further into one in which the central components exchange and replicate data regularly. It could also be developed in a direction in which there is one central component that hosts all the data (cf. KanTA above). This would be in that respect similar to the first choice, that the problems with establishing the central component would be the same. Local storage contains a subset of the data from the global data storage, which can also be implemented as a PostgreSQL database. A synchronization module allows interchange of the data with the central data storage. Local storage also provides user interface (UI), which can be used by the clients. Local storage does not need to communicate with central storage persistently, and might carry out data refresh at rather long time intervals, e.g., overnight. This would function under the assumption of low inter-hospital mobility.

4.5   Envisioned Deployment

The Kumba District Hospital is a "district reference" hospital for an estimated population area of about 300,000 inhabitants (The Kumba Health District) [20]. It is the largest health district in the southwest region of Cameroon. The hospital has 148 beds and is run by six physicians of various specialties: ophthalmology, obstetrics and gynecology, general surgery, radiology, and general medicine (family practice) [20]. The hospital receives daily about 150 patients for consultation and supports about 145 deliveries in a month. Supervisory reports produced by the Kumba Health District reveal that there are many unauthorized medical settings in the health district, with a huge quantity of drugs sold in clandestine "medicine stores" in the central market [20]. The most prevalent medical condition is malaria infection with *Plasmodium falciparum*, and all clinical variants are reported.

5   Conclusions

The current paper describes requirements for the medical data storage system for Cameroon. The paper aims at elaborating the requirements via designing potential scenarios and subsequent requirements elicitation. The paper considers the realities of Cameroon such as frequent electricity shortages and low Internet penetration rate and high mobile handset penetration. In addition, we present and discuss two architectural solutions: centralized and decentralized. Further we plan to verify and validate requirements using surveys of potential user groups in Cameroon. In addition, we plan to pilot a prototype of the system in a Kumba local hospital, applying the most suitable architecture option above.

References

1. The World Fact Book, https://www.cia.gov/library/publications/the-world-factbook/geos/cm.html
2. MTN Cameroon SA, http://www.mtncameroon.net/LoadedPortal
3. World Health Organization, http://www.who.int/countries/cmr/en/
4. Anokwa, Y., Ribeka, N., Parikh, T., Borriello, G., Were, M.C.: Design of a Phone-Based Clinical Decision Support System for Resource-Limited Settings. In: ICTD 2012, Atlanta, GA, USA, March 12-15 (2012), doi:10.1145/2160673.2160676
5. Vo, K.A.T.: Challenges of Health Information Systems Programs in Developing Countries: Success and Failure. M.Sc. thesis, Univ. of Oslo (2009), http://urn.nb.no/URN:NBN:no-23652
6. Vanessa, C.W.T., Huimin, M.L., Rodricks, R.M., Jiao-Lei, C.Q., Chib, A.: Adoption, Usage and Impact of Family Folder Collection (FFC) on a Mobile Android Tablet Device in Rural Thailand. In: ICoCMTD, Istanbul, Turkey, May 9-11 (2012)
7. Hutchings, M.T., Dev, A., Palaniappan, M., Srinivasan, V., Ramanathan, N., Taylor, J.: mWASH: Mobile Phone Applications for the Water, Sanitation, and Hygiene Sector (2012), Accessed online at http://www.pacinst.org/reports/mwash/full_report.pdf
8. Freifeld, C.C., Chunara, R., Meraku, S.R., Chan, E.H., Kass-Hout, T., Iacucci, A.A., Brownstein, J.S.: Participatory Epidemiology: Use of Mobile Phones for Community-Based Health Reporting. PLoS Med. 7(12), e1000376 (2010)

9. Cellular-news, Cameroon Publishes Short-List for 3G License Award, Accessed online at http://www.cellular-news.com/story/56157.php
10. Berg, M., Wariero, J., Modi, V.: Every Child Counts—The Use of SMS in Kenya to Support the Community Based Management of Acute Malnutrition and Malaria in Children Under Five (2009), Accessed online at http://www.mobileactive.org/files/file_uploads/ChildCount_Kenya_SMS.pdf
11. Littman-Quinn, R., Chandra, A., Schwartz, A., Chang, A.Y., Fadlelmola, F.M., Ghose, S., Armstrong, K., Bewlay, L., Digovich, K., Seymour, A.K., Kovarik, C.L.: mHealth Applications for Clinical Education,Decision Making and Patient Adherence in Botswana. In: IST-Africa Conference Proceedings (2011)
12. mHealth in Low-Resource Settings, http://www.mhealthinfo.org/projects_table
13. EpiSurveyor Mobile Health Data Collection, http://www.mhealthinfo.org/project/episurveyor-mobile-health-data-collection
14. Expedited Results System to Improve Early Infant Diagnosis, http://www.mhealthinfo.org/project/expedited-results-system-improve-early-infant-diagnosis
15. Fitun Warmline AIDS Hotline, http://dev.globalhealthmagazine.com/cover_stories/aids_hotline_for_ethiopian_health-care_workers
16. Wiegers, K.: Software Requirements: Practical Techniques for Gathering and Managing Requirements Throughout the Product Development Life Cycle. Karl Wiegers (2009)
17. Preiss, O., Wegmann, A.: Stakeholder Discovery and Classification Based on Systems Science Principles. J. IEEE (2001)
18. Sharp, H., Finkelstein, A., Galal, G.: Stakeholder Identification in the Requirements Engineering Process. J. IEEE (1999)
19. Kansallinen Terveysarkisto (KanTa), http://www.kanta.fi
20. Kumba District Hospital Report No.1 for Performance-Based Finances (PBF) supervision and initiation (2012) (unpublished)
21. Istepanian, R.S., Zitouni, K., Harry, D., Moutosammy, N., Sungoor, A., Tang, B., Earle, K.A.: Evaluation of a Mobile Phone Telemonitoring System for Glycaemic Control in Patients with Diabetes. J. Telemed. Telecare 15, 125–128 (2009)
22. Foster, K.R.: Telehealth in Sub-Saharan Africa: Lessons for Humanitarian Engineering. IEEE Technology and Society Magazine 29, 42–49 (2010)
23. Littman-Quinn, R., Chandra, A., Schwartz, A., Fadlelmola, F.M., Ghose, S., Luberti, A.A., Tatarsky, A., Chihanga, S., Ramogola-Masire, D., Steenhoff, A., Kovarik, C.: mHealth applications for telemedicine and public health intervention in Botswana. IST-Africa
24. Thirumurthy, H., Lester, R.T.: mHealth For Health Behaviour Change in Resource-Limited Settings: Applications to HIV Care and Beyond. BOWH 90, 390–392 (2012)
25. Nyemazi, J.P.: TRACnet: sustaining mHealth at scale in Rwanda. Sexually Transmitted Infections 87, A322 (2011), doi:10.1136/sextrans-2011-050108.542
26. Gruber, H., Wolf, B., Reiher, M.: Status, Barriers and Potential of Telemedical Systems in African Countries. In: AFRICON (2011), doi:10.1109/AFRCON.2011.6072022

Towards a Mobile Implementation of Waaves for Certified Medical Image Compression in E-Health Applications

Imen Mhedhbi[1], Khalil Hachicha[1], Patrick Garda[1], Yuhui Bai[2], Bertrand Granado[2], Sébastien Topin[3], and Sylvain Hochberg[3]

[1] UPMC, LIP6, CNRS UMR 7606; 4 Place Jussieu, 75252 PARIS Cedex 05, France
[2] ETIS, CNRS UMR 8051, ENSEA, Université Cergy Pontoise; 6 avenue du Ponceau, 95014 CERGY Cedex, France
[3] CIRA, 38 Boulevard Henri Sellier, 92156 SURESNES, France

Abstract. In this article, we present two studies that pave the way towards a mobile implementation of the WAAVES certified medical image compression encoder. On the algorithmic side, we compared three techniques to increase the compression rate. The obtained results show a significant bit-rate reduction, around 40% with respect to the WAAVES encoder, while keeping the same visual quality. On the architectural side, we describe the HW/SW co-design of an architecture implemented in a FPGA platform. By using code profiling, critical portions of the code were identified, then two methods for hardware acceleration were used to implement the critical part of the coder. The tests were done on a StratixIVGX230 FPGA and the results showed that HW/SW co-design could achieve up to 20x performance gain in the critical portion. The combination of these results demonstrates the feasibility of a mobile implementation of the WAAVES certified medical image coder suitable for e-health applications.

Keywords: Medical images, Image compression, Motion detection, Markov Models, SSIM, FPGAs, NIOS II, HW/SW co-design, Medical devices.

1   Introduction

Nowadays, medical images are becoming an important source of information for a medical expert to realize a diagnosis. But their size is growing continuously to provide more accurate information. In addition, some examination such as endoscopy or angiography, use video imaging, thus increasing tremendously the amount of data and hence the need for their compression. Fortunately, there is a clinically validated compression algorithm that reduces with a big ratio the volume of images while ensuring sufficient quality for medical diagnosis: this is the WAAVES coder developed by CIRA [1]. The basic steps used in its compression scheme include Discrete Wavelet Transformation (DWT) and quantization followed by entropy coding to encode the resulting coefficients. This solution is compatible with DICOM (Digital Communications in Medicine). It was certified as a Medical Device.

B. Godara and K.S. Nikita (Eds.): MobiHealth 2012, LNICST 61, pp. 79–87, 2013.
© Institute for Computer Sciences, Social Informatics and Telecommunications Engineering 2013

The challenge today is to give access to these medical images remotely on embedded terminals with low computing power through low bandwidth networks. On the one hand, to address the network bandwidth limitation, we propose to improve the compression performance of the original WAAVES algorithm. Specifically, in the case of video imaging, our approach is to divide the medical images flow into images of reference and images of difference that are then compressed by the WAAVES coder. On the other hand, to address the low computing power of embedded platforms, we propose a dedicated architecture and we developed an efficient HW/SW co-design technique for real time execution of MMWAVES on embedded terminals.

This article is organized as follow: section 2 presents our masking algorithm principle. Next, we describe MMWAVES and give the compression performances results. In section 3, we describe the real-time image acquisition hardware interface and the HW/SW co-design architecture for WAAVES encoder. Next, we present the optimization of performance by using NIOS Custom Instructions and Hardware Accelerator IPs. The implementation results in terms of time partition are discussed in section 8. Finally, we conclude the paper and present future work.

2   MMWaaves

To increase the compression rate for video sequences, our approach is to combine a motion detection algorithm with WAAVES to create the MMWaaves coder (Motion Mask WAAVES) as shown in Figure 1. More specifically, we divide the medical images flow into images of reference and images of difference and we use a masking technique based on Markov models to reduce the difference images noise. This technique was introduced, patented and validated in previous works [2][3] with different video coders (MJPEG2000, H264) and it achieved good results for generic video benchmarks. We describe the motion detection in section 2.1.

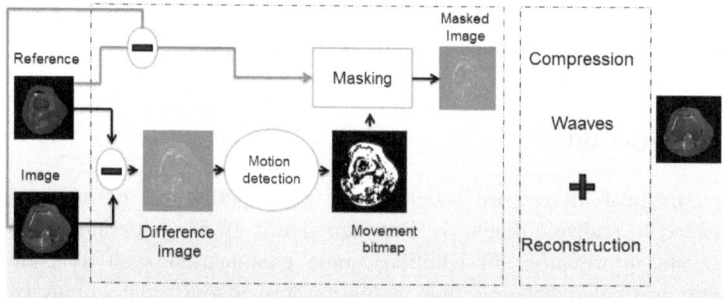

Fig. 1. Mask Motion Waaves

For the masking algorithm, three techniques were studied: the *difference*, *substitution* and *Exclusive-or*. The *difference* means that, when we get a "1" pixel in the binary mask map, we write in the output image the difference between the same pixel in the reference and in the current image. The *substitution* means that, when we get a "1" pixel in the binary mask map, we write in the output image the same pixel in the current image. The *Exclusive-or* means that, when we get a "1" pixel in the binary mask map, we write in the output image the exclusive-or between the same pixel in the reference and in the current image. The performances achieved for these three techniques on a set of medical images will be given in the following.

At first, we reworked a model using the potential functions foreseen by the detection of motion combining the spatial and temporal information [5][6][7]. It is composed of two distinct steps: the first consists of a preprocessing phase through which the variance is determined. The absolute value of the difference matrix is then calculated and binarized by setting a threshold.

The second grouping algorithm of the ICM to update the binary state of the pixels of difference (moving or not) which is made site by site in the sense that every change in state is taken immediately into account in the relaxation of the neighboring site. In this way, it will allow the convergence to the first minimum of the energy function. In order to calculate the energy, one must know the state of the pixels belonging to a neighborhood defined by eight spatial neighbors and two temporal neighbors. The principle of this algorithm is presented in Figure 2.

To choose one of these three techniques, we proposed a multi-criteria performance evaluation based on an objective measure (PSNR, SNR) and a psycho visual measure (SSIM index). Tests were carried out using 512x512 images. We applied a subtraction

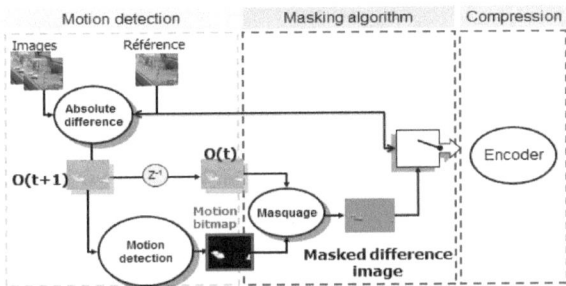

Fig. 2. Masking technique

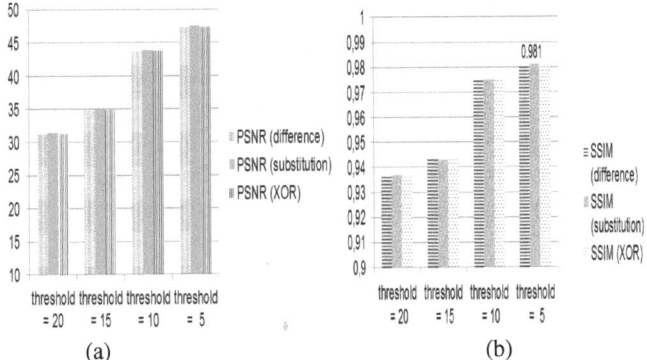

Fig. 3. (a) Threshold impact on PSNR (b) Threshold impact on SSIM

operation between the reference image and the current image and we computed the mask using the Markov model. To measure the performance of the quality of the image, we applied these two metrics.

Figure 3(a) summarizes the impact of the binarization on the PSNR evolution. Firstly, we notice that we find the best PSNR, equal to 46, using a threshold equal to 5. Secondly, we remark that PSNR's values are almost identical for the various techniques. This is due to the use of the same motion bitmap.

However, for medical images, PSNR metric does not accurately reflect image quality as perceived by a clinician. Thus we used the index of structural similarity SSIM[8][9] as a metric measuring the psycho visual quality of image. SSIM has a value between 0 and 1 that indicates the correlation with respect to the source, where 1 indicates a perfect correlation. The diagram in Figure 3(b) summarizes the results giving the impact of the binarization threshold on the evolution of the SSIM index. We showed that the reconstructed images using a threshold equal to 5 got the best quality. This confirms the measurements obtained previously using the PSNR metric.

Finally, we made a comparison between the compression of masked images (difference, substitution, Or Exclusive) and the compression of the original images (Figure 4(a)).

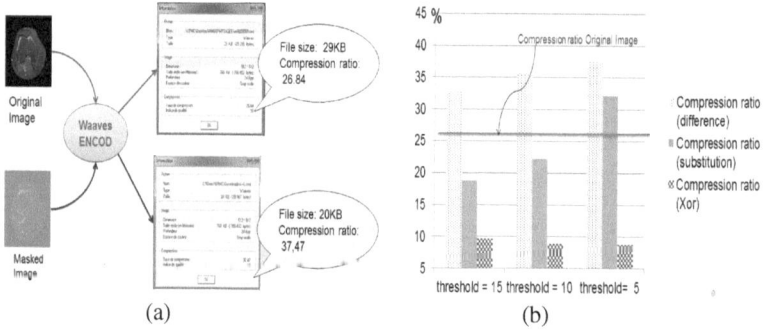

(a)   (b)

Fig. 4. (a) Waaves compression (b) Threshold Influence on evolution of compression ratio

The diagram in Figure 4(b) shows the impact of the binarization threshold on the compression ratio of the different images. We note that we got a loss of compression performances using the exclusive-or technique. However, we got a gain that varied between 21% for the substitution technique and 42% for the difference technique using a threshold equal to 5. The gain could reach 50% for other sets of test images.

In conclusion, the results demonstrate that a significant gain in compression rate can be achieved while preserving the image quality performances.

3   Embedded Encoding System

To embed the Waaves and MMWaaves algorithms, we need to accelerate their execution on an embedded terminal. To realize this task, we preliminary use an experiment platform with a camera and a FPGA Altera StratixIV GX230 that was chosen for its outstanding benchmarking in terms of density, performance and power consumption among 40-nm FPGA family.

The diagram of our camera system platform is briefly presented in Figure 5(a), the FPGA is connected with off-chip devices trough GPIO, such as a 5-megapixel CMOS camera that provides digital raw image data and a VGA monitor to display the compressed then uncompressed images. The camera controller component provides an interface between the Cmos camera and the FPGA to send the acquired real time image data to the memory buffer and further to an external DDR, while the VGA controller allows transferring data from the memory buffer to the VGA monitor for visualization. The DDR controller is composed of two DMA modules which allow circular transfer between the on chip FIFO and the external DDR memory.

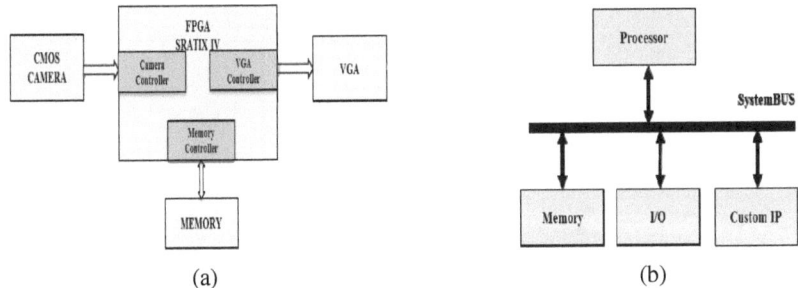

(a)   (b)

Fig. 5. (a) Camera system (b) A generic SOC system

4   HW/SW Co-design Encoding System

A generic system on chip is illustrated in Figure 5(b) in order to develop hardware and software in parallel. The processor, memory and peripherals, along with hardware IPs, are connected with a NoC (Network on Chip) interface to ease function re-use and system co-design.

Our SoC co-design is conducted using Altera's design flow with the SOPC builder tool. Instead of using fixed hardware cores, the NIOS II Soft-core processors are designed to fit and run inside an FPGA. The core is a 32-bits scalar RISC Processor that allows the designer to add user-defined instructions [11] in addition to pre-specified features to give a highly focused, programmable processor solution. Here, NIOS II soft-core processor is used as an experiment processor to validate the HW/SW codesign and the acceleration of both algorithms with techniques like user defined instruction and IP based accelerator.

The Waaves wavelet-based image encoding algorithms were first coded in C++ and validated on a PC host. The tested code was then compiled for the Nios II Integrated Device Electronics (IDE) and deployed in the development board. The standard HW/SW co-design process can consist of three main steps [10], which include the implementation of the Algorithm into software, followed by an analysis of the program with profiling to detect the critical parts of Algorithm, then efficiently implement the algorithm in hardware. The detection of critical part of the software and the optimization will be discussed in the next section.

4.1   Timing Analysis of Application

In order to optimize and achieve the best performance in terms of real-time operation of the image encoder, we identified the critical portions in the software by using Altera Performance Counters [16], which allow measuring the number of processor clock cycles for the execution time.

As illustrated in Figure 6, DWT (Discrete Wavelet Transform) and Encoder (Entropy Encoder), which use respectively 60 % and 30 % of the execution time, are the two primary computationally intensive components. Thus, two methodologies were adopted to accelerate the critical component.

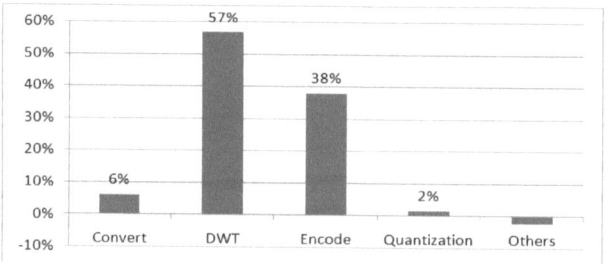

Fig. 6. Execution time distribution for image encoder

4.2   Optimization of the DWT Module with Custom Instructions

The 2D DWT module is used for decomposition of the images with high-pass and low-pass filtering and a factor of two sub sampling, the operations are applied in row and column wise direction and are implemented in floating point. Since Nios II does not have a floating point unit (FPU), like many processors in embedded systems, the processing of DWT becomes expensive. Altera provides an efficient way of adding small custom instructions in the Nios II processor using its Sopc/Qsys tools. Custom instructions is a straightforward option for accelerating software in FPGAs, which allows increasing system performance by offloading portions of the software code to hardware functions [11][12]. The custom instruction presents a data path in parallel to the CPU's arithmetical logical unit (ALU). During system generation, special assembler instructions are generated to access the additional component. Nios Embedded Design Suites directly generates a macro in to simplify the access to the hardware component; each custom component can transfer at most 64 bits of data. Thus the simple operations can be replaced by several custom instructions. With the Nios II floating point custom instructions, we can accelerate arithmetic functions executed on float variable types and are able to take full advantage of the flexibility of the FPGA to optimize the system performance.

4.3   Optimization of Encoder Module with Hardware Accelerator IP

The wavelet based coding scheme is used in several image coding methods, among which the state of art coding algorithm EZW [13] and SPIHT [14] both proposed the progressive sub-band coding based on the frequency and spatial correlation after sub-band transform, to encode separately each resolution level of the image in an progressive way. In our application, the Encoder module, that takes 30% of total execution time, consists of an adaptive scanning algorithm which reorganizes the wavelet coefficients of each sub-band to get a better compression rate [15].

This algorithm is inefficient in software because the manipulated coefficients are accessed with two linked list and a memory block. The linked list needs to be updated frequently to select the wavelet coefficients. The utilization of linked list requires extremely random memory access. In order to reduce the random memory access, our hardware accelerator is designed by using a structure of grouped linked for accelerating the adaptive scanning algorithm. Instead of using 3 memory blocks to separately store the indexes, one memory block, which is three times larger, is used to store the coefficients. Thus the DMA could use memory burst to reduce the number of random memory access, which leads to more time efficiency. The IP is designed in Verilog and it is connected to the processor via the Avalon bus interface. Due to the stand-alone design of the hardware component, a simple re-use of the design files in different architectures is supported.

5   Implementation Results

Results were obtained with the implementation of the wavelet-based image encoder in FPGA. The DWT module was optimized with floating point custom instruction set and the Encoder module was optimized with hardware accelerator IP. The prototyping board operated at 100 MHz. The system received images from the camera and restituted processed images on the VGA monitor. Our implementation on the prototype showed up to 20 times speed improvement for the DWT module and 10 times speed improvement for the Encoder module compared to the software based solution. The results before and after timing optimization are presented in Figure 7.

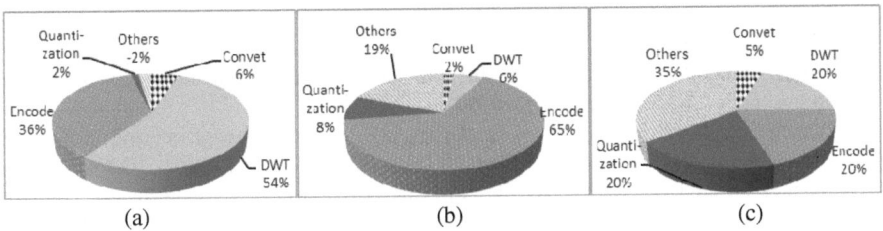

(a)   (b)   (c)

Fig. 7. CPU time partition before and after optimization : (a) Average coding time before using Custom Instructions (b) Average coding time after using Custom Instructions (c) Average coding time after using Hardware Accelerator

6   Conclusion

In this work, we proposed to combine the WAAVES coder with a mask motion detection algorithm based on Markov Model (MMWAAVES). We developed three techniques to create masked images and we evaluated the image quality based on two measures: objective (PSNR, SNR) and Psycho visual (SSIM index). We demonstrated that masking the image differences gives the best results and allows a compression gain up to 42%. We also described the HW/SW co-design architecture of WAAVES based on FPGA platform. We proposed two methods for hardware acceleration, which led to 20x speedup for the critical part of the encoder compared to pure software based solution. Our future work will focus on the improvement of the masking process and building hardware acceleration IP for the critical parts.

Acknowledgments. This work takes part in the WARM project with the support from the FEDER/FUI funds. The authors thank the HEGP and PARTELEC partners of the project for fruitful exchanges.

References

1. Created in 1998, CIRA has developed WAAVES, a digital imaging compression technology offering a paradigm shift in compression, transfer and recovery quality performance. Based on a major professional and social potential impact the technology may have in public healthcare, CIRA has developed an initial strategic focus in medical imaging. WAAVES has been partnered with a growing number of medical applications, such as Apicrypt, MacDent, Medistory, PDB, SantNet and, recently, Dentalvia. A number of French University hospitals have adopted WAAVES as their imaging technology standard (1998), http://www.waaves.com,
2. Bouthemy, P., Lalande, P.: Recovery of moving object masks in an image sequence using local spatiotemporal contextual information. Optical Engineering 32, 1205–1212 (1993)
3. Lohier, F., Garda, P., Lacassagne, L.: Procédé et dispositif de traitement de séquences d'images avec masquage. Brevet Français UPMC FR2804777 (Août 10, 2001), Brevet Européen EP1297494 (Avril 2, 2003)
4. Hachicha, K., Garda, P.: Accelerating the multiple reference frames compensation in the H.264 video coder. Journal of Real-Time Image Processing 4(1) (March 2009) ISSN1861-8200
5. Luthon, F., Caplier, A.: Motion detection and segmentation in image sequences using Markov Random Field Modeling. In: 4th Eurographics Animation and Simulation Workshop, pp. 265–275 (September 1993)
6. Hachicha, K., Faura, D., Romain, O., Garda, P.: Noise-robustness improvement of the H.264 video coder. Journal of Electronic Imaging, SPIE and IS&T 17(03), 033019 (2008)
7. Lohier, F., Garda, P., Lacassagne, L.: Procédé et dispositif de traitement de séquences d'images avec masquage. Brevet Français UPMC FR2804777 (Août 10, 2001), Brevet Européen EP1297494 (Avril 2, 2003)
8. Wang, Z., Bovik, A.C., Sheikh, H.R., Simoncelli, E.P.: Image quality assessment: From error visibility to structural similarity. IEEE Transactions on Image Processing 13(4), 600–612 (2004)

9. Taubman, Marcellin, M.W.: JPEG 2000: Image Compression Fundamentals, Standards, and Practice. Kluwer Academic Publishers (November 2001)
10. Atitallah, A.B., Kadionik, P., Ghozzi, F., Nouel, P., Masmoudi, N., Levi, H.: An FPGA implementation of HW/SW codesign architecture for H.263 video coding. AEU – International Journal of Electronics and Communications (December 2006)
11. Altera nios custom instructions User Guide – Altera
12. Altera SOPC Builder User Guide – Altera
13. Shapiro, J.M.: Embedded image coding using zerotrees of wavelet coefficients. IEEE Trans. Signal Process. 41, 3445–3462 (1993)
14. Said, A., Pearlman, W.A.: A new fast and efficient image codec bsed on set partitioning in hierarchical trees. IEEE Trans. Circuits Syst. Video Technol. 6, 243–250 (1996)
15. Haapala, K., Lappalainen, V., Hämäläinen, T.D.: Experimental parallel implementation of a wavelet-based still image encoder. Microprocessors and Microsystems 29(4), 155–167 (2005)
16. Profiling Nios II Systems – Altera

DAPHNE: A Disruption-Tolerant Application Proxy for e-Health Network Environments

Emmanouil G. Spanakis[1] and Artemios G. Voyiatzis[2]

[1] Institute of Computer Science, Foundation for Research and Technology, Hellas (FORTH/ICS), Heraklion, Crete, Greece
[2] Industrial Systems Institute, Athena Research and Innovation Center (ISI/RC Athena), Platani, Patras, Greece
spanakis@ics.forth.gr, bogart@isi.gr

Abstract. Future health informatics for personalized e-Health services rely on innovative technologies and systems for transparent and continuous collection of evidence-based medical information at any time, from anywhere, and despite the coverage and availability of communication means. We explore Disruption and Delay Tolerant Networking (DTN) as a novel approach for next-generation e-Health information exchange where end-to-end homogeneous networking connectivity is not available. This setting can occur in both rural and urban environments and in both disaster events and normal day-to-day life. The ability of DTN to provide in-transit persistent information storage allows the uninterruptible provision of crucial e-Health services overcoming network instabilities, incompatibilities, or even absence for a long duration. We further describe the integration efforts for a DTN proxy on an e-Health application and discuss experiences and lessons learned.

Keywords: Health Informatics, Delay Tolerant Networks, Biomedical Informatics, Telemedicine, Health Monitoring.

1   Introduction

E-health stands for the application of Information and Communication Technologies (ICT) to improve the access efficiency, effectiveness, and quality of clinical and business processes utilized by healthcare organizations, medical personnel, practitioners, patients, and consumers in an effort to improve the health status of patients [1]. Personalized e-Health, based on best practices and evidence-based medicine, provisions the delivery of key information services and the facilitation and integration of healthcare allowing local and remote access to health information [2].

The healthcare environment is evolving, with increased emphasis on prevention and early detection of disease, primary care, home care, and intermittent healthcare services provided by medical centers of excellence. Part of the care responsibility is shifting to the hands of the citizen, focusing on wellness and health maintenance, forming a social health network among different actors (patients, healthcare professionals, and careers). The traditional care of *single* doctor-patient relationship is gradually transforming

B. Godara and K.S. Nikita (Eds.): MobiHealth 2012, LNICST 61, pp. 88–95, 2013.
© Institute for Computer Sciences, Social Informatics and Telecommunications Engineering 2013

towards *shared* or *integrated care*, where a team of healthcare professionals spanning across organizational boundaries is responsible for an individual's healthcare. These trends are accompanied by a significant growth in the development and deployment of e-Health services with increased sophistication, facilitated by intelligent sensors, monitoring devices, handheld or wearable technologies, and the Internet. In this dynamic and diverse environment, information exchange holds a leading role and has a significant impact on the practice of e-Health.

In this paper, we explore disruption-/delay-tolerant networking (DTN), an innovative and promising network technology, as an approach for e-Health information exchange in multiple settings, including those where end-to-end connectivity cannot be realized. We present a prototype Disruption-Tolerant Network Application Proxy for e-Health Network Environments (DAPHNE) and its integration with modern e-Health applications. We discuss trends, challenges and advantages of e-Health on how future e-Health services can be built using DTN technologies.

2   Networking for e-Health Applications

An important challenge for e-Health is to shift the entire system of healthcare, including medical education, evident based predictive medicine, and patient empowerment to a proactive model of care. A clear benefit can be obtained through the use of sophisticated telecommunication services, ubiquitous computing, social user interfaces and wireless communication technologies to create intelligent health spaces accelerating the deployment of future e-Health services [3, 4]. Existing e-Health applications allow monitoring by using several proprietary hardware, software, networking technologies, and medical protocols [5].

The research efforts focus on providing solutions for e-Health services and applications that can: i) provide interoperability among medical information systems through different networking technologies, ii) preserve confidentiality with a high level of security, iii) facilitate mobility and extend monitoring spaces beyond areas with ample connectivity, towards making e-Health services available for anyone, anywhere, anytime, and anyhow, and iv) manage the vast amount of information healthcare services generate and transfer from one repository to another.

There is an apparent need for a new networking paradigm able to integrate multiple sensor streams of medical and environmental devices, responsible for collecting local and global state indicator variables that need to be queried and monitored on regular basis from a dense heterogeneous e-Health enabled network [6]. This new communication environment, a common networking architecture, must be easy to deploy; free of network related disruptions; scalable to hundreds or thousands of devices; allow progressive deployment over time; provide processing, filtering, and aggregation of data; and support remote data collection, accessibility, security, and privacy. The capability to collect clinical information from dispersed points is becoming an urgent need and requirement especially in environments with lack of end-to-end connectivity for both rural and urban settings. The DTN paradigm discussed in the next sections can act as a unifying middleware embedded in the network stack to address the aforementioned issues.

3   Disruption- and Delay-Tolerant Networking

Disruption/Delay-Tolerant Networking (DTN, term used depending on environment context) is a new communication paradigm that addresses issues arising in challenged environments, such as the ones with extremely large delays, intermittent connectivity, and severe disruptions [7]. Originally designed for deep-space communications, it was soon realized that it can support application scenarios in terrestrial environments with heterogeneous networks and harsh connectivity [8]. The two main design characteristics of DTN are a) its ability to span across networks with different network protocol stacks (for example, a TCP/IP and IEEE 802.15.4 network) and b) its ability to support communication between nodes that have no end-to-end connectivity at any given time point. The latter is achieved thanks to DTN's concept of *in-transit persistent storage*, transforming the classical "store-and-forward" networking approach into a "store-*carry*-forward" one [7].

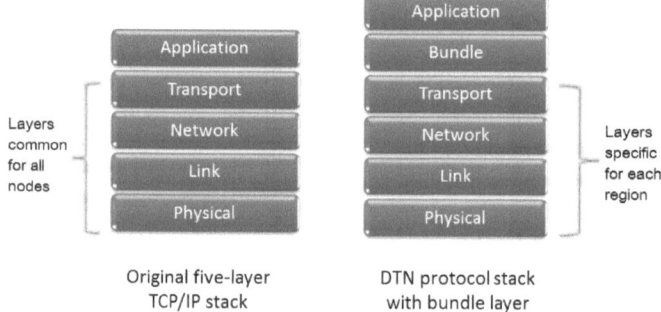

Fig. 1. DTN layering over the Internet model

The IETF RFC 4838 and RFC 5050 define the DTN architecture and the Bundle Protocol (BP) that is used for exchange of information (bundles) among DTN nodes [8, 9]. Figure 1 depicts the placement of the bundle layer over the classical Internet model. In general, the bundle layer exists on top of the transport layer and beyond the application layer. The adaptation of the BP to the specific network stack implemented in a DTN node is realized via a convergence layer (CL) placed among them. This architecture allows bundles encapsulated in BP to transparently travel across regions with different network protocol stacks. Convergence layers have been implemented for a wide range of network protocols, such as HTTP, TCP, UDP, TCP-TLS, NORM, LTP, Ethernet, Bluetooth, AX.25, RS232, and IEEE 802.15.4 LR-WPAN [10].

Applications have been developed for a wide range of devices, including computers, embedded systems, TinyOS-based sensors, and smartphones running Google Android and Apple iOS [10, 11]. Most terrestrial applications target low-resource settings with infrequent communication opportunities, such as Internet connection of remote villages in Africa, wildlife monitoring, communication in mines, and military operations. Experiments were also held on exploring opportunistic or scheduled connectivity using social interactions, vehicular networks, and public transportations. The DTN technology was also demonstrated in e-Health applications, such as a teleconsultation service utilizing diaspora professionals in Ghana [12-14] and a sentinel surveillance application in Tanzania [15].

4   Design of DTN-enabled e-Health Applications

The traditional approach for developing e-Health applications assumes the existence of continuous communication albeit with low bandwidth. If an end-to-end connection is not available, then it is the responsibility of the application to retain the information until such a connection is available. Also, if multiple Internet connections are available (e.g., a WiFi and a 3G one), the application has little control on which one to utilize for a more efficient transmission of the information. Finally, it may be required to implement all the network intelligence within the e-Health application using different platforms and/or for multiple applications. In this case, it is clear that a cross-platform middleware layer can be rather useful.

The DTN architecture can provide a unifying view of e-Health endpoints (proxies), irrespective of the underlying communication technologies and networks they must transverse in order to establish communication. A *common network application programming interface* (API) can provide the necessary middleware adaptation layer as to liberate the e-Health application development from interfacing with different networking technologies. The Bundle Protocol is capable of interfacing with both rich network protocols, as is the case of Internet-based communications, but also with light, non-IP protocols, such as ZigBee and Bluetooth. Furthermore, the bundle protocol specification is open and, if deemed necessary, convergence layers for other protocols can be developed by interested parties. This ability to interface transparently multiple network protocol stacks can be beneficial also in disaster relief operations, where infrastructure cannot be guaranteed and multiple communication technologies may need to co-exist and collaborate [16].

The DTN paradigm works equally well when connectivity exists and when it does not, thanks to its ability of *in-transit persistent storage*. In both cases, the programmer interfaces with one API, independently of underlying networking technology and existence or lack of end-to-end connectivity. The DTN approach *liberates e-Health applications from handling any disconnections* that span delays beyond what current networking technologies can tolerate. This can be beneficial for urban settings, as for example in case of emergencies or when navigating in areas lacking connectivity or when large crowds collect in same space struggling for network access. The availability of an already-deployed application in the field with the inherent capability to communicate in such an environment can be a matter of life and death. Indeed, it may not be possible to deploy after the cause event an e-Health application compatible with the then-available network stacks exactly due to the lack of network infrastructure to support such an operation.

The DTN *late binding approach* allows to *route traffic between e-Health endpoints* that span across different regions, where in each region different network technologies are used and different naming/addressing/binding/routing is used. The DTN approach allows *implanting network intelligence in transferring health related information and medical data.* The bundle layer can have knowledge of link quality and quantitate characteristics. It can also have knowledge about the criticality of the information to be transmitted, realizing smart routing. Such routing considers both current network state *and future connectivity opportunities* in deciding which network connection (existing or future) is more appropriate for transmitting the information efficiently and on time.

Not all e-Health information is time-critical; some may be transmitted later on or stored on a device and retrieved on demand at a later time. Even when network coverage exists, it may not be optimal to transmit collected information at a given time moment due to cost, available bandwidth, or required energy. A *smart bundle routing algorithm* can consider all the aforementioned parameters and choose the optimal transmission schedule and/or switch communication networks based on bundle expiration. This complexity is totally hidden from the e-Health application, which needs only to designate the criticality of information to transfer and an expiration date (i.e., "deliver until this date") and can then pass the responsibility to the DTN layer. The advantage of this approach is that the application is liberated from the complexities of network connectivity management.

The unique ability of DTN to explore not only current but also *future* connectivity opportunities can be very useful in urban settings with multiple connectivity options, as the following example demonstrates. A rich set of sensory media may be collected while commuting from home to work. Given that network connectivity does exist, a traditional e-Health application will try to transmit the information as soon as possible. Using a DTN approach, the application can pass this information to the bundle layer for transmission, designating an expiration date. The bundle layer exploits this information and the fact that a high-speed connection will be available through the office network in a few minutes, based on past connectivity events. Thus, it *defers the transmission of the media-rich sensory data* until then. Suppose now that due to a sad event, the future connection is not realized on time. In this case, the bundle layer activates the alternative, lower-quality links in order to transfer the necessary information before its expiration. It is important to emphasize that in this urban-setting scenario, the *e-Health application is unaware of the entire intelligence planted in the network layers*; the application just delivers the data to be transmitted and never deals with the end-to-end network connection availability.

Last but not least, *security* is addressed in DTN by the already agreed Bundle *Security Protocol* (BSP), described in RFC 6257 [17]. Thus, secure communication between two e-Health DTN endpoints can be implemented across different networks and independently of available networks. From an application designer's point of view, secure links at the bundle layer can be available no matter what the underlying network offers or lacks. Intelligence may be implanted in the networking stack as to avoid double security, or as to implement secure edges in specific points of the network that may be considered more vulnerable.

5   DAPHNE: An Implementation of a DTN Application Proxy

We implemented DAPHNE, an e-Health application proxy as a proof-of-concept for the applicability and advantages of the DTN technology in such an environment. In our scenario, there is an e-Health application that utilizes medical devices to collect patient's data and transmit them to a remote location for further processing.

We realized DAPHNE on a FitPC Slim computer with a 500 MHz CPU, 512 MB RAM, and 60 GB storage running the Linux operating system and the DTN2 reference implementation of the Bundle Protocol. The computer has an Ethernet, a WiFi, and a Bluetooth interface for connectivity with medical devices. It is connected to the Internet and may face disconnections for multiple reasons. An e-Health application runs as a server component on this computer and acquires data from nearby medical devices using the Continua[1] standard. The collected information is then transmitted for display to a remote host. We used two medical devices in our tests: a commercial SpO_2 device (Onyx® II Model 9560) and a 12-lead ECG (Welch Allyn PRO ECG) connected through a USB interface with the patient unit. The application supports connections from multiple remote ends and broadcasts the information to all connected remote hosts. It also allows the user to configure the frequency of transmission measurements independently of the collection rate and the device-specific biomedical parameters related to sensing. The remote host connects with the server application and is able to display any medical data received on a monitor canvas (i.e., running on a light tablet device). If a disconnection, a delay, or a broken link occurs, then the application is responsible for re-establishing the connection when the problem is resolved.

We bridged the two e-Health application ends with the "*dtntunnel*" proxy available in the DTN2 implementation. This proxy allows the creation of a DTN tunnel over a network that can sustain any delay or disruption, thanks to the in-network storage of the DTN architecture. In the near-end host, the tunnel application receives data from the medical devices and transforms them to bundles. These bundles are stored in the computer until a connection is available with the remote end of the tunnel. In the display application host, the tunnel application receives the bundles from the network and provides a continuous stream of information to the application. In this setup, the two ends of the e-Health applications have an always-on, uninterrupted connection (albeit without data) with the local end of the DTN tunnel. In this way, the two applications need not handle any network connectivity issues at all since their connection is local to the host. We established a testbed between two locations. The medical devices, the sensor application, and the near end of the DTN tunnel were installed at the premises of the Computational Medicine Lab of FORTH-ICS in Crete. The far end of the DTN tunnel and the display application were installed in the premises of the Industrial Systems Institute in Patras. Both systems access the Internet through noisy and unstable wireless connections.

The first set of experiments involved no DTN tunnels. The applications initially established connection and exchanged information (SpO_2 and ECG measurements). After a few seconds, the connection was dropped due to network instabilities and they ceased operation until restarted

The second set of experiments involved the DTN tunnels. In this case, the two applications retained connectivity for prolonged time. Figure 2 depicts a screenshot of the successful experiment. The instable connectivity was apparent, as there were

---

[1] http://www.continuaalliance.org/

periods of silence (no connection between the two ends of the tunnel). However, once network connectivity was recovered, the tunnel was reestablished automatically and the pending bundles were forwarded transparently to the e-Health application. The DTN network handled all medical-data-related transmissions rendering this simple e-Health application for this urban-setting scenario, unaware of the entire intelligence planted in the network layers; the application just delivered the data to be transmitted and never dealt with the network availability.

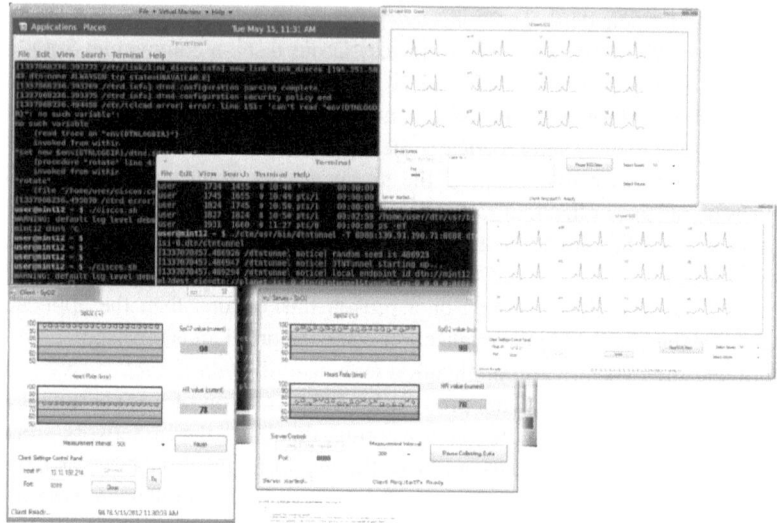

Fig. 2. DAPHNE – DTN Application Proxy for e-Health Network Environments

6   Conclusions and Future Work

The emerging area of e-Health is influenced by factors such as biomedical and clinical incentives, advances in mobile telecommunications and information technology developments, and the socio-economic environment. It aims to the delivery of complex healthcare services enabling personalization, patient inclusion and empowerment with the expectation that such systems will enhance traditional care provision in a variety of situations where remote consultation and monitoring can be implemented despite the lack of end-to-end connectivity.

In this paper, we explored the applicability of delay-tolerant networking as a viable approach to transport information for next-generation e-Health services. We seconded this by presenting an example of a personalized health service provision using medical sensors and e-Health DTN enabled proxies. The diversity of already deployed or envisioned e-Health applications and the heterogeneity of network environments, where the guaranteed end-to-end connectivity assumption cannot be valid, creates an ideal setting for utilizing this promising technology as to allow future e-Health services to overcome the limitations and capabilities of available communication technologies. We aim to further explore this approach and experiment on technology integration in future e-Health services.

Acknowledgement. This work is partially supported by the European Commission under the project "p-medicine: From data sharing and integration via VPH models to personalized medicine" (FP7-ICT-2009.5.3, No 270089).

References

1. Marconi, J.: E-Health: Navigating the Internet for Health Information Healthcare. Advocacy White Paper. Healthcare Information and Management Systems Society (2002)
2. Saranummi, N.: IT Applications for Pervasive, Personal, and Personalized Health. IEEE Transactions on Information Technology in Biomedicine 12(1), 1–4 (2008)
3. Spanakis, M., Lelis, P., Chiarugi, F., Chronaki, C., Tsiknakis, M.: R&D challenges in developing an ambient intelligence eHealth platform. In: 3rd European Medical and Biological Engineering Conference, IFMBE (2005)
4. Lymberis, A.: Wearable health systems and applications: the contribution of information & communication technologies. In: 27th Annual IEEE Engineering Conference in Medicine and Biology (2005)
5. DTN Reference Implementation v2, http://www.dtnrg.org/wiki/Code
6. Wartena, F., Muskens, J., Schmitt, L., Petković, M.: Continua: The reference architecture of a personal telehealth ecosystem. In: 12th IEEE International Conference one-Health Networking Applications and Services, Healthcom 2010 (July 2010)
7. Fall, K.: A Delay-Tolerant Network Architecture for Challenged Internets. In: Proceedings of the 2003 Conference on Applications, Technologies, Architectures, and Protocols for Computer Communications (SIGCOMM 2003), pp. 27–34. ACM Press (2003)
8. Cerf, V., Burleigh, S., Hooke, A., Torgerson, L., Durst, R., Scott, K., Fall, K., Weiss, H.: Delay-tolerant networking architecture. IETF RFC 4838 (April 2007)
9. Scott, K.L., Burleigh, S.: Bundle protocol specification. IETF RFC 5050 (2007)
10. Voyiatzis, A.G.: A Survey of Delay- and Disruption-Tolerant Networking Applications. Journal of Internet Engineering 5(1), 331–344 (2012)
11. Khabbaz, M.J., Assi, C.M., Fawaz, W.F.: Disruption-Tolerant Networking: A Comprehensive Survey on Recent Developments and Persisting Challenges. IEEE Communications Surveys & Tutorials 14(2), 607–640 (2012)
12. Luk, R., Ho, M., Aoki, P.M.: Asynchronous Remote Medical Consultation for Ghana. In: ACM SIGCHI Conference on Human Factors in Computing Systems, CHI (2008)
13. Luk, R., Zaharia, M., Ho, M., Levine, B., Aoki, P.M.: ICTD for Healthcare in Ghana: two parallel cases. In: IEEE/ACM Conference on Information and Communication Technologies and Development, ICTD (2009)
14. Luk, R.L., Ho, M., Aoki, P.: A Framework for Designing Teleconsultation Systems in Africa. In: International Conference on Health Informatics in Africa, HELINA (2007)
15. Ntareme, H., Zennaro, M., Pehrson, B.: Delay Tolerant Network on smartphones: Applications for communication challenged areas. In: Extremecom 2011, Brazil (2011)
16. Fall, K., Iannaccone, G., Kannan, J., Silveira, F., Taft, N.: A disruption-tolerant architecture for secure and efficient disaster response communications. In: 7th International Conference on Information Systems for Crisis Response and Management (2010)
17. Symington, S., Farrell, S., Weiss, H., Lovell, P.: Bundle Security Protocol. IETF RFC 6257 (May 2011)

A Novel Method for Feature Extraction in Vocal Fold Pathology Diagnosis

Vahid Majidnezhad and Igor Kheidorov

Department of Computer Engineering, Shabestar Branch,
Islamic Azad University, Shabestar, Iran
vahidmn@yahoo.com, ikheidorov@sakrament.com

Abstract. Acoustic analysis is a proper method in vocal fold pathology diagnosis so that it can complement and in some cases replace the other invasive, based on direct vocal fold observation, methods. There are different approaches for vocal fold pathology diagnosis. These algorithms usually have two stages which are Feature Extraction and Classification. While the second stage implies a choice of a variety of machine learning methods, the first stage plays a critical role in performance of the classification system. In this paper, three types of features which are Energy and Entropy resulting from the Wavelet Packet Tree and Mel-Frequency-Cepstral-Coefficients (MFCCs), and also their combination are investigated. Finally a new type of feature vector, based on Energy and Mel-Frequency-Cepstral-Coefficients, is proposed. Support vector machine is used as a classifier for evaluating the performance of our proposed method. The results show the priority of the proposed method in comparison with other methods.

Keywords: Vocal fold pathology diagnosis, Wavelet Packet Decomposition, Mel-Frequency-Cepstral-Coefficients (MFCCs), Energy, Entropy, Support Vector Machine (SVM).

1 Introduction

Vocal signal information often plays an important role for specialists to understand the process of vocal fold pathology formation. In some cases vocal signal analysis can be the only way to analyze the state of vocal folds. Nowadays diverse medical techniques exist for direct examination and diagnostics of pathologies. Laryngoscopy, glottography, stroboscopy, electromyography and videokimography are most frequently used by medical specialists. But these methods possess a number of disadvantages. Human vocal tract is hardly-accessible for visual examination during phonation process and that makes it more problematic to identify a pathology. Moreover, these diagnostic means may cause patients much discomfort and distort the actual signal, that may lead to incorrect diagnosis as well [1-4].

Acoustic analysis as a diagnostic method has no drawbacks, peculiar to the above mentioned methods. It possesses a number of advantages. First of all, acoustic analysis is a non-invasive diagnostic technique that allows pathologists to examine

B. Godara and K.S. Nikita (Eds.): MobiHealth 2012, LNICST 61, pp. 96–105, 2013.

many people in short time period with minimal discomfort. It also allows pathologists to reveal the pathologies on early stages of their origin. This method can be of great interest for medical institutions.

In recent years a number of methods were developed for segmentation and classification of speech signals with pathology. The general scheme of vocal fold pathology diagnosis is illustrated in Fig. 1.

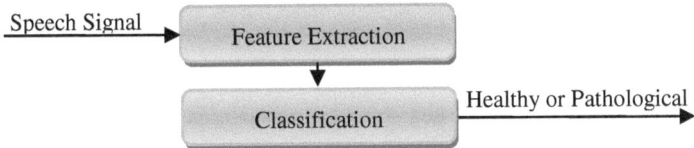

Fig. 1. The general scheme of vocal fold pathology diagnosis

The wavelet transform, as was shown in [5], is a flexible tool for time-frequency analysis of speech signals, especially for short data frames, like separate phonemes. In Fig.2 wavelet transform of a stressed vowel [a:], pronounced by a healthy speaker, is shown. But the situation changes in case of pathological voices. In Fig. 3, Fig. 4 and Fig. 5 wavelet transforms of the same vowel are given, but in these cases it is pronounced by speakers with different voice pathologies. The instability of the formant frequency is obviously seen.

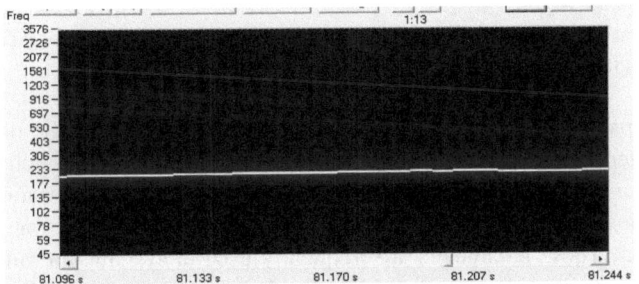

Fig. 2. Wavelet transform of a stressed vowel [a:] pronounced by a healthy speaker

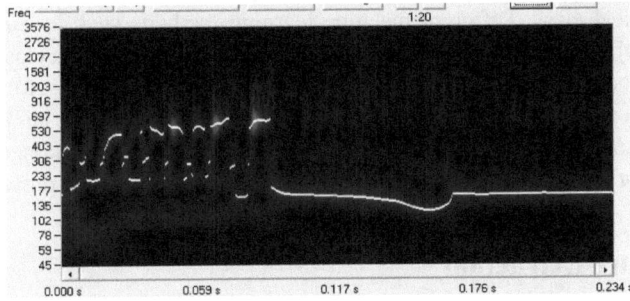

Fig. 3. Wavelet transform of a stressed vowel [a:] pronounced by the speaker with hypertrophic laryngitis

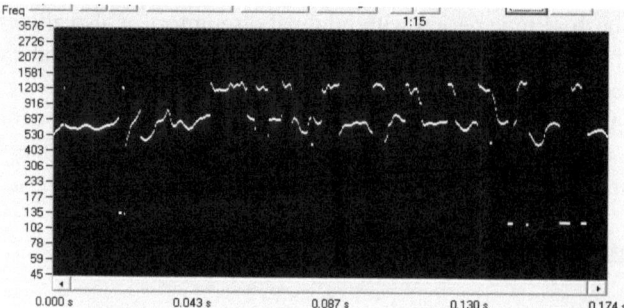

Fig. 4. Wavelet transform of a stressed vowel [a:] pronounced by the speaker with hypertonic dysphonia

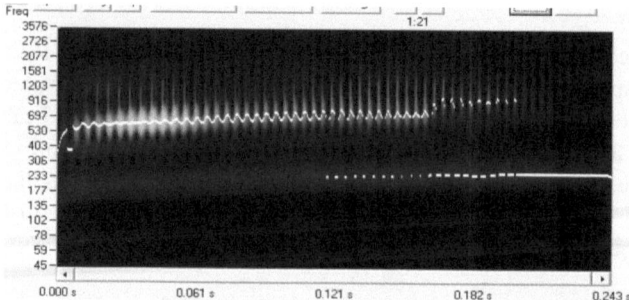

Fig. 5. Wavelet transform of a stressed vowel [a:] pronounced by the speaker with chronic catarrhal laryngitis

Different parameters for feature extraction are used. Traditionally, one deals with such parameters like pitch, jitter, shimmer, amplitude perturbation, pitch perturbation, signal to noise ratio, normalized noise energy [5] and others [6-9]. Feature extraction, using the above mentioned parameters, has shown its efficiency for a number of practical tasks. These parameters are frequently used in systems for automatic vocal fold pathology diagnosis, in speaker identification systems or in multimedia database indexing systems.

Finally, the extracted features are used for speech classification into the healthy and pathological class. Different machine learning methods such as Support Vector Machines [10], Artificial Neural Networks [11], etc. can be used as a classifier.

The presence of a pathology in a vocal tract inevitably leads to voice signal distortion. Depending on pathology severity the distortion may be more or less significant. Among all sounds that are produced by vocal tract, sustained vowels and some sonorant consonants are most easily distorted if a pathology is present.

2   Feature Extraction

In the first stage of the proposed method, as it is shown in Fig. 1, features extraction must be done. For this purpose, first, by the use of cepstral representation of the input signal, 13 Mel-Frequency-Cepstral-Coefficients (MFCC) are extracted. Then the wavelet packet decomposition in 5 levels is applied on the input signal to make the wavelet packet tree. Then, from the nodes of resulting wavelet packet tree, 63 energy features along with 63 Shannon entropy features are extracted. Finally, these three types of features and all possible states of their combination are considered and investigated to find the best state for constructing the proposed feature vector.

2.1   Mel-Frequency-Cepstral-Coefficients (MFCCs)

MFCCs are widely used features to characterize a voice signal and can be estimated by using a parametric approach derived from linear prediction coefficients (LPC), or by the non-parametric discrete fast Fourier transform (FFT), which typically encodes more information than the LPC method. The signal is windowed with a hamming window in the time domain and converted into the frequency domain by FFT, which gives the magnitude of the FFT. Then the FFT data is converted into filter bank outputs and the cosine transform is found to reduce dimensionality. The filter bank is constructed using 13 linearly-spaced filters (133.33Hz between center frequencies,) followed by 27 log-spaced filters (separated by a factor of 1.0711703 in frequency.) Each filter is constructed by combining the amplitude of FFT bin. The Matlab code to calculate the MFCC features was adapted from the Auditory Toolbox (Malcolm Slaney). The MFCCs are used as features in [12] to classify the speech into pathology and healthy class. Reduction of MFCC information has been used by averaging the sample's value of each coefficient.

2.2   Wavelet Packet Decomposition

Recently, wavelet packets (WPs) have been widely used by many researchers to analyze voice and speech signals. There are many out-standing properties of wavelet packets which encourage researchers to employ them in widespread fields. The most important, multi resolution property of WPs is helpful in voice signal synthesis [13-14].

The hierarchical WP transform uses a family of wavelet functions and their associated scaling functions to decompose the original signal into subsequent sub-bands. The decomposition process is recursively applied to both the low and high frequency sub-bands to generate the next level of the hierarchy. WPs can be described by the following collection of basic functions:

$$W_{2n}(2^{p-1}x-1)=\sqrt{2^{1-p}}\sum_{m}h(m-2l)\sqrt{2^p}W_n(2^p x-m) \qquad (1)$$

$$W_{2n+1}(2^{p-1}x-1)=\sqrt{2^{1-p}}\sum_{m}g(m-2l)\sqrt{2^p}W_n(2^p x-m) \qquad (2)$$

where p is scale index, l the translation index, h the low-pass filter and g the high-pass filter with

$$g(k) = (-1)^k h(1-k) \tag{3}$$

the WP coefficients at different scales and positions of a discrete signal can be computed as follows:

$$C_{n,k}^p = \sqrt{2^p} \sum_{m=-\infty}^{\infty} f(m)W_n(2^p m - k) \tag{4}$$

$$C_{2n,l}^{p-1} = \sum_m h(m-2l)C_{n,m}^p \tag{5}$$

$$C_{2n+1,l}^{p-1} = \sum_m g(m-2l)C_{n,m}^p \tag{6}$$

for a group of wavelet packet coefficients, energy feature in its corresponding sub-band is computed as

$$Energy_n = \frac{1}{N^2} \sum_{k=1}^{n} \left| C_{n,k}^p \right|^2 \tag{7}$$

The entropy evaluates the rate of information which is produced by the pathogens factors as a measure of abnormality in pathological speech. Also, the measure of Shannon entropy can be computed using the extracted wavelet-packet coefficients, through the following formula

$$Entropy_n = -\sum_{k=1}^{n} \left| C_{n,k}^p \right|^2 \log \left| C_{n,k}^p \right|^2 \tag{8}$$

In this study, mother wavelet function of the tenth order Daubechies has been chosen and the signals have been decomposed to five levels. The mother wavelet used in this study is reported to be effective in voice signal analysis [15-16] and is being widely used in many pathological voice analyses [14]. Due to the noise-like effect of irregularities in the vibration pattern of damaged vocal folds, the distribution manner of such variations within the whole frequency range of pathological speech signals is not clearly known. Therefore, it seems reasonable to use WP rather than DWT or CWT to have more detail sub-bands.

3   Classification by Support Vector Machine

For classification, a statistical learning algorithm called support vector machine (SVM) is used. SVMs which were proposed by Vapnik [17], have become an acknowledged classification method in the task of musical genre recognition. Their usage in this task was already justified by works of Li et al. [18] were SVMs outperformed other commonly used classification methods (Gaussian Mixture models, K-Nearest Neighbors classifier, Hidden Markov Models, etc.). We will consider the basic theory of SVM below.

Given a set of training vectors belonging to two separate classes, $(x_1,y_1),...,(x_l,y_l)$, where $x_i \in R^N$ and $y_i \in \{-1,...,1\}$, one wants to find a hyper-plane $wx + b = 0$ to separate the data. In fact, there are many possible hyper-planes, but there is only one that maximizes the margin (the distance between the hyper-plane and the nearest data point of each class). The solution to the optimization problem of SVM is given by the saddle point of the Lagrange functional

$$L(w,b,\alpha) = \frac{1}{2}\|w\|^2 - \sum_{i=1}^{l} \alpha_i \{ y_i[(w.x_i)+b]-1\} \tag{9}$$

where α_i are the Lagrange multipliers. Classical Lagrangian duality enables the primal problem (15) to be transformed to its dual problem, which is easier to solve. The solution is given by

$$\overline{w} = \sum_{i=1}^{l} \overline{\alpha}_i y_i x_i, \overline{b} = -\frac{1}{2}\overline{w}.[x_r + x_s] \tag{10}$$

where x_r and x_s are any two support vectors with $\overline{\alpha}_i, \overline{\alpha}_s > 0$, $y_r=1$, $y_s=-1$.

To solve the non-separable problem slack variables $\xi_i > 0$ and a penalty function, $f(\xi_i) = \sum_i \xi_i$, where the ξ_i are measures of the misclassification error. The solution is identical to the separable case except for a modification of the Lagrange multipliers as $0 \le \alpha_i \le C$, $i=1,..l$. The choice of C is not strict in practice.

The SVM can realize nonlinear discrimination by kernel mapping [17], when the samples in the input space cannot be separated by any linear hyper-plane, but can be linearly separated in the nonlinear mapped feature space. Of course in the proposed method, linear function is used as the kernel function of the SVM.

4 Experiments and Results

In this section, seven experiments have been designed. These experiments are simulated in Matlab 7.11.0. For displaying and comparing the results, four indicators (TP, FN, TN and FP) have been used.

True positive rate (TP), also called sensitivity, is the ratio between pathological files correctly classified and the total number of pathological voices. False negative rate (FN) is the ratio between pathological files wrongly classified and the total number of pathological files. True negative rate (TN), sometimes called specificity, is the ratio between normal files correctly classified and the total number of normal files. False positive rate (FP) is the ratio between normal files wrongly classified and the total number of normal files.

The final accuracy of the system is the ratio between all the hits obtained by the system and the total number of samples. Also for displaying the results, the ROC curve (AUC) has been used which is a very common way in medical decision systems.

4.1   Database Description

The database was created by specialists from the Belarusian Republican Center of Speech, Voice and Hearing Pathologies. 40 pathological speeches and 40 healthy speeches, which are related to sustained vowel "a", have been selected randomly. All the records are in PCM format, 16 bits, mono, with 16 kHz sampling frequency. A random partition is also created for applying the holdout validation on the dataset. This partition divides the dataset into a training set with 40 records and a test (or holdout) set with 40 records.

4.2   Results

In the first experiment, only the MFCC is used to make the final feature vector. In the second experiment, only the energy resulting from the wavelet packet tree is used to make the final feature vector. In the third experiment, only the entropy resulting from the wavelet packet tree is used to make the final feature vector. In the fourth experiment, the MFCC along with the energy resulting from the wavelet packet tree are used to make the final feature vector. In the fifth experiment, the MFCC along with the entropy resulting from the wavelet packet tree are used to make the final feature vector. In the sixth experiment, the energy along with the entropy resulting from the wavelet packet tree are used to make the final feature vector. In the seventh experiment, the MFCC along with the energy and entropy resulting from the wavelet packet tree are used to make the final feature vector. Finally, in all experiments, for each speech signal the samples according its feature vector are extracted and fed to the SVM classifier. The classification results are shown in table 1. Also the comparison diagrams, including ROC curves and accuracy charts, are illustrated in Fig. 6 and Fig. 7.

Table 1. The results of experiments

Feature Extraction Method	TP	TN	FP	FN	Accuracy
MFCC	85%	100%	0%	15%	92.5%
Energy	85%	100%	0%	15%	92.5%
Entropy	85%	95%	5%	15%	90%
MFCC + Energy	95%	100%	0%	5%	97.5%
MFCC + Entropy	85%	100%	0%	15%	92.5%
Energy + Entropy	95%	90%	10%	5%	92.5%
MFCC + Energy + Entropy	90%	100%	0%	10%	95%

With considering the results, it is clear that the feature vector base on the combination of MFCC and energy of wavelet packet tree nodes has more potential and accuracy for using in the classification in comparison with other types. So, it is suggested to use the combination of MFCC and energy of wavelet packet tree nodes as the final feature vector.

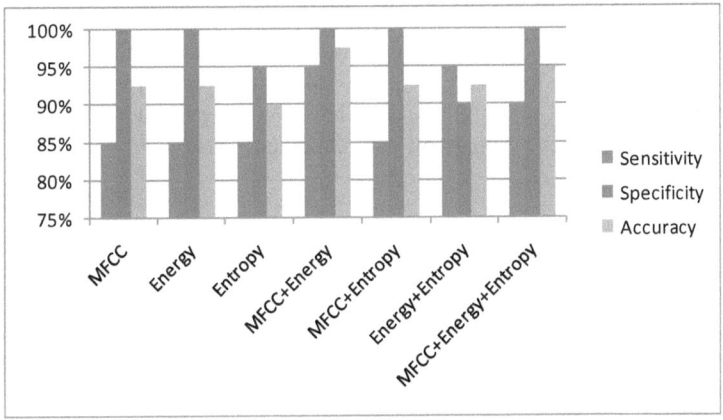

Fig. 6. The comparative results of different feature extraction methods

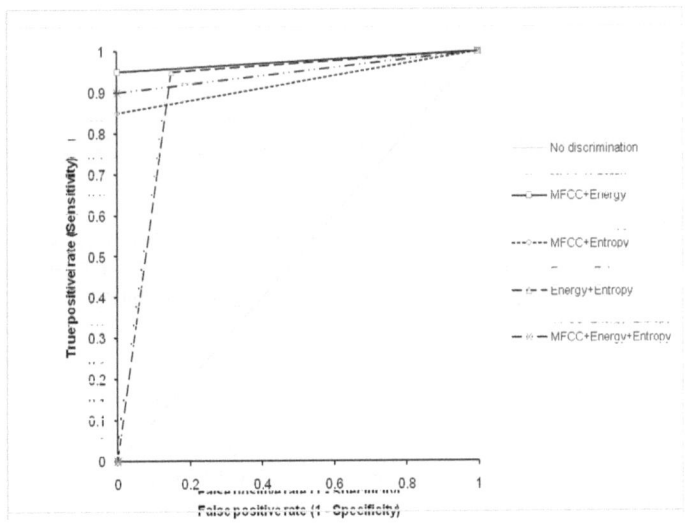

Fig. 7. The ROC curves of different feature extraction methods

4.3   Discussion

In pervious works, different parameters are used as the feature vector. For example, in [9] amplitude perturbation, pitch perturbation, etc. are used as the features and an average classification rate of 85.8% is reported. In [7] jitter, peak of autocorrelation, etc. are used as the features and an accuracy of 54.79% is reported for clustering of voice types.

But in this article, utilizing of the MFCC and the energy of the wavelet packet tree nodes as the features are proposed. The classification results in Fig. 6 show the accuracy of 97.5% and the sensitivity of 95% and the specificity of 100% for the proposed method.

Moreover, this fact can be seen in Fig. 7 that the AUC obtained with other types of features are decreased, while with the proposed feature vector (MFCC + Energy) the expected performance of system increases. This fact shows better performance of the proposed feature vector in comparison with the other types.

5 Conclusion

In this article, it is shown that features based on wavelet transformation have potential for detection of vocal fold pathology. So, three types of features which are energy and entropy resulting from the wavelet packet tree and the Mel-Frequency-Cepstral-Coefficients (MFCCs) and also their combination are investigated.

Also, a novel feature vector base on the combination of MFCC and energy of the wavelet packet tree nodes is proposed. By the means of SVM classifier, seven experiments are designed to investigate the efficiency of the proposed feature vector. The results of experiments show better performance of the proposed feature vector in comparison with other types.

Although it may be possible to try to build a complete multi-class classification system with a hierarchy of support vector machines so that detection of different type of pathological speech will be possible. For further research, it is suggested to work on the more sophisticated feature extraction phase.

Acknowledgments. This work was supported by the speech laboratory of NASB in Belarus. The authors wish to thank the Belarusian Republican Center of Speech, Voice and Hearing Pathologies by its support in the speech database.

References

1. Alonso, J.B., Leon, J.D., Alonso, I., Ferrer, M.A.: Automatic Detection of Pathologies in the Voice by HOS Based Parameters. EURASIP Journal on Applied Signal Processing 2001(4), 275–284 (2001)
2. Ceballos, L.G., Hansen, J., Kaiser, J.: A Non-Linear Based Speech Feature Analysis Method with Application to Vocal Fold Pathology Assessment. IEEE Trans. Biomedical Engineering 45(3), 300–313 (2005)
3. Ceballos, L.G., Hansen, J., Kaiser, J.: Vocal Fold Pathology Assessment Using AM Autocorrelation Analysis of the Teager Energy Operator. In: Proc. of the ICSLP 1996, pp. 757–760 (1996)
4. Adnene, C., Lamia, B.: Analysis of Pathological Voices by Speech Processing. In: 2003 Proc. of the Signal Processing and Its Applications, vol. 1(1), pp. 365–367 (2003)

5. Manfredi, C.: Adaptive Noise Energy Estimation in Pathological Speech Signals. IEEE Trans. Biomedical Engineering 47(11), 1538–1543 (2000)
6. Llorente, J.I.G., Vilda, P.G.: Automatic Detection of Voice Impairments by Means of Short-Term Cepstral Parameters and Neural Network Based Detectors. IEEE Trans. Biomedical Engineering 51(2), 380–384 (2004)
7. Rosa, M.D.O., Pereira, J.C., Grellet, M.: Adaptive Estimation of Residue Signal for Voice Pathology Diagnosis. IEEE Trans. Biomedical Engineering 47(1), 96–104 (2000)
8. Mallat, S.G.: A Theory for Multi-resolution Signal Decomposition: the Wavelet Representation. IEEE Trans. Pattern Analysis and Machine Intelligence 11(7), 674–693 (1989)
9. Wallen, E.J., Hansen, J.H.: A Screening Test for Speech Pathology Assessment Using Objective Quality Measures. In: Proc. of the ICSLP 1996, pp. 776–779 (1996)
10. Chen, W., Peng, C., Zhu, X., Wan, B., Wei, D.: SVM-based identification of pathological voices. In: Proceedings of the 29th Annual International Conference of the IEEE EMBS, pp. 3786–3789 (2007)
11. Ritchings, R.T., McGillion, M.A., Moore, C.J.: Pathological voice quality assessment using artificial neural networks. Medical Engineering & Physics 24(8), 561–564 (2002)
12. Lee, J.-Y., Jeong, S., Hahn, M.: Classification of pathological and normal voice based on linear Discriminant analysis. In: Beliczynski, B., Dzielinski, A., Iwanowski, M., Ribeiro, B. (eds.) ICANNGA 2007. LNCS, vol. 4432, pp. 382–390. Springer, Heidelberg (2007)
13. Herisa, H.K., Aghazadeh, B.S., Bahrami, M.N.: Optimal feature selection for the assessment of vocal fold disorders. Computers in Biology and Medicine 39(10), 860–868 (2009)
14. Fonseca, E.S., Guido, R.C., Scalassarsa, P.R., Maciel, C.D., Pereira, J.C.: Wavelet time frequency analysis and least squares support vector machines for identification of voice disorders. Computers in Biology and Medicine 37(4), 571–578 (2007)
15. Guido, R.C., Pereira, J.C., Fonseca, E.S., Sanchez, F.L., Vieirra, L.S.: Trying different wavelets on the search for voice disorders sorting. In: Proceedings of the 37th IEEE International Southeastern Symposium on System Theory, pp. 495–499 (2005)
16. Umapathy, K., Krishnan, S.: Feature analysis of pathological speech signals using local discriminant bases technique. Medical and Biological Engineering and Computing 43(4), 457–464 (2005)
17. Vapnik, V.N.: Statistical Learning Theory. Wiley, New York (1998)
18. Li, T., Oginara, M., Li, Q.: A comparative study on content based music genre classification. In: Proc. of the 26th Annual Int. ACM SIGIR Conf. on Research and Development in Information Retrieval, pp. 282–289 (2003)

Using Support Vector Regression for Assessing Human Energy Expenditure Using a Triaxial Accelerometer and a Barometer

Panagiota Anastasopoulou[1,2], Sascha Härtel[2,3], Mirnes Tubic[3], and Stefan Hey[2]

[1] Institute for Information Processing Technology, Karlsruhe Institute of Technology, Karlsruhe, Germany
[2] House of Competence, Karlsruhe Institute of Technology, Karlsruhe, Germany
[3] Institute of Sport and Sports Science, Karlsruhe Institute of Technology, Karlsruhe, Germany
{panagiota.anastasopoulou,sascha.haertel,stefan.hey}@kit.edu,
mirnes_tuba@hotmail.com

Abstract. Physical inactivity is nowadays defined as the fourth leading risk factor for global mortality. These levels are rising worldwide with major aftereffects on the prevention of several diseases and the general health of the population. Energy expenditure (EE) is a very important parameter usually used as a dimension in physical activity assessment studies. However, the most accurate methods for the measurement of the EE are usually costly, obtrusive and most are limited by laboratory conditions. Recent technological advancements in the sensor technology along with the great progress made in algorithms have made accelerometers a powerful technique often used to assess everyday physical activity. This paper discusses the use of support vector regression (SVR) to predict EE by using a single measurement unit, equipped with a triaxial accelerometer and a barometer, attached to the subject´s hip.

Keywords: accelerometers, barometers, energy expenditure, physical activity monitoring, support vector regression.

1 Introduction

During the last decade several studies have shown the positive affect of adequate exercise on the health of people and the correlation between the lack of exercise and the risk of developing various diseases such as cardiovascular diseases, colon and breast cancers, Type 2 diabetes and osteoporosis [7]. According to the World Health Organisation (WHO), physical inactivity (lack of physical activity) has been identified as the fourth leading risk factor for global mortality (6% of deaths globally) leading to approximately 3.2 million deaths each year [10] (Fig. 1).

Energy expenditure (EE) is one of the most widely used quantitative measures in studies that try to assess people's everyday life physical activity. Doubly labeled water and indirect calorimetry are considered to be the gold standard measures to measure EE. Nevertheless those methods are rather obtrusive and require high operating costs. Other methods like questionnaires or diaries have on the other hand

B. Godara and K.S. Nikita (Eds.): MobiHealth 2012, LNICST 61, pp. 106–113, 2013.

limited accuracy. Due to the improvements in sensor technology and algorithms, accelerometry has become the mostly used technique to assess everyday life physical activity.

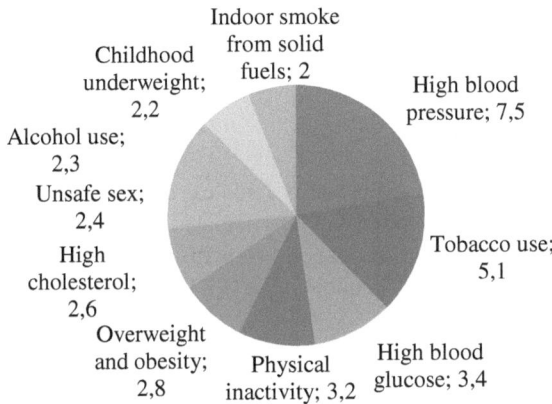

Fig. 1. 10 leading risk factors causes of death in millions per year

Jatobá et al. [3] proposed an acceleration-based EE prediction process. The activity-based linear models were developed by using the intensity of the acceleration together with some other subject-related features (such as age, weight, height).

Su et al. [8] proposed the use of SVR in order to predict EE during walking by using an acceleration sensor attached to the lower back close to the subject's center of gravity.

A well-known limitation of those devices is that they are not able to assess the increase in energy cost of walking upstairs or uphill, since the acceleration pattern remains unchanged under these conditions, although increased effort is required.

Yamazaki et al. [9] and Voleno et al. [4] introduced, along with the accelerometer, the use of an additional air pressure sensor in order to capture the movement in the vertical axis and used linear regression models for the EE estimation.

The purpose of this paper is to discuss the use of SVR to predict EE for different everyday life activities by using a single measurement unit, which consists of a triaxial accelerometer and a barometer, placed on the subject´s right side hip.

2   Measurement Setup and Data Collection

2.1   Measurement System

The Move II sensor (movisens GmbH, Karlsruhe, Germany) was used for the data collection. Move II consists of a triaxial acceleration sensor with a range of ±8 g, a resolution of 12 bit and a sampling frequency of 64 Hz. The measuring unit has an additional air pressure sensor with a sampling frequency 8 Hz and a resolution of 0.03hPa (corresponds to 15 cm at sea level). The recorded raw data were saved using the unisens format [5] and were transferred on a computer for further analysis via a USB 2.0 interface.

The assessment of the reference for the EE was performed by using the portable indirect calorimeter Meta Max 3B (Cortex Biophysics GmbH, Leipzig, Germany). The indirect calorimeter measures the breath by breath energy consumption and transmits the measured data wirelessly to a laptop.

2.2   Subject Characteristics

Twenty healthy subjects (12 male and 8 female), all students or employees of the Karlsruhe Institute of Technology (KIT) participated in the data collection study. The data collection was performed in cooperation with the Institute of Sport and Sports Science, Karlsruhe Institute of Technology (KIT). Descriptive data of the subjects can be found in Table 1.

Table 1. Subject characteristics

Subject parameter	Males (N=12)	Females (N=8)	All subjects (N=20)
Age (yrs.)	30.1 ± 8.8	30.8 ± 8.6	30.4 ± 8.7
Height (cm)	179.8 ± 8.0	167.3 ± 4.3	174.8 ± 9.2
Weight (kg)	81.9 ± 12.9	64.9 ± 9.2	75.1 ± 14.2
BMI (kg·m^{-2})	25.3 ± 3.3	23.2 ± 3.1	24.5 ± 3.3

2.3   Measurement Procedure

In our study all the subjects were equipped with the measurement unit, placed over the right anterior axillary line (Fig. 2) and the indirect calorimeter. The indirect calorimeter was both used to assess the reference data for the EE and to set the markers at every transition between the different activities. The markers where later on synchronized with the acceleration and air pressure signals.

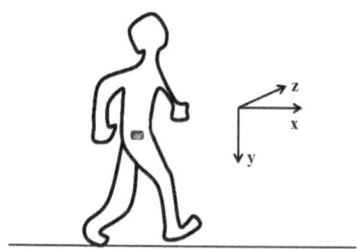

Fig. 2. Position of the sensor and direction of the acceleration axes

For the training and the evaluation of the algorithms a study with a variety of different activities (10 in total) was carried out. The data collection protocol of the study can be seen in Table 2.

Table 2. Study- Data Collection Protocol

Activity	Duration	Frequency x Distance
sitting	5 min	
standing	5 min	
walking slow		1 x 415 meter
walking fast		1 x 415 meter
jogging		2 x 415 meter
cycling	app. 5min	
walking up- /downhill		4 x130 meter
walking upstairs		3 x 84 stairs
walking downstairs		3 x 84 stairs

3   Signal Processing

3.1   Signal Preprocessing

The signal processing for the development of the EE prediction models was done with MATLAB (R2010a). Both the acceleration and the air pressure signals were preprocessed in two steps.

During the first step the acceleration signals were band-pass (0.25 Hz - 10 Hz) filtered to suppress DC-response (static acceleration due to gravity) and high frequencies that cannot arise from human movement respectively. Using the barometric formula, the air pressure signal was converted into altitude and the noise was suppressed using a Butterworth low-pass filter.

In the second step the activity was classified in intervals of 4 seconds. The activity recognition process is discussed in [6]. The classification algorithm differentiated between the following 7 activities: lying, rest (sitting/standing), cycling, up-hill/-stairs, down-hill/-stairs, level walking and jogging.

The reference for the EE was the output from the mobile indirect calorimeter. The indirect calorimeter measures the breath by breath energy consumption. Due to the non-uniform sampling frequency of the indirect calorimeter, linear interpolation was used in order to resample the EE reference to a uniform 1 Hz sampling frequency.

3.2   Parameter Extraction

The key step for the preparation of the data for the modeling is the parameter extraction. Each second of the acceleration and the air pressure data is transformed into a feature vector. The feature vector is the input for the EE modeling and estimation. The features that were extracted are as follows:

Acceleration Magnitude. The acceleration magnitude represents the intensity of the movement in each interval and is proven to be highly correlated to the EE. The acceleration magnitude was calculated using the AC part of each acceleration component as follows:

$$EEAC(i) = mean(sqrt (ax_{AC}^2(i) + ay_{AC}^2(i) + az_{AC}^2(i))) . \tag{1}$$

Altitude Change. The altitude change corresponds to the direction of the vertical movements. Therefore the altitude change (Δh) at every segment was calculated. The altitude change was split into two separate features, the positive and the negative altitude change (Δh_{pos} and Δh_{neg} respectively). By means of this value, it is possible to estimate the intensity of the movement in the vertical axis, and therefore a better estimate of the energy consumption when walking up- or downhill.

Subject Related Data. Besides the features extracted from the acceleration and the air pressure signal, other subject-related features, which are determinant for the person's EE (body height, body weight age and sex), were used in the model development as well.

3.3   Support Vector Regression (SVR)

Support vector machine (SVM) was firstly developed in the sixties but it has been further developed during the last four decades and is nowadays one of the widely used techniques to solve classification problems. Support vector regression (SVR) is a technique based on the SVM used when the predicted values are not discrete but continuous values. SVR can be used to learn complex nonlinear relationships between predictor and predicted values.

SVR tries to find a function f(x), which given the training data $\{(x_1,y_1),..., (x_l,y_l)\}$ has at most ε deviation from the actually obtained targets y_i and at the same time is as flat as possible. SVR approximates the function in the following form:

$$f(x) = w \cdot \varphi(x) + b . \tag{2}$$

Where w and b are coefficients and φ maps the original data x to a high dimensional feature space. This optimization problem can be transformed by applying Lagrangian theory into:

$$f(x) = \Sigma_{i=1}^l (\alpha_i^* - \alpha_i) \cdot k(x_i,x) + b . \tag{3}$$

Where α_i and α_i^* are Lagrange multipliers and the function $k(x_i,x)$ is called the kernel function and is defined as a linear dot product of the nonlinear mapping, i.e.,

$$k(x_i,x) = \varphi(x_i) \cdot \varphi(x) .$$

(4)

The types of kernel functions mostly used are: linear, polynomial, radial basis and sigmoid. Here the use of radial basis function was investigated and compared with the traditional linear regression (LR).

All calculations were done using the library LIBSVM [2].

3.4   Estimation of Energy Expenditure

For the estimation of the EE, the activities were divided into groups. The activity-based EE prediction included 3 groups. The first group included all passive activities (lying, sitting and standing), all walking activities (walking fast, slow, up-/downhill, up-/downstairs and jogging) in the second and cycling in the third.

For the first activity-group, the EE estimation was done using the basal metabolic rate (BMR) formulas as published in [1]. BMR is defined as the minimal rate of energy expenditure compatible with life. It is measured in the supine position under standard conditions of rest, fasting, immobility and represents the calories the body needs only for the functioning of the vital organs (e.g. heart, lungs, nervous system). The EE for the passive activities was defined as 25% above the BMR. For the other 2 groups, SVR- and LR-based models were developed. The EE estimation models were further separated into 2 groups according to the gender.

4   Results

For the validation of the EE prediction models we chose the leave-one-subject-out cross validation method. Using this method, the generalization of the models can be tested. The difference between the reference and the predicted values of the EE was computed for each subject and each activity and compared with the results of the LR.

Table 3 summarizes the results of the EE estimation, showing the mean percent error of the second-by-second estimation of EE for each activity and the mean error in kcal for the whole activity. Fig. 3 shows the measured and the estimated EE for the whole protocol for one subject.

The results suggest that the use of SVR improves the estimation of EE. The mean percent error for all the activities was reduced from -1.8 ± 12.0 %, when using LR to -1.4 ± 10.5 %, when using SVR. For some specific activities like walking slowly and fast the prediction errors were reduced significantly from -10.1 ± 14.8 % and -7.7 ± 17.5 % to -6.0 ± 14.8 % and -2.2 ± 17.1% respectively. Only during walking up-/downhill there was a slight increase in the prediction error. This might be due to the short time period. Generally the biggest errors were observed during the movement transitions; the time needed for the stabilization of the energy expenditure.

Table 3. Prediction errors (mean ± SD) for the energy expenditure

Activity	LR		SVR	
	Mean error [kcal]	Percent error [%]	Mean error [kcal]	Percent error [%]
all activities	-0.7 ± 26.2	-1.8 ± 12.0	-1.0 ± 22.8	-1.4 ± 10.5
sitting / standing	0.6 ± 2.3	2.0 ± 12.4	0.6 ± 2.3	2.1 ± 12.4
walking slow	-2.3 ± 3.5	-10.1 ± 14.8	-1.3 ± 3.3	-6.0 ± 14.8
walking fast	-1.3 ± 3.3	-7.7 ± 17.5	-0.1 ± 3.5	-2.2 ± 17.1
jogging	3.6 ± 6.3	5.5 ± 12.1	1.7 ± 7.8	2.0 ± 13.9
cycling	0.3 ± 8.5	-1.3 ± 31.4	0.6 ± 7.9	0.5 ± 26.5
walking up- / downhill	-1.3 ± 4.7	-3.5 ± 11.5	-2.1 ± 4.1	-4.9 ± 10.5
walking upstairs	-0.6 ± 2.5	4.4 ± 15.8	-0.6 ± 2.8	4.4 ± 17.7
walking downstairs	0.4 ± 1.3	4.1 ± 13.2	0.2 ± 1.2	3.2 ± 12.1

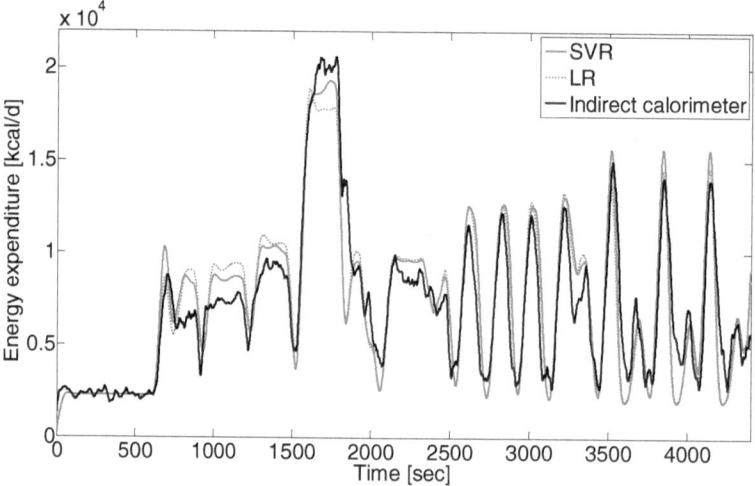

Fig. 3. Energy expenditure. The gray line is the estimated EE using the SVR, the gray dashed line is the estimated EE using the LR and the black solid line is the smoothed gold standard measure obtained by the portable indirect calorimeter.

5   Conclusion

A novel method for the estimation of human everyday activity EE has been presented and evaluated. The algorithm uses the acceleration and the air pressure signals assessed at the subject's hip and with the developed SVR-based models, it predicts the EE with high accuracy. The biggest errors were observed during the activities-transitions. This is due to the fact that the time to arrive at the steady state depends mostly on the fitness index of the subject, which was not included in the model parameters.

Future work will focus on the evaluation of the method in other population groups such as the elderly or people suffering from obesity, where physical activity monitoring is needed.

Acknowledgments. The authors would like to thank the company movisens GmbH and all the people that supported the data collection study as well as all the subjects that voluntarily participated in it.

References

1. Energy and protein requirements: Report of a joint FAO/WHO/UNU expert consultation. WHO Technical Report Series No. 724. Geneva (1985)
2. Chang, C.-C., Lin, C.-J.: LIBSVM: A Library for Support Vector Machines. ACM Transactions on Intelligent Systems and Technology 2(3), Article 27 (2011)
3. Jatobá, L.C., Großmann, U., Ottenbacher, J., Härtel, S., Haaren, B., Stork, W., Müller-Glaser, K.D., Bös, K.: Obtaining Energy Expenditure and Physical Activity from Acceleration Signals for Context-aware Evaluation of Cardiovascular Parameters. In: CLAIB 2007. IFMBE Proceedings, vol. 18, pp. 475–479 (2007)
4. Voleno, M., Redmond, S.J., Cerutti, S., Lovell, N.H.: Energy Expenditure Estimation Using Triaxial Accelerometry and Barometric Pressure Measurement. In: 32th Annual International Conference of the Engineering in Medicine and Biology Society, pp. 5185–5188 (2010)
5. Krist, M., Ottenbacher, J.: Open Source Data Format unisens (universal data format for multi sensor data), http://www.unisens.org
6. Anastasopoulou, P., Tansella, M., Stumpp, J., Shammas, L., Hey, S.: Classification of Human Physical Activity and Energy Expenditure Estimation by Accelerometry and Barometry. In: 34th Annual International Conference of the Engineering in Medicine and Biology Society, pp. 6451–6454 (2012)
7. Physical Activity Guidelines Advisory Committee. Physical Activity Guidelines Advisory Committee Report, Washington, DC, USA: Department of Health and Human Services (2008)
8. Su, S.W., Wang, L., Celler, B.C., Ambikairajah, E., Savkin, A.V.: Estimation of Walking Energy Expenditure by Using Support Vector Regression. In: 27th Annual International Conference of the Engineering in Medicine and Biology Society, pp. 3526–3529 (2005)
9. Yamazaki, T., Gen-No, H., Kamijo, Y.-I., Okazaki, K., Masuki, S., Nose, H.: A New Device to Estimate V˙O2 during Incline Walking by Accelerometry and Barometry. Medicine & Science in Sports & Exercise 12, 2213–2219 (2009)
10. World Health Organisation. Global health risks: Mortality and burden of disease attributable to selected major risks (2009)

Monitoring Respiratory Sounds: Compressed Sensing Reconstruction via OMP on Android Smartphone

Dinko Oletic, Mateja Skrapec, and Vedran Bilas

University of Zagreb, Faculty of Electrical Engineering and Computing, Unska 3,
Zagreb HR-10000
{dinko.oletic,mateja.skrapec,vedran.bilas}@fer.hr
http://www.fer.unizg.hr/aig

Abstract. We present a novel respiratory sounds monitoring concept based on compressive sensing (CS). Respiratory sounds are streamed from a body-worn sensor node to a smartphone where processing is conducted. CS is used to simultaneously lower sampling frequency on the sensor node and over-the-air data rate. In this study we emphasize compressed sensing reconstruction via orthogonal matching pursuit (OMP) on Android smartphone. Accuracy of the reconstruction and execution speed are investigated using synthetic signals. We demonstrate applicability of the technique in real-time reconstruction of at least 10 components of compressible DCT spectrum of respiratory sounds containing asthmatic wheezing, acquired at 4x lower sampling rate.

Keywords: asthma, m-health, compressive sensing, orthogonal matching pursuit, smartphone, Android.

1 Introduction

Concept of patient-centric solution for long-term self-monitoring of chronic respiratory diseases, such as asthma was shown in [8]. The system featured monitoring of physiological functions via body-worn sensor nodes. Smartphone was proposed as an access point for the sensor nodes and for convenient interaction with the patient.

Seizures related to different chronic respiratory disorders exhibit occurrence of specific pathological sounds superimposed to the sound of normal breathing. In asthma, these are wheezes, signals continuous in duration, exhibiting concentration of energy into discrete sets of spectral crests (peaks) in frequency band of normal respiratory sound (100-1000 Hz) [7]. Purpose of long-term physiological function monitoring is quantification of occurrence and durations of portions of respiratory cycles occupied by wheezing.

Capture of such information consists of acquisition of respiratory sounds via microphone or accelerometer and signal processing in order to classify breathing sounds into a normal or pathological class. In order to fulfil the requirement

B. Godara and K.S. Nikita (Eds.): MobiHealth 2012, LNICST 61, pp. 114–121, 2013.

of long-term operation, energy consumption needs to be minimized. Analysis of energy consumption of the sensor node [9] identified two feasible approaches. The first includes intensive signal processing on body-worn node at the signal acquisition site, and transmission of the classification result to the smartphone for logging and/or presentation. Advantage of such approach is reduced load on the communication subsystem. Disadvantages are the higher energy consumption of the sensor node and higher cost of software maintenance/upgrade.

The alternative approach is streaming the signal to smartphone where processing is performed. Such approach enables lower power design of the sensor node and simplifies maintenance of software by moving signal processing into the domain of smartphone mobile applications development. On the other side, in this approach the quality of information is heavily dependent on the communication link between the sensor node and the smartphone. Also, energy costs of both communication and signal processing on the smartphone can be high.

Compressive sensing (CS) enables simultaneous reduction of energy cost in both acquisition and communication part on the sensor side by lowering data rate, as seen in [3] where CS is applied in a wireless sensor network for frequency-sparse signal detection. Implementations of CS reconstruction algorithms for popular smartphone platforms can be found in [4]. [6] and [5] have shown reconstruction of streamed CS electrocardiogram signal. In this article, we present our work on reconstruction of respiratory sounds on an Android smartphone, part of the CS-based asthma monitoring system shown in Fig. 1. So far, we experimented with "orthogonal matching pursuit" (OMP) iterative reconstruction algorithm [10].

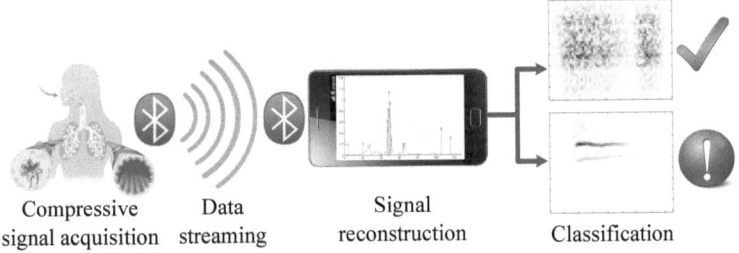

| Compressive signal acquisition | Data streaming | Signal reconstruction | Classification |

Fig. 1. Architecture of the asthma monitoring system

2 Methods and Materials

2.1 Compressed Sensing Paradigm

Let $\mathbf{x} = \{x_1, ..., x_N\}^T$ be an N-dimensional column vector representing samples of time-discrete signal acquired by the sensor node. Suppose that x can be represented by only $K << N$ non-zero components $\{\theta_1, ..., \theta_K\}$ when transformed by suitable transformation matrix $\mathbf{\Psi}$, as shown by (1):

$$\theta = \Psi x. \tag{1}$$

Compression of N-dimensional signal x to the M-dimensional vector y, $M < N$ is performed on the sensor node by inner product of rows (i.e. *measurement vectors*) of $M \times N$ dimensional measurement matrix Φ and signal x:

$$y = \Phi x = \Phi \Psi^{-1} \theta. \tag{2}$$

Vectors of compressed data y are streamed over a wireless link to the smartphone. The original signal, represented by its sparse coefficients estimates $\hat{\theta}$, is obtained by solving an undetermined system (3). Compressive sensing theory states that the good estimate of a sparse solution is the one with minimal $l1$-norm:

$$\hat{\theta} = argmin||z||_1, \ subject \ to \ y = \Phi \Psi^{-1} z. \tag{3}$$

2.2   Orthogonal Matching Pursuit Algorithm

The premise of the algorithm is that as θ is K-sparse, only K of N columns-vectors $\{\varphi_1, ..., \varphi_N\}$ of $\Phi \Psi^{-1}$ participate in the compressed signal y. Algorithm searches for the column φ_j most highly correlated to y and uses it to calculate a signal estimate $\hat{\theta}$ by solving associated over-determined system by least-squares method. Residual of y is found and the algorithm advances to the next iteration until K components are found.

We evaluate straight-forward implementation described in [10] on Android smartphone, using Java and Android SDK. Matrix operations, including least-squares algorithm were implemented using Efficient Java Matrix Library (EJML) [1]. All tests described in the following sections were performed on a Samsung Galaxy S2 device running Android OS v2.3.5 and were compared against referent implementation in Matlab [2].

2.3   Testing

Testing was conducted in three parts. In the first part we evaluated the accuracy of signal reconstruction. Secondly, the execution speed was tested. Finally, the algorithm was tested on respiratory sound signals.

Reconstruction Error. Reconstruction error was evaluated against signal sparsity K, and compressed signal lengths M for the fixed signal block length of $N = 256$ samples. Similar test-setup as in [10] was used: 1-s on random indices were used as sparse input signal. As a measurement matrix, a dense random matrix of uniformly distributed ± 1 values was used. Identity transformation matrix was used, because input signal was already sparse. Experiment was repeated 100 times for different combinations of N, M and K.

Two metrics for reconstruction error evaluation were used. First was the percentage of reconstructed signal blocks in which all samples have been reconstructed on correct indices. Goal was to measure the similarity to referent OMP algorithm by evaluating occurrence of estimates at incorrect indices when sparsity K becomes too large or compressed signal length M too short compared to original signal length N. The second metric was the accuracy of amplitude reconstruction, measured by normalized $l2$-error (4), averaged over all repetitions of the experiment.

$$Err = \frac{||\hat{x} - x||_2}{||x||_2} \qquad (4)$$

Execution Speed. OMP guarantees deterministic execution time. It breaks down the problem of solving an under-determined system of M equations and N unknowns to a set of K least squares problems of order t which is increasing by each iteration $t_1, ..., t_K$.

Dependency of execution time was verified for signal length $N = \{128, 256, 1024\}$, signal compression ratios of $4\times$ and $8\times$ and signal sparsity of $K = \{2, ...30\}$. Android method $System.nanoTime()$ was used for time measurement. Results were averaged over 300 repetitions.

Respiratory Sounds. In order to test recovery of both compressible spectrum of wheezing and broadband spectrum of normal breathing, $N \times N$ inverse discrete cosine transform (IDCT) matrix Ψ was used as a transformation matrix. Sparse measurement matrix Φ containing uniformly distributed discrete set of $\{0, 1\}$ was used, effectively defining a mask for random selection of M out of N rows of IDCT matrix. At the same time, indices of 0-s in Φ define which of the (discrete) time-domain samples can be omitted from sampling.

Pre-recorded respiratory sounds acquired from various Internet sources (such as R.A.L.E.) were used as input signals. The dataset consisted of 10 recordings N01...N10 of normal respiratory sounds (total duration 76 s), and 12 recordings W01...W12 of wheezing (in total 44 s). Each recording originated from a different patient. Intervals of intra-respiratory silence and normal breathing were removed from W01...W12 in order to produce continuous sections of signal compressible in frequency. All recordings were bandpass-filtered to 100-1000 Hz, resampled to Nyquist frequency of 2048 samples/s, normalized by amplitude, and segmented into blocks of $N = 256$ samples.

This test was repeated 100 times on each N-block of every recording, with combinations of parameters $M = \{64, 128\}$ and $K = 10$. Results were evaluated by three metrics. The first was the accuracy of reconstruction of amplitudes, measured by normalized $l2$-error as already described by (4). Remaining two metrics address frequency-locations (indices) of reconstructed spectral samples: percentage of indices reconstructed within set of frequencies containing 90 % of energy of original DCT spectrum, and percentage of reconstructed samples exhibiting grouping of two or more indices in an uninterrupted sequence. Results were averaged over all repetitions of the same signal-block, and furthermore over all blocks within each recording.

3   Results

3.1   Accuracy

Fig. 2(a) shows good fit between our implementation and the referent OMP from Matlab. On the other hand, Fig. 2(b) shows worse fit when examining $l2$-error (4). For the case of relaxed conditions of reconstruction, (lower signal sparsity K, lower compression rate/higher M), $l2$-error of our algorithm converges to a value of around 10 %. Nevertheless, relations between N, M and K obey terms stated by CS theory. It can be seen that at 30 % reconstruction error, maximum obtainable compression rate $N/M = 4$ with 8 components recovered, or alternatively 16 components can be recovered at $N/M = 2$.

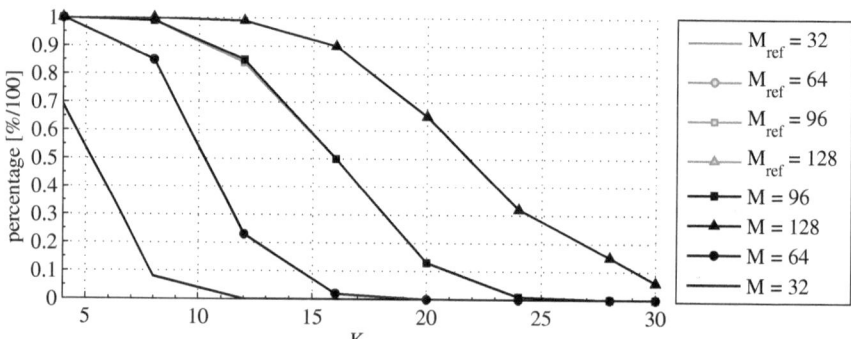

(a) Percentage of blocks with all data reconstructed at correct indices, $N = 256$.

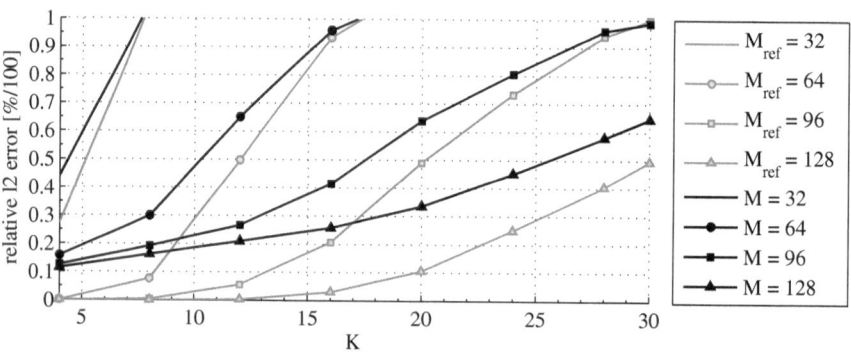

(b) Error of amplitude estimation, $N = 256$.

Fig. 2. Accuracy of signal reconstruction by our version of OMP executed on Android, compared to referent OMP implementation, both tested on an identical data set

3.2   Execution Speed

Results corroborating the expected theoretical relations are visualized in Fig. 3. It is interesting to notice that higher compression ratios N/M, apart from increasing energy saving in communication, also shorten execution of reconstruction of the same targeted number of components K proportionally.

Let's evaluate constraints for real-time operation on respiratory sounds. If the sampling rate of the original time-domain signal was 2 kHz, block-size was $N = 256$ and a 50 % block overlap was used, duration between subsequent blocks would be 64 ms. As seen from Fig. 3, at most $K = 10$ components could be recovered in real-time at $N/M = 4$. The time for real-time construction of measurement matrix is not considered.

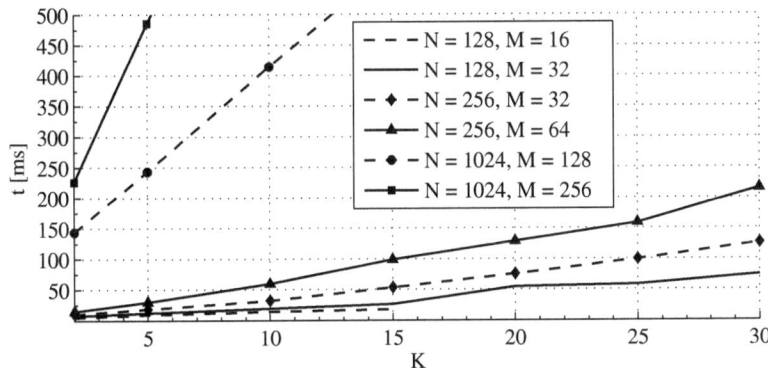

Fig. 3. Duration of execution versus N, M and K, measured on Samsung Galaxy S2

3.3   Reconstruction of Respiratory Signals Spectra

Characteristic reconstruction examples of DCT spectrum blocks originating from normal and wheezy signals shown in Figs. 4(a) and 4(b) can be compared in Figs. 4(c) and 4(d). Several effects can be observed, justifying the choice of three metrics described in Section 2.3. Most obvious is the grouping of reconstructed samples at spectral crest frequencies of the wheeze, and less evident for broadband normal breathing. Also, two side-effects arise: reconstruction of frequencies beyond those containing most of signal block energy, and error of amplitude/ energy estimation.

Overall results are shown in Fig. 5. Percentage of indices reconstructed within 90 % of the energy of an original DCT block decreases with M for both normal and wheezy respiratory signals. Relative $l2$-error ceases with increase of M, with wheezes exhibiting lower error, as a consequence of higher accuracy of estimation of high energy wheeze crests. Percent of grouped indices rises with M, and is higher for compressible spectrum of wheezing.

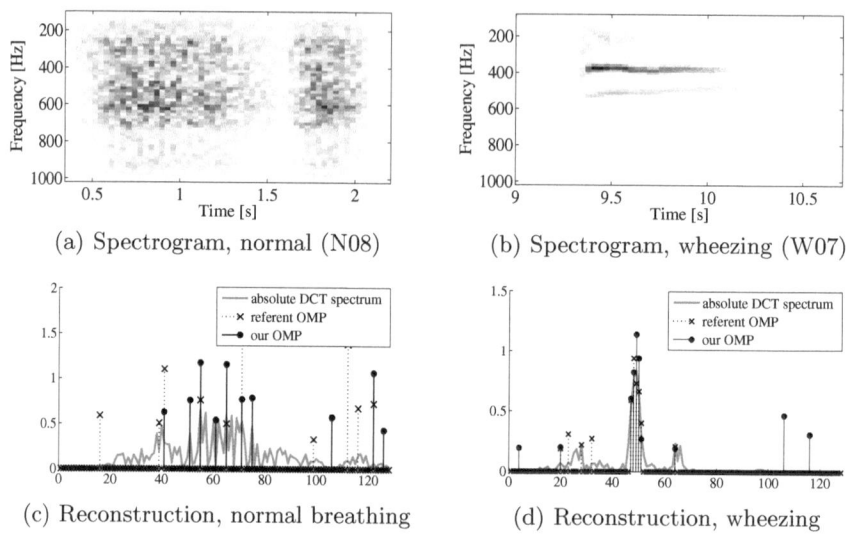

(a) Spectrogram, normal (N08)

(b) Spectrogram, wheezing (W07)

(c) Reconstruction, normal breathing

(d) Reconstruction, wheezing

Fig. 4. Examples of DCT reconstructed by OMP for single block of normal respiratory signal and block with wheezing ($N = 128$, $M = 32$, $K = 10$)

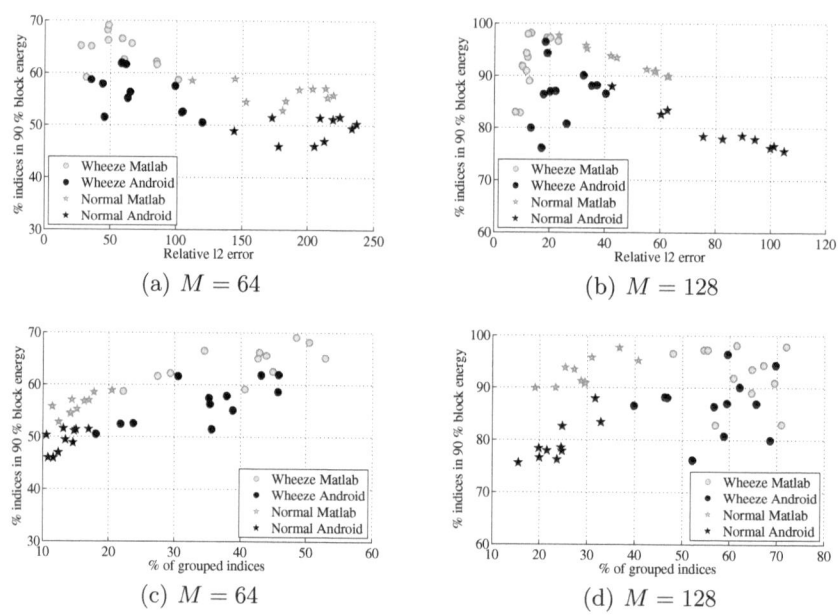

(a) $M = 64$

(b) $M = 128$

(c) $M = 64$

(d) $M = 128$

Fig. 5. Overall comparison of DCT spectrum reconstruction accuracy on data sets N01...N10 and W01...W12, $N = 256$, $K = 10$

4 Conclusion

Our implementation of OMP algorithm was shown. Results were compared to referent OMP algorithm in Matlab. Compression ratio of at least 4× can be achieved in reliable reconstruction of 10 frequency components for signal-block lengths of 256 samples in real-time on a smartphone, as demonstrated on spectrum of frequency-compressible respiratory signals. Drawbacks of current implementation are low accuracy of amplitude estimation, and operation on real matrices only. In the future we plan to extensively evaluate CS sampling setups and further investigate tradeoff between accuracy and execution speed of other CS algorithms. Reconstruction algorithm is to be accompanied by a suitable classification algorithm using features drawn from the reconstructed spectrum.

Acknowledgment. This study is supported by RECRO-NET through the *Biomonitoring of physiological functions and environment in management of asthma* project conducted at University of Zagreb, Faculty of Electrical Engineering and Computing.

References

1. Ejml, http://code.google.com/p/efficient-java-matrix-library/
2. Matlab central file exchange - cosamp and omp for sparse recovery, http://www.mathworks.fr/matlabcentral/fileexchange/32402
3. Charbiwala, Z., Kim, Y., Zahedi, S., Friedman, J., Srivastava, M.B.: Energy efficient sampling for event detection in wireless sensor networks. In: Proceedings of the 14th ACM/IEEE International Symposium on Low Power Electronics and Design, ISLPED 2009, pp. 419–424. ACM, New York (2009)
4. Drori, I.: Sparselab 2 omp in java for android (2010), http://www.cs.tau.ac.il/~idrori/sparselab2/Android/ (July 2012)
5. Faust, O., Acharya, U.R., Ma, J., Min, L.C., Tamura, T.: Compressed sampling for heart rate monitoring. Comput. Methods Programs Biomed. (2012)
6. Kanoun, K., Mamaghanian, H., Khaled, N., Atienza, D.: A real-time compressed sensing-based personal electrocardiogram monitoring system. In: Design, Automation Test in Europe Conference Exhibition (DATE), pp. 1–6 (March 2011)
7. Moussavi, Z.: Fundamentals of respiratory sounds and analysis. Synthesis Lectures on Biomedical Engineering 1(1), 1–68 (2006)
8. Oletic, D., Arsenali, B., Bilas, V.: Towards continuous wheeze detection body sensor node as a core of asthma monitoring system. In: Nikita, K.S., Lin, J.C., Fotiadis, D.I., Arredondo Waldmeyer, M.-T. (eds.) MobiHealth 2011. LNICST, vol. 83, pp. 165–172. Springer, Heidelberg (2012)
9. Oletic, D., Bilas, V.: Wireless sensor node for respiratory sounds monitoring. In: Anton, F. (ed.) IEEE I2MTC 2012, pp. 28–32. IEEE (2012)
10. Tropp, J.A., Gilbert, A.C.: Signal recovery from random measurements via orthogonal matching pursuit. IEEE Transactions on Information Theory 53(12), 4655–4666 (2007)

Performance of Miniature Implantable Antennas for Medical Telemetry at 402, 433, 868 and 915 MHz

Asimina Kiourti and Konstantina S. Nikita

National Technical University of Athens, School of Electrical and Computer Engineering
akiourti@biosim.ntua.gr, knikita@ece.ntua.gr

Abstract. In this paper, we compare the performance of implantable antennas for integration into implantable medical devices and telemetry in the MICS (402.0–405.0 MHz) and ISM (433.1–434.8, 868.0–868.6 and 902.8–928.0 MHz) bands. A parametric model of a miniature (volume of 32.7 mm^3) patch antenna is proposed for skin–implantation, and further refined for each frequency set–up. Implantation inside canonical models of the human head, arm and trunk is considered, and the antenna resonance, radiation and safety performance is compared. Results indicate enhanced bandwidth and improved radiation and safety performance at higher frequencies because of the increased copper surface area. Implantation of a specific antenna inside different parts of the human body is shown to insignificantly affect its performance.

Keywords: arm, Finite Element (FE), head, implantable antenna, Implantable Medical Device (IMD), Industrial Scientific and Medical (ISM) band, Medical Implant Communications Service (MICS) band, medical telemetry, trunk.

1 Introduction

Medical telemetry permits the measurement of physiological signals at a distance, through either wire or wireless communication technologies. One of its latest applications is in the field of Implantable Medical Devices (IMDs), which are used to perform an expanding variety of diagnostic and therapeutic functions (e.g. pacemakers [1], Functional Electrical Stimulators (FES) [2], blood glucose sensors [3] etc). In the past, wireless medical telemetry for IMDs relied on inductive coil coupling [4]. To overcome the inherent drawbacks of low data rate (1–30 kb/s), restricted communication range (less than 10 cm), and sensitivity to coils' positioning, research is currently oriented towards antenna–enabled medical telemetry for IMDs (e.g. [5]–[7]).

The ITU–R Recommendation SA.1346 [8] has outlined the use of the 402–405 MHz frequency band for Medical Implant Communications Systems (MICS). The MICS band attracts high scientific interest because of its advantages to be internationally available and feasible with low power circuits, reliably support high data rate transmissions, fall within a relatively low noise portion of the spectrum, and propagate acceptably through human tissue. The 433.1–434.8, 868.0–868.6 and 902.8–928.0 MHz Industrial Scientific and Medical (ISM) bands are also suggested for IMD telemetry in some countries [9].

B. Godara and K.S. Nikita (Eds.): MobiHealth 2012, LNICST 61, pp. 122–129, 2013.
© Institute for Computer Sciences, Social Informatics and Telecommunications Engineering 2013

In this study, we propose a parametric model of a miniature patch antenna for skin–implantation [10], and tune its parameters inside a canonical head model to obtain antennas at 402, 433, 868 and 915 MHz. Implantation inside canonical models of the human arm and trunk is also considered, and antenna performance is compared in terms of resonance (bandwidth), radiation (far–field radiation pattern and exhibited gain) and safety (conformance with the IEEE C95.1–1999 and C95.1–2005 [11] safety guidelines). Numerical simulations are carried out using the Finite Element (FE) method.

The paper is organized as follows. Section 2 describes the models and numerical method used in this study. Numerical results are presented and discussed in Section 3. The paper concludes in Section 4.

2   Models and Numerical Method

2.1   Antenna and Tissue Models

The parametric antenna model of Fig. 1 is proposed for designing the 402, 433, 868 and 915 MHz implantable antennas of this study. The model is a modified version of the one presented by the authors in [7], emphasizing on miniaturization and biocompatibility. Miniaturization techniques including patch stacking, meandering and addition of a shorting pin are applied to reduce the antenna volume to 32.7 mm^3. Biocompatible alumina (dielectric constant, $\varepsilon_r = 9.4$, and loss tangent, $\tan\delta = 0.006$), which has long been used in implantable antenna design [12], [13], is chosen as the dielectric material. Throughout this paper, the origin of the coordinate system is located at the center of the antenna ground plane, as shown in Fig. 1.

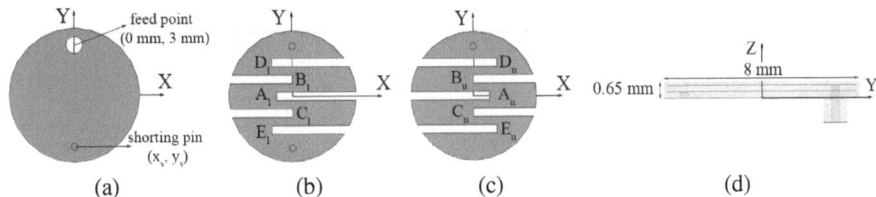

Fig. 1. Proposed parametric antenna model: (a) ground plane, (b) lower patch, (c) upper patch, and (d) side view

The antenna model consists of a 4 mm–radius ground plane and two 3.9 mm–radius vertically–stacked meandered patches, which are both fed by a 50–Ohm coaxial cable ($x = 0$ mm, $y = 3$ mm). Patches are printed on 0.25 mm–thick substrates, while a 0.15 mm–thick superstrate covers the structure to preserve its biocompatibility and robustness. Meanders are equi–distant by 1 mm, their width is fixed to 0.5 mm, and their lengths are considered variable (denoted by the x coordinate (x_{ij}), where the subscripts {ij, i = A–F, j = L, U} identify the meander in Fig. 1(b) and (c)). A variably–positioned shorting pin ($x = x_s$, $y = y_s$) connects the ground plane with the lower patch. Tuning the x_{ij}, x_s and y_s variables alters the effective dimension of the antenna and helps achieve the desired resonance characteristics.

Antenna performance is evaluated inside the skin–tissue of canonical head, arm, and trunk models for applications such as intra–cranial pressure, blood pressure, and glucose monitoring, respectively. The following tissue models are considered:

(a)   a spherical head model consisting of skin (thickness of 5 mm), bone (thickness of 5 mm), and grey matter tissues (Fig. 2(a) [7],

(b)   a cylindrical arm model consisting of skin (thickness of 5 mm), muscle (thickness of 25 mm), and bone tissues (Fig. 2(b)) [14], and

(c)   an ellipsoidal trunk model consisting of skin (thickness of 5 mm), fat (thickness of 10 mm), and muscle tissues (Fig. 2(c)) [15].

Tissue electric properties at f_0 (f_0 = 402, 433, 858, 915 MHz) are considered (Table 1 [16]), and approximated as constant inside a ±100 MHz frequency range around f_0 [7]. Tissue mass densities are also provided in Table 1. Effect of the tissue anatomy and dielectric parameters is expected to be of minor importance, as indicated by the authors in [17].

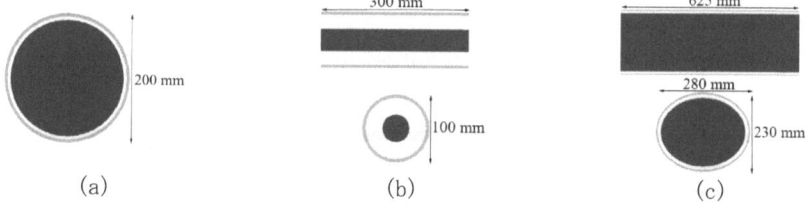

(a)   (b)   (c)

Fig. 2. Canonical models of the human: (a) head [7], (b) arm [14], and (c) trunk [15]

Table 1. Electric properties (permittivity, ε_r, and conductivity, σ) [16] and mass density of the tissues used in this study

Tissue type	402 MHz		433 MHz		868 MHz		915 MHz		Mass Density
	ε_r	σ [S/m]	ε_r	σ [S/m]	ε_r	σ [S/m]	ε_r	σ [S/m]	[kg/m^3]
skin	46.74	0.689	46.08	0.702	41.58	0.856	41.33	0.872	1100
bone	13.10	0.090	13.07	0.094	12.48	0.139	12.44	0.145	2200
grey matter	57.39	0.738	56.83	0.751	52.88	0.929	52.65	0.949	1030
muscle	57.11	0.797	56.87	0.805	55.11	0.932	54.99	0.948	1040
fat	5.58	0.041	5.57	0.042	5.47	0.050	5.46	0.051	920

2.2   Numerical Method

Simulations are carried out using the Finite Element method [18], which has been extensively used in the literature to study the design and performance of implantable antennas (e.g. [5], [7]). The mesh is automatically refined by the FE solver in an iterative way. A maximum perturbation of 30% is performed between each iteration, and the mesh refinement procedure stops when the maximum change in the magnitude of the reflection coefficient ($|S_{11}|$) between two consecutive iterations is less than 0.02, or when the number of iterations exceeds 10. Radiation boundaries are set $\lambda_0/4$ (λ_0 is the free–space wavelength, f_0 = 402 MHz) away from all simulation set–ups in order to extend radiation infinitely far and guarantee stability of the numerical calculations.

3   Numerical Results

3.1   Antenna Design and Resonance Performance

The parametric antenna model of Fig. 1 is implanted by 2.5 mm under the skin–tissue of the canonical head model (Fig. 2(a)), and its parameter (x_{ij}, x_s, and y_s) values are manually updated in an iterative way, until the magnitude of the reflection coefficient ($|S_{11}|$) at the desired resonance frequency (f_0) is adequately low, as dictated by:

$$|S_{11}|_{@ f_0} \leq -20 \text{ dB} \tag{1}$$

In this way, four antennas are obtained for scalp–implantation and medical telemetry at 402, 433, 868, and 915 MHz, respectively, as shown in Fig. 3 and Table 2. Longer meanders increase the length of the current flow path on the antenna, decreasing, in turn, the exhibited resonance frequency. The patch surface area of the 433, 868 and 915 MHz antennas is found to be increased by 2.2%, 24.9% and 25.4% as compared to that of the 402 MHz antenna.

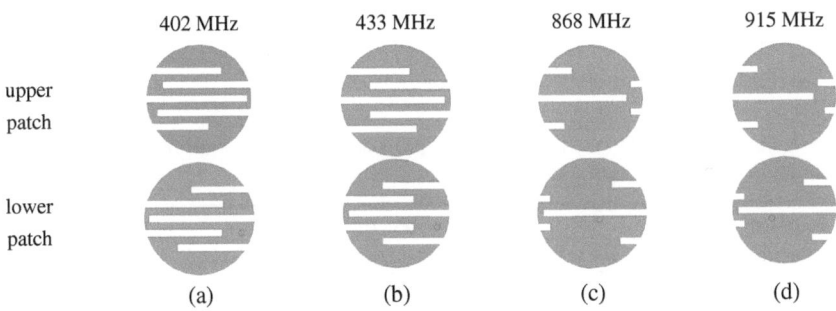

Fig. 3. Geometries of the proposed antennas at: (a) 402, (b) 433, (c) 868, and (d) 915 MHz

The reflection coefficient frequency responses of the proposed antennas inside the head model (Fig. 2(a)) are shown in Fig. 4(a). Further implantation of these designs by 2.5 mm under the skin–tissue of the arm (Fig. 2(b)) and trunk (Fig. 2(c)) models causes insignificant changes in the exhibited resonance performance, as shown in Fig. 4(b) and Fig. 4(c). The computed values for the 10 dB–bandwidth (i.e. the bandwidth defined at a return loss of 10 dB) of the antennas are indicated in Table 3 for all frequency set–ups and implantation scenarios of this study. Original values are recorded, while percent changes from the values of the 402 MHz antenna are given in parentheses. Bandwidth improvement with increasing frequency is attributed to the larger current surface area of the patches, as shown in Fig. 3.

Table 2. Variable values of the proposed antenna designs

Var.	Values [mm]			
	402 MHz	*433 MHz*	*868 MHz*	*915 MHz*
x_{Al}	−3.6	−3.5	−3.5	−3.4
x_{Bl}	1.7	1.3	−3	−3
x_{Cl}	1.6	1.3	−3	−3
x_{Dl}	−0.6	−1	1.4	1.4
x_{El}	−1.6	−1	2	2
x_{Au}	3.6	3.5	2.6	2.2
x_{Bu}	−2.7	−1.9	3	2.5
x_{Cu}	−3.1	−1.9	3	3
x_{Du}	1.7	1	−1.4	−2
x_{Eu}	0.7	1.5	−2	−2
(x_s, y_s)	(3, −1)	(3, −1)	(0.5, −0.5)	(−1, −0.6)

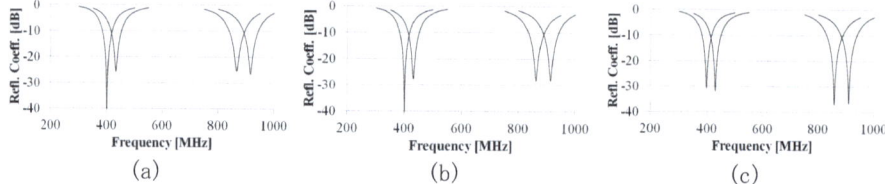

(a)   (b)   (c)

Fig. 4. Reflection coefficient frequency responses of the proposed antennas inside the human: (a) head (Fig. 2(a)), (b) arm (Fig. 2(b)), and (c) trunk (Fig. 2(c))

Table 3. 10 dB–Bandwidth (in [MHz]) of the proposed antennas for all frequency set–ups and implantation scenarios of this study

Implantatio Scenario	Frequency Set–Up			
	402 MHz	*433 MHz*	*868 MHz*	*915 MHz*
Head	35.2	38.4 (+9.1%)	53.3 (+51.4%)	54.3 (+54.3%)
Arm	35.3	38.7 (+9.6%)	53.7 (+52.1%)	55.1 (+56.1%)
Trunk	35.4	39.3 (+11.0%)	54.7 (+54.5%)	56.1 (+58.5%)

3.2   Radiation Performance

The three–dimensional far–field gain radiation patterns of the proposed antennas are shown in Fig. 5 for all frequency set–ups and implantation scenarios of this study. A near–zone to far–field transformation is used to speed–up calculations. Since the antennas are electrically very small, they radiate nearly omni–directional, monopole–like radiation patterns. The maximum exhibited far–field gain values are given in Table 4. Original values are recorded, while percent changes from the values of the 402 MHz antenna are given in parentheses. Low gain values are computed because of the miniaturized antenna dimensions. Higher gain values with increasing frequency are attributed to the larger current surface area of the patches, as indicated in Fig. 3.

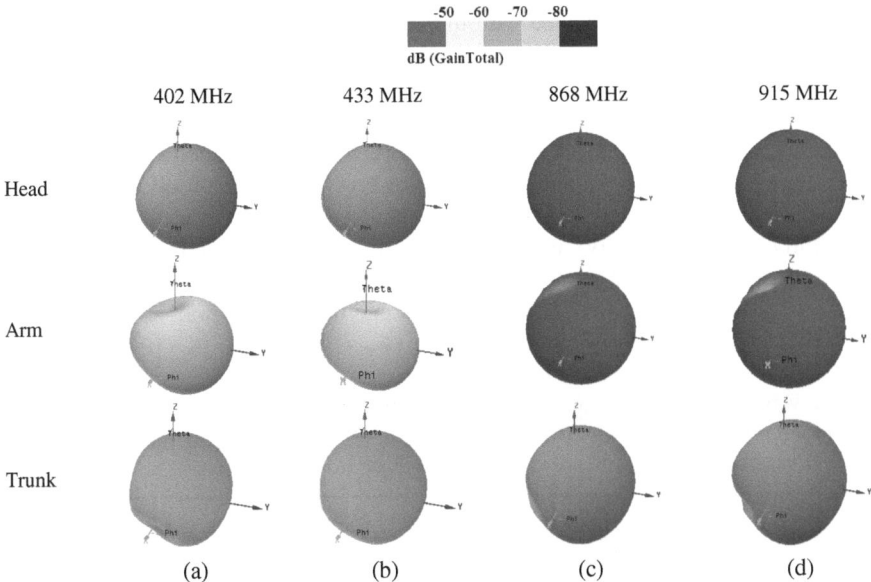

Fig. 5. Far–field gain radiation patterns of the proposed antennas for all implantation scenarios, at: (a) 402, (b) 433, (c) 868, and (d) 915 MHz

Table 4. Maximum far–field gain values (in [dB]) exhibited by the proposed antennas for all frequency set–ups and implantation scenarios of this study

Implantatio	Frequency Set–Up			
Scenario	402 MHz	433 MHz	868 MHz	915 MHz
Head	−50.98	−50.25 (+1.4%)	−41.90 (+17.8%)	−41.36 (+18.9%)
Arm	−54.16	−53.74 (+0.8%)	−42.56 (+21.4%)	−41.96 (+22.5%)
Trunk	−53.26	−52.69 (+1.1%)	−41.35 (+27.5%)	−40.07 (+28.4%)

3.3   Safety Performance

Issues related to patient safety limit the maximum allowable power incident to an implantable antenna. The Specific Absorption Rate (SAR) (rate of energy deposited per unit mass of tissue) is generally accepted as the most appropriate dosimetric measure, and compliance with international guidelines is assessed. For example, the IEEE C95.1–1999 standard restricts the SAR averaged over any 1 g of tissue in the shape of a cube to less than 1.6 W/kg, while the IEEE C95.1–2005 standard restricts the SAR averaged over any 10 g of tissue in the shape of a cube to less than 2 W/kg [11].

In order to determine the maximum allowable net–input power levels to the proposed implantable antennas, an SAR numerical analysis is carried out for all frequency set–ups and implantation scenarios of this study. The net–input power is initially set to 1 W and the maximum 1 g– and 10 g–averaged SAR values are computed, based on numerical computational procedures recommended by IEEE [19]. In order to guarantee conformance with the IEEE C95.1–1999 and the IEEE C95.1–2005 standards [11], the power incident to the antenna should be decreased to the levels indicated as P_{1999} and P_{2005} in Table 5, respectively. Original values are recorded, while percent changes from the values of the 402 MHz antenna are given in parentheses. The old IEEE C95.1–1999 standard is found to be much stricter, limiting the net–input power to more than 10 times lower than that imposed by the recent IEEE C95.1–2005 standard. At higher operation frequencies, electric field, or, equivalently, current density, is more uniformly distributed across an increased surface area of the radiating patches, as indicated in Fig. 3. Lower maximum SAR values, or equivalently, higher maximum allowable net–input power levels are, thus, computed.

Table 5. Maximum allowable net–input power to the proposed antennas which guarantees conformance with the IEEE C95.1–1999 (P_{1999}) and C95.1–2005 (P_{2005}) [11] standards (in [mW]), for all frequency set–ups and implantation scenarios of this study

Implantation Scenario	Frequency Set–Up							
	402 MHz		*433 MHz*		*868 MHz*		*915 MHz*	
	P_{1999}	P_{2005}	P_{1999}	P_{2005}	P_{1999}	P_{2005}	P_{1999}	P_{2005}
Head	1.664	20.853	1.672	20.927	1.685	21.338	1.714	21.409
			(+0.48%)	(+0.35%)	(+1.26%)	(+2.33%)	(+3.00%)	(+2.67%)
Arm	1.676	20.951	1.680	21.008	1.724	21.470	1.727	21.531
			(+0.24%)	(+0.27%)	(+2.86%)	(+2.48%)	(+3.04%)	(+2.77%)
Trunk	1.678	20.962	1.686	21.033	1.726	21.559	1.729	21.529
			(+0.48%)	(+0.34%)	(+2.86%)	(+2.85%)	(+3.04%)	(+2.71%)

4   Conclusion

A parametric model of a skin–implantable antenna was proposed, emphasizing on size miniaturization and biocompatibility, and further refined for implantation inside the skin–tissue of a canonical head model and medical telemetry at 402, 433, 868 and 915 MHz. Implantation of the same antenna inside different implantation scenarios (head, arm, trunk) was shown to cause minor changes to the exhibited resonance, radiation and safety performance. On the other hand, the operation frequency of the antenna was found to be relatively significant: antennas at higher frequencies were shown to exhibit enhanced bandwidths, higher gains, and increased maximum allowable input power levels imposed by international safety guidelines. Results are attributed to the enhanced patch surface area of the antennas at higher frequencies.

References

1. Wessels, D.: Implantable pacemakers and defibrillators: Device overview and EMI considerations. In: IEEE Int. Symp. Electromagn. Compat. Conference (2002)

2. Guillory, K., Normann, R.A.: A 100–channel system for real time detection and storage of extracellular spike waveforms. J. Neurosci. Methods 91, 21–29 (1999)
3. Shults, M.C., Rhodes, R.K., Updike, S.J., Gilligan, B.J., Reining, W.N.: A telemetry–instrumentation system for monitoring multiple subcutaneously implanted glucose sensors. IEEE Trans. Biomed. Eng. 41, 937–942 (1994)
4. Tang, Z., Smith, B., Schild, J.H., Peckham, P.H.: Data transmission from an implantable biotelemeter by Load-Shift Keying using circuit configuration modulator. IEEE Trans. Biomed. Eng. 42, 524–528 (1995)
5. Karacolak, T., Hood, A.Z., Topsakal, E.: Design of a dual–band implantable antenna and development of skin mimicking gels for continuous glucose monitoring. IEEE Trans. Microw. Theory Techn. 56, 1001–1008 (2008)
6. Sánchez–Fernández, C.J., Quavado–Teruel, O., Requena–Carrión, J., Inclán–Sánchez, L., Rajo–Iglesias, E.: Dual–band microstrip patch antenna based on short 0 circuited ring and spiral resonators for implantable medical devices. IET Mikrow. Antennas Propag. 4, 1048–1055 (2010)
7. Kiourti, A., Nikita, K.S.: Miniature Scalp–Implantable Antennas for Telemetry in the MICS and ISM Bands: Design, Safety Considerations and Link Budget Analysis. IEEE Trans. Antennas Propag. 60, 3568–3575 (2012)
8. International Telecommunications Union-Radiocommunications, radio regulations, SA.1346, ITU, Geneva, Switzerland, http://itu.int/home
9. International Telecommunications Union-Radiocommunications, radio regulations, section 5.138 and 5.150, ITU, Geneva, Switzerland, http://itu.int/home
10. Kiourti, A., Nikita, K.S.: A Review of Implantable Patch Antennas for Biomedical Telemetry: Challenges and Solutions. IEEE Antennas Propag. Mag. 54, 210–228 (2012)
11. IEEE Standard for Safety Levels with Respect to Human Exposure to Radiofrequency Electromagnetic Fields, 3kHz to 300 GHz, IEEE Standard C95.1 (1999) (2005)
12. Capello, W.W., D'Anthonio, J., Feinberg, J., Manley, M.: Alternative Bearing Surfaces: Alumina Ceramic Bearings for Total Hip Arthroplasty. In: Benazzo, F., Falez, F., Dietrich, M. (eds.) Bioceramics and Alternative Bearings in Joint Arthroplasty, pp. 87–94. Springer (2005)
13. Kiourti, A., Christopoulou, M., Nikita, K.S.: Performance of a novel miniature antenna implanted in the human head for wireless biotelemetry. In: IEEE Int. Symp. Antennas Propag. (2011)
14. Wegmueller, M.S., Oberle, M., Kuster, N., Fichtner, W.: From dielectrical properties of human tissue to intra–body communications. In: World Congress Med. Physics Biomed. Eng. (2006)
15. Shiba, K., Nukaya, M., Tsuji, T., Koshiji, K.: Analysis of current density and specific absorption rate in biological tissue surrounding transcutaneous transformer for an artificial heart. IEEE Trans. Biomed. Eng. 55, 205–213 (2008)
16. Gabriel, C., Gabriel, S., Corthout, E.: The dielectric properties of biological tissues. Phys. Med. Biol. 41, 2231–2293 (1996)
17. Kiourti, A., Nikita, K.S.: Numerical Assessment of the Performance of a Scalp-Implantable Antenna: Effects of Head Anatomy and Dielectric Parameters. Wiley Bioelectromagnetics (to appear), doi:10.1002/bem.21753
18. Sadiku, M.N.O.: Numerical techniques in electromagnetic. CRC Press (2001)
19. IEEE Recommended Practice for Measurements and Computations of Radio Frequency Electromagnetic Fields with Respect to Human Exposure to such Fields, 100 kHz to 300 GHz, IEEE Standard C95.3–2002 (2002)

A Personalized Model for Galvanic Coupling in Intrabody Communication Systems

M. Amparo Callejón[1], David Naranjo[2,1],
Javier Reina-Tosina[3,2], and Laura M. Roa[1,2]

[1] Biomedical Engineering Group, University of Seville, Seville, Spain
[2] CIBER de Bioingeniería, Biomateriales y Nanomedicina (CIBER-BBN), Spain
[3] Dept. of Signal Theory and Communications, University of Seville, Seville, Spain
{mcallejon,dnaranjo,jreina,lroa}@us.es

Abstract. Intrabody communication (IBC) uses the human body as a transmission medium for electrical signals, providing an efficient channel to interconnect devices in Body Sensor Networks. For IBC galvanic coupling, the signal path is accomplished through two pairs of electrodes deployed on the skin, which suggest the dependence of the attenuation signal on the subject's electrophysiological skin properties. With the purpose of gaining an insight into the attenuation differences observed for diverse subjects, a simple transmission line-based model has been used for the identification of those personalized parameters that best emulate the attenuation behavior. Experimental results for two different subjects have been carried out using a harmonized measurement set-up. Model simulations have shown to match measurement data more accurately when individualized instead standard skin parameters were used, thus highlighting the need to deal with personalized models in IBC research.

Keywords: electrophysiological properties, galvanic coupling, intrabody communication, measurement set-up, pathloss, personalized parameters, transmission line model.

1 Introduction

Pervasive monitoring along with Body Sensor Networks (BSN) have been established as the technological basis for the delivery of preventive and personalized health systems, which aim to improve patients' quality of life [1]. Nevertheless, some technical challenges regarding the design of small-size, power-saving and miniaturized intelligent wearable devices are yet to be solved [2]. In this sense, a promising technique called Intrabody Communications (IBC), which uses the human body as a transmission medium for electrical signals, allows low frequencies and low power signals to be used, thus reducing consumption, permitting miniaturization and avoiding interferences [3]. One key issue involving IBC research is the human body characterization as a communication channel. For this purpose, different models, which have shed light on signal propagation mechanisms through the human body, have been proposed in the literature [4–7].

B. Godara and K.S. Nikita (Eds.): MobiHealth 2012, LNICST 61, pp. 130–137, 2013.

However, an accurate validation has not always been possible due to the great dependence of the experimental results on both the measurement conditions and the test subject [4, 6, 8]. In this way, significant differences in pathloss data have been found due to each subject's particular anthropometrical characteristics (e.g., diameter and length of the arm, weight, sex,...) and the position of electrodes through the body [4, 6]. For instance, previous results reported by the authors evidenced that the frequencies at which the minimum attenuation was obtained did not match for different subjects [9], thus highlighting the need for personalized models. In spite of the fact that all existing IBC models in the literature use the widely accepted parameters reported in [10], there is evidence that these models have not always been able to emulate the complex frequency behavior of attenuation, with discrepancies existing among diverse authors' outcomes and different subjects. In addition, in the case of galvanic coupling, the dependence of the attenuation results on the subject's physiological parameters has been found to be even higher [4, 9], which could be explained by the fact that the signal path is confined to the skin when sensors are deployed on it.

In this work, a skin transmission line model previously reported by the authors [11] has been used in order to identify the personalized parameters that best match the frequency behavior of the pathloss found for different subjects. Consequently, the objective of this work has been to show that a better agreement can be accomplished by considering personalized instead of generalized parameters. In order to assess these parameters, galvanic coupling attenuation experiments for different subjects have been carried out using a harmonized set-up [12]. For the purpose of validation, a set of measurements over different distances between electrodes were obtained and a satisfactory agreement between the model's predicted behavior and the experimental data was found. Finally, the results of the personalized model and those obtained by using generalized parameters were compared in order to show the need to deal with personalized models in IBC research.

2   Material and Methods

2.1   Distributed Transmission Line Model

The model used in this work, which can be seen in Fig. 1, is based on a skin transmission line model [11]. It consists in the distributed insertion of skin cross-sectional admittances, $Y_{skin}(\omega)$, and skin longitudinal impedances, $Z_{skin}(\omega)$, along a longitudinal plane. Specifically, $Y_{skin}(\omega)$ is formed by a shunt circuit composed of a conductance $G(\omega)$ that represents the conductive pathways of the skin (sweat glands and the ionic channels that cross the cell membrane), and a susceptance $B(\omega)$ that accounts for the keratinized cells of the stratum corneum (SC) and the lipid bilayer [13]. In addition, $Z_{skin}(\omega)$ corresponds to a resistive characteristic $R(\omega)$ that emulates the signal propagation between adjacent admittances. Finally, Z_e, whose frequency response was taken from [14], models the electrode impedance, and Z_l represents the input impedance of the receiver.

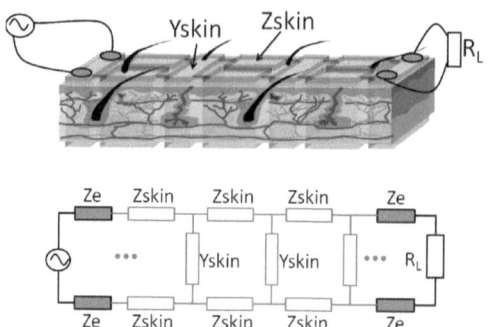

Fig. 1. Galvanic coupling transmission line model

A propagation constant $\gamma(\omega)$ can be found through

$$\gamma(\omega) = \sqrt{2Z_{skin}(\omega)Y_{skin}(\omega)} = \sqrt{2R(G(\omega) + jB(\omega))}, \tag{1}$$

where the constant factor of 2 is due to the differential characteristic of galvanic coupling.

In order to take into account the electrode effect through the Z_e impedances, which could cause an impedance mismatch, a reflection coefficient $\Gamma_l(\omega)$ was introduced in the model to obtain the total pathloss of the IBC system,

$$L(\text{dB}) = 20 \log_{10} \frac{1 + \Gamma_l(\omega)e^{-2\gamma(\omega)l}}{(1 + \Gamma_l(\omega))e^{-\gamma(\omega)l}}, \tag{2}$$

where l is the length between electrodes.

The electrophysiological properties of the skin were addressed by means of $G(\omega) = K\sigma'(\omega)$, $R(\omega) = 1/G(\omega)$ and $B(\omega) = \omega\varepsilon_r'(\omega)\varepsilon_0 G(\omega)/\sigma'(\omega)$, where $K = A/d$, d is the transverse distance between the same pair of electrodes and A is the electrode measurement area. On the other hand, $\varepsilon_r'(\omega)$ and $\sigma'(\omega)$ are the real part of the permittivity $\hat{\varepsilon}_r(\omega)$ and the conductivity $\hat{\sigma}(\omega)$ of the skin, respectively. For the sake of simplicity, these were modeled by means of a single-pole Cole-Cole model given by (3) and (4), instead of the usual two-pole model reported in [10]. This simplification was validated within a limited frequency range, taking into account that galvanic coupling usually operates at frequencies up to 1 MHz, where a single-dispersion model is accurate enough.

$$\hat{\varepsilon}_r(\omega) = \varepsilon_\infty + \frac{\triangle\varepsilon_1}{1 + (j\omega\tau_1)^{1-\alpha_1}} + \frac{\sigma_s}{j\omega\varepsilon_0}, \tag{3}$$

$$\hat{\sigma}(\omega) = j\omega\varepsilon_0\hat{\varepsilon}_r(\omega), \tag{4}$$

where ε_0 is the permittivity of vacuum. Subsequently, the rest of parameters in (3)-(4), were personalized for different subjects, instead of using the usual parameters reported in [10].

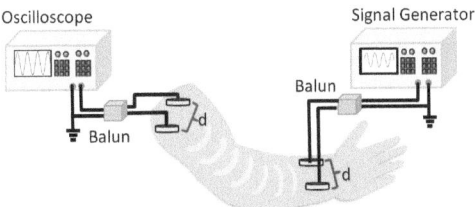

Fig. 2. Galvanic coupling measurement set-up

2.2 Galvanic Coupling Measurement Set-Up

The galvanic coupling measurement set-up, shown in Fig. 2, consisted of a GFG-8015G function generator of GW Instek to provide the signal, an MSO6032A digital oscilloscope of Agilent Technologies Inc. ($R_{input} = 1$ MΩ) to acquire it, a pair of PT4 balun transformers of Oxford Electrical Products and four electrodes. The baluns were used to remove the effect of the internal ground of both the signal generator and the oscilloscope, in order to obtain a realistic IBC galvanic coupling transmission path. Commercial round pregelled silver/silverchloride Swaromed ECG electrodes (0.5 cm-radius) were chosen. The two transmitter electrodes were attached to the skin near the wrist and the two receiving electrodes were moved along the forearm using two distances: 5 and 10 cm. At the same time, a distance of 9 cm between the two electrodes of the same pair was chosen, according to [12]. A sinusoidal signal with a peak-to-peak current amplitude of 0.5 mA was applied. Twelve frequency points from 20 kHz up to 1 MHz were considered. This limited frequency range was chosen because of the evidence that the human body acts as an antenna for higher frequencies [15, 16] and, in addition, some other non-deterministic effects, such as radiation from cables and electrodes, become non-negligible as frequency increases [17]. Finally, some anthropometrical characteristics such as sex, age, height, weight, arm length and arm diameter were taken into account, and are summarized in Table 1, for two subjects A and B. Finally, it must be noted that the amplitude levels considered in this work were established well in the bounds of the International Commission on Non-Ionizing Radiation Protection's (ICNIRP) regulations [18].

Table 1. Test subjects' anthropometrical characteristics

Subject	Sex	Age	Height	Weight	Arm length	Arm diameter
A	Male	33	1.82 m	100 kg	65 cm	9.5 cm
B	Female	27	1.57 m	50 kg	50 cm	4.3 cm

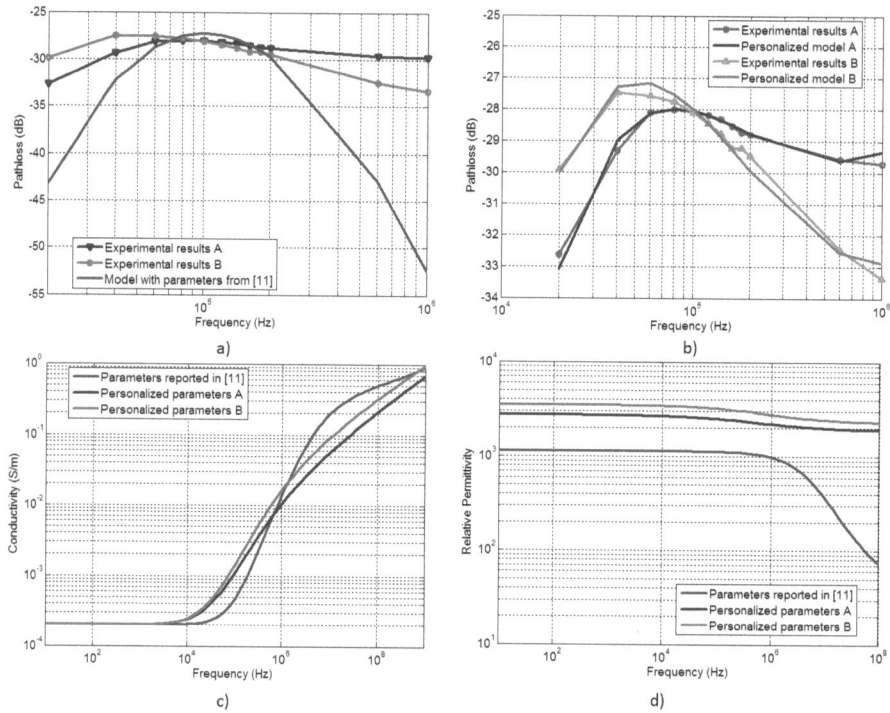

Fig. 3. (a) Comparison between experimental results and model simulations for subjects A and B. (Marks: measurement data; solid line: model with generalized parameters and $K = A/d$; dashed line: model with generalized parameters and $K = 0.7A/d$) (b) Comparison between experimental results and model simulations by using personalized parameters for subjects A and B. (c) Comparison between conductivity model by using generalized and personalized parameters for subjects A and B. (d) Comparison between permittivity model by using generalized and personalized parameters for subjects A and B.

Table 2. Personalized Parameters for (3)

Parameter set	ε_∞	$\triangle\varepsilon_1$	τ_1 (ns)	α_1	σ_s
Dry skin	37	1122	32.51	0.18	0.0002
Subject A	1855.81	876.32	325.11	0.49	0.0002
Subject B	2225.81	1246.32	230.61	0.45	0.0002

3   Results

We first implemented a Least-Mean-Square (LMS) algorithm to find the parameters from which the simplified single-pole Cole-Cole model was able to accurately

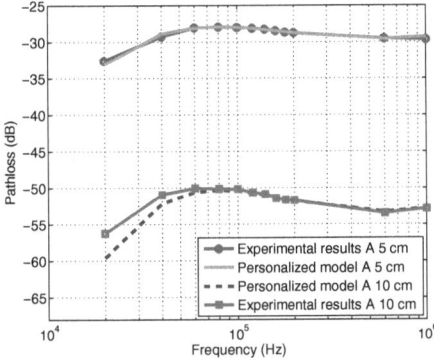

Fig. 4. Experimental results and model simulations obtained for subject A and two different distances of 5 and 10 cm between electrodes

reproduce both skin permittivity and conductivity reported in [10]. These parameters, whose values are given in Table 2 (Dry Skin), showed to be valid up to 1 GHz, which is much higher than the usual galvanic coupling frequency band (up to 1 MHz) [4,6,9]. Once the validity of this simplification was proven, we subsequently used the same LMS algorithm to identify the personalized parameters that best match the model's pathloss curve to that obtained experimentally, for both subjects A and B. These parameters are also listed in Table 2 (Subjects A and B). The pathloss curves obtained by using the generalized parameters in [10] are shown in Fig. 3a, whereas those obtained by using personalized parameters are shown in Fig. 3b. It can be seen that in the former case, personalization was addressed through the parameter K, considering a smaller measurement area (parameter A) for subject B, whose arm diameter was lower. The characteristics obtained for $\hat{\varepsilon}_r(\omega)$ and $\hat{\sigma}(\omega)$ using the single-pole Cole-Cole model along with the personalized parameters found for each subject are shown in Fig. 3c and 3d. Furthermore, in order to validate the model with personalized parameters, other experimental samples by changing the distance between the electrodes were considered. Therefore, once the personalized parameters were found for the given subjects, they were subsequently applied to the model in order to predict the experimental results obtained with a separation of 10 cm between the electrodes. The results for subject A and two different distances are shown in Fig. 4.

4   Discussion

The attenuation results obtained from using generalized parameters in Fig. 3a show that only a satisfactory agreement is obtained within 50-250 KHz, as was previously evidenced in [9]. This could be due to the fact that the signal path is primarily accomplished through the skin within this frequency range, and out of which other signal paths begin to be dominant. In fact, the signal could even penetrate through the skin towards the muscle or the fat, notwithstanding that there also exist other external phenomena such as off-body radiation that could affect at higher frequencies. On the other hand, it must be noticed how the maximum peak of the pathloss curve is located at different frequencies for different subjects, as can be seen in Fig. 3b. It can also be noticed how the use of personalized parameters yields to a better fit between model and experimental results in the galvanic coupling approach. This may be explained by the fact that they are capable of reproducing the dominant effect of different tissues within a wider frequency range. In much the same way, these parameters address some underlying issues related not only to the subjects' anthropometrical characteristics, but also to the electrophysiological properties of the skin. In fact, skin admittance varies considerably between different people and different environmental conditions. Changes in hydration mechanisms due to sweat gland activity and temperature can be manifested in large variations of skin admittance [19]. Nevertheless, the trends observed for the dielectric properties of skin by using personalized parameters were found to be quite similar to those reported for skin in [10], thereby producing a response within a physiological range, as can be seen in Fig. 3c and 3d. Finally, the results for subject A shown in Fig. 4 highlight that there exists a satisfactory agreement for both distances, thus showing the validity of the model using personalized parameters.

5   Summary and Conclusion

In order to gain an insight into the differences observed for diverse subjects, a simple IBC galvanic coupling model has been used in this paper. With this objective in mind, an LMS algorithm was implemented in order to find those personalized parameters that best adapt the model's response to the experimental results. In fact, we have shown that it is necessary to personalize the models not only regarding anthropometrical characteristics but also skin dielectric properties. In addition, the conductivity and permittivity obtained by means of these parameters showed to have a similar trend to that reported in [10]. Finally, experimental results considering another distance between electrodes were used in order to validate such personalized parameters. The satisfactory agreement between the model's response and the experimental results shows the validity of the proposed approach and suggests the use of personalized models in order to overcome some of the discrepancies observed between authors' outcomes in IBC literature.

Acknowledgments. The authors are grateful to E.C. Wiegers, G. Barbarov and D. Plant for their useful comments and help. This work was supported in part by the Consejería de Economía, Innovación y Ciencia, Government of Andalucía, under Grants P08-TIC-04069 and P10-TIC-6214.

References

1. Maglaveras, N., Bonato, P., Tamura, T.: Guest Editorial Special Section on Personal Health Systems. IEEE Trans. Inf. Technol. Biomed. 14, 360–363 (2010)

2. Li, S., Hu, F., Li, G.: Advances and Challenges in Body Area Network. In: Zhang, J. (ed.) ICAIC 2011, Part III. CCIS, vol. 226, pp. 58–65. Springer, Heidelberg (2011)
3. Zimmerman, T.G.: Personal area networks: Near-field intrabody communication. IBM Systems Journal 35(3.4), 609–617 (1996)
4. Song, Y., Qun Hao, Q., Zhang, K., Wang, M., Chu, Y., Kang, B.: The Simulation Method of the Galvanic Coupling Intrabody Communication With Different Signal Transmission Paths. IEEE Trans. Instrum. Meas. 60, 1257–1266 (2011)
5. Xu, R., Hongjie Zhu, H., Yuan, J.: Electric-Field Intrabody Communication Channel Modeling With Finite-Element Method. IEEE Trans. Biomed. Eng. 58, 705–712 (2011)
6. Pun, S.H., Gao, Y.M., Mak, P.U., Vai, M.I., Du, M.: Quasi-Static Modeling of Human Limb for Intra-Body Communications With Experiments. IEEE Trans. Inf. Technol. Biomed. 15(6), 870–876 (2011)
7. Bae, J., Cho, H., Song, K., Lee, H., Yoo, H.-J.: The Signal Transmission Mechanism on the Surface of Human Body for Body Channel Communication. IEEE Trans. Microw. Theory Tech. 60(3), 582–593 (2012)
8. Lucev, Z., Krois, I., Cifrek, M.: Effect of body positions and movements in a capacitive intrabody communication channel from 100 kHz to 100 MHz. In: IEEE International Instrumentation and Measurement Technology Conference (I2MTC), pp. 2791–2795 (2012)
9. Callejón, M.A., Naranjo, D., Reina, J., Roa, L.M.: Distributed Circuit Modeling of Galvanic and Capacitive Coupling for Intrabody Communication. IEEE Trans. Biomed. Eng. PP(99), 1 (2012); early access article
10. Gabriel, S., Lau, R.W., Gabriel, C.: The dielectric properties of biological tissues: III. Parametric models for the dielectric spectrum of tissues. Physics in Medicine and Biology 41, 2271 (1996)
11. Callejón, M.A., Roa, L.M., Reina, J., Naranjo, D.: Study of Attenuation and Dispersion through the Skin in Intra-Body Communications Systems. IEEE Trans. Inf. Technol. Biomed. 16(1), 159–165 (2012)
12. Callejón, M.A., Naranjo, D., Reina-Tosina, L.J., Roa, L.M.: A First Approach to the Harmonization of Intrabody Communications Measurements. In: Long, M. (ed.) World Congress on Medical Physics and Biomedical Engineering May 26-31, 2012 Beijing, IFMBE Proceedings, vol. 39, pp. 704–707. Springer, Heidelberg (2013)
13. Grimnes, S., Martinsen, Ø.G.: Bioimpedance and bioelectricity basics, pp. 105–109. Ed. Academic Press (2000)
14. Hachisuka, K., Takeda, T., Terauchi, Y., Sasaki, K., Hosaka, H., Itao, K.: Intrabody data transmission for the personal area network. Microsystem Technologies 11, 1020–1027 (2005)
15. Cho, N., Yoo, J., Song, S.-J., Lee, J., Jeon, S., Yoo, H.-J.: The Human Body Characteristics as a Signal Transmission Medium for Intrabody Communication. IEEE Trans. Microw. Theory Tech. 55, 1080–1086 (2007)
16. Koutitas, G.: Multiple Human Effects in Body Area Networks. IEEE Antennas Wireless Propag. Lett. 9(5), 1080–1086 (2007)
17. Xu, R., Ng, W., Zhu, H., Shan, H., Yuan, J.: Environment Coupling and Interference on the Electric-Field Intrabody Communication Channel. IEEE Trans. Biomed. Eng. 59(7), 2051–2059 (2012)
18. International Commission on Non-Ionizing Radiation Protection: Guidelines for Limiting Exposure to Time-Varying Electric, Magnetic, and Electromagnetic Fields (up to 300 GHz). Health Physics 74(4), 494–522 (1998)
19. Tronstad, C., Johnsen, G.K., Grimnes, S., Martinsen, Ø.G.: A study on electrode gels for skin conductance measurements. Physiol. Meas. 31, 1395 (2010)

Switching from Traditional Medical Applications to Mobile Devices: Cardiac and Cochlear Implants

Claudia C. Gutiérrez Rodríguez and Anne-Marie Déry-Pinna

University of Nice Sophia-Antipolis, I3S Laboratory
Sophia Antipolis, France
cgutierr@i3s.unice.fr, pinna@polytech.unice.fr

Abstract. Designing HCI in a medical context is not trivial. It needs to provide patients and medical experts with essential information for the tasks to be performed while ensuring the safety of operations. In this paper, we tackle this issue focused on the HCI requirements and expectations revealed by the use of mobile devices (Smartphone for patients/Tablet for specialists) on the assistance of cochlear or cardiac implanted patients. To illustrate the feasibility of our research work, we report several experiments and evaluations attempting to guarantee the safety of operations on adjusting cochlear implants and supporting the monitoring of patients with cardiac implants. This work is carried out as part of an academic and industrial research project.

Keywords: Human Computer Interaction, IT and Healthcare, Mobile and Medical Applications, Medical Data Visualization.

1 Introduction

In the last decade, technological enhancement increasingly motivates medical domain to discover new ways to improve the quality of healthcare. By means of adapted information systems and exploiting new visualization techniques, patients and medical professionals are progressively better supported and assisted [1,2]. Indeed, visualization techniques in this domain extends to a variety of application cases, such a consulting an EHR (Electronic Health Record) [3], providing a diagnosis [4] or monitoring patients with chronic pathologies [5].

However, designing the HCI in the medical domain is not trivial. This is particularly due to the significance of providing essential information to the intended tasks for a given user (i.e. practitioners, specialists, patients...), meeting clarity and ease of use criteria (depending on type of user, for example a disabled patient) [6], guaranteeing safety of operations and ensuring trustable data discovering.

The study that we conduct in this paper refers to the HCI challenges revealed by the future generation of medical implants (cochlear and cardiac) and implying the migration of medical applications to mobile devices. More specifically, we are interested in two main issues: one related to the specificities of patients with cochlear and cardiac implant interacting through a Smartphone (i.e. visualization choice, available functionalities...) and another one concerning the visualization requirements of specialists to easily correlate medical data by using a Tablet. In both cases, the

B. Godara and K.S. Nikita (Eds.): MobiHealth 2012, LNICST 61, pp. 138–145, 2013.

rapidity of execution, safety of operations and the confidence on the applications must be guaranteed. For this paper, our solutions are described in terms of safety of operations and its impact on the HCI design and development.

The rest of the paper is organized as follows. Section 2 describes the specificities and HCI challenges of our study cases: cardiac monitoring and cochlear implant adjustment. Section 3 details our   approach and finally, we conclude in Section 4.

2   Monitoring and Assisting Implanted Patients: Cochlear and Cardiac Visualization Requirements

In the following paragraphs, we describe the specificities of the traditional procedures for cochlear adjustment and cardiac monitoring. Together, we underline their resulting evolution and its consequences on the HCI design and implementation.

2.1   Adjusting Cochlear Implants: Patients and Medical Experts

Cochlear implants are intended for profound deafness or hard-of-hearing people from infants to elderly[1]. An implant is mainly composed of two parts: an inner part and an outer part (prosthesis) (Figure 1a). The inner part is implanted by a surgical procedure and it is composed by several electrodes (currently 24 electrodes) connected directly to the patient's auditory nerve. The prosthesis sits behind the ear and requires a battery and a processor to correctly process sound signals and convert them into electric impulses. These two parts are connected by magnetization and a transceiver system through the skin.

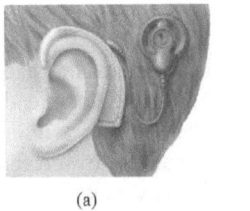 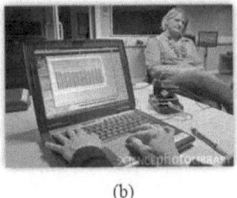

(a)   (b)

Fig. 1. Cochlear implant and implant adjusting

A cochlear implant is adjusted by an audiologist with a fitting software (on PC, Figure 1b). Audiologist sets several parameters like the minimum and maximum band frequency threshold for each electrode. Also, the audiologist (with patients) can create and set programs matching four different listening situations. These programs enable the patient to dynamically adjust the settings of the implant (i.e. transition from silent to noisy environment) and are accessible via few buttons placed on the prosthesis. Actions performed over these buttons, involve an immediate adaptation of the implant.

---

[1] http://www.nidcd.nih.gov/Pages/default.aspx

2.2   Monitoring Patients with Cardiac Implants

The monitoring of patients implanted with Cardiovascular Electronic Implantable Devices (CEIDs) like defibrillators or pacemakers (Figure 2a) implies a continuous monitoring and regulation of the heart activity and by transmitting electrical impulses to stimulate it, only if it is necessary. Such a monitoring can be performed at specialized clinics, by transferring data to the specialist, initiated by the device or by the patient (remote monitoring), or even by the combination of both monitoring modes. Traditionally, portable defibrillators are developed to analyze data from cardiac implants and interact with. Recently, labs monitoring and recording systems (over a PC, Figure 2b) are used to analyze heart activity and other associated parameters (i.e. blood pressure).

The heart activity or cardiac signal analysis is specially based on an Electrocardiogram (ECG). The ECG is a measurement of the electrical activity of the hearth and is traditionally represented or traced over 12-lead, where each lead points to a specific part of the hearth (Figure 2c).

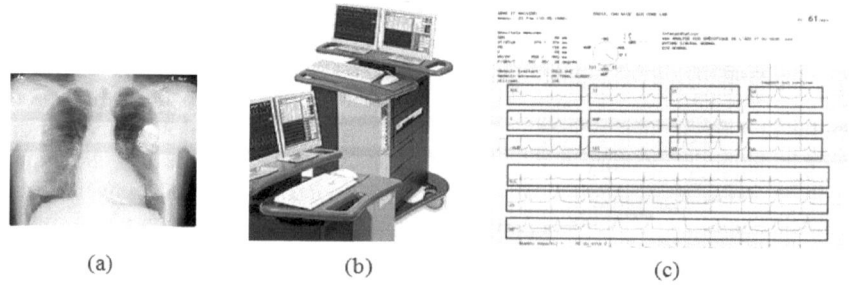

(a)   (b)   (c)

Fig. 2. Cardiac implant and ECG representation

When the specialist analyzes the ECG, he/she examines the size and length of each part of the ECG. Indeed, the size and length variations of each lead may be significant to determine a problem with a specific part of the heart. In a monitoring context, the ECG can be discovered in different ways, for example by performing a random or programmed recording of the heart's electrical activity as well as recording only when a given situation occurs (i.e. arrhythmia, blood pressure variations, etc.).

2.3   Cochlear and Cardiac Implants: New Visualization Challenges

Until now, most of the medical applications are deployed on PCs or on dedicated medical equipment; their interfaces are developed as user-friendly environments, with icons and menus, images or multimedia. More recently, Web 2.0 technologies have offered patients and healthcare professionals with more interactive and attractive graphical interfaces for displaying medical information such as patient's medication control, consultations boards, etc. Further, thanks to mobile devices patient information can be also integrated with medical sensors such as ECG, glucose, temperature, etc [5,7]. Applications for remotely monitor patients with chronic diseases [5] are focus on simple but very specific data (i.e. heart rate) often associated with a timestamp and representing patient's behavior. Besides, applications assisting diagnosis through medical imagining manipulate more complex data which are processed and discovered by features like zoom, scale, color, 3D... [4] and where a migration to mobile devices is not already conceived.

The evolution of cochlear and cardiac implants requires adapted visualization design over new interaction devices such as mobile devices. In both cases, our goal is to provide patients and experts with HCI ensuring the quality required for such applications: in any case we should not compromise patients' safety.

The new generation of cochlear implants deals with issues related to the disappearance of the prosthesis and the migration of the adjusting software (PC) to mobile devices. As a result, patients would be capable to adjust their implant via a Smartphone and the audiologists will switch over Tablets in order to achieve cochlear setting. Besides, the future generation of CEIDs addresses new challenges related to the accessibility, autonomy and performance, aiming to better assist and support patients and specialists. For example: patients will be able to visualize their heart condition and the implant status on their personal Smartphone and specialists will have the possibility to interact with an electronic ECG through a Tablet.

3   Towards Medical Mobile Applications: Patient and Specialists Oriented Visualizations

Switching traditional applications for cochlear and cardiac implants to mobile devices requires adequate visualization solutions while ensuring the safety of operations in terms of patients' safety and quality of healthcare. For the cochlear implant adjustment as well as for the cardiac monitoring, the richness of information to be transmitted to medical specialists can be summarized in *correlated data visualization* for a given task. For example, adjusting a cochlear implant requires a simultaneous visualization and interaction with the implanted electrodes, and for cardiac monitoring, several visualizations of *EVi* values (in real-time or in periods of time) are required to isolate possible malfunctions and provide better diagnostic (Figure 2c).

For both cases, the new visualizations and interactions should be based on the existing correlated data visualizations and which have been proven through the years by the medical domain. Such visualizations ensure implants adjustment and diagnostic without compromise patients' safety and thus, migrating to a mobile device like a Tablet, must preserve such visualizations which specialists are used to interact with. Also, in order to avoid inconsistencies, we have to take into account aspects like device's screen size (17" for a PC to 10" for a Tablet) and the diversity of interactions (mouse for a PC to tactile functions for a Tablet).

Switching to mobile devices opens also new interaction perspectives for patients. Actually, the operations are constrained by the current medical equipment: the prosthesis enabling to adjust listening profiles and the alert button for the cardiac implanted devices. Our survey of users' requirements conducted through patient interviews reveals their concern about to maintain a limited interface on the mobile phone. In fact, they estimate that traditional interfaces may frustrate patients who ask for more interaction functionalities. However, considering the *safety of operations* as a fundamental requirement, it is important to define the interactions and visualizations adaptable to the patient requirements but in agreement with medical procedures. In the rest of this section, we describe several solutions provided to satisfy the application requirements.

3.1   Correlated Data Visualizations for Specialists

In this paragraph, we detail our prototype proposal oriented to medical specialists and targeting Tablets as medical support equipment.

For a specialist, two main factors are essentials: rapidity of execution and the safety of operations. Until now, there are not specific visualization techniques that allow user to improve their rapidity of execution as this strongly depends on the sequence of tasks to be performed. However, inspired on [4] we provide an approach basing the visualization on three main aspects: *support navigability in the main tasks*, *facilitate data reading and changes*, and if necessary *provide access to secondary tasks*(i.e. patient records consulting). In the description of our prototypes, we particularly focus on the data reading and their changes by using views illustrating the visualizations of correlation data adapted to the main tasks to perform.

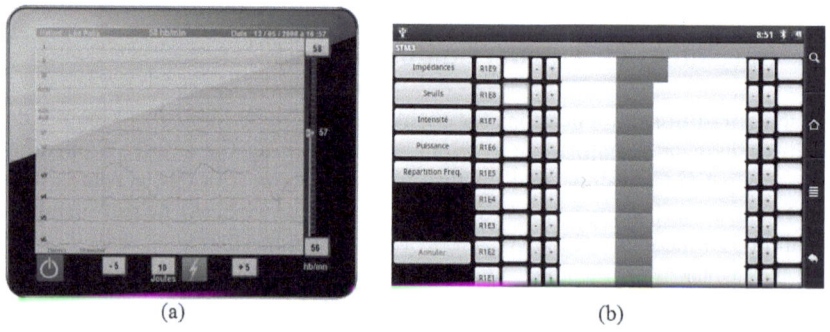

Fig. 3. Prototype for an ECG view and for a Cochlear implant adjustment

These prototypes (Figure 3) have been defined according to the existing PC-based HMI and are intended for audiologists who carry out the cochlear implants adjustment and for cardiologists who examine the condition of a patient with a cardiac implant. They have been tested by domain experts and incorporate the first feedbacks regarding the safety of operations. In both cases, our evaluations were performed with three testers: two experts on (cardiac/cochlear) implants and one specialist (cardiologist/audiologist).

The evaluation was characterized by three phases: (i) Overview of the scenario (i.e. you must adjust the implant of M. Dupont according to the pathologies indications and the type of implant in accordance with several associated medical guidelines), (ii) task achievement (i.e. observing the user in the sequence of performed tasks), and (iii) feedback (questionary about the strengths and weaknesses of the prototype). Due to the lack of space we only detail in this paper the evaluation and results obtained for the cardiac monitoring study case.

Evaluation and Results: The first model (Figure 3a) provides a real-time display of an ECG and tests only the representation of the data correlations by simulation of transmitted data.

During the patient examination or diagnosis, the specialist can traditionnally act on the implant by providing heart-shocks or stopping the implant operation when necessary. Our view is thus complemented by actuators that perform emergency settings. Testers feedback contributed to select the adapted colors and organize the prototype visualization. They prefer a classic ECG at the center with the available operations be performed around it. Together, tests hightlight the necessity to provide cardiologist with secondary tasks like *zoom* or *markers* enabling to focus or isolate segments of the ECG and compare the measures differently to the traditional (cf. Figure 2c).

The difficulties concerning the migration to mobile devices are essentially related to the relevance of the information displayed, especially considering the screen size limitation. Also, the real-time management requires easily browse the graph (if necessary) by moving tactilely. The zoom areas identification requires extensive reliability and confidence testing. This is part of our work in progress.

3.2   Visualizations for Patients: Ensuring Safety of Operations

This paragraph introduces our prototype proposal oriented to implanted patients and targeting Smartphone as medical support equipment (Figure 4).

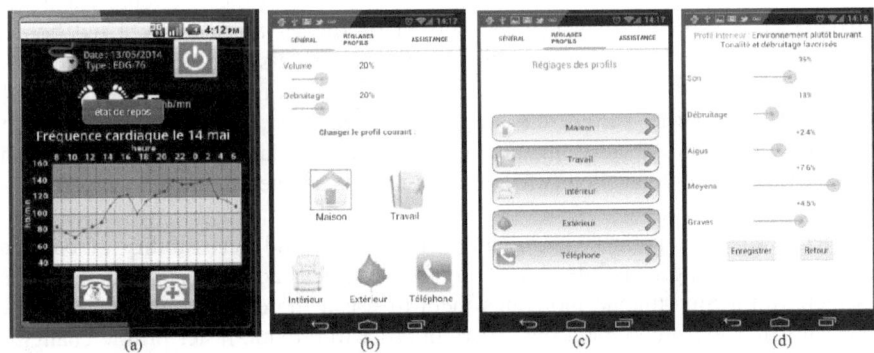

Fig. 4. Prototypes for implanted patients (Cochlear and Cardiac implants)

For patients, two main factors are necessary: simplicity of usage and the safety of operations. Indeed, the specificities of the selected device to interact with their implants arises new usage perspectives which must be approved by the medical specialists in order to guarantee patients' safety. Beyond the well known security issues (e.g. user authentication and data privacy) not covered in this paper, it is necessary to provide an adequate level of functionalities adapted to the pathology in question. Furthermore, studies have also shown that providing adapted tools for patients and their families, we obtain better results both for patients' health condition as for clinical procedures [8].

These prototypes have been defined according to a cross analysis of the user requirements and the medical constraints addressed to a panel of patients and the concerned experts of implants. Such prototypes were tested (according to the same evaluation phases than for specialists, see Section 3.1) over two experts of each domain and by several patients chosen by the experts themselves. They have incorporated the first feedbacks regarding the safety of operations. For example, in order to reassure patient (for both use cases), we provide a feature enabling the patient to call a specialists when a doubt or problem arise. The scope of this paragraph tackles only the description of the cochlear implant prototype (Figure 4b,c,d).

Evaluation and Results. The prototypes proposed in Figure 4b,c,d expand the possibilities of cochlear adjustment for patients. For example, on the current generation of implants, the only way to interact with is by the four buttons placed on the prosthesis. Such specificity is ergonomically compatible with the hardware constraint (implant's size and area accessible by the patient). Also, it is possible to modify or adjust listening profiles during the visits to the specialist.

In particular, switching to a mobile device lifts the limit of the number of embedded listening profiles. Thus, in order to better assist patient in their regular life, it is important to provide the possibility to easily change their current listening profile and/or adjust several parameters (i.e. volume o noise) several times per day.

As a result, our prototype privilege a task menu based on a Dashboard including icons and a sequence of screens adapted to the usage frequency. Considering this design, the patient is allowed to change (anytime, anywhere) his/her current listening profile among those programmed by the specialist. Such profiles are represented with standard icons (Figure 4b) where the current profile is indicated by a red border. Together, a summary of the settable profile parameters and functionalities (i.e. volume, noise, lower, frequencies…) to adjust the implant is also provided (Figure 4c and Figure 4d). These parameters are strictly supervised by specialists during the configuration stage. Actually, medical experts must validate the available functions and ensure safe and controlled percentage thresholds adapted to the patient pathology and needs.

After evaluation, patients highlighted the comfort and accessibility of cochlear adjustment by using a mobile device. In fact, cochlear adjustment becoming more discreet with a Smartphone motivates them to use it more frequently and probably being in better listening conditions. Also, in order to provide faster profile changing, we suggested the use of GPS for Smartphones. For example, automatically switch to "office" or "home" listening profile according to their location. However, practitioners are concerned about the automatic listening profile adaptation; they estimate this function as a dangerous for patient safety and recommend rather provide suggestions such as:*"It seems you are in a noisy place. Consider to activate your outside profile if necessary"*. This new feature will be tested soon.

4   Conclusion

In this paper, we have highlighted the HCI challenges related to the specificities of the future generation of cochlear and cardiac implants being monitored and managed through mobile devices. In this study, we emphasized the importance to guarantee safety of operations in particular for patient's care and safety. For specialists, the migration to mobile devices implies a strictly respect of safety criteria based and especially guided by the current medical software on PC. However, for the patients switching to a new device holds new needs and expectations that involve a thoughtful approach to provide adapted functionalities while respecting safety criteria.

For these first prototypes, we made design choices concerning visualization and task organizations accordingly. Such design has been evaluated and validated by potential users. The current proposal still needs further validation steps before it can be completely accepted.

Our ongoing work address also issues such a compare the impact of new interactions, for example switching from mouse to tactile functions, especially considering specialists requirements (rapidity of execution and reliability on implant data). Also, we plan to perform more scalable tests of our prototypes under limited time and delicate operations. Such tests should enable the estimation of the confidence and safety level of the prototypes.

References

1. AHIMA e-IHM Personal Health Record Work Group: Defining the Personal Health Record. Journal of AHIMA 76(6), 24–25 (2005)
2. Andry, F., Freeman, L., Gillson, J., Kienitz, J., Lee, M., Naval, G., Nicholson, D.: Highly-Interactive and User-Friendly Web Application for People with Diabetes. In: IEEE HEALTHCOM 2008, pp. 118–120 (2008)
3. Andry, F., Naval, G., Nicholson, D., Lee, M., Kosoy, I., Puzankov, L.: Data Visualization in a Personal Health Record using Rich Internet Application Graphic Components. In: Azevedo, L., Londral, A.R. (eds.) 'HEALTHINF', INSTICC 2009, pp. 111–116 (2009)
4. Hû, O., Cavaro-Ménard, C., Cooper, L.: Analyse de la tâche de diagnostic et évaluation d'IHM en imagerie médicale. In: 23rd French Speaking Conference on Human-Computer Interaction (IHM 2011), 4 p. ACM (2011)
5. Kanoun, K., Mamaghanian, H., Khaled, N., Atienza Alonso, D.: A Real-Time Compressed Sensing-Based Personal Electrocardiogram Monitoring System. In: IEEE/ACM 2011 Design, Automation and Test in Europe Conference, DATE 2011 (2011)
6. Cronin, C.: Personal Health Records: An Overview of What Is Available To The Public. Tech. Rept. AARP (2006)
7. Lyles, C.R., Harris, L.T., Le, T., Flowers, J., Tufano, J., Britt, D., Hoath, J., Hirsch, I.B., Goldberg, H.I., Ralston, J.D.: Qualitative evaluation of a mobile phone and web-based collaborative care intervention for patients with type 2 diabetes. Diabetes Technol. Ther. 13(5), 563–569 (2011)
8. Stroetmann, K.A., Pieper, M., Stroetmann, V.N.: Understanding Patients: Participatory Approaches for the User Evaluation of Vital Data Presentation. In: ACM Conference on Universal Usability, pp. 93–97 (2003)

Modelling User Acceptance
of Wireless Medical Technologies

Katrin Arning, Sylvia Kowalewski, and Martina Ziefle

Human Computer Interaction Center (HCIC), RWTH Aachen University
Theaterplatz 14, 52062 Aachen, Germany
{arning,kowalewski,ziefle}@humtec.rwth-aachen.de

Abstract. Wireless medical technologies (WMT) offer an enormous potential to improve healthcare, e.g. by a continuous monitoring of patients' vital health parameters. As user acceptance is a key factor for WMT success, a model of acceptance for WMT-users and non-users was developed and empirically tested by applying structural equation modelling techniques (PLS). Based on a sample of N=305 participants the impact of different system architecture elements (device vs. wireless infrastructure) as well as user factors (knowledge, risk perception, and perceived control) on WMT acceptance was analysed. Perceived benefits and barriers as determining elements of WMT acceptance were quantified and guidelines for WMT system development, training and marketing were derived.

Keywords: technology acceptance, wireless, medical technologies, benefits, barriers, user factors, structure equation modelling, PLS.

1 Introduction

Wireless medical technology (WMT) offers an enormous potential to improve healthcare and to reduce financial pressure on healthcare systems. Medical sensor networks are a typical example of a medical application of mobile communication network technologies. They allow for a continuous monitoring and wireless data transfer of vital health parameters over a long period of time. However, in order to fully exploit the potential of WMT, user acceptance should be considered as a key factor, as it is vital for both, patient's well-being and market success of a technology.

1.1 Acceptance of Medical Technologies

In information system research, the technology acceptance model (TAM [1]) and its successors (e.g. UTAUT [2]) are widely used to explain the acceptance of technical systems. The TAM assumes that the decision to use a technical system is determined by the behavioural intention to use the system, which is in turn influenced by the perceived ease of use and its perceived usefulness. Since the TAM was developed for a specific *technology type* with a less complex *system architecture* (mainly stationary desktop computing) in a specific *application context* (job-related computer usage),

B. Godara and K.S. Nikita (Eds.): MobiHealth 2012, LNICST 61, pp. 146–153, 2013.

covering specific *user groups* (computer-experienced workforce), it is increasingly doubted to be sufficient for a valid prediction of WMT acceptance (e.g. [3]).

Considerable research effort has been made to extend the scope of the TAM. In order to account for novel technology types such as wireless technologies, the Mobile Wireless Technology Acceptance Model (MWTAM) was proposed [4]. However, the MWTAM constructs still focus on a job-related ICT context, whereas the application context of medical technologies activates different acceptance patterns of usage drivers and barriers [5], related to trust, privacy and security issues [6]. Moreover, the characteristics of more heterogeneous user groups of WMT have to be considered. ICT-research identified demographic variables, experience, cognitive abilities, cultural factors, and personality factors as influential factors [7, 8]. Referring to WMT users, who might suffer from multiple physical and psychological restraints, an even stronger impact of individual factors on acceptance is expected. Regarding system architecture complexity, integrated wireless system architectures of WMT comprise a broader scope of technical elements (e.g. cellular networks, WLAN, RFID, GPS, devices). In contrast to well-accepted mobile devices, infrastructure elements of wireless technologies (e.g. base stations) often raise concerns or even fear about negative health effects [9]. This implies, that not only medical devices and interfaces, but also the underlying technical infrastructure should be considered in WMT acceptance research. As a final methodological aspect, the TAM constructs are too generic to provide concrete guidelines for WMT system design. Although the significance of constructs such as "usefulness" in explaining system acceptance was repeatedly proven, specific system characteristics, which actually make a system useful, were often not identified.

The present study therefore pursues a broader approach of investigating WMT acceptance, explicitly focusing on differential effects of WMT system architecture (devices and infrastructure), analysing underlying usage benefits and barriers in the medical application context as well as the impact of individual user factors on WMT acceptance. More specifically, the following research aims were aspired:

1. Quantification of WMT acceptance and investigation of system-architecture-related differences in WMT acceptance
2. Explanation of WMT acceptance by underlying usage benefits and barriers
3. Contrast of WMT acceptance for medical technology users and non-users
4. Analysis of user factors and their impact on WMT acceptance
5. Derivation of guidelines for WMT system development, trainings and marketing campaigns

2   Method

2.1   Questionnaire

The first part of the questionnaire assessed demographic data (age, sex, education, medical technology usage), the following parts assessed the items for our research model. Items for usage benefits and barriers of WMT were developed based on the findings of a focus-group study [5]. In order to familiarize participants with WMT, a detailed introduction into a WMT scenario of a blood pressure monitoring system, which automatically monitors and transfers data to medical care centres via mobile communication networks, was given. Multiple-choice items had to be answered on a six-point Likert scale ranging from 1 (do not agree at all) to 6 (fully agree).

2.2   Sample

The sample consisted of users and non-users of medical technologies (MedTec). According to diffusion of innovation theories [10], the non-user group can be regarded as "pre-adopter" or future user group of WMT in contrast to MedTec users. A total of 8.5% (N=24) participants reported to own and use a medical device (MedTec-users: M = 38.6 years, SD = 13.9, range 20-71 years, 58.3% female; MedTec non-users years: M = 33.9, SD = 11.8, range 17-72, 50.2% female). Since PLS allows to model rather small sample sizes, we contrasted MedTec users and non-users in order to investigate differences in acceptance patterns in both groups.

2.3   Statistical Analysis

ANOVAS and Partial Least Squares (PLS), a component-based structural equation modelling (SEM) technique, was employed. In contrast to covariance-based SEM techniques, PLS has less strict requirements on sample size and residual distribution [11], but allows for statistical modelling with formative and reflective constructs [12].

2.4   Research Model and Hypotheses

The following hypotheses were investigated in our research model:

H1 (User factors)
H1a: Knowledge is positively related to usage benefits, and negatively correlated to device threat and infrastructure threat.
H1b: Perceived control is positively related to usage benefits, and negatively related to usage barriers, device threat, and infrastructure threat.
H1c: Risk perception is positively related to device threat and infrastructure threat.
H2 (System Evaluation)
H2a   Usage benefits are positively related to device acceptance and infrastructure acceptance.
H2b   Usage barriers are positively related to device threat and infrastructure threat.
H2c   Device threat is negatively related to device acceptance.
H2d   Infrastructure threat is negatively related to infrastructure acceptance.
H3 (Acceptance)
H3a   Device acceptance is positively related to infrastructure acceptance.

3   Results

3.1   PLS Model Quality

The analysis of the PLS measurement models demonstrated that all constructs and items had acceptable measurement properties. For the two formative constructs "usage barriers" and "usage benefits" the variance inflation factor varied from 1.01 to 2.3; therefore validity problems due to multicollinearity could be ruled out [11]. All reflective constructs met reliability criteria (Cronbach's alpha > 0.7, Table 1) and discriminant validity criteria (Fornell-Larcker-Criterion, [10]).

3.2   Construct Measurement Results for MedTec-Users and Non-users

Descriptive statistics for measured constructs are presented in Table 1 and 2, along with the results of ANOVA analyses to assess differences between MedTec-users and non-users. Due to the small sample size of the *MedTec-user* sample there were no statistical differences on a 5% significance level, but the following descriptive results provide interesting result tendencies in user ratings.

User factors. MedTec users and *non-users* did not differ with regard to the user factors knowledge, risk perception and perceived control (Table 2).

Table 1. Reflective constructs characteristics and ANOVA results for group differences

Construct	Group	M	SD	Cronbachs' s alpha	p
Knowledge about wireless	MedTec-user	4.04	2.85	-	n.s.
technologies (1 Item)	Non-user	4.11	2.11		
Perceived Control	MedTec-user	3.62	1.36	.95	n.s.
(3 Items)	Non-user	3.54	1.03	.80	
Risk Perception	MedTec-user	2.80	1.38	.86	n.s.
(2 Items)	Non-user	2.47	1.21	.87	
Threat - Device	MedTec-user	2.33	0.67	.75	n.s.
(2 Items)	Non-user	2.69	0.94	.87	
Threat - Infrastructure	MedTec-user	3.36	1.22	.88	n.s.
(2 Items)	Non-user	3.02	1.09	.91	
Acceptance - Device	MedTec-user	4.30	1.40	.95	n.s.
(2 Items)	Non-user	4.09	1.42	.95	
Acceptance- Infrastructure	MedTec-user	4.41	1.20	.99	n.s.
(2 Items)	Non-user	4.45	1.04	.91	

System evaluation. The most important *usage benefit* for both user groups is the aspect of faster medical help in emergencies (Table 2). While *MedTec-users* judge improved safety as second important criterion, n*on-users* perceive higher mobility and flexibility as second most important benefit of using WMT. This benefit is, in contrast, the least important one for *MedTec-users*. Overall, results show that *MedTec-users* favour benefits that concern safety and security aspects regarding their own health status.

Table 2. Formative construct characteristics and ANOVA results by groups

	MedTec-user (N = 24)		Non-user (N=281)		
Usage Benefits	M	SD	M	SD	p
increased awareness of own health status	4.00	1.53	3.69	1.35	n.s.
improved safety due to medical monitoring	4.21	1.47	4.06	1.25	n.s.
faster medical help in emergencies	4.43	1.47	4.48	1.20	n.s.
higher mobility and flexibility	3.78	1.73	4.18	1.19	n.s.
Usage Barriers	M	SD	M	SD	p
surveillance due to medical monitoring	2.87	0.97	3.10	1.23	n.s.
loss of privacy	2.63	1.28	3.10	1.37	n.s.
data abuse	2.88	1.39	3.31	1.41	n.s.
dependency on technology	3.58	1.44	3.52	1.48	n.s.

Regarding WMT *usage barriers* two aspects turn out to be very interesting. Based on a six-point Likert-scale mean values above three can be seen as general compliance. Hence, Table 2 clearly shows that *non-users* in general agree with all barriers, i.e. perceive more usage barriers than *MedTec-users*. Second, the sole significant barrier for *MedTec-users* is "dependency of technology". Nevertheless, high standard deviations on barriers of privacy and data security in the *MedTec-user-group* indicate a great amount of heterogeneity concerning these two barriers.

Referring to the evaluation of infrastructure and device we found an interesting result pattern. *MedTec-users* perceive a lower device threat than *non-users,* whereas perceived infrastructure threat is higher in *MedTec users* than in *non-users.* ANOVAs with the factors "technology level" (device vs. infrastructure) and "MedTec-usage" (user vs. non-user) confirmed this statistical interaction ($F(1,251) = 8.41$, $p < 0.01$).

Acceptance. Regarding acceptance ratings, we found that WMT was perceived positively on the device and on the infrastructure level. *MedTec-users* tend to show a greater acceptance of WMT on the device level than *non-users* do, whereas there is no difference in WMT infrastructure acceptance. Both user groups perceived a higher usefulness of WMT infrastructure than of WMT devices. For acceptance ratings no interaction was found in ANOVAs.

3.3   Structural Model Results for MedTec-Users and Non-users

The PLS analysis yielded path coefficients for the structural models of MedTec users (Fig. 1) and non-users (Fig. 2). Levels of significance were estimated using t-statistics derived from a bootstrapping procedure with 1000 re-samples.

Most of our research hypotheses were supported, at least for *non-users.* Overall, the *MedTec-user* model explained major proportions of device (87%) and infrastructure (77%) acceptance, the non-user model explained 55% of device acceptance and 49% of infrastructure acceptance.

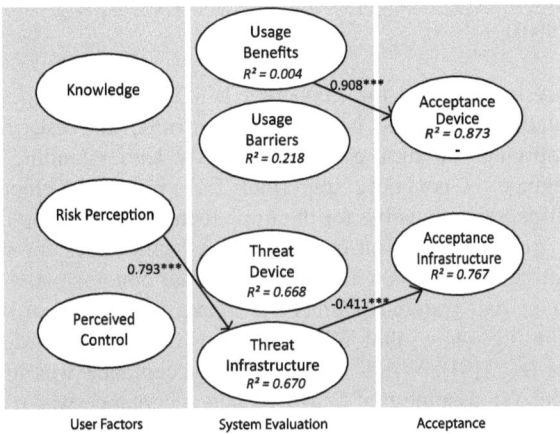

Fig. 1. WMT acceptance model for MedTec-users (*** = p < 0.001)

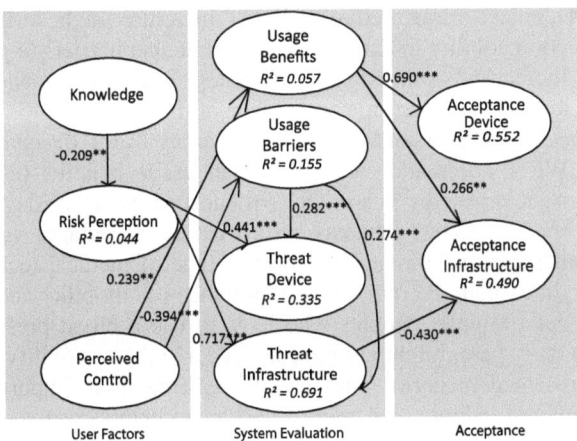

Fig. 2. WMT acceptance model for non-users (** = p < 0.01, *** = p < 0.001)

User factors. Knowledge has a negative effect on risk perception for *non-users*, but no effect on usage benefits or for *MedTec-users* at all (H1a). Risk-perception has a significant positive influence on device threat and infrastructure threat in the *non-user* model and is only positively related to infrastructure threat in the *MedTec-user* model (H1c). Whereas perceived control is only relevant for explaining usage barriers and benefits of *non-users* (H1b).

System Evaluation. Usage benefits are the most important predictor of device acceptance in both groups (H2a). In contrast, usage barriers are only relevant for device threat and for infrastructure threat in the *MedTec-user* model (H2b). However, infrastructure threat is a significant predictor for infrastructure acceptance in both groups (H2d), whereas device threat does not affect device acceptance at all (H2c).

Acceptance. Device acceptance has no impact on infrastructure acceptance in both user groups (H3).

4   Conclusion

The present study investigated the impact of WMT system-architecture (device vs. infrastructure), underlying usage benefits and barriers, and user factors on WMT acceptance by applying structural equation methods. Understanding the determinants of WMT acceptance is not only important for system developers but also for healthcare practitioners responsible for the implementation and employment of WMT. Therefore, apart from a discussion of our findings, guidelines for system designers, training or marketing campaigns will be derived in our conclusion.

WMT acceptance and system-architecture-related differences in WMT acceptance. In general, our findings show, that WMT were positively perceived. Contrary to ICT research findings (e.g. [9]), WMT infrastructure acceptance was higher than WMT device acceptance. We assume that WMT device acceptance was reduced due to the stigmatized image of MedTec device usage. On the other side, WMT infrastructure might be perceived more positively as it gives a general feeling of medical safety. Interestingly, WMT device and infrastructure acceptance were found to be independent from each other, without positive or negative moderating effects. Since the expanding technical infrastructure of WMT in future might influence perceived usefulness (e.g. compatibility to existing devices) but also barriers (e.g. growing sense of control by a increasingly autonomous technology), researchers should not neglect one technology level while analyzing acceptance of the other.

Underlying usage benefits and barriers explaining WMT acceptance. Regarding the sources of WMT acceptance we found, that usage benefits (especially "faster medical help in emergencies") are the strongest drivers of device acceptance, especially for *MedTec users*, whereas infrastructure acceptance is predominantly influenced by infrastructure threat. The specific type of medical technology used in our scenario might explain the rather low importance of "mobility and flexibility" for MedTec-users. For example, patients who have to use a blood pressure or diabetes monitoring on a daily base, might not have noticed a higher flexibility potential due to WMT in the presented scenario. This aspect might be more important for patients who are e.g. confined indoors or bound to healthcare centres at fixed points in time. Interestingly, usage barriers play a minor role in WMT acceptance; they only have an indirect effect on perceived threat in *non-users*. MedTec usage experience leads to a further decrease of perceived barriers. Even though usage barriers act only indirectly in *non-users* on acceptance, they should nevertheless be considered: Enhancing WMT acceptance could be accomplished for example by focusing on problems of "technical reliability" or "data safety" in system design or addressing the aspects of "increased safety due to WMT" or "dependency of technology" in marketing.

Impact of MedTec usage experience and user factors on WMT acceptance. Our findings emphasize the need to differentiate between *MedTec-users* and *non-users*, especially in the context of healthcare. Apparently, MedTec usage experience not only affects the perception of benefits and barriers, but also mitigates the effect of individual user factors such as knowledge, risk perception or perceived control. However, as the (young) *non-users* of today can be regarded as potential future WMT users, the impact of individual user factors on acceptance patterns is highly important for the commercial launch of WMT as well as for compliance-related issues. Knowledge was found to directly affect risk perception in *non-users*, which considerably influences perceived threats of WMT device and infrastructure. In order to enhance WMT acceptance in *non-users* by trainings or marketing activities it is therefore necessary to a) impart knowledge about wireless technology and b) to specifically address risk perceptions and health fears associated with this technology.

Limitations and future research. Future studies will have to examine larger samples with a higher proportion of actual MedTec-users in order to validate our findings. In order to investigate the causes of the "reversed" WMT acceptance pattern (higher infrastructure than device acceptance), we will contrast wireless technology acceptance in different application contexts (ICT vs. MedTec usage context). Finally, the specific impact and the relationship of device and infrastructure acceptance on actual WMT acceptance and compliance should be studied in more detail.

Acknowledgments. Thanks to Barbara Zaunbrecher for research support.

References

1. Davis, F.D.: Perceived usefulness, perceived ease of use, and user acceptance of information technology. MIS Quarterly 13(3), 319–340 (1989)
2. Venkatesh, V., Morris, M.G., Davis, G.B., Davis, F.D.: User acceptance of information technology: Toward a unified view. MIS Quarterly 27(3), 425–478 (2003)
3. Holden, R.J., Karsh, B.T.: The technology acceptance model: Its past and its future in health care. Journal of Biomedical Informatics 43, 159–172 (2010)
4. Kim, S., Garrison, G.: Investigating mobile wireless technology adoption: An extension of the technology acceptance model. Information Systems Frontiers 11(3), 323–333 (2009)
5. Arning, K., Gaul, S., Ziefle, M.: Same same but different. How service contexts of mobile technologies shape usage motives and barriers. In: Leitner, G., Hitz, M., Holzinger, A. (eds.) USAB 2010. LNCS, vol. 6389, pp. 34–54. Springer, Heidelberg (2010)
6. Wilkowska, W., Ziefle, M.: Perception of privacy and security for acceptance of E-health technologies: Exploratory analysis for diverse user groups. In: User-Centred-Design of Pervasive Health Applications (UCD-PH 2011), held in Conjunction with the 5th ICST/IEEE Conference on Pervasive Computing Technologies for Healthcare, pp. 593–600 (2011)
7. Czaja, S.J., Sharit, J.: Age Differences in Attitudes Toward Computers. Journal of Gerontology 5, 329–340 (1998)
8. Arning, K., Ziefle, M.: Understanding age differences in PDA acceptance and performance. Computers in Human Behavior 23, 2904–2927 (2007)
9. Siegrist, M., Earle, T.C., Gutscher, H., Keller, C.: Perception of Mobile Phone and Base Station Risks. Risk Analysis 25, 1253–1264 (2005)
10. Rogers, E.: Diffusion of innovations. Free Press, New York (1995)
11. Weiber, R., Mühlhaus, D.: Strukturgleichungsmodellierung: Eine anwendungsorientierte Einführung in die Kausalanalyse mit Hilfe von AMOS, SmartPLS und SPSS. 1 Auflage. Springer, Heidelberg (2009)
12. Petter, S., Straub, D., Rai, A.: Specifying formative constructs in information systems research. MIS Quarterly 31(4), 623–656 (2007)

Persuasive Design in Mobile Applications for Mental Well-Being: Multidisciplinary Expert Review

Ting-Ray Chang, Eija Kaasinen, and Kirsikka Kaipainen

VTT Technical Research Centre of Finland
{firstname.lastname}@vtt.fi

Abstract. Smartphones are a promising channel for health promotion interventions. Mobile applications can track behaviour and provide real-time guidance and support. Research on mobile interventions has mainly focused on physical health and disease management, whereas promotion of mental well-being has received less attention. This paper presents results of a multidisciplinary expert review of twelve currently available mobile applications for mental well-being. The aim of the study was to identify what kinds of engaging and persuasive features are used in the applications and to assess how well the features were implemented. The expert reviews were carried out from user acceptance, mobile intervention design, and persuasive design points of view. Current applications were assessed moderately good from all three perspectives but improvement needs were identified in more versatile utilisation of mobile technology, leveraging social support, and providing a wider range of personalized intervention features.

Keywords: Mobile Applications, Mental Well-being, Persuasive Design, Expert Reviews, TAMM, Technology Acceptance Model.

1 Introduction

Wide-reaching interventions that support and encourage healthy habits are essential to prevent diseases and improve life quality among general population. Mobile devices are considered especially promising tools for pervasive and unobtrusive well-being management, because mobile phones are usually personal and people carry them most of the time [1]. Thus, they are often present in daily situations when people make health related decisions, providing opportunities for timely interventions to support behaviour change [2]. Furthermore, the technical capabilities of smartphones enable not only collecting user data but also its real-time analysis and interpretation to support situational decision making [3].

Promotion of mental well-being is crucially important because subjective well-being influences overall health and longevity [4]. Mood problems and low self-efficacy can be significant barriers for behavioural changes. Many mobile applications have been developed for physical health monitoring and lifestyle interventions [5], such as weight management [6] and exercise [7, 8]. Recently, more research has started to emerge on applications that also address mental health and

B. Godara and K.S. Nikita (Eds.): MobiHealth 2012, LNICST 61, pp. 154–162, 2013.
© Institute for Computer Sciences, Social Informatics and Telecommunications Engineering 2013

well-being [5, 9]. Recently an abundance of mobile applications for mood monitoring or general well-being have become available. In order to develop or identify engaging and effective mobile interventions, it can be beneficial to learn from relevant existing mobile applications [10].

The purpose of this study was to identify engaging and persuasive features in a sample of existing mobile applications that target mental well-being. We screened relevant twelve applications out of the hundreds of available applications for an in-depth analysis. The selection process is described in section 2. Section 3 describes the expert review methodology to evaluate the applications from three different perspectives: user acceptance, mobile intervention design, and persuasive design. The results are presented in section 4. Finally in section 5 we analyse and conclude the results.

2   Application Selection Process

Search for relevant mobile applications in the stores of two main platforms, Android and iOS, was carried out during May-July 2011 by browsing through the following categories (Android Market): health & fitness, medical, lifestyle, social, productivity, education, entertainment, communication, and (iPhone App Store): the top 50 applications in all categories, as well as top 300 free and top 150 paid applications in health and fitness; and by entering keywords (Android market): mood, social, mental, behavio(u)r, and (App Store): mood, stress, happiness, training, monitor(ing), smoke, behavio(u)r, mental and awareness. 85 applications from App Store and 26 from Android market were selected based on their relevance and having an average rating of at least 3 in the scale 0-5 in the application store.

Applications were placed on a map with two axes: social-individual usage, and mental-physical focus. The aim was to identify applications that had a holistic approach to well-being. Finally, two researchers reviewed the map of applications and tagged promising applications based on the following criteria:

1. Including any kinds of social functions;
2. Connected to web services;
3. Purpose to track or improve mood;
4. Interactivity (user input and/or data interpretation);
5. Focus on mental well-being and lifestyle, not sports or specific diseases.

The final selection consisted of twelve applications (Table 1), nine from App Store and three from Android Market.

Table 1. Selected twelve mobile applications

	Application name	Description
iPhone	miMood (miM)	Mood tracking over time. Option to email mood history.
	Mood Runner (MoR)	For female users. Tracking emotional patterns with diet, exercise, sleep, stress, energy, sex drive and menstrual cycles.
	LiveHappy (LiH)	Surveys, therapeutic guides for happiness and mood, option to connect to Twitter and Facebook. Based on positive psychology.

Table 1. (*continued*)

	Healthy Habits (HeH)	Self-tracking new/old habits, reminders, high customizability.
	SeemyCity (SmC)	Recommends ways to explore a city based on user mood type.
	Anger Coach (AnC)	Survey input, therapeutic guide for anger management.
	Moodkit (Mok)	Survey input of social, sport, productivity, enjoyment & diet. Committing to actions. Based on Cognitive Behaviour Therapy.
	Awareness Lite (AwL)	Mood lifting by rehearsing mindfulness and reading aphorisms.
	My Balance (MyB)	Self-monitoring life balance with nutrition, fitness and lifestyle.
Android	Mood Meter (MoM)	Collects data automatically, presents mood scores and motivational messages based on time and social interaction.
	My CalmBeat (MCB)	Stress reduction through a guided breathing exercise.
	T2 Mood Tracker(T2M)	Self-monitoring anxiety, depression, general well-being, head injury, post-traumatic stress, or stress based on daily events.

3   Expert Review Methods

After the twelve applications were selected, we studied them further from three viewpoints: user acceptance, mobile intervention design, and persuasive design. Because multidisciplinary guidelines or heuristics that would cover all the three viewpoints do not exist, we decided to carry our three separate expert reviews with three different experts. The method was based on usage simulation as proposed by [11]. In usage simulation the reviewers who have wide experience of different applications aim to see the applications from an ordinary user's viewpoint. Each of our three experts had 5-15 years of research experience on their field (user acceptance of mobile services, mobile intervention design, and persuasive design).

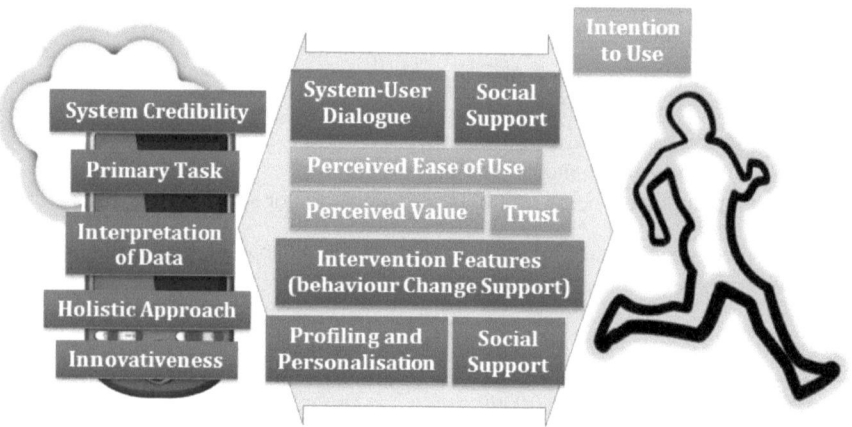

Fig. 1. A diagram combine three relevant theoretical models of user acceptance (green), mobile intervention (purple), and persuasive design (red)

With this expert group we studied whether the applications fulfilled basic user acceptance criteria for mobile services, whether the applications included features for effective attitude or behaviour change and whether the applications included persuasive features (Figure 1). Each expert defined individually their review criteria and carried out the review individually. The aim of the reviews was to assess the applications from user point of view and to identify applications that would be suitable for further evaluations with real-world users. Another aim of the reviews and the earlier selection process was to identify the strengths and shortcomings of current persuasive mental well-being applications. The reviewers are also co-authors of this paper. The review criteria and the expert review methods are described in the following sub sections.

3.1   User Acceptance of Mobile Services

Expert review on user acceptance was based on the Technology Acceptance Model for Mobile Services [12]. The model covers perceived value, ease of use, trust and ease of adoption. The model is intended for user evaluations but in here it was used as a framework to analyse the applications from potential users' points of view based on the evaluator's expertise on other mobile services. The model was interpreted as described in Table 2.

Table 2. User acceptance expert review criteria

Criterion	Description
Ease of use	How effortless it is to use the application? Are functions easy to identify, find and use? Is information provided to the user easy to understand?
Ease of start-to-use	How easy it is to get an overview of the functionality as a first time user? Any specific tricks to do before you can use application?
Value to user	What is the targeted value of the application to the user? Is the proposed value credible?
Trust	Does the information and feedback provided to the user seem reliable? Are there threats related to privacy or safety?
Overall	Overall grade, focusing especially on the persuasive features of the application and the suitability of the application to user evaluation.

3.2   Mobile Intervention Design

The criteria were formed based on various existing guidelines about mobile and technology-based intervention design for health behaviour change [13]. User engagement and effectiveness of mobile interventions can be optimized by using evidence-based intervention methods, profiling and personalization, data interpretation, holistic approach to well-being rather than a narrow focus, and overall expected novelty for the user. The review criteria from mobile intervention design perspective and the theoretical background are presented in Table 3.

Table 3. Mobile intervention expert review criteria

Criterion	Description
Profiling and personalization	Does application collect information to profile the user and tailor output based on user needs and characteristics? [14]
Interpretation of data	Does application interpret the data it collects? Is data abstraction rather than raw data used to display information? [15]
Intervention & behaviour change support	Are there features which actively support behaviour and/or attitude change with the aim of improving well-being of the user?
Holistic approach	Are all sides of well-being covered (mental, physical, social)? [16].
Social support	How much application leverages social support to improve psychosocial well-being [17] and/or increase user engagement? [18]
Novelty	How novel, innovative and interesting the application feels?

3.3   Persuasive Design in Mobile Applications

The criteria were built mainly based on Persuasive System Design model [19] but modified specifically for this review (Table 4). Twenty-nine principles of persuasive design were used as heuristics. The principles were in four categories: primary task support, system credibility, dialogue support, and social support [19]. In addition, goal setting was used as an additional principle [20]. Persuasiveness was defined as the set of attributes that bear on the ability of software to support change in its users' attitudes and/or behaviour. The applications were assessed based on the number of occurrences of the persuasive design principles. A similar but more detailed persuasive design evaluation of the applications is described by Langrial et al [21].

Table 4. Persuasive application design expert review criteria

Primary task	System credibility	Dialogue support	Social support
Reduction	Trustworthiness	Praise	Social facilitation
Tunnelling	Expertise	Rewards	Social comparison
Tailoring	Surface- credibility	Reminders	Normative influence
Personalisation	Real-world feel	Suggestion	Social learning
Self-monitoring	Authority	Similarity	Cooperation
Simulation	Third-party endorsements	Liking	Competition
Rehearsal	Verifiability	Social role	Recognition
Goal-setting			

4   Results of the Expert Reviews

The grades of **user acceptance** review are presented in Table 5. The ease of use of all the applications was at least moderate and crucial usability problems were not identified. Problems in starting to use were identified in two applications and the value to the user was doubtful with two applications. The overall grade was lower than 3 only with 2 applications, so from user acceptance point of view the selection was quite successful. Quite a few applications were basically life style books transferred to mobile applications, thus they did not utilize the measurement and monitoring possibilities of mobile technology.

Table 5. Ratings from user acceptance expert review (1-5)

App	miM	MoR	LiH	HeH	SmC	AnC	Mok	AwL	MyB	MoM	MCB	T2M
Ease of use	4	3	4	3	3	3	3	4	4	4	5	3
Ease of start-to-use	4	3	4	2	2	4	3	4	4	3	4	3
Value	3	4	3	4	2	3	4	3	3	2	3	5
Trustworthy	3	3	3	4	3	4	4	3	3	2	3	4
Overall	**3**	**3**	**4**	**4**	**2**	**3**	**3**	**3**	**3**	**2**	**4**	**4**

The grades of **mobile intervention design** review are presented in Table 6. Live Happy, Moodkit and Healthy Habits incorporated the widest variety of tools and exercises to encourage users to make actual changes in their lives, such as guided exercises or committing to actions. They addressed several life domains and provided explanations for the recommended actions, attempting also to profile users and personalize their output. Also MoodRunner, MyBalance and T2 Mood Tracker allowed tracking of several factors. However, they did not apply intervention techniques beyond reminders and graphical comparisons. The rest of the applications were either fairly simple mood trackers, or otherwise focused on one specific thing such as dealing with anger (Anger Coach) or practising breathing (MyCalmBeat).

The results of the **persuasiveness** review are presented in table 7. From the four categories of the PSD model, the principles in primary task support were the most popular ones whereas the principles in social support category were used the least. Generally, the applications did not use persuasive design principles very widely.

Table 6. Ratings from mobile intervention expert review (1-5)

App	miM	MoR	LiH	HeH	SmC	AnC	Mok	AwL	MyB	MoM	MCB	T2M
Profiling	2	2	4	3	2	2	3	1	1	2	2	2
Interpretation	2	3	3	2	2	2	3	2	2	2	2	3
Intervention	1	2	4	3	1	3	4	2	1	2	2	2
Holistic	2	4	4	4	1	2	4	1	3	1	1	3
Soc-support	2	1	3	2	1	2	2	1	1	2	1	1
Novelty	2	3	4	3	1	2	3	3	2	3	3	2
Overall	**2**	**2**	**4**	**3**	**1**	**2**	**4**	**2**	**2**	**2**	**2**	**2**

Table 7. Occurences of persuasive principles (maximum scores given in brackets)

App	miM	MoR	LiH	HeH	SmC	AnC	Mok	AwL	MyB	MoM	MCB	T2M
Primary task (8)	1	2	5	3	2	2	5	3	1	1	3	1
Credibility (7)	0	1	2	2	1	1	1	1	0	2	0	1
Dialogue (7)	0	0	5	0	0	4	5	2	0	0	0	0
Social support (7)	1	0	1	0	0	0	1	0	0	0	0	0
Total (29)	**2**	**3**	**13**	**5**	**3**	**7**	**12**	**6**	**1**	**3**	**3**	**2**

5   Conclusions

From user acceptance point of view, all the selected applications were at least moderately good. However, many applications were basically life style guide books transformed to mobile applications, and were not utilizing the monitoring capabilities of the mobile devices.

Our selection included both applications focused on a specific issue such as breathing correctly and applications with a more versatile focus. Applications with a sharp focus and simple functions can perform well in providing short-term support for immediate needs and improving self-awareness in small steps. Mood trackers may be sufficient for people who are just curious but for more permanent use, the applications need to include support for behaviour change. In general, the reviewed applications were not using persuasive design principles very widely. The two applications this utilised more than ten persuasive design principles (LiveHappy and Moodkit), were also identified as the most versatile applications in the intervention evaluation. However, it has to be kept in mind that the occurrence of the principles alone does not guarantee the success of the application, the persuasive features also need to be well implemented and the application as a whole needs to be acceptable.

Especially social support features were generally scarce in applications. Live Happy allowed users to send questions to the psychologist who had helped in the design, and Anger Coach offered access to online community resources. Mood-related data may be too sensitive to share in public, but emotional support from peers can have a great impact on well-being and motivation to make lifestyle changes [22].

We identified three major areas of improvement in the applications: 1) Utilising mobile technology more for measures and interactivity. Many of the applications were based on textual input and passive reading by the user instead of actual sensor measures and multimodal interactions. 2) Social support mechanisms that allow users connect and share with a selected group of friends or peers with similar goals. 3) Wider range of intervention features to promote actual behaviour change, tailored to the user. Most of the applications merely collected data without interpretation and suggestions, or provided static information without personalized approach.

When assessing the results of this study it has to be kept in mind that expert reviews do not replace user studies. Long term user studies will be needed e.g. to study how well the applications manage in changing user behaviour. Our future plans include gathering users' insights about their actual preferences and usage behaviour with the applications.

Acknowledgments. The study was supported by SalWe Research Program for Mind and Body (Tekes - the Finnish Funding Agency for Technology and Innovation grant 1104/10). The work of Ting-Ray Chang has been supported by VTT graduate school from 2010 to 2014. Special thanks to Marja Harjumaa for her contribution to persuasive design knowledge and expertise.

References

1. Atienza, A.A., Patrick, K.: Mobile Health: The Killer App for Cyber infrastructure and Consumer Health. American Journal of Preventive Medicine 40(5S2), S151–S153 (2011)
2. Fogg, B.J.: Persuasive Technology. Using Computers to Change What We Think and Do, p. 318. Morgan Kaufmann, San Francisco (2003)
3. Patrick, K., Griswold, W.G., Raab, F., Intille, S.S.: Health and the Mobile Phone. American Journal of Preventive Medicine 35(2), 177–181 (2008)
4. Diener, E., Chan, M.Y.: Happy people live longer: Subjective well-being contributes to health and longevity. Applied Psychology: Health and Well-Being 3(1), 1–43 (2011)
5. Harrison, V., Proudfoot, J., Wee, P.P., Parker, G., Pavlovic, D.H., Manicavasagar, V.: Mobile mental health: Review of the emerging field and proof of concept study. J. Ment. Health 20(6), 509–524 (2011)
6. Mattila, E., Lappalainen, R., Pärkkä, J., Salminen, J., Korhonen, I.: Use of a Mobile Phone Diary for Observing Weight Management and Related Behaviours. Journal of Telemedicine and Telecare 16, 260–264 (2010)
7. Consolvo, S.E., Everitt, K., Smith, I., Landay, J.A.: Design Requirements for Technologies that Encourage Physical Activity. In: Proceedings of the SIGCHI Conference on Human Factors in Computing Systems, vol. 1, pp. 457–466. ACM, Montreal (2006)
8. Toscos, T., Faber, A., An, S., Gandhi, M.P.: Chick Clique: Persuasive Technology to Motivate Teenage Girls to Exercise. In: CHI 2006 Extended Abstracts on Human Factors in Computing Systems, pp. 1873–1878. ACM (2006)
9. Morris, M.E., Kathawala, Q., Leen, T.K., Gorenstein, E.E., Guilak, F., Labhard, M., Deleeuw, W.: Mobile Therapy: Case Study Evaluations of a Cell Phone Application for Emotional Self-awareness. Journal of Medical Internet Research 12(2), e10 (2010)
10. Fogg, B.J.: Creating Persuasive Technologies: An Eight-Step Design Process. In: Proceedings of Persuasive 2009, Claremont, California, USA, April 26-29 (2009)
11. Preece, J., Rogers, Y., Sharp, H., Benyon, D., Holland, S., Carey, T.: Human-Computer Interaction. Addison Wesley (1994)
12. Kaasinen, E.: User Acceptance of Mobile Services. International Journal of Mobile Human Computer Interaction 1(1), 79–97 (2009)
13. Honka, A., Kaipainen, K., Hietala, H., Saranummi, N.: Rethinking Health: ICT-Enabled Services to Empower People to Manage Their Health. IEEE Reviews in Biomedical Engineering 4 (2011)
14. Noar, S.M., Harrington, N.G., Van Stee, S.K., Aldrich, R.S.: Tailored health communication to change lifestyle behaviors. Am. J. Lifestyle Med. 5, 112–122 (2011)
15. Consolvo, S., McDonald, D.W., Landay, J.A.: Theory-driven design strategies for technologies that support behavior change in everyday life. In: CHI 2009 Proceedings, pp. 405–414 (2009)
16. WHO. Constitution of the World Health Organization, Basic Documents, 45th edn., Supplement (October 2006)
17. Hogan, B.E., Linden, W., Najarian, B.: Social support interventions: do they work? Clinical Psych. Rev. 22, 381–440 (2002)
18. Schubart, J.R., Stuckey, H.L., Ganeshamoorthy, A., Sciamanna, C.N.: Chronic health conditions and Internet behavioral interventions: a review of factors to enhance user engagement. CIN 29(2), 81–92 (2011)
19. Oinas-Kukkonen, H., Harjumaa, M.: Persuasive Systems Design: Key Issues, Process Model, and System Features. Communications of the Association for Information Systems 24, Article 28, 485–500 (2009)

20. Nawyn, J., Intille, S.S., Larson, K.: Embedding behavior modification strategies into a consumer electronic device: A case study. In: Dourish, P., Friday, A. (eds.) UbiComp 2006. LNCS, vol. 4206, pp. 297–314. Springer, Heidelberg (2006)
21. Langrial, S., Lehto, T., Oinas-Kukkonen, H., Harjumaa, M., Karppinen, P.: Native mobile applications for personal well-being: a persuasive systems design evaluation. In: The 16th Pacific Asia Conference on Information Systems, PACIS 2012 (2012)
22. Munson, S.: Beyond the share button: Making social network sites for health and wellness. IEEE Potentials, 42–47 (September/October 2011)

Securing Legacy Mobile Medical Devices*

Vahab Pournaghshband, Majid Sarrafzadeh, and Peter Reiher

Computer Science Department
University of California, Los Angeles
{vahab,majid,reiher}@cs.ucla.edu

Abstract. Millions of people use mobile medical devices—more every day. But our understanding of device security and privacy for such devices is incomplete. Man-in-the-middle attacks can be performed on typical Bluetooth-enabled mobile medical devices, compromising the privacy and safety of patients. In response, we developed the *Personal Security Device*, a portable device to improve security for mobile medical systems. This device requires no changes to either the medical device or its monitoring software, and offers protection for millions of existing devices. We evaluate our defense mechanism to show that it adds insignificant overhead and analyze its robustness against various attacks.

Keywords: medical device security, man-in-the-middle attack.

1   Introduction

Studies show that by 2015, over 500 million people will be using mobile health applications [1]. There were approximately 245,000 insulin pump users in 2005, and the market for insulin pumps is expected to grow at a rate of 9% from 2009 to 2016 [3]. Hanna et al. reports that in the U.S. alone there are 25 million people with wireless implantable medical devices (IMD), and about 300,000 of these IMDs are implanted every year [10].

In 2003, the U.S. Food and Drug Administration (FDA) approved a Bluetooth-enabled medical device for the first time [14]. Since then, dozens of such devices have been introduced to the U.S. market for uses ranging from life-sustaining to life-supporting.

While the need for secure mobile medical systems is widely recognized [9,4,11,13], many manufacturers have not addressed the security risks of such devices, and thus have provided little security for either the devices themselves, or for the data they create and transmit.

Communications security is one critical aspect of protecting these devices. Mobile medical devices typically communicate to an intermediate computer that forwards its signals to a healthcare facility. Since such devices are typically used with little or no configuration by a user or healthcare provider, there is ample opportunity for attackers to mislead the device into communicating with a hacker's machine instead of its intended intermediary. The communication between the

---

* This work is supported by NSF grant CNS-1116371.

device and its intermediary (real or malicious) typically is wireless, making it more susceptible to eavesdropping and injections.

The consequences of attacks can be extreme, potentially allowing attackers to cause the devices to operate in a life-threatening manner. As an example, consider a heart rate monitor carried by a patient that communicates via Bluetooth to the patient's home computer, which in turn, forwards heart rate data to the patient's doctor in real time. If an attacker can alter the data to fake a heart attack, the doctor may institute unnecessary emergency measures. Even worse, if the attacker conceals the actual signs of an impending heart attack, the doctor will be unaware of the need for immediate action.

In this paper we demonstrate a successful man-in-the-middle (MITM) attack and its consequences on a commercially deployed pulse oximeter system; we then propose a defense approach against this and similar attacks. After discussing potential security and privacy failures that can result from an MITM attack, we demonstrate such an attack, showing that the device discloses sensitive information unencrypted. This attack shows that these Bluetooth-enabled mobile medical devices can be made to communicate with an unauthenticated intermediary. This attack can be performed by an unauthorized party equipped with a Bluetooth-enabled laptop.

Our study examines the Nonin Onyx II 9550 fingertip pulse oximeter, a typical Bluetooth mobile medical device introduced to the U.S. market in 2008. It measures pulse rate and blood oxygen saturation levels continuously or on demand, and communicates with an access point (AP) to pass this data at a range of several meters. With only the user's manual and some publicly available information, we were able to launch a successful MITM attack. Although our experiment used the pulse oximeter, the attacks presented can be performed on other devices, such as the A&D Medical UA-767PBT blood pressure monitor, with little modification.

Our approach to reducing this risk does not require rebuilding or altering legacy devices. We propose a personal area network security device designed to interoperate with mobile medical devices. This security device recognizes the security properties and risks associated with a particular patient's existing devices, and takes measures to lower those risks. Our defense solution works with existing devices and requires no modification to either the device or the monitoring software installed on the AP; it also offloads security from the medical device, reserving the medical device's resources for only medical functions. Our proposed defense mechanism is designed for generality and wide applicability for this class of medical devices.

The organization of this paper is as follows: Section 2 presents related work, followed by an overview of Bluetooth-enabled medical devices in Section 3. Our attack assumptions and threat model, active MITM attacks, defending against these attacks, and evaluation are in Sections 4, 5, 6, and 7 respectively. Future work is presented in Section 8, and Section 9 concludes this paper.

2   Related Work

The security of mobile medical devices is a generally recognized problem that has received special attention in recent years [9,4,11,13]. As a result, there has been some work on demonstrating attacks against various mobile medical devices [8,12]. As complementary research, some work focused on implementing or recommending defensive approaches against these kinds of attacks [7,18,15,8,12]. Among the proposed defense approaches, IMDGuard [18], Amulet [17], and Shield [7] are three defense mechanisms against attacks on mobile medical devices that require a special-purpose third-party device to facilitate security. Also, Denning et al. [6] propose a class of devices called communication cloakers that would share secret keys with an IMD and act as a third-party mediator in the IMD's communications with external programmers.

IMDGuard proposes changes in the design of future IMDs for a more secure system and does not work with legacy devices. Also, Amulet, by definition, does not work with existing devices since it requires changes to the existing mHealth system including the medical device. For example, it requires the medical sensor to verify that it is indeed the right Amulet before connecting. Shield, however, is the only solution that is designed to work with existing and even already implanted IMDs by requiring no changes to the device. Shield protects an IMD by jamming its IMD messages, preventing others from decoding them, while the authorized intermediary is able to decode them. It also jams unauthorized commands to protect the patient. However, the idea behind Shield may not be applicable to many mobile medical devices that operate on widely used radio technologies such as Bluetooth or 802.11; this is due to both the nature of the radio technology and the potential legal issues of jamming their signals.

3   Bluetooth-Enabled Mobile Medical Devices Overview

In our work emphasis is placed on a class of Bluetooth-enabled mobile medical devices that communicate with an AP. An AP is a cellphone, a home PC or a hospital monitoring system. This is a broad class of medical devices with common characteristics. In a common Bluetooth authentication mechanism, a predefined PIN is required for pairing the two parties. These devices are usually configurable by the AP. Depending on the device, the AP can set a wide range of parameters on the device, from changing date and time, frequency rate and data format, to setting specific therapy management. Moreover, these devices may store the patient's identity information. Normally, some proprietary software is installed on the AP that organizes and visualizes the data, and may report it to the patient and doctor for therapy management.

4   Attack Assumptions and Threat Model

4.1   Attack Assumptions

We first assume that the PIN used in standard Bluetooth pairing is known to the attacker. This is not an ambitious assumption since it is known that the PIN can be deduced by carefully observing the Bluetooth pairing process [16]. However, alternatively for some devices, there are even easier ways to figure out the PIN than exploiting the existing vulnerability in the Bluetooth pairing process. For instance, the pulse oximeter's static PIN is included in its advertised service name, hence, making it publicly available ("Nonin_Inc_XXXXXX" where the X's indicate its six-digit PIN). In some other devices, such as the the blood pressure monitor, a common default PIN is used for all shipped units and is available in a publicly disclosed specification. Secondly, we assume that the attacker is in the proper range to launch the attack (up to 10 m in this case), meaning that it can communicate with both the AP and the device via Bluetooth. Finally, we assume that the attacker knows the type and model of the device the patient is using.

4.2   Threat Model

In this section we enumerate the possible attacks on mobile medical devices that can be leveraged from MITM attacks.

1. Confidentiality: An MITM eavesdropper listens to the communication between the device and the AP. An attacker can also retrieve private identity information by sending bogus requests to the device on behalf of the AP.

2. Integrity: MITM attackers can modify data packets sent by the device to the AP, thus misleading the AP with false data. They can also perform replay attacks and generate fake data or commands.

3. Availability: Attackers can interrupt the communication by simply refusing to pass the data through. More cleverly, the attacker can send unauthorized configuration commands to the device to either keep the device in a state of elevated energy consumption (e.g., by setting it to a higher data transmission rate) or disrupt the connection establishment process (e g , by changing the PIN).

5   Active Man-in-the-Middle Attacks on Wireless Links

In this section we discuss the technical details of how to perform MITM attacks on Bluetooth-enabled mobile medical devices. We first need to successfully position the man-in-the-middle, and here, we discuss the steps to do it: (1) Jamming Bluetooth: the first step is to force the existing connection to be dropped, making both the device and the AP discoverable and available to pair up. (2) Pairing with the device: the attacker's machine pairs itself with the device, providing the correct PIN. (3) Pairing with the AP: to deceive the AP into pairing with the attacker's machine, that machine needs to masquerade exactly as the device. Hence, the attacker's machine should advertise the identical service name and available services, as well as using the same PIN as the one used in the device and spoofing the device's MAC address.

Once MITM is in place, then the attacker can perform the attacks described listed in Section 4.2, given that the protocol used in the device is understood.

Since the entire protocol for the pulse oximeter is not publicly available, before performing the attacks we had to deduce the necessary information about it by using reverse-engineering, as described below.

1. Transmission from the Device: After capturing and inspecting the Bluetooth transmissions from the mobile medical device, we discovered the key aspects of the device's protocol and the data that it sends to the AP. Our analysis of the captured traffic revealed some useful information. We observed that the data is sent from the device as 4-byte long packets. The second and third bytes are pulse rate and oxygen level, respectively. Additionally, we conjectured that the first and last byte are indicating some sort of status. This is because their values rarely change, and when they change, they seem to be independent of data or its fluctuation (Fig. 1). Similar analysis allowed us to reverse-engineer data coming from the blood pressure monitor.

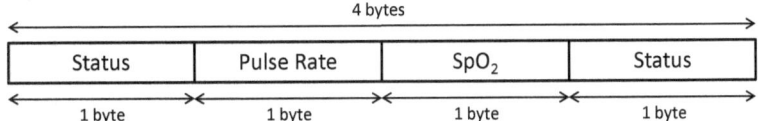

Fig. 1. Proposed format of the communication packet in the pulse oximeter

2. Transmission from the AP: For reverse-engineering packets coming from the AP, we issued commands from the device with different settings and looked at the packet generated from the software. In doing so we observed that the structure of the packet and the contents would only change with packets containing variables (e.g., setting date and time), allowing us to replay previously sent commands. We also learned that there were no packet-specific fields in the packet, such as checksum, packet length or timestamps.

6 Defending against MITM Attacks

We begin this section with enumerating the characteristics of a desirable defense solution. We then present our proposed solution for preventing such attacks, along with assumptions underlying our solution.

6.1 Desirable Characteristics of a Defense Mechanism

1. Security vs. Responsiveness: An effective mechanism for security should not introduce a significant increase (in medical terms) in the transmission time.
2. Security vs. Availability: A robust defense mechanism should not decrease the functionality of the system. Also, it should not provide new avenues for an unauthorized person to drain a device's battery. Furthermore, the mechanism itself should not introduce significant power or memory requirements that threaten the availability of the device itself.

3. No Changes to the Medical Device: To secure existing medical devices, the defense mechanism should not require any changes to the device.

4. No Changes to the Monitoring Software: The defense mechanism should not require changes to the implementation of the proprietary monitoring software running on the AP. This, coupled with the previous requirement for "no changes to the medical device," would improve the security of the existing systems. Note that minor changes to the operating system running on the AP are still acceptable.

6.2   Personal Security Device

In our solution, we propose that a separate wireless mobile device augments the security of mobile medical device systems. As envisioned, this Personal Security Device (PSD) will be small, portable, inexpensive, and easy to use. It can be small enough to clip on a belt or fit in a pocket. The PSD would work with other wireless medical devices to enhance their security and monitor their environment.

The PSD is aware of the suite of wireless mobile medical devices used by the owner, and it has a built-in knowledge of their security properties and vulnerabilities. The PSD takes steps to augment the security of the owner's devices, such as adding authentication and encryption to data streams.

The PSD can be used as an overlay, changing the transmission path from device→AP to device→PSD→AP (Fig. 2). In this case, even though the PSD could secure the link to the AP, the link from the device to the PSD remains unsecured. This is because we are constrained by not changing the device. In Section 7.2 we discuss possible improvements on the security of this link.

Even if the PSD cannot ask the device to transmit its data stream through the PSD, it may be able to improve the security of the system. For example, if the medical device always pairs with any device knowing its protocol, service name, and PIN, the PSD cannot prevent this device from pairing with others, but it can listen to the signals sent by the device. The PSD can create a parallel data stream containing authentication information (signed by a secret key known only to the PSD) to vouch for the data stream to other machines further along in the data flow of the overall system. This way, integrity attacks leveraged from MITM attacks are substantially harder for attackers to achieve without being detected.

For our PSD system to work, some assumptions must hold. We assume that the medical device pairs with only one AP at a time. Note that in the absence of this assumption, and since we cannot make any changes to the device, we cannot prevent the device from connecting to the attacker's machine. Moreover, we assume that the device and the AP are not compromised, meaning that the attacker has not been able to alter the hardware or software of the device or the AP, so they behave exactly as specified. We further assume that the PSD is located close to the device. And finally, we assume that the adversary does not physically try to remove the PSD, or damage it, or remotely hack it.

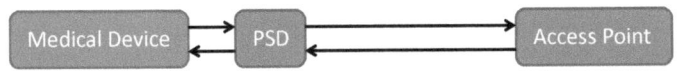

Fig. 2. Illustration of the mobile medical system when using the PSD

6.3 Required Changes at the AP

The AP needs to understand the new authentication and augmented encryption to be able to communicate securely with the PSD. On the other hand, as discussed in Section 6.1, we want to be able to use the monitoring software as it is, without imposing any changes. Therefore, the AP needs to ensure that the monitoring software still sends and receives the data unencrypted. To accomplish this we installed a virtual machine on the AP and installed the monitoring software on the guest operating system. The host OS, on the other hand, is basically used as a gateway for all traffic coming from or going to the monitoring software, leaving all authentication and encryption to be done on the host OS. For the monitoring software to communicate transparently with the device, we manually created two serial COM ports on the guest OS to emulate both incoming and outgoing Bluetooth communication. Accordingly, we configured two pipes on the virtual machine to redirect unencrypted traffic to and from the serial COM ports.

Our proposed changes at the AP rely on the fact that most modern operating systems either have native facilities for supporting virtual machines of the style we used, or can be easily augmented with other software to do so.

6.4 Discussion

1. In our proposed defense mechanism, we left major security components out of the medical device by introducing the PSD. While this decision was made to secure existing devices by requiring no change to their current design, there are also benefits to this design choice that make it attractive, even for designing other devices in the future:

a) Mobile medical devices have the unique property that they must fail-open when unbounded access is needed in emergency situations. Simply put, security in life-critical medical devices should never come ahead of accessibility. For instance, if a patient with an implantable defibrillator collapses, the treating doctor would need to be able to communicate with the device to retrieve the patient's information and history and issue necessary commands for treatment. Denying access to the doctor in such a situation is unacceptable. For life-critical medical devices, our defense mechanism approach complies with the fail-open property since unbounded access to the device can be always granted by simply turning off the PSD.

b) Resource constraints such as limited memory and battery pose a challenge for security implementation in mobile medical devices. Leaving expensive cryptographic computations to another device would make the device resources more available to life-sustaining functionalities.

2. Our approach requires a less detailed understanding of the device and its protocols, limited to certain security issues, than required by others [17].

3. Our defense solution makes it possible for the PSD-AP link to use any radio technology other than Bluetooth if desirable. With this, the PSD and the AP could agree on using a different radio technology that is more suitable for that particular environment.

4. Although we presented this defense solution only on Bluetooth, the idea can be extended to medical devices of other radio technologies. In order to implement this for another radio technology, on one end the PSD needs to be equipped with that particular radio technology capability to connect to the device. On the other end, at the AP, the host OS needs to virtualize the radio interface so that it communicates with the monitoring software running on the guest OS via a pipe. In Bluetooth, as described earlier, we have accomplished this by creating serial COM ports emulating a Bluetooth connection. For 802.11 for instance, one can perhaps modify the implementation of wireless card virtualization so that it communicates via a pipe created in the host OS rather than the actual wireless card on the AP. Chandra et al. [5] provides an implementation of virtualizing a single wireless card.

7   Evaluation

7.1   Performance

Our implementation introduced 783 ± 136 ms delay for every data packet sent by the device and received by the monitoring software when we used a Python implementation [2] of the 128-bit key AES encryption algorithm. This delay is insignificant, even in life-critical medical systems.

7.2   Robustness Analysis

1. Security of PSD-AP link: Since we have complete control over this link, given the availability of resources, we can make it arbitrarily secure by using a strong authentication and encryption, as well as an entirely different radio technology other than Bluetooth, if it is more suitable for our environment.

Bluetooth jamming is one source of denial of service attacks on this link. Even though the PSD does not protect against this attack, this attack is easily detected. Alternatively, the PSD and the AP can switch to using a radio technology that remains unaffected by Bluetooth jamming.

2. Security of Device-PSD link: This link is arguably vulnerable to MITM attacks. This is because an attacker can potentially perform MITM attacks on the link between the PSD and the device, making the entire security system introduced in this paper ineffective. The fundamental challenge to securing this link is that we cannot implement an additional security that requires altering or rebuilding the device. Here we present some recommendations that, while not completely eliminating the possibility of an attack, represent a substantial improvement in minimizing the risk.

a) *Configuring the device to low power transmission:* If it is feasible for the transmit power of the medical device to be set very low, then it could only communicate with devices that are very close to the medical device, perhaps only to those worn by the patient—namely the PSD.
b) *Designing an alert PSD:* Unlike the device and the monitoring software, the PSD is designed for security. Hence, an alert PSD would watch for signs of attacks such as MITM and other suspicious events, and would raise an alarm accordingly.

8   Future Work

The PSD idea could be developed into either a self-contained, specialized device, or into a smart phone as an application. Having it as a special-purpose piece of hardware theoretically has some advantages over the smart phone application idea: it makes the system harder to hack, it is less battery-consumptive, and there is no resource contention with other applications. On the other hand, having it implemented as a smart phone application makes it more convenient and readily available to the user. Future work could involve careful investigation of advantages and disadvantages of either option.

We designed the PSD so that it prevents MITM attacks. The other element of the PSD's behavior could be to observe the local environment for signs of attacks on its devices. For example, if the personal security device observes improper attempts by unauthorized devices to pair with the medical device over Bluetooth, it can raise an alert that there is a heightened risk of man-in-the-middle or data stream alteration attacks. A further study could look into feasibility of extending the current PSD to employ more sophisticated security tools, such as medical telemetry anomaly detection and detecting, not just preventing, man-in-the-middle attacks.

Work is needed to find ways to make the use of the PSD acceptable to the class of users it would most benefit.

9   Conclusion

This paper addresses the problem of communication security and privacy for the class of mobile medical devices that communicate via Bluetooth. We presented the steps we used to launch an MITM attack on such devices. Then, we introduced our Personal Security Device, a separate wireless device that augments security to the existing mobile medical devices to defend against MITM attacks.

References

1. Mobile Health Apps: What Do You Use?, http://www.cbc.ca/news/pointofview/2010/12/mobile-health-apps-what-do-you-use.html
2. PyCrypto: The Python Cryptography Toolkit, http://www.pycrypto.org
3. Insulin pumps - global pipeline analysis, opportunity assessment and market forecasts to 2016, globaldata. Global Data (2010)
4. Avancha, S., Baxi, A., Kotz, D.: Privacy in mobile technology for personal healthcare. ACM Computing Surveys (2012)
5. Chandra, R., Bahl, P.: Multinet: Connecting to multiple ieee 802.11 networks using a single wireless card. In: INFOCOM 23rd Annual Joint Conference of the IEEE Computer and Communications Societies, vol. 2, pp. 882–893 (2004)
6. Denning, T., Fu, K., Kohno, T.: Absence makes the heart grow fonder: New directions for implantable medical device security. In: Proceedings of the 3rd Conference on Hot Topics in Security, p. 5. USENIX Association (2008)
7. Gollakota, S., Hassanieh, H., Ransford, B., Katabi, D., Fu, K.: They can hear your heartbeats: non-invasive security for implantable medical devices. In: Proc. of the ACM SIGCOMM Conference, New York, NY, USA, pp. 2–13 (2011)
8. Halperin, D., Heydt-Benjamin, T.S., Ransford, B., Clark, S.S., Defend, B., Morgan, W., Fu, K., Kohno, T., Maisel, W.H.: Pacemakers and implantable cardiac defibrillators: Software radio attacks and zero-power defenses. In: IEEE Symposium on Security and Privacy, pp. 129–142. IEEE (2008)
9. Halperin, D., Kohno, T., Heydt-Benjamin, T., Fu, K., Maisel, W.: Security and privacy for implantable medical devices. In: Pervasive Computing (2008)
10. Hanna, K. Innovation and invention in medical devices: workshop summary. National Academies Press (2001)
11. Kotz, D.: A threat taxonomy for mHealth privacy. In: 3rd International Conference on Communication Systems and Networks (COMSNETS), pp. 1–6. IEEE (2011)
12. Li, C., Raghunathan, A., Jha, N.K.: Hijacking an insulin pump: Security attacks and defenses for a diabetes therapy system. In: 13th IEEE International Conference on e-Health Networking Applications and Services, pp. 150–156 (2011)
13. Maisel, W.: Safety issues involving medical devices. JAMA: the Journal of the American Medical Association 294(8), 955–958 (2005)
14. Ott, L. The evolution of Bluetooth in wireless medical devices. Socket Mobile, Inc. White Papers (2010)
15. Rasmussen, K., Castelluccia, C., Heydt-Benjamin, T., Capkun, S.: Proximity-based access control for implantable medical devices. In: Proc. of 16th ACM Conference on Computer and Communications Security (2009)
16. Shaked, Y., Wool, A.: Cracking the Bluetooth PIN. In: Proc. of 3rd International Conference on Mobile systems, Applications and Services (2005)
17. Sorber, J., Shin, M., Peterson, R., Cornelius, C., Mare, S., Prasad, A., Marois, Z., Smithayer, E., Kotz, D.: An amulet for trustworthy wearable mHealth. In: HotMobile, pp. 7:1–7:6. ACM, New York (2012)
18. Xu, F., Qin, Z., Tan, C., Wang, B., Li, Q.: IMDguard: Securing implantable medical devices with the external wearable guardian. In: INFOCOM (2011)

Fundamental Study for Optical BAN

Koichi Shimizu, Takeshi Namita, and Yuji Kato

Graduate School of Information Science and Technology,
Hokkaido University, Sapporo, Japan
{shimizu,tnamita,kato}@bme.ist.hokudai.ac.jp

Abstract. For a new optical body area network (BAN) technique, a fundamental study was conducted of optical data transmission through a human body using diffusely scattered light. The frequency bandwidth for data transmission was restricted by the effect of strong scattering inside body tissues. In experiments using human bodies, the possibility of the transmission up to 100 MHz was confirmed. Using the linear equalization process, we can transmit an 800 MHz square wave signal. Data transmission of around 200 mm distance in a human hand was possible. To overcome problems of noise, multipath transmission, and the instantaneous interruption of data transmission, the space diversity (SD) technique was applied to stabilize data communications. The SD technique effectiveness was confirmed through analysis using real optical impulse responses. The feasibility of BAN using diffusely scattered light in the body was verified through these analyses.

Keywords: BAN, body area network, optical BAN, optical communication, data transmission, scattering, diffusion, space diversity.

1   Introduction

Recently, the usefulness of wearable computer has been widely recognized. Many reports describe the body area network (BAN) [1]. In most studies, the signal carrier for BAN is an electrical signal such as electric field, electric current, or electromagnetic wave [2]. Many attempts have been undertaken to use the electric BAN in medical practice [3]. However, related to the use of electrical signals for BAN, there have been restrictions of signal bandwidth, problems of electromagnetic interference, and difficulties controlling information leakage by electromagnetic radiation.

To overcome these problems, we propose the use of light as a signal carrier [4]. Few reports describe optical signal transmission through the human body for BAN. We can find few practical applications of optical BAN for medicine. When light enters our body, it is scattered diffusely. If we can use this scattered light for data transmission, then we can realize a new optical technique for BAN.

In this study, we analyzed characteristics of light transmission through body tissues and attempted a new detection technique to examine the feasibility of the optical BAN in practical applications.

B. Godara and K.S. Nikita (Eds.): MobiHealth 2012, LNICST 61, pp. 173–178, 2013.
© Institute for Computer Sciences, Social Informatics and Telecommunications Engineering 2013

2   Optical BAN from Wrist to Fingertip

When we illuminate near-infrared (NIR) light on our body surface, some light propagates diffusely in the body tissue. When we illuminate the light on the wrist area for example, the light propagates widely in the hand area and part of it reaches the fingers. Therefore, we can make the BAN from/to a wristwatch type device to/from the fingertips. Figure 1 presents the optical BAN principle. For example, we can identify the individual with the wristwatch by just touching the door-knob with no action of the personal authentication such as fingerprint imaging or iris scanning. If another person wears the watch, then it cannot be operated by the authentication function built-in the watch. Many other applications are possible with this optical BAN from the wrist to the fingertips.

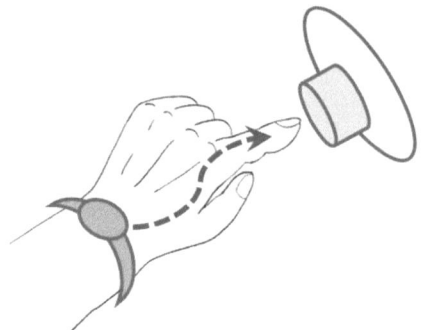

Fig. 1. Optical BAN principle

3   Data Transmission Rate

In the BAN using diffusely scattered light, the propagation path of light is spread in a wide area in the body tissue, which brings pulse broadening in the light propagation through the body. This pulse broadening restricts the data transmission rate.

To evaluate the transmission rate, the optical responses of a human arm and a human hand were measured. Short pulses of laser light (Ti:Sapphire, wavelength 786 nm, pulse width 20 ps FWHM, optical power 200 mW) were illuminated on one side of the body. The light transmitted through the body was received at the other side of the body with an optical fiber. The light was led to a streak camera (temporal resolution < 15 ps, repetition rate 2 MHz) and the broadened pulse shape was measured [5].

Table 1 shows results of pulse broadening. From this result, we can expect the signal transmission in the order of 100 MHz. With signal processing techniques such as the linear equalizing process, we were able to transmit an 800 MHz square wave signal in our experiment [5].

Table 1. Pulse broadening through living body tissue

	Thickness [mm]	Pulse width [ns FWHM]	Freq. band [MHz]
Palm	27	0.78	130
Arm	46	0.98	100

4   Data Transmission Range

Attenuation of an optical signal in our body is much higher than the electric signal, which makes the control of information leakage through unnecessary radiation easier than the electric signal. However, if the range is too small, then it is not practically useful. Consequently, the data transmission range was analyzed using a model phantom and a human body.

Figure 2 depicts the experimental setup schematically. The light beam from the laser (Ti:Sapphire, wavelength 800 nm, optical power 1 W) was made intermittent with a mechanical chopper for the lock-in detection of received light. It was illuminated on the surface of a model phantom which simulated the human hand tissue. The agar phantom was produced with intralipid and black ink added to simulate the respective scattering and absorption coefficients of mammalian tissues: μ_s'=1.0 /mm and μ_a=0.01 /mm. The light

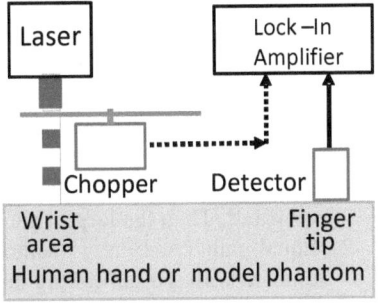

Fig. 2. Measurement of transmission range

propagated through the phantom was detected using a Si photodiode placed at a specific distance away from the light incident point. The intensity of the received light was measured using a lock-in-amplifier. The noise unsynchronized with the chopper was eliminated in the process of phase-sensitive detection.

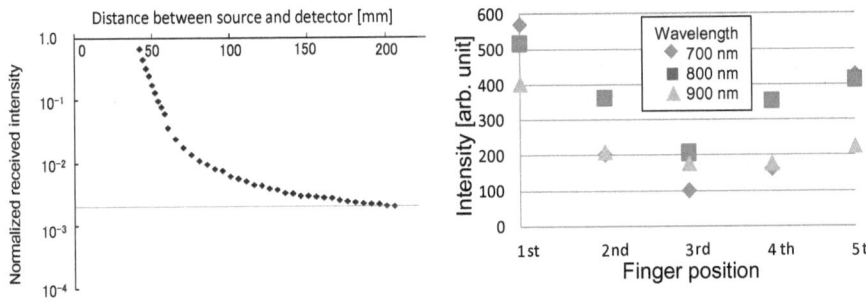

Fig. 3. Attenuation of optical signal with source-detector distance: horizontal line indicates a noise level

Fig. 4. Received optical signal intensity at different fingers and wavelengths

Figure 3 presents measurement results, which suggest that the transmission around 200 mm surface distance was possible. Using the same experimental setup, the transmission range was evaluated using a human hand. To reduce the optical power density on the body, the incident light beam (optical power 250 mW) was expanded to 40 mmφ using an optical beam expander. The received light intensity at the tip of each finger was measured using different wavelengths in the NIR range. Figure 4 shows the result of measurements. Results show that optical data transmission from the wrist is possible to all fingers. Among the wavelengths examined, the highest performance was obtained with the 800 nm wavelength.

5   Application of Space Diversity Technique

In optical BAN, signal attenuation attributable to the strong scattering in the body is severe, and data transmission is vulnerable to optical and electrical noises. To address this problem, we introduced the space diversity (SD) technique. For this technique, we placed some detectors on the body surface at separate positions, and applied an operation to the outputs of some detectors. For the SD operation, the following three methods were used.

1) Selection method: Instantaneous signal intensities from all detectors are compared. Then the largest signal is selected.
2) Equal-gain combining method: Signal intensities from all detectors were summed with the same weights.
3) Maximum-ratio combining method: Signal intensities from all detectors were summed with the weight of each signal intensity.

To compare the performance of SD operation methods described above, noise of different kinds was added to the signal. Table 2 presents different noises, and Figures 5 and 6 show them. Figure 7 portrays the arrangement of the detectors. Five detectors were aligned along a line with 20 mm separation. The distance of the line from the light-incident point was 100 mm.

Table 2. Different type of noises

#	Distribution	Synchronism	Appearance
1-1	Uniform distribution (0-1)	Asynchronous	Fig. 5(a)
1-2			Fig. 5(b)
1-3			Fig. 5(c)
1-4		Synchronous	Fig. 5(c)
2-1	Normal distribution (m=0.5, σ^2=0.5)	Asynchronous	Fig. 6(a)
2-2			Fig. 6(b)
2-3			Fig. 6(c)
2-4		Synchronous	Fig. 6(c)

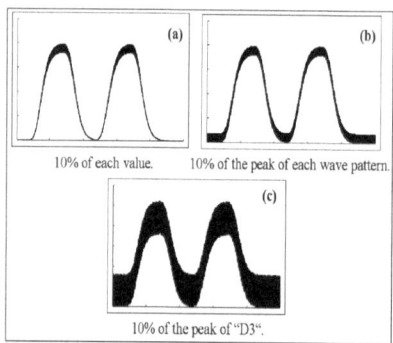

Fig. 5. Noise-added wave shape (uniform distribution noise)

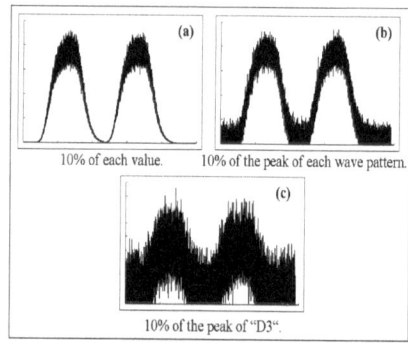

Fig. 6. Noise-added wave shape (normal distribution noise)

The impulse response of light propagation from the incident point to each detector was measured using a laser (Ti:Sapphire, wavelength 800 nm, pulse width 20 ps FWHM, optical power 1 W) and a streak camera. As a scattering medium, chicken breast meat was used. Figure 8 shows the measured pulse shapes at different detectors. These were regarded as impulse responses. The waveform received at each detector was calculated as the convolution of the impulse response and the input rectangular waveform. Figure 9 presents the signal waveform deformed by the scattering effect. Noises of different kinds shown in Table 2 were added to these deformed signals, and the three kinds of SD operations described above were applied.

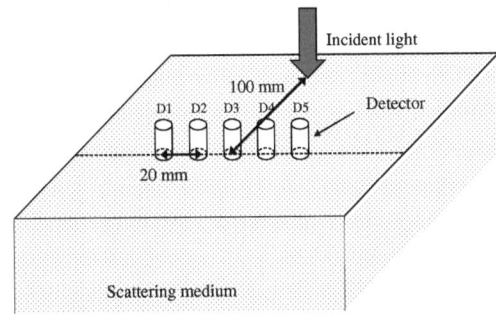

Fig. 7. Arrangement of photodetectors for space diversity techniques

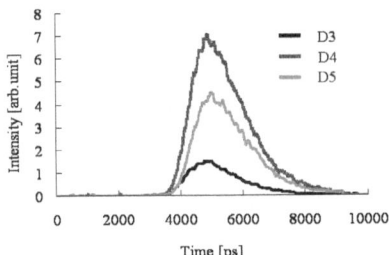

Fig. 8. Measured pulse shapes

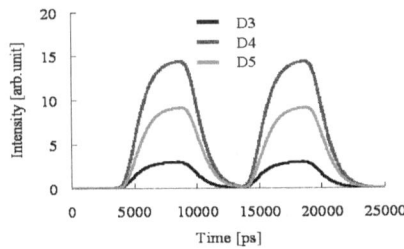

Fig. 9. Signal waveforms obtained from measured impulse response

Table 3. Comparison of signal-to-noise ratio for different synthesis methods of space diversity [rms dB]

#	Selection	Equal-gain combining	Max-ratio combining
1-1	24.8	24.9	**25.6**
1-2	**19.5**	16.5	18.7
1-3	20.8	20.9	**21.7**
1-4	**19.5**	15.5	17.8
2-1	21.3	23.5	**24.0**
2-2	17.3	19.6	**20.1**
2-3	16.0	15.2	**17.3**
2-4	**16.0**	11.9	14.2

Table 3 presents the signal-to-noise ratio of the resultant waveform after the SD operations. Bold figures denote the largest signal-to-noise ratio in the noise category.

As expected, the SD performance differed for different noise types. Results suggest that the maximum-ratio combining method had superior noise suppression ability to that of other methods.

6   Conclusions

An optical BAN technique was proposed using near-infrared light as a data transmission carrier. It offers different merits over conventional BANs with electrical carriers.

The frequency bandwidth for data transmission was evaluated in the experiment with a human arm and a human hand. The possibility of the transmission on the order of 100 MHz was confirmed. Using the linear equalizing process, we were able to transmit an 800 MHz square wave signal.

The transmission range through body tissue was analyzed in experiments. Data transmission around 200 mm surface distance was possible. The data transmission from the wrist area to each fingertip was confirmed. The feasibility of the optical BAN from the wristwatch-type device to the fingertips was verified.

To overcome problems in practical use, the space diversity (SD) technique was applied to stabilize data communication. The SD technique effectiveness was confirmed in the analysis using real optical impulse responses. For the SD technique, data-synthesis methods of different kinds were compared. Among them, the maximum-ratio combining technique was found to be the most appropriate for the SD method of this purpose. Results of these analyses verified the feasibility of optical communication through the human body using diffusely scattered light.

This study was conducted with the approval of the Ethics Committee of Graduate School of Engineering, Hokkaido University.

Acknowledgements. The authors thank Mr. Toshihide Saito, Mr. Shun Kakita, and Mr. Junkichi Akiyama for their efforts to obtain data when they were in Graduate School of Information Science and Technology, Hokkaido University. This research was supported in part by a Grant-in-Aid for Scientific Research from the Japan Society for the Promotion of Science.

References

[1] Hanson, M.A., Powell, H.C., Barth, A.T., Ringgenberg, K., Calhoun, B.H., Aylor, J.H., Lach, J.: Body area sensor networks: challenges and opportunities. Computer 42, 58–65 (2009)
[2] Cao, H., Leung, V., Chow, C., Chan, H.: Enabling technologies for wireless body area networks: a survey and outlook. IEEE Comm. Mag. 47, 84–93 (2009)
[3] Khan, J.Y., Yuce, M.R., Bulger, G., Harding, B.: Wireless body area network (WBAN) design techniques and performance evaluation. J. Med. Syst. 1, 199–216 (2010)
[4] Shimizu, K.: Optical biotelemetry. In: Lin, J.C. (ed.) Advances in Electromagnetic Fields in Living Systems, vol. 4, pp. 131–154 (2005)
[5] Saito, T., Kakita, S., Kato, Y., Shimizu, K.: Feasibility of transcutaneous data transmission using scattered light. Tech. Rep. IEICE, 107, 57–60 (2008)

Spectrum Sensing Improvement in Cognitive Radio Networks for Real-Time Patients Monitoring

Dramane Ouattara[1], Francine Krief[1], Mohamed Aymen Chalouf[2], and Omessaad Hamdi[1]

[1] Université de Bordeaux, LaBRI, 351 cours de la Libration
33405 Talence Cedex, France
{dramane.ouattara,francine.krief,ohamdi}@labri.fr
[2] Université de Rennes 1, IRISA, IUT de Lannion, Rue Edouard Branly
22300 Lannion, France
mohamed-aymen.chalouf@irisa.fr

Abstract. Regular monitoring of vital signs guarantees a preventive treatment of common diseases ensuring better health for people. Most of the proposed solutions in e-health context are based on a set of heterogeneous wireless sensors, fitting the patient and his environment. Often, these sensors are connected to a local smart node acting as a gateway to the outside (contacts, servers). When the patient is mobile, one of the issues we may face is the guarantee of a permanent connectivity between local smart node and the outside. To overcome this problem, we need to define a robust communications architecture able to benefit from different technologies and standards. This provides equipments with the ability to dispose of free-bands to perform their transmission anytime and anywhere. Cognitive radio, although appropriate technology, requires taking into account the interdependence between the patient's mobility and frequency band changes. Our proposal, is an anticipation model, a decision-making function that predicts the state of frequency bands occupancy. The model combines the machine learning techniques to the Grey Model system to provide low cost algorithm for spectral prediction which facilitates or guarantees permanent connectivity.

Keywords: Cognitive radio networks, e-health, patients monitoring, connectivity, Grey Model, Machine Learning, spectral prediction.

1 Introduction

The emergence of new health risks, requires the design of new solutions able to assume a preventive role. These solutions must provide more autonomy to the patient with an anywhere and any-time monitoring capabilities. This requires a permanent connectivity and therefore, the spectral availability. In the context of communications rise in wireless networks, leading to the spectrum scarcity, cognitive radio is seen as a reliable alternative technology. However, remains a set

B. Godara and K.S. Nikita (Eds.): MobiHealth 2012, LNICST 61, pp. 179–188, 2013.

of issues concerning spectrum sensing, spectrum sharing, spectrum decision and spectrum mobility to be solved for this technology. Concerning the spectrum mobility, issues related to permanent connectivity for mobile cognitive radio equipments are less explored. In this paper, we address the connectivity problem that could result from the patient's mobility. At this purpose, we propose a function that facilitates the detection of free-bands by the mobile cognitive radio equipment dedicated to the real-time patient's monitoring. This solution is based on machine learning techniques and the Grey Model system for performing a spectral prediction. The remainder of this paper is a definition of cognitive radio in section 2, a state of the art on this technology used in e-health context in section 3, the patients monitoring principle description in section 4 , the proposed prediction model in section 5. Finally, the section 6 presents the experimental results and the section 7 concludes.

2 The Cognitive Radio Networks

2.1 Definition and Principle of Cognitive Radio Networks

The Cognitive Radio [1] is a paradigm for wireless networks where a node is able to automatically modify its transmitting parameters in order to communicate efficiently, while avoiding interference with other users. This self-configuration and self-adaptation of parameters is based on a set of modules and several factors in the internal or the external environment of the radio such as radio frequency, user behaviour and the network state.

2.2 The Modules of the Cognitive Radio

Figure 1.1 summarizes the modules and the structure of the cognitive functions.

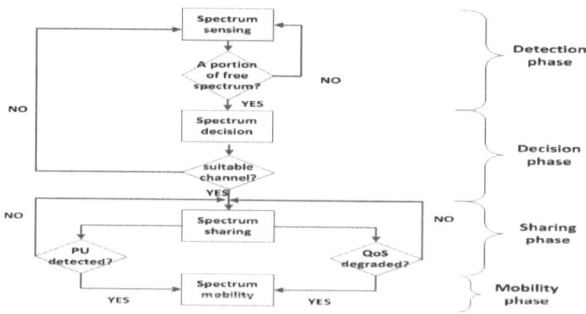

Fig. 1. Operating diagram of a cognitive radio node

The spectrum sensing: The spectrum sensing is defined as the ability to measure, examine, learn and be aware of the parameters related to the charac-teristics of the radio channel. This module measures the availability of spectrum, the signal strength, the interference and noise, scans operating environment of the radio, estimates the needs of the users and applications, checks the availability of networks and nodes, learn about the local policies and other operators restrictions.

The spectrum decision: The decision-making is based on the appropriate communication channel choice, justifying the quality of service required for the data or the collected information transmission.

The spectrum sharing: The channel sharing has to comply with the requirement of synchronized access to the detected free-bands portions. This scheduling is done between the secondary[1] users on the one hand, and between these users and the primary[2] users on the other.

The spectrum mobility: Spectrum mobility reflects the fact that each transceiver, must be able to change frequency band if the initial band becomes busy. Moving to a new frequency band could happen also when the initial band fails to provide the desired quality of service to the data transmission applications.

3   Cognitive Radio Used in e-health Context

Cognitive radio technology used for patients monitoring is increasingly considered in the literature. An example of an e-health wireless communication system based on cognitive radio, deployed in a hospital setting is described in [2]. This article suggested answerers to the interferences caused by wireless transmissions to various medical devices. The proposal presented in [3], demonstrates the ability of cognitive radio to improve Wireless Body Area Networks (WBAN) performances. Another approach [4] proposes a parallel detection of vital signs and communication signals through the cognitive radio sensing module. From these different proposals and seen the cognitive radio technology capabilities, emerge the evidence, that dispose of a high channel availability by free-bands detection is essential for achieving the patients monitoring.

The patient monitoring requirements: The collected data by medical sensors followed by their transmission to a local or remote node are a range of services focused on communications. The emergency of medical data transmission and the need to have a robust communications architecture requires technologies that are able to provide a low cost communication links (bands) for ensuring reliable connectivity any-time and anywhere.

4   The Scenario Addressed in Patient Monitoring

Vital signs monitoring leads to data collecting by the medical sensors, a minimal treatment performed by the local smart node (fixed: Medical Box or mobile: Smart-phone, PDA) and a set of exchanges generated as shown at Figure 1.2.

---

[1] Cognitive radio users, who do not have any band-use license, such as the patient's equipments in our context.

[2] Users that have the band-use license.

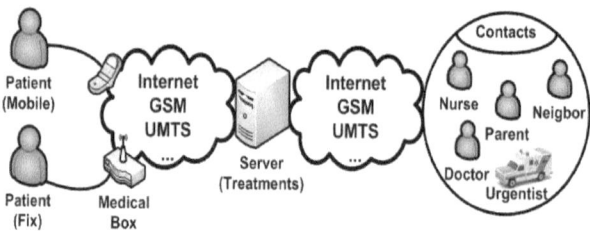

Fig. 2. The communication description scheme

Thus, the dissemination of the alerts and the medical data updates, increase demands of frequency bands. To ensure a continuous connectivity between the monitored patient in his environment and external actors (contacts, servers), the cognitive radio technology is well suited. According to the need for medical application, and depending on communication urgency and the frequency availability, the cognitive radio selects the appropriate channel, and the adequate technology to ensure transmissions. For this purpose, the communication protocol proposed in [5], based on a centralized architecture where a cognitive radio node (server) is responsible for the management of all transmissions (primary users and secondary users) by a queuing packets mechanism, provides partial response. In fact, this solution, is focused on the access synchronization to a single channel for the data transmission, explores the same technology and is limited to a hospital environment. Adapting this idea to our anywhere and any-time patient monitoring context, requires improvements to integrate multi-technologies and multichannel exploration capabilities. Thus, in addition to a distributed solution, our proposal offers an opportunity to explore all available technologies, to transmit on different channels and is adapted to the patient mobility context.

The spectrum sensing problematic: The spectrum sensing is the most expensive operation in terms of processing time and energy consumption for a mobile cognitive radio equipment. The energy autonomy to maximize for all mobile medical equipments can not tolerate an inefficient and inappropriate perpetual sensing. A spectrum prediction mechanism, measuring the channels states (free or occupied) probabilities, would significantly reduce the sensing frequency by ensuring a rational choice of the band to be sensed.

The limitations of existing prediction algorithms : The handover prediction is the most studied in the literature, leaving less-explored the spectral prediction in mobile environment. Spectral prediction studies using the game theory approaches and machine learning [6][7] are also proposed but in a static environment where there is no cell change. Others standard prediction model less considered in cognitive radio networks using the statistical techniques [8] such as AR (Auto Regressive), MA (Moving Average), ARMA (Auto Regressive Moving Average), ARIMA (Auto Regressive Integrated Moving Average) are also explored. However, these models require complete and representative data. The studies, whose aim is to reduce the cell change impact on connectivity in cognitive radio networks by the design of prediction model, will ensure permanent transmissions required by the mobile patients monitoring process.

5   The Proposed Solution

The proposed solution is to add a prediction function to the spectrum sensing module as illustrated in Figure 1.1. This function combines the machine learning techniques with the Grey Model system to assess the probability of the channel occupancy and thus, guide the choice of the band to be sensed. Figure 1.3 represents a description of the prediction function operating mode and is more detailed in section 1.5.1. The goal is to have a low cost prediction algorithm with a learning module well trained but also compensate training time with Grey Model module predictions. This idea could enhance the current solutions, which consist in a set of multiple sensing to create free-bands data base. Our prediction proposal allows us to limit the number of sensing operations, and especially to achieve a timely sensing with significant reduction of computational cost.

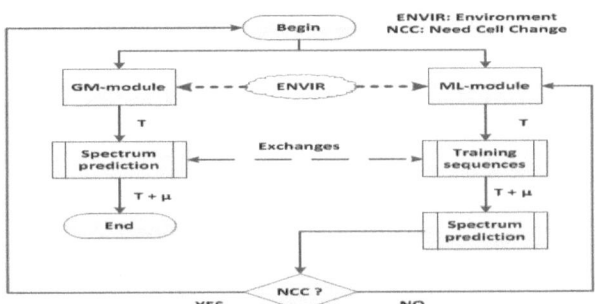

Fig. 3. Prediction function operating mode

5.1   The Details of the Prediction Process

The Grey Model theory [9], is known for the analysis of problems with incomplete or uncertain information. Its main advantage on the statistical prediction techniques such as AR, MA, ARMA, ARIMA, is the ability to settle for a minimum input data to achieve its predictions. Our solution is based on the ability to predict, on the basis of incomplete data, provided by the Grey Model and the low cost processing offered by the machine learning algorithms when well trained. Indeed, the smart node runs with the two modules, Machine Learning (ML) and Grey Model (GM) in a new cell or at the beginning of its activity. The Grey Model at this stage makes predictions while the learning module executes training sequences. The prediction process returned to the ML-module, once its effectiveness is proved by the relevance of its prediction results and none Need of Cell Change (NCC) is detected as defined at figure 1.3.

5.2   The Model Input Data

We are particularly interested to the 2.4 GHz frequency band (WIFI). This is justified by characteristics of our platform GNU-Radio, but the principle is similar for the other channel types (GSM, Bluetooth, Zigbee etc.). Our goal being to achieve a probability distribution of the channel status on the future periods, leads to base the reasoning on the following parameters :

The energy on each sub-band : The energy detected on a channel could be used to identify a signal type [10]. A comparison of the received signal (energy) by the radio equipment to a predefined threshold depending on the type of channel, could determine a primary user signal status as shown at figure 1.4. The principle is based on two assumptions, H_0 (OFF) for channel is free and H_1 (ON) for channel is busy such that : $H_O : y(t) = n(t)$ and $H1 : y(t) = x(t) + n(t)$ Where t = 1, 2, ..., N represents the received signal sample periods, y(t) the received signal, n(t) the Gaussian noise and x(t) the detected signal.

The other data : The other data to be taken into account are dynamic and static data. The dynamic data, much more random and scalable, includes energy, transmission power, number of primary users and number of free-channels. The static data can be defined as the number of channels, the band type, the location and the type of area (heavily urban, rural), the central frequency, the energy threshold.

The energy distribution on the channel : The patient's cognitive radio equipment makes periodic measurements of the channel energy. Our solution is a distribution of this data and its likelihood estimation on future periods.

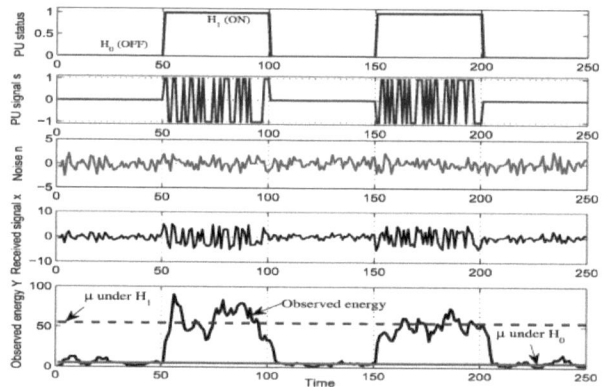

Fig. 4. Spectrum usage description

Figure 1.4 shows the links between the received signal and the energy of the band, the primary users signal distinction to Gaussian noise. the signal strength determines the presence (H_1 ON) or the absence (H_0 OFF) of a primary user. The mobile (Smart-phone) or the Medical Box equipment as described in figure 1.2, exploits these periods (ON/OFF) for their medical data transmissions.

5.3   Machine Learning and Grey Model Description

For the model simulation, we have opted for Hidden Markov Models (HMM) as learning module associated with the GM (1,1). As objective, we have two quantities to optimize namely, minimize the cost and maximize the precision; Hence, the choice of GM for its reasonable cost and the HMM for its errors-correcting ability.

The Hidden Markov Models (HMM): The error-correcting technique is based on the observation of a trend curve and only the most recent values of the series are pertinent in predicting the future values. For a set of sampling data X (1), X (2), X (3), ..., X (N), an adjustment function applied to the values, predicts the future trends by assessing weight to previous values as follow : $Xhat(k) = p_1 x_k + p_2 x_{k-1} + p_3 x_{k-2} + ... + p_n x_{k-n+1}$, with $p_1, p_2, ..., p_n$, the weigths assigned to previous observations, where the most recent values have higher weight such as :

$$Xhat(t) = \alpha * [x_{t-1} + (1-\alpha)x_{t-2} + (1-\alpha)^2 x_{t-3} + (1-\alpha)^3 x_{t-4} + ...] + (1-\alpha)^{t-1} x_1$$

and α the adjustment coefficient, $(1, (1-\alpha), (1-\alpha)^2, (1-\alpha)^3, (1-\alpha)^4$ the weights. The α value is thought of as a Markov chain which takes on a number of 'fuzzy' states. The m-step transition probabilities p(i,j) of the chain are calculated by observing for each state i, the number of observed α-values that drift state j, in m quanta of time. The initial distribution of the chain is calculated by observing the number of points in the cluster(state). Given this initial distribution and the transition probabilities, the evolution of the chain is fully determined. Thus, the probability of transition from state i to state j, denoted P_{ij} is evaluated as follows : $P_{ij} = Q_{ij}/Q_i$, with Q_i, representing the number of times α remains in the state i and P_{ij}, the number of transitions occurrences between the state i and the state j.

To the initial distribution is associated an initial vector : $\pi^{(0)} = [\pi_1^{(0)} \pi_2^{(0)} \pi_3^{(0)} \pi_4^{(0)} \pi_5^{(0)}]$, the transition probabilities. The probabilities distribution of future transition (t+1) states from $\pi^{(0)}$ is obtained by : $\pi^{(t+1)} = \pi^{(0)} M^{(i)}$.

The Grey Model GM(1,1) : The GM (1,1) is the most used in prediction systems [11].

The GM(1,1) modelling process :

- The system takes as input a sequence of values (energy), with $X^0 = [x^0(1), x^0(2), x^0(3), ..., x^0(n)]$, the initial sequence, where $x^0(t)$ corresponds to the output of the system at time t.
- From the initial sequence, a new sequence X^1 is generated by the system with new values $X^1 = [x^1(1), x^1(2), x^1(3), ..., x^1(n)]$.
- The first order differential equation obtained from X^1 is given by : $\frac{dx^1(t)}{dt} + ax^1(t) = b$, a is the coefficient that reflects the trend and b is the predictive control coefficient expressing the portion of the information known and unknown part of the information model.

- The parameter estimation or coefficients of the matrix $[a, b]^T$ can be obtained by the method of least squares knowing that $[a, b]^T = (B^T B)^{-1} B^T y_N$, where

$$B = \begin{bmatrix} -\frac{1}{2}(x^1(1) + x^1(2)) & 1 \\ -\frac{1}{2}(x^1(2) + x^1(3)) & 1 \\ \ldots\ldots\ldots & . \\ -\frac{1}{2}(x^1(n-1) + x^1(n)) & 1 \end{bmatrix}$$

and $y_N = [x^0(2), x^0(3), x^0(4), ..., x^0(n)]^T$; n being the size of the sequence defined by the model.
- The prediction function becomes : $\hat{x}^1(t) = (x^1(1) - \frac{b}{a})e^{-at} + \frac{b}{a}$
- The predicted value at time t+1 is obtained by : $\hat{x}^0(t+1) = \hat{x}^1(t+1) - \hat{x}^1(t)$.

6   The Experimentation

Our study is based on an observation/analysis of the spectrum through cognitive radio platform and simulation results.

The cognitive radio platform : We set up a cognitive radio platform using GNU-Radio and the USRP1 of Ettus[12]. The ultimate goal is to transmit and receive through the platform, all radio standard (AM, FM, DAB, GSM, Wifi, GPS, TV) and also to analyse spectrum and medical signals.

The sample data and predicted values : On the basis of results described in [13], the ability of Grey Model to achieve predictions without any prior training (see figure 1.5) is proved. The simulation results (figure 1.6) are only the ML-module outputs. Based on the real-time measured values, adjustments are made by the learning function for taking into account the errors for future predictions. The values (X) generated as our learning sample represent the energy on a sub-channel at different slot-time.

$$X = \begin{bmatrix} 48 & 70 & 50 & 40 & 90 & 46 & 72 & 48 & 39 & 91 & 49 & 71 & 49 & 37 & 88 & 45 & 70 & 51 & 38 & 95 & 47 & 75 \\ 50 & 36 & 93 & 42 & 76 & 60 & 40 & 98 & 41 & 77 & 55 & 39 & 97 & 42 & 73 & 50 & 38 & 99 & 41 & 76 & 53 & 37 \end{bmatrix}$$

The predictions results :
Figure 1.6(a) shows that with adequate samples and training, the algorithm is able to control stationary events such as high activity moments of primary users and their low attendance times. The stationary behaviour of primary users allows obtaining better prediction results.

Figures 1.6(b) and (c) show that the behaviour of primary users may be random and non-stationary and require more training time and sample data. In this case, the objectivity of the predictions is limited to one predicted value (t+1). The predicted values distribution for the future periods ($\geq$ t +2), becomes less and less relevant. These results reveal the importance of the GM-module as an alternative prediction tool during the ML-module training periods.

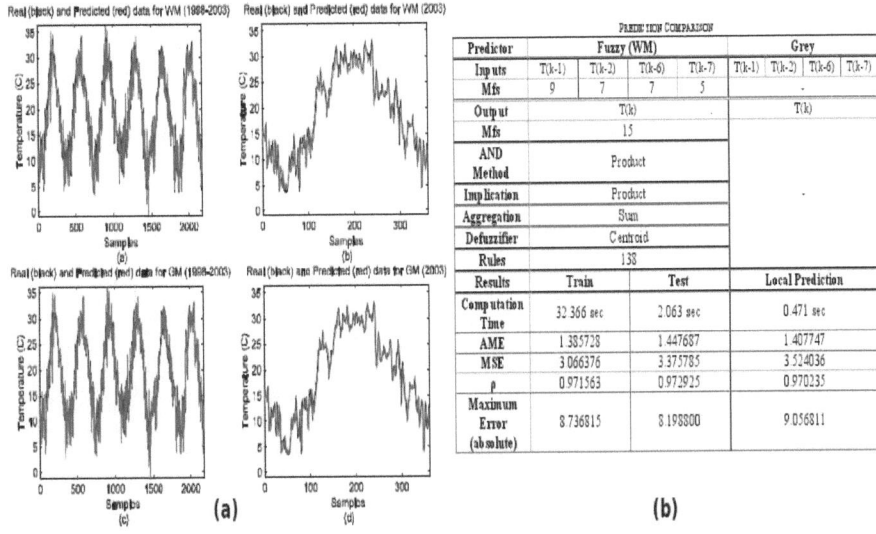

Fig. 5. Result of GM(1,1) predictions [13]

The table shown in Fig. 5(b):

PREDICTION COMPARISON								
Predictor	Fuzzy (WM)				Grey			
Inputs	T(k-1)	T(k-2)	T(k-6)	T(k-7)	T(k-1)	T(k-2)	T(k-6)	T(k-7)
Mfs	9	7	7	5	-			
Output	T(k)				T(k)			
Mfs	15							
AND Method	Product							
Implication	Product				-			
Aggregation	Sum							
Defuzzifier	Centroid							
Rules	138							

Results	Train	Test	Local Prediction
Computation Time	32.366 sec	2.063 sec	0.471 sec
AME	1.385728	1.447687	1.407747
MSE	3.066376	3.375785	3.524036
ρ	0.971563	0.972925	0.970235
Maximum Error (absolute)	8.736815	8.198800	9.056811

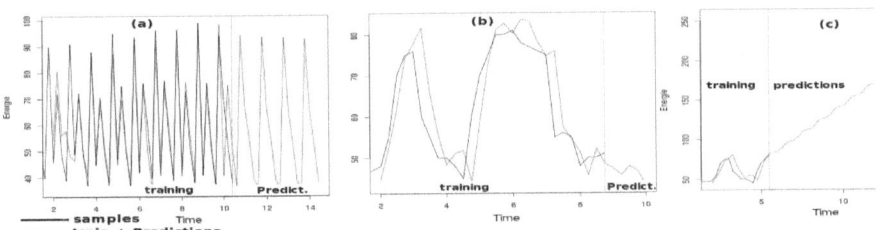

Fig. 6. Result of ML-module predictions

7   Conclusion

The problems for achieving the anywhere, any-time and real-time monitoring of vital signs, call for development of ambitious technologies able to overcome any lack of connection. In this paper, we have presented the concept of cognitive radio networks, seen as a solution to ensure constant connectivity for patient monitoring. We have also proposed a module, whose implementation would improve the sensing process for cognitive radio networks, crucial for the ongoing transmission of medical data. The spectral prediction model that we propose combines the Grey Model techniques to machine learning technology to ensure connectivity and facilitate channel change with low processing cost. Finally, we performed simulations based on machine learning to evaluate the prototype. The development of the Grey Model module for measuring the real performance of the complete model is part of our future works.

References

1. Palicot, J.: Cog. Radio: An Enabling Technology for the Green Radio Communications Concept, Leipzig, Germany, June 21-24 (2009)
2. Phunchongharn, P., Hossain, E., Niyato, D.: A cognitive radio system for e-health applications in a hospital environment 17, 20–28 (2010)
3. Feng, J., Liu, W., Li, Y.: Performance Enhancement of Wireless Body Area Network System Combined with Cognitive Radio 3, 313–317 (2010)
4. Wang, F., Li, C., Hsiao, C.: An injection-locked detector for concurrent spectrum and vital sign sensing. In: IEEE MTT-S Int. (MTT), pp. 768–771 (2010)
5. Phun, P., Hossain, E., Niyato: A cognitive radio system for e-health applications in a hospital environment. IEEE 17, 20–28 (2010)
6. Li, Y., Dong, Y., Hui, Z.: Spectrum Usage Prediction Based on High-order Markov Model for Cognitive Radio Networks. In: IEEE 10th Intern. Conf. (July 2010)
7. Liu, Y., Reddy, T.B., Manoj: On Cognitive Network Channel Selection and the Impact on Transport Layer Performance. In: IEEE Global Telecom. Conf., pp. 1–5 (December 2010)
8. Xu, Y.: The Application of ARIMA Model in Chinese Mobile User Prediction. In: IEEE Intern. Conf. G. Comput, GrC (August 2010)
9. Deng, J.: The Basis of Grey Theory. Huazhong University of Science and Technology Press (2002) (in Chinese)
10. Zhang, L.-L., Huang, J.-G., Tang, C.-K.: Novel energy detection scheme in cognitive radio. In: IEEE Int. Conf., Sig. Proc., pp. 1–4 (September 2011)
11. Chen, S., Ye, L., Zhang, G., Zeng, C., Dong, S., Dai, C.: Short-term wind power prediction based on combined grey-Markov model 3, 1705–1711 (2011)
12. http://gnuradio.org/redmine/projects/gnuradio/wiki
13. Dounis, A.I., Tseles, D., Nikolaou, G.: A Comparison of Grey Model and Fuzzy Predictive Model for Times Series, 176–181 (2006)

Theoretical Analysis and Modeling of Link Adaptation Schemes in Body Area Networks

Wen-Bin Yang and Kamran Sayrafian-Pour

Information Technology Laboratory
National Institute of Standards and Technology
Gaithersburg, Maryland, USA
{wyang,ksayrafian}@nist.gov

Abstract. Considering the medical nature of the information carried in Body Area Networks (BAN), interference from coexisting wireless networks or even other nearby BANs could create serious problems on their operational reliability. As practical implementation of power control mechanisms could be very challenging, link adaptation schemes can be an efficient alternative to preserve link quality while allowing more number of nodes to operate simultaneously. This paper provides theoretical analysis and Markov chain modeling of interference mitigation schemes such as adaptive modulation and adaptive data rate for body area networks. These schemes are relatively simple and well-suited for low power nodes in body area networks that might be operating in environments with high level of interference.

Keywords: Link adaptation, Interference mitigation, Body area networks, Markov chain, Interference mitigation factor.

1   Introduction

Body Area Networks (BANs) consist of multiple wearable (or implantable) radio-enabled sensors that can establish two-way wireless communication with a controller node that could be either worn or located in the vicinity of the body [1]. These potentially mobile networks are expected to coexist with other wireless devices that are operating in their proximity. Considering the medical nature of the data carried in a BAN, interference from coexisting wireless networks or even other nearby BANs could create a serious problem on the reliability of the network operation. The interference among nodes of a single BAN can be avoided by using multiple access techniques, e.g., TDMA. However, as no coordination exists across multiple BANs, interference may occur when several individuals wearing BAN are within close proximity of each other. This inter-BAN interference could result in performance degradation of the communication link within one network.

To maintain the link quality (e.g. desired received signal strength level or signal to interference and noise ratio (SINR)) in such varying communication channels, efficient power control mechanisms have been proposed [2, 3]. However, practical implementation of such mechanisms for BAN applications could be very challenging,

B. Godara and K.S. Nikita (Eds.): MobiHealth 2012, LNICST 61, pp. 189–198, 2013.

particularly in fast changing scenarios when the SINR is varying due to the unpredictable movement of multiple nearby BANs.

Advanced signal processing using interference cancellation techniques [4] has also been proposed to minimize the impact of interference. However, there are two main problems with such techniques especially when it comes to their application in BAN. First is the high complexity of the receiver which makes the implementation of interference cancelation impractical unless the number of nodes is very small. Complexity is especially a critical issue in body area networks. As nodes mainly rely on battery power, prolonging their lifetime is of prime importance. The second problem is that some interference cancellation schemes require knowledge of the channel condition (such as attenuation, phase, and delay) between each of the interferers and the receiver. Obtaining accurate estimates of the channel condition is extremely difficult for body area networks. To overcome the two main problems, a low complexity algorithm was proposed in our previous work [10, 11].

Interference mitigation schemes [5, 6] can be an attractive alternative to interference cancellation particularly in an environment with a high interference level. The principle of the interference mitigation is basically to reduce transmit power by using link adaption schemes. Lowering the transmit power decreases the interference on other networks and therefore allows the possibility of having more networks operating simultaneously. The trade-off in achieving this gain is degradation in other performance measures such as throughput or data rate. In this paper, we focus on theoretical analysis and modeling of our proposed schemes [6] using Markov chain.

The remainder of this paper is organized as follows. The overall system is described in Section 2. Algorithms for the proposed multi-BAN interference mitigation are provided in Section 3. Theoretical analysis and modeling of interference mitigation for multiple BANs are presented in section 4. Finally, simulation results and conclusions are discussed in Sections 5 and 6 respectively.

2   System Description

In a BAN, several nodes form a network with a star topology. These nodes could share the same spectrum in a time-division multiple access manner based on the IEEE 802.15.6 standard. Therefore, there is no interference among the nodes within a single BAN. However, interference may come from other sources, such as nearby BANs or other coexisting non-BAN wireless networks. In the analysis, we focus on the performance at the controller (or master) node of the desired BAN. The Signal to Interference plus Noise Ratio (SINR) [7] at the controller node of BAN i is defined as:

$$SINR_i = \frac{S_i}{N + \sum_{j \neq i} S_j},$$ (1)

where S_i is the received power from the desired transmitter at the controller node of BAN i, S_j is received power from interferer j, and N is additive noise power.

The interference signal may come from any coexisting wireless network including other BANs that are not coordinated with the BAN i. Analyzing a special scenario with pre-specified node locations will not provide sufficient information in order to judge effectiveness of the mitigation schemes. Here, we assume that the desired received signal and total interference plus noise power information are available at the controller node of the considered BAN. Based on the available SINR, the controller node may command other nodes to select appropriate interference mitigation scheme.

3   Interference Mitigation for Multiple BANs

The purpose of interference mitigation is to lower the average transmit power using link adaptation schemes while maintaining link quality. Although, this might lead to lower throughput or data rate, it will allow for more number of active networks that can reliably coexist in possible interference rich environment. In low interference scenarios (i.e. normal operational status), all nodes can operate in their default (i.e. normal) mode. For higher levels of interference, one of the interference mitigation schemes will be activated. Here, we propose Interference Mitigation Factor (IMF) as a measure of the effectiveness of such schemes. The IMF is defined as the reduction of transmit power level using a mitigation scheme compared with the normal operational mode. In the next section, we will briefly review our proposed algorithms outlined in [6].

3.1   Adaptive Modulation

We consider a set of MPSK schemes (such as Ω={BPSK, QPSK, 8PSK}) for adaptive modulation due to their similar detection mechanism at the receiver. These modulation schemes can be easily implemented with minor modifications for link adaption. Given a pre-specified BER, the required SINR may be determined based on channel conditions. For higher SINR (i.e. normal operation), the 8PSK scheme is chosen in order to achieve higher bit rate. With an adaptive modulation scheme, QPSK or BPSK may be used to maintain the same BER. This will lower the required transmit power level, which will result in less interference to all other nodes in the neighboring BANs.

Two thresholds $\{\gamma_H, \gamma_L\}$ are considered to determine the range of adaptation within the set of modulation schemes. When SINR is higher than the higher threshold (i.e. γ_H), 8PSK scheme is used. Likewise, BPSK is chosen when SINR is lower than the lower threshold (i.e. γ_L). QPSK is used when the SINR is between the two thresholds. Since SINR may be changing rapidly in practice, a weighting factor α_M is introduced to maintain a running average of SINR over a fast changing channel. The algorithm for adaptive modulation scheme was presented in [6]. For adaptive modulation, the interference mitigation factor, when 8PSK is used as the normal mode, is defined as:

$$IMF(dB) = P_{8PSK}(dBm) - P_S(dBm) = 10\log\left(P_{8PSK}(watt)/P_S(watt)\right), \qquad (2)$$

where P_{8PSK} and P_S are the required transmit power for 8PSK and the chosen modulation scheme, S, respectively. The IMF is a function of SINR and channel condition.

3.2   Adaptive Data Rate

The second mitigation scheme is adaptive data rate. The data rate is divided into M steps between the maximum and minimum values R_{max} and R_{min}. The data rate is operated at R_{max} in the normal mode and is changed by comparing the weighted sum of SINR with the target SINR. The weighted sum (with an appropriate weighting factor $0 < \alpha_R < 1$) is used to smooth significant variation and fluctuation of SINR. A hysteresis factor Δ_R is also used to minimize possible ping-pong effect between the two data rates. The algorithm for interference mitigation using adaptive data rate was proposed in [6]. The relationship between the transmit power (S) and data rate (R) is:

$$\frac{E_b}{I_o + N_o} = \frac{S}{I_o + N_o}\frac{1}{R} \qquad (3)$$

where E_b, I_o, and N_o are bit energy, interference and noise spectral density, respectively. To keep the same required $E_b/(I_o + N_o)$, the transmit power and the data rate must be proportional. The higher the data rate, the more transmit power is required. Therefore, the instantaneous interference mitigation factor, when R_l is the data rate in the normal mode, is defined as:

$$IMF = 10 \cdot \log\frac{S_1}{S_f} = 10 \cdot \log\frac{R_1}{R_f} \text{ (dB)}, \qquad (4)$$

where S_l and S_f are the corresponding transmit powers for the rates R_l and R_f, respectively.

4   Theoretical Analysis

4.1   Autoregressive Process of Order 1 for SINR

As shown in Algorithms 1-2 [6], a weighted sum of SINR is used for the proposed adaptive schemes. This weighted sum of SINR may be rewritten in general form as below.

$$\bar{\gamma}_i = \alpha \cdot \gamma_i + (1-\alpha) \cdot \bar{\gamma}_{i-1}, \qquad (5)$$

where γ_i is assumed to have independent and identical distributions (*i.i.d.*) at discrete time $i \in \{-\infty, \dots -1, 0, 1, 2, \dots \infty\}$ and α is a weighting scalar. Thus $\bar{\gamma}_i$ is a recursive form of an autoregressive process of order 1 (i.e. AR(1)) [8]. If $|1-\alpha| < 1$, the process of $\bar{\gamma}_i$ is stationary. Practically, the weighting scalar is chosen between 0.5 and 1. (Note that the discrete random process $\bar{\gamma}_i$ remains identically distributed for all i, but not independent except when $\alpha = 1$.) If γ_i has a common mean μ and variance σ^2, the mean and variance of $\bar{\gamma}_i$ (unconditional case) are constant and independent of i and may be obtained as below.

$$\mu_{un} = E(\bar{\gamma}_i) = \mu \text{ and } \sigma_{un}^2 = Var(\bar{\gamma}_i) = \alpha\sigma^2/(2-\alpha) \tag{6}$$

On the other hand, the mean and variance of $\bar{\gamma}_i$ given $\bar{\gamma}_{i-1}$ (conditional case) can be expressed by:

$$\mu_c = E(\bar{\gamma}_i \mid \bar{\gamma}_{i-1} = z) = \alpha\mu + (1-\alpha)z, \text{ and } \sigma_c^2 = Var(\bar{\gamma}_i \mid \bar{\gamma}_{i-1} = z) = \alpha^2\sigma^2 \tag{7}$$

Note that the SINR measurements γ_i is not necessarily a Gaussian process. However, if γ_i is a Gaussian process, then $\bar{\gamma}_i$ will also be a Gaussian process for both unconditional and conditional cases. In other non-Gaussian cases, the central limit theorem indicates that $\bar{\gamma}_i$ will be approximately Gaussian when α is close to zero. The theoretical analysis under the Gaussian assumption has been provided in the following two subsections (4.2 and 4.3). For the non-Gaussian case with given distribution $\bar{\gamma}_i$, the formula can also be derived in a similar way.

4.2   Model for Adaptive Modulation

From the discussion in the previous section, we realize that $\bar{\gamma}_i$ has an identical distribution for each i. In this approach, a modulation scheme is chosen at any time instant i according to the predefined thresholds and the distribution of $\bar{\gamma}_i$ as shown in Algorithm 1 [6]. Therefore, the steady state probabilities of having BPSK, QPSK or 8PSK may be easily obtained as below.

$$\begin{aligned}
\pi(BPSK) &= P_r\{\bar{\gamma}_i < \gamma_L\} \\
\pi(8PSK) &= P_r\{\bar{\gamma}_i > \gamma_H\} \\
\pi(QPSK) &= P_r\{\gamma_L \leq \bar{\gamma}_i \leq \gamma_H\}
\end{aligned} \tag{8}$$

If $\bar{\gamma}_i$ has a Gaussian distribution with mean and standard deviation as shown in Eq. (6), then the steady state probabilities are given by:

$$\pi(BPSK) = P_r\{\bar{\gamma}_i < \gamma_L\} = 1 - Q\{(\gamma_L - \mu_{un})/\sigma_{un}\} \tag{9}$$

$$\pi(8PSK) = P_r\{\bar{\gamma}_i > \gamma_H\} = Q\{(\gamma_H - \mu_{un})/\sigma_{un}\} \tag{10}$$

where

$$Q(x) = \int_x^\infty \frac{1}{\sqrt{2\pi}} e^{-u^2/2} du \; . \tag{11}$$

From Equations (2) and (8), the average IMF for the adaptive modulation is obtained as.

$$IMF_{avg}(dB) = 10\log\left(\frac{P_{8PSK}(watt)}{\sum_{s\in\Omega}\pi(s)P_s(watt)}\right) \tag{12}$$

4.3   Model for Adaptive Data Rate

From Algorithm 2 [6], and when $\alpha = 1$, the adaptive data rate forms a finite state Markov process. For $\alpha \neq 1$, this will not be the case since the distribution of $\bar{\gamma}_i$ will depend on the prior events. However, given the conditional distribution of $\bar{\gamma}_i$, the process of adaptive data rate will still be a Markov process, and more specifically, a birth-death process. If $\bar{\gamma}_i$ has a Gaussian distribution, its mean and variance may be obtained from Eq. (7). And, its conditional distribution will be $i.i.d.$ As a result, the birth and the death rates will be independent of the state as shown in Fig. 1. In other words, the transition probabilities of the birth-death process (p and q) are constant and can be calculated by:

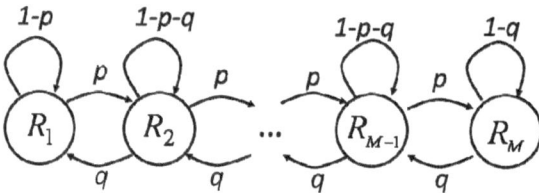

Fig. 1. Markov Process Model for Adaptive Data Rate

$$p = P_{m,m+1} = P_r\{\bar{\gamma}_i < \hat{\gamma} - \Delta_R\} = 1 - Q\left\{(\hat{\gamma} - \Delta_R - \mu_c)\Big/\sqrt{\frac{\alpha}{2-\alpha}} \cdot \sigma_c\right\} \tag{13}$$

$$q = P_{m,m-1} = P_r\{\bar{\gamma}_i > \hat{\gamma} + \Delta_R\} = Q\left\{(\hat{\gamma} + \Delta_R - \mu_c)\Big/\sqrt{\frac{\alpha}{2-\alpha}} \cdot \sigma_c\right\} \tag{14}$$

Given p and q in Equations (13) and (14), the conditional steady state probability of R_m, given $\bar{\gamma}_{i-1} = z$, is $\pi_z(R_m)$ and may be obtained by solving the following set of equations.

$$\begin{cases} \pi_z(R_j) = \sum_{m=1}^{M} p_{m,j} \cdot \pi_z(R_m) \\ \sum_{m=1}^{M} \pi_z(R_m) = 1 \end{cases} \tag{15}$$

The first equation of this set may be rewritten in matrix form as below.

$$\begin{bmatrix} \pi_z(R_1) \\ \pi_z(R_2) \\ \vdots \\ \pi_z(R_{M-1}) \\ \pi_z(R_M) \end{bmatrix} = \begin{bmatrix} 1-p & q & \cdots & 0 & 0 \\ p & 1-p-q & \cdots & 0 & 0 \\ \vdots & \vdots & \ddots & \vdots & \vdots \\ 0 & 0 & \cdots & 1-p-q & q \\ 0 & 0 & \cdots & p & 1-q \end{bmatrix} \begin{bmatrix} \pi_z(R_1) \\ \pi_z(R_2) \\ \vdots \\ \pi_z(R_{M-1}) \\ \pi_z(R_M) \end{bmatrix} \tag{16}$$

From (15), the conditional steady state probabilities $\pi_z(R_m)$, $m=1,2,...,M$, of the Markov process are given by

$$\pi_z(R_m) = \frac{(p/q)^{m-1}}{\sum\limits_{i=1}^{M}(p/q)^{i-1}} = \begin{cases} \dfrac{(p/q)^{m-1}-(p/q)^m}{1-(p/q)^M} & \text{if } p \neq q \\ 1/M & \text{if } p = q \end{cases} \tag{17}$$

With a Gaussian assumption and Eq. (6), the distribution of $\bar{\gamma}_{i-1}$ is given by

$$P_r(\bar{\gamma}_{i-1} = z) = \frac{1}{\sqrt{2\pi}\sigma_{un}} \exp\left(\frac{-(z-\mu_{un})^2}{2\sigma_{un}^2}\right). \tag{18}$$

Thus, the unconditional steady state probabilities $\pi(R_m)$, $m=1,2,...,M$, of the Markov process are given by

$$\pi(R_m) = \int_{-\infty}^{\infty} \pi_z(R_m) \frac{1}{\sqrt{2\pi}\sigma_{un}} e^{-(z-\mu_{un})^2/2\sigma_{un}^2} du. \tag{19}$$

The average IMF for adaptive data rate may be obtained by combining Equations (4) and (19) as below.

$$IMF_{avg} = 10 \cdot \log \frac{R_1}{\sum\limits_{m} R_m \cdot \pi(R_m)} \text{ (dB)} \tag{20}$$

From Equations (13), (14) and (17), the following special scenarios can be observed.
   (i) if $\hat{\gamma} = \mu_c$, then $p=q$ and the steady state probabilities are equal to $1/M$ for all data rates of R_m. Also the average IMF is a constant and independent of σ.

(ii) if $\hat{\gamma} = \mu_c$, the value of p (and q) decreases while Δ_R increases.

(iii) if $\Delta_R = 0$, then $p + q = 1$.

(iv) if $p > q$, the steady state probability of R_m increases with m. That is, the data rate becomes lower in order to decrease interference level.

5   Simulation Results

The channel model used is that of body surface to external nodes at 2.4 GHz as outlined in [7]. The effect of shadowing has been considered by a lognormal distribution with standard deviation of 3.80 dB for a hospital room [7]. Assume that there exists co-channel interference from other BANs as well as other non-BAN networks. Also, assume that each one of the BAN interferers is causing the same level of interference. Due to higher transmit power; the non-BAN interferer usually causes higher levels of interference. We also assume that the distribution of shadowing for all interferers is identical (i.e. lognormal distribution with the same standard deviation). Therefore, the SINR values can be generated based on the lognormal distributions. Note that the distribution of total interference plus noise is not log-normal. However, an approximation of lognormal distribution may be used if one of the interference signals is dominant. In our simulation, we have not used this approximation. In the theoretical analysis, however, the lognormal distribution assumption was made for interference plus noise. The comparison between simulation and theoretical results will therefore highlight the validity of this assumption. The average IMF will be evaluated in terms of signal to other BAN interference ratio plus noise, S / I_{BAN} and non-BAN to BAN interference ratio, $I_{non-BAN} / I_{BAN}$.

5.1   Adaptive Modulation

The adaptive modulation schemes considered in our simulation include BPSK, QPSK, and 8PSK. To select the thresholds γ_H and γ_L, BER performance of modulation schemes over AWGN channel is used. At BER=0.1%, the required SNR values are 6.8 dB, 9.8 dB and 14.8 dB for BPSK, QPSK and 8PSK, respectively [9]. Therefore, we choose $\gamma_H = 12dB$, $\gamma_L = 8dB$. These threshold values may be adjusted with channel conditions if necessary. The interferers include 3 other close-by BANs and one non-BAN interferer. Let S be the desired received signal power. Define I_{BAN} to be the received interference power from each BAN interferer; likewise, define $I_{non-BAN}$ to be the received interference power from a non-BAN source. The results shown in Fig. 2 indicate a good agreement between simulation and theoretical analysis. As expected, given the same S / I_{BAN} , higher non-BAN interference levels will lead to higher average IMF. And under those circumstances, BPSK is the choice for the modulation scheme since it requires lower transmit power for a given BER. Higher average IMF is also observed at lower values of S / I_{BAN} .

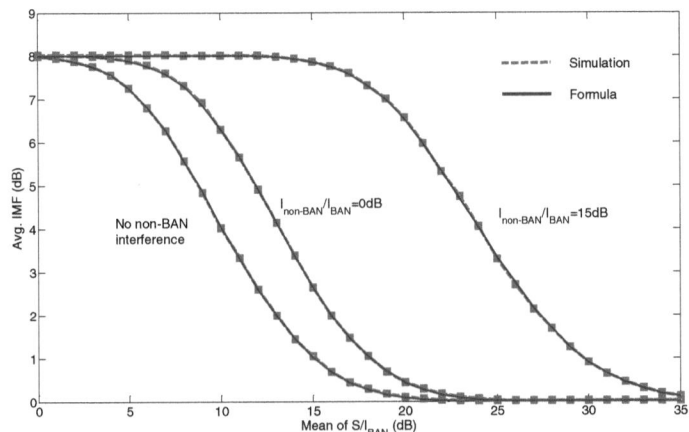

Fig. 2. Interference mitigation using adaptive modulation at $\alpha_M = 0.8$

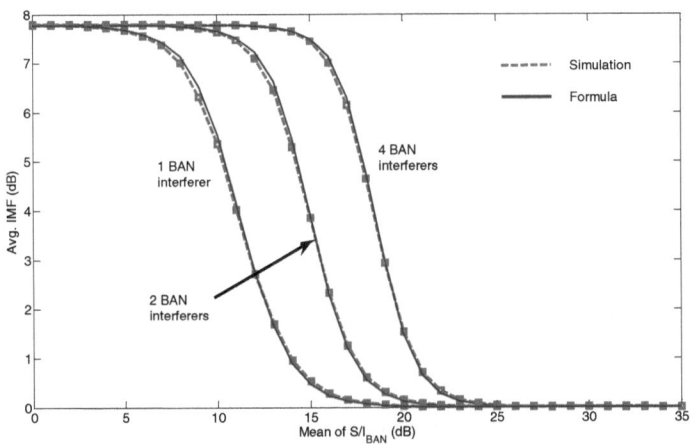

Fig. 3. Interference mitigation using adaptive data rate

5.2   Adaptive Data Rate

Average interference mitigation factors in terms of mean of SINR and number of BAN interferers using adaptive data rate scheme are shown in Fig. 3. The mean of S/I_{BAN} at the x-axis is the ratio of signal to one BAN interference. All the BAN interfering signals have statistics with the same mean and standard deviation. The total interference power is calculated by summing total interference power, where the number of BAN interferers is from 1, 2 and 4. The data rates may be chosen in accordance with the quality of service (QoS) requirements. The set of data rates in the simulation is assumed to be {600, 400, 200, 100} kbps while $\alpha_R = 0.8$, $\Delta_R = 2.0\,\mathrm{dB}$

and $\hat{\gamma} = 12dB$. As expected, the more BAN interferers, the more the average IMF, which requires a lower data rate. For lower mean of SINR cases, higher average IMF values are observed. This effectively means a lower data communication rate for the link at the lower mean of SINR cases. Again, the results shown in Fig. 3 using simulation and theoretical formula match very well.

6   Conclusion

In this paper, we have proposed and analyzed two interference mitigation schemes including adaptive modulation and adaptive data rate. A quantitative measure called the interference mitigation factor was used to evaluate the effectiveness of these schemes in body area networks applications. These schemes are relatively simple and well-suited for very low power nodes in body area networks that might be operating in environments with high interference level. Theoretical analysis to assess the performance of these schemes has also been provided. Results of the theoretical analysis show a close match with simulations. This theoretical analysis is particularly helpful to determine or optimize the parameters used in the adaptive schemes.

References

1. Yang, G.: Body sensor networks. Springer-Verlag London Limited (2006) ISBN 1-84628-272-1
2. Xiao, S., et al.: Transmission power control in body area sensor networks for healthcare monitoring. IEEE Journal on Selected Areas in Communications 27(1) (January 2009)
3. Kazemi, R., et al.: Inter-Network Interference Mitigation in Wireless Body Area Networks Using Power Control Games. In: 10th International Symposium on Communications and Information Technologies, Tokyo, Japan (2010)
4. Fantacci, R.: Proposal of an interference cancellation receiver with low complexity for DS/CDMA mobile communication systems. IEEE Trans. Vehicular Technology 48, 1039–1046 (1999)
5. Zhang, H., Dai, H.: Design Fundamentals and Interference Mitigation for Cellular Networks. In: Min, G., Pan, Y., Fan, P. (eds.) Advances in Wireless Networks: Performance Modeling, Analysis and Enhancement. Nova Science Publishers (2008)
6. Yang, W.-B., Sayrafian-Pour, K.: Interference Mitigation for body area networks. In: IEEE PIMRC 2011, Toronto, Canada, pp. 2201–2207 (2011)
7. Yazdandoost, K.Y., Sayrafian-Pour, K.: Channel Models for Body Area Network (BAN). IEEE P802.15-08-0780-10-0006 (2010)
8. Hamilton, J.: Time Series Analysis. Princeton Press (1994)
9. Proakis, J.: Digital Communications, 4th edn. McGraw-Hill (2001) ISBN 0-07-232111-3
10. Yang, W.-B., Sayrafian-Pour, K.: A DS-CDMA interference cancellation technique for body area networks. In: IEEE PIMRC 2010, Istanbul, Turkey, pp. 751–755 (2010)
11. Yang, W.-B., Sayrafian-Pour, K.: A low complexity interference cancellation technique for multi-user DS-CDMA communication. In: ICC 2010, Cape Town, South Africa (2010)

Remote Programming of Biomedical Smart Sensors

David Naranjo[2,1], Laura M. Roa[1,2], Javier Reina-Tosina[3,2],
and Miguel A. Estudillo-Valderrama[2,1]

[1] Biomedical Engineering Group, University of Seville, Seville, Spain
[2] CIBER de Bioingeniería, Biomateriales y Nanomedicina (CIBER-BBN), Spain
[3] Dept. of Signal Theory and Communications, University of Seville, Seville, Spain
{dnaranjo,lroa,jreina,m.estudillo}@us.es

Abstract. This paper proposes a processing architecture and a programming framework for the remote and seamless update of the algorithms used in the context of biomedical smart sensors. The generic processing architecture provides, among others, the following facilities to a Body Sensor Network in a seamless way to the user beyond functional modularity: 1) direct and immediate update with new and improved versions of the algorithms, 2) personalization of algorithms, 3) adaptability to the user context, 4) remote test of algorithms, 5) hardware reusability and sustainability, 6) parallel execution of several monitoring applications in one device, 7) structural modularity. Due to its simplicity, the proposed technique takes advantage over other solutions employed in applications that impose severe limitations on hardware/software resources of the devices, which may result in lower cost and size of them. The results obtained on two heart monitoring applications shows the viability of the proposed scheme.

Keywords: Biomedical smart sensor, Body Sensor Network, code dissemination, remote programming, structural modularity.

1 Introduction

Population ageing and the rise of chronic diseases [1] make necessary the application of new technologies for the improvement of patients welfare and the sustainability of the associated costs. Body Sensor Networks (BSN) are a promising solution in this context, because they make possible the real-time unobstructive ubiquitous monitoring of patient's health status and the detection of emergencies [2, 3]. This kind of sensor networks pose important restrictions in terms of size, computation, communication, energy consumption and data storage, related with the requirements of portability, transparency and long battery lifetime, which are even more evident when dealing with implanted sensors [4,5].

In order to reduce consumption in communications, many authors propose diverse functional modularity approaches like an initial processing within the intelligent sensors so as to reduce the number of data sent [2,6–8]. For this purpose,

B. Godara and K.S. Nikita (Eds.): MobiHealth 2012, LNICST 61, pp. 199–206, 2013.
© Institute for Computer Sciences, Social Informatics and Telecommunications Engineering 2013

it is necessary to provide the customization of BSNs to adapt its functionality to changes in patient's medical condition, context, activity, individual needs or lifestyles [3, 6, 9]. However, despite the fact that the spread of code technique is widely used in generic wireless sensor networks [10, 11], there are few authors who have considered the possibility of a remote and user-seamless update of the software in the context of BSNs.

The vast majority of the solutions for BSNs are developed in *motes* and use frameworks based on the TinyOS operating system to support dynamic modification of code with different levels of abstraction [2, 6, 12]: A model-driven development in which the models are translated into platform-dependent code, virtual machines with byte code interpreters running on TinyOS, or programming abstractions free of low level details. However, when the restrictions of size, cost and energy limit the use of microcontrollers with the ability to integrate an operating system, even as light as TinyOS, the functional modularity faces poor performance due to the structural hardware/ software (HW/SW) constraints of the arquitecture, and many times other architectures are required for the remote programming of sensors. In such situations, a possible solution could be the sending of firmware with a very reduced set of instructions [13], which has the disadvantage that they are limited to the specific application for which they have been developed and may fail to provide sufficient flexibility to develop algorithms out of the functional domain of the instruction set.

In the present paper, it is proposed a processing architecture and programming framework designed to consume the fewest resources in smart sensors with very limited hardware-software capabilities. This architecture provides the ability to remotely upgrade the software of intelligent sensors (dissemination code) transparently to the user, a framework for running multiple applications in parallel within a single device, and the minimization of energy consumption in communications. As a proof-of-concept, the proposed scheme has been validated in a laboratory setup on an ECG virtual sensor, since both the processing and the definition of the observed characteristics of such signals are necessary to make a customization and adaptation to the activity and user context [3, 9].

1.1   Distributed Processing Architecture

In the proposed approach, smart sensors are devices able to send, wirelessly and unobtrusively, the monitored physiological information. The smart sensors perform a first information processing, in order to distribute the processing load among all the devices, abstract and compress the captured information to send only the relevant data and execute a first detection of events related with the physiological variables under monitorization. A wearable device with more computational and energy resources, referred to as Decision-Analysis Device (DAD), manages the information provided by all sensors and connects, if necessary, with the Remote Telehealthcare Center (RTC) [14] (see Figure 1).

The design of the smart sensors follows a modular scheme in order to facilitate the integration of new technologies in the devices, both for processing and communications tasks:

1. Sensor device: it constitutes the acquisition element of the physiological monitoring signals.
2. Communications module: Unit responsible for the transmission of biomedical information that releases the processing module from all the tasks associated with communications.
3. Processing unit: The intelligence of the sensor device is provided by the processing modules (PMs) that are executed in real-time and in parallel within the processing unit of the smart sensor. Each PM is capable of transmitting the captured information or the result of its processing. This data are structured into information samples generated with a given sampling frequency, which can be set via commands. In the normal operating modes of the PMs, no data are sent until the sensor device detects an alert event after processing the monitored physiological variables. This way, the overall system consumption is minimized [14].

2   Remote Programming Mechanism

Taking into account that PM interfaces are perfectly defined, the addition or removal of a new module does not affect to the rest of them, and thus the system integrity is not affected. In addition, these modules are designed to work in parallel, therefore they can cooperate easily. The developed modular scheme also allows updating the devices functionalities in order to adapt them to the user information needs. In the case of the smart sensor, the addition, update or removal of PMs can be developed by means of a firmware update of the PMs within the smart sensor (adaptable functionality, personalization and medium and context adaptation) which could be remotely performed in real time. In order to enable these characteristics, without forgetting that the smart sensor processing capabilities are limited by the device size and power consumption, a software architecture that allows the execution and the optimum management of the PMs has been researched and developed.

According to the proposed paradigm, the data memory (related to microcontroller RAM) is divided into the following blocks (see Figure 1):

1. DAT_G: related to the global variables for the device performance management.
2. DAT_I: this data block stores the information needed to manage the queues of data employed by the PMs. DAT_I is divided in turn into several subblocks, one per queue, each of which consists of the initial and final address of the queue in the data memory, the address where the next data will enter in the queue and the number of items in the queue.
3. DAT_C: area of memory where different data queues are implemented.

The information is organized into queues to facilitate its transference in this modular architecture. Several procedures to extract data from the queues, read indexed information or enter new data are also considered. The proposed scheme uses the following queues:

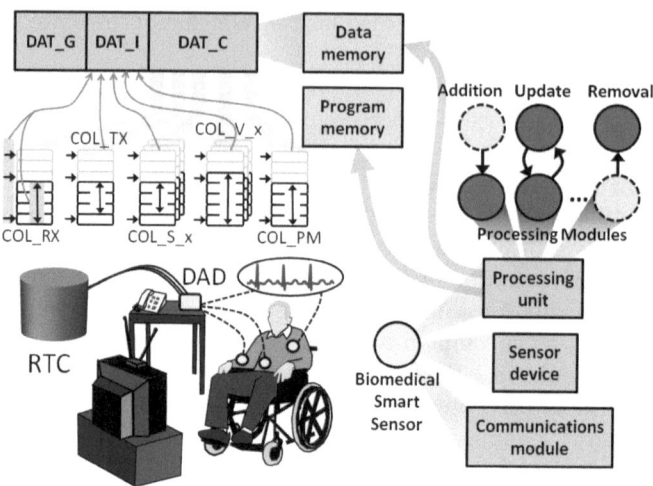

Fig. 1. Structural modularity in the proposed distributed monitoring system and data memory of the processing unit

1. *COL_RX*: a queue that stores the data received from the DAD.
2. *COL_TX*: a queue that stores the information to be sent to the DAD.
3. *COL_S_x* ($x = 1..N\_PM$, N_PM defined below) a queue for each PM where the information samples associated with the PM are stored.
4. *COL_V_x* ($x = 1..N\_PM$): a queue for each PM that stores the current values of the variables used by the PM. At the beginning of the PM execution, the data are transferred to the spaces reserved for the auxiliary variables. Then, these updated data return to the queue at the end of the execution. Since the PMs work only with auxiliary variables, the generic use of the device's memory capacity is powered.
5. *COL_PM*: this queue stores the information needed for the implementation of the different processing modules. It consists of a first field that indicates the number of PMs (N_PM), followed by N_PM blocks which are broken down into the following elements: the PM identifier (unique for each PM development), the initial program memory address of the PM, the number of 8 bytes blocks that compound the PM, the memory data address where the *DAT_I* information sub-block of the *COL_S_x* queue associated with the PM starts, and the address of the data memory where the *DAT_I* information sub-block of the *COL_V_x* queue starts.

On the other hand, the program memory (nonvolatile) is organized into the following blocks to facilitate the implementation of the modular software (see Figure 2):

1. *PROG_Gen*: related to the non-modifiable generic code of the device, which is responsible for the administration and management of its overall operation as well as the PMs implemented on it.

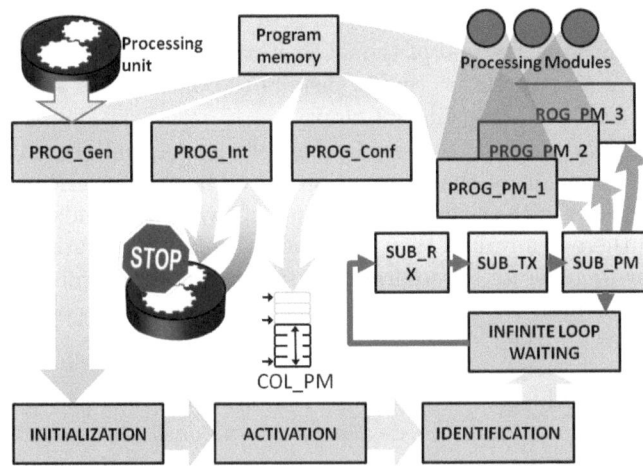

Fig. 2. Structural modularity in program memory and processing unit operation

2. *PROG_Int*: where the non-modifiable interrupt routines that control the peripheral of the smart sensor processing unit are implemented (timers, sensor data capture, transmissions, etc.).
3. *PROG_Conf*: where the code responsible for the setting of the appropriate parameters in the *COL_PM* queue after a device reset is placed, to ensure the correct management of the PMs. This code is remotely changed every time a PM is added, modified or deleted.
4. *PROG_PM_x* $(x = 1..N\_PM)$: the N_PM modifiable memory blocks are subsequently located containing the operation code of the PMs, one per block.

The device operation is based on the execution of the following operating system algorithm corresponding to the generic code stored in *PROG_Gen*:

1. INITIALIZATION: setup of initial global parameters and device peripherals initialization.
2. ACTIVATION: activation of the executing code stored in *PROG_Conf* for the configuration of *COL_PM* queue.
3. IDENTIFICATION: process in which the smart sensor transmits the contents of the *PROG_Conf* queue to the DAD. Thus, the DAD knows the device memory map and identifies the PMs implemented in the smart sensor. This identification can also be activated through a command.
4. INFINITE LOOP WAITING: where the following subroutines are activated whenever a data from the sensor is received:
   (a) *SUB_RX*: subroutine that receives data from the DAD, which are stored in the *COL_RX* queue. The transceiver develops a low-power transmission protocol that enables the smart sensor PM to transparently communicate with the DAD. A detailed explanation of this communication protocol exceeds the scope of this paper. If the reception of a command

is completed, its processing starts. If the command is for a PM, it is introduced at the end of the COL_V_x queue associated with the PM.

(b) SUB_TX: subroutine that transmits the data to the DAD in the case that COL_TX queue is not empty.

(c) SUB_PM: subroutine responsible for the sequential execution of the PMs by means of the information stored in the COL_PM queue. Each PM begins with the execution of the received commands associated with it, if there is any, and then continues with the information processing in order to generate the information samples and perform the detection of events. Finally, it ends with the storage of the data to be transmitted to the DAD in the COL_TX queue, if necessary.

The procedure to add, edit or delete a PM is initiated by sending a programming command, which suspends the device operation until the end of the writing process in program memory. Afterwards, the smart sensor is reset.

3   Validation of the Proposed Technique

In order to validate the proposed framework a virtual ECG sensor has been implemented consisting of a PIC18F2431 microcontroller from Microchip as the processing unit, a CC2430 Chipcom transceiver that corresponds to the communications module and an algorithm in the microcontroller core that simulates the periodical reception of ECG signals. A processing module for the detection of heartbeats has been developed, which is an important parameter for the detection of tachycardia, bradycardia and fibrillation, and a processing module to estimate PQ interval duration, which is of relevance in the detection of auricle-ventricular conduction defects, atrioventricular blocks or blocks of His bundle branches [9]. Both modules generate data samples at a rate of 500 Hz and transmit data continuously. The following experimental setup was developed:

1. A transceiver located 3m apart from the virtual sensor wirelessly sent the processing module to detect the heartbeat (about 400 bytes).
2. After about 4 seconds, the device began sending information samples of heart rate.
3. Afterwards, the processing module to estimate the duration of PQ interval was wirelessly sent (about 1 Kbyte).
4. After about 7 seconds, the device began sending information samples of heart rate and the estimated duration of the PQ interval.
5. Later on, a command was wirelessly sent to remove the processing module for detecting the heartbeat, and almost immediately, the device began sending only information samples corresponding to PQ interval.

These update times are comparable to others obtained by other authors with similar code sizes and greater resources in the devices [3, 15], including generic Wireless Sensor Networks [10] (see Table 1).

Table 1. Comparison of the results obtained with related works

	Code size	Update time	Description	Resources
This work	1 KB	7 sec	Parallel processing modules managed by a generic code	ROM: 984 B RAM: 46 B (Generic code)
[3, 15]	9 KB	10 sec	Command interpreter (MedOS) that acts as a virtual machine upon FreeRTOS	ROM: 6 KB (MedOS + FreeRTOS)
[10]	10 KB	30 sec	Code dissemination system (Seluge) for wireless sensor networks running TinyOS	ROM: 45258 B RAM: 2278 B (only Seluge)

4 Conclusion

The results show the feasibility of the processing architecture and programming framework proposed as a method for updating remotely software from intelligent sensors (code dissemination) transparently to the user and to the execution of multiple applications in parallel within one device. The addition, update or removal of new functionalities does not affect to the rest of them, or the system integrity. Due to its simplicity and compared to other proposals, the proposed scheme allows to be used for smart sensors with very limited HW/SW resources, such as the case of implants. Furthermore, the approaches of other authors address the problem through a functional modularity, whereas in the present work goes further, also establishing a structural modality that affects to the system architecture. In addition, the referred generic processing architecture provides, among others, the following facilities to a BSN in a seamless way to the user: 1) update capability of the processing algorithms to include any improvement or modification that may arise as a result of future research; 2) personalization of algorithms to remotely fit the particular characteristics of the user; 3) adaptability to the context in which the user is monitored or his/her vital signs; 4) remote test of algorithms; 5) hardware reusability for different applications so as to obtain lower development costs and a greater sustainability of the devices.

Future works will be the development of security mechanisms to prevent malicious software modification, and guarantee data protection and error-free and robust execution of processing algorithms. Once established such mechanisms, the system will undergo a comprehensive experimental study to verify and validate the operation of the programming and processing architecture, detect errors, correct and document them, in accordance with the regulations for medical devices (FDA or European Commission). Furthermore, the proposed system enables the software update to correct problems identified a posteriori, according to the regulations, but with the advantage of being performed immediately.

Acknowledgments. This work was supported in part by the CIBER de Bioingeniería, Biomateriales y Nanomedicina (CIBER-BBN) and the intramural Grant

PERSONA, in part by the Instituto de Salud Carlos III under Grants PI082023 and PI11/00111, and in part by the Dirección General de Investigación, Tecnología y Empresa, Government of Andalucía, under Grants P08-TIC-04069 and TIC6214. CIBER-BBN is an initiative funded by the 6th National R&D&i Plan 2008-2011, Iniciativa Ingenio 2010, Consolider Program, CIBER Actions and financed by the Instituto de Salud Carlos III with assistance from the European Regional Development Fund.

References

1. Thorpe, K., Philyaw, M.: The Medicalization of Chronic Disease and Costs. Annu. Rev. Public Health 33, 409–423 (2012)
2. Raveendranathan, N., et al.: From Modeling to Implementation of Virtual Sensors in Body Sensor Networks. IEEE Sensors J. 12(3), 583–593 (2012)
3. de Barbosa, T.A., da Rocha, A.: A Smart System to Program Body Sensor Networks. In: 5th IEEE Int. Conf. on Intelligent Systems, pp. 168–172 (2010)
4. Ghasemzadeh, H., Loseu, V., Ostadabbas, S., Jafari, R.: Burst Communication by means of Buffer Allocation in Body Sensor Networks. IEEE J. Sel. Areas Commun. 28(7), 1073–1082 (2010)
5. Mitsch, S., Kurschl, W., Schoenboeck, J.: Modeling Distributed Signal Processing Applications. In: 6th Int. Workshop on Wearable and Implantable Body Sensor Networks, pp. 103–108 (2009)
6. Zhu, Y., Keoh, S.L., Sloman, M., Lupu, E.: A Lightweight Policy System for Body Sensor Networks. IEEE Trans. Netw. Service Manag. 6(3), 137–148 (2009)
7. Mondal, N., Zaman, S., Al Masud, A., Alam, J.: Comparisons of Maximum System Lifetime in Diverse Scenarios for Body Sensor Networks. In: 11th Int. Conf. on Computer and Information Technology, pp. 73–78 (2008)
8. Nabar, S., Walling, J., Poovendran, R.: Minimizing Energy Consumption in Body Sensor Networks Via Convex Optimization. In: Int. Conf. on Body Sensor Networks (BSN), pp. 62–67 (2010)
9. Augustyniak, P.: Autoadaptivity and Optimization in Distributed Ecg Interpretation. IEEE Trans. Inf. Technol. Biomed. 14(2), 394–400 (2010)
10. Hyun, S., Ning, P., Liu, A., Du, W.: Seluge: Secure and DoS-Resistant Code Dissemination in Wireless Sensor Networks. In: Int. Conf. on Information Processing in Sensor Networks, pp. 445–456 (2008)
11. Miller, C., Poellabauer, C.: Paler: A Reliable Transport Protocol for Code Distribution in Large Sensor Networks. In: 5th IEEE Conf. on Sensor, Mesh and Ad Hoc Communications and Networks, pp. 206–214 (2008)
12. Kowalczuk, J., Vuran, M., Perez, L.: A Dual-Network Testbed for Wireless Sensor Applications. In: IEEE Global Telecommunications Conf., pp. 1–5 (2011)
13. Passama, R., Andreu, D., Guiraud, D.: Computer-Based Remote Programming and Control of Stimulation Units. In: 5th Int. IEEE/EMBS Conf. on Neural Engineering, pp. 538–541 (2011)
14. Naranjo, D., Roa, L., Reina, J., Estudillo, M.: Personalization and Adaptation to the Medium and Context in a Fall Detection System. IEEE Trans. Inf. Technol. Biomed. 16(2), 264–271 (2012)
15. Barbosa, T., Sene, I., da Rocha, A., Nascimento, F., Carvalho, H., Camapum, J.: Application-Oriented Programming Model for Sensor Networks Embedded in the Human Body. In: 28th Int. IEEE Conf. on Engineering in Medicine and Biology Society, pp. 6037–6040 (2006)

Mobile Multi-parametric Sensor System for Diagnosis of Epilepsy and Brain Related Disorders

Panagiota Anastasopoulou[1], Christos Antonopoulos[2], Hatem Shgir[1],
George Krikis[2,3], Nikolaos S. Voros[2], and Stefan Hey[1]

[1] Karlsruhe Institute of Technology,
Fritz-Erler-Str. 1-3, 76133 Karlsruhe, Germany
{panagiota.anastasopoulou,hatem.sghir,stefan.hey}@kit.edu
[2] Technological Educational Institute of Mesolonghi,
Department of Communication Systems and Networks
National Road Antiriou Nafpaktou, Varia, Nafpaktos 30300, Greece
{cantonopoulos,voros}@teimes.gr
[3] Noesis Technologies, L.P. Suite B5,
Patras Science Park Stadiou Str, Platani Rion 26504, Greece
gkrikis@noesis-tech.com

Abstract. Epilepsy is the commonest serious brain disorder, affecting 1-2% of the general population. Epileptic seizures are usually expressed with a wide range of paroxysmal recurring motor, cognitive, autonomic symptoms and EEG changes. Therefore reliable diagnosis requires state of the art monitoring and communication technologies providing real-time, accurate and continuous brain and body multi-parametric data measurements. The purpose of this paper is to present an adequate mobile system comprising all required sensor types for the everyday life monitoring of patients with epilepsy.

Keywords: epilepsy monitoring, biosensors, security and privacy.

1 Introduction

Epilepsy is one of the most common and devastating of the incurable neurological disorders, affecting about 1-2% of the general population. Due to its multifactorial causes and paroxysmal nature, epilepsy needs multi-parametric monitoring for purposes of accurate diagnosis, alerting, prevention, treatment follow-up and pre-surgical evaluation.

State of the art for the monitoring of epilepsy includes a series of laboratory tests. These tests can only be done in a specific unit of a specialized hospital, they are rather expensive (about 1,500 euros per day) and their diagnostic yield depends on whether the clinical event of interest occurs during the period of the monitoring (typically less than a week). Current diagnosis relies either on video EEG that records the habitual suspected event or ambulatory EEG without video. Recent research has shown that while ECG monitoring is used for real-time epileptic seizure detection [2], activity monitoring via accelerometry and GSR monitoring can also be used as extra context parameters [7-8], while monitoring epileptic patients.

B. Godara and K.S. Nikita (Eds.): MobiHealth 2012, LNICST 61, pp. 207–214, 2013.
© Institute for Computer Sciences, Social Informatics and Telecommunications Engineering 2013

Therefore reliable diagnosis requires technologies that provide real-time, accurate and continuous brain and body multi-parametric monitoring. The assessment of those physiological signals should be ambulatory and not affect the patient's everyday life. Furthermore extra attention on security aspects should be paid.

During the past years, several hardware and software solutions for multi-parametric assessment of physiological signals have been developed. However, none of them was able to provide an integrated platform for the assessment of all the parameters needed. Furthermore the proposed systems were not appropriate to be used in everyday life. Our goal is the development of an unobtrusive sensor platform, aiming to design and develop a Personal Health System (PHS) for monitoring and analysis of epilepsy-relevant multi-parametric data, emphasizing in convenience and security issues.

In section 2 of this paper, the architecture of the whole system is introduced. The focus of this section is the description of the mobile sensor-platform for multiparametric monitoring of different vital signals related to epilepsy and the description of encryption unit for secure transmission of the data. Section 3 presents the processing of the acquired signals and their role in diagnosis of epilepsy. Then section 4 presents the initial performance results, while section 5 concludes indicating the main objectives and directions of this on-going effort.

2   System

Depending on the type of epilepsy, different brain and body parameters need to be assessed in order to have a better understanding of the patient's state of health and to adapt the medical treatment accordingly. Therefore our goal is to develop a personalized system that assists in diagnosis, prognosis and treatment of the disease. Such system should fulfill the following criteria; it should be non-invasive, mobile, continuous, unobtrusive and all possible security and privacy aspects should be taken into account. Fig. 1 shows an overview of the system.

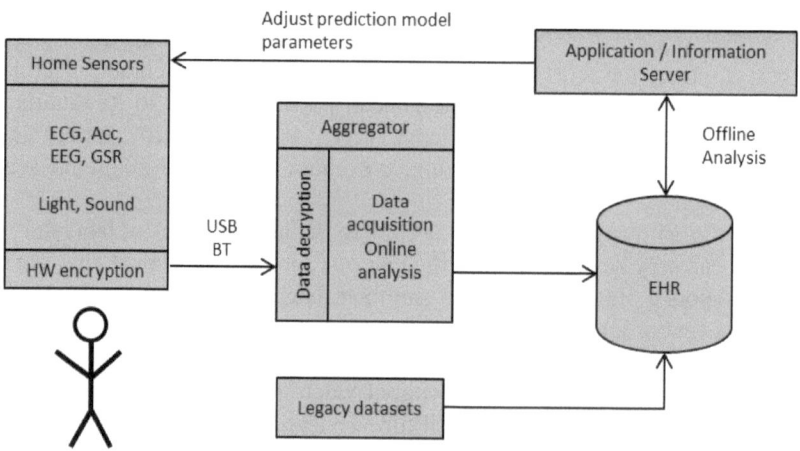

Fig. 1. System overview

The sensor platform performs the following actions: data logging, data preprocessing, data encryption and wireless transmission of the assessed data to an aggregator for further analysis. A Laptop used as an aggregator performs the data decryption (needed for the online analysis), processing and transmission to the Electronic Health Record (EHR) database. The transmission to the EHR is realized by a standardized SSL secure internet connection. EHR includes all the legacy datasets of the patient as well. The offline analysis of the data is realized on the information server. Based on the offline analysis, the prediction models may be adjusted, thus creating a personalized monitoring system.

2.1   Data Acquisition Unit

The measurement of the autonomic functions should be done by light-weight, portable, low-power sensors, specially developed for the assessment in everyday life.

Our main platform (Fig. 2) is based on a sensor platform developed by movisens (movisens GmbH, Karlsruhe, Germany) and consists of an ultra-low-power microcontroller (MSP430F1611, Texas Instruments) with an AD/DA converter, 2 UART interfaces, a 48 kB flash and a 10 kB RAM. The assessed data is encrypted and then transmitted wirelessly to the aggregator by using the Bluetooth interface. Due to the big amount of data to be transmitted, data reduction on the sensor side is fundamental. The transmitted data, following appropriate processing, are no longer raw data, thus reducing the amount of data to be transmitted. To avoid data loss in case the data transmission is not possible, the raw data is in parallel stored in a 2 GB micro SD card. The stored data can then be saved on the computer by using the USB 2.0 interface that is available. The charging of the power supply of the sensors is recognized by the USB interface as well.

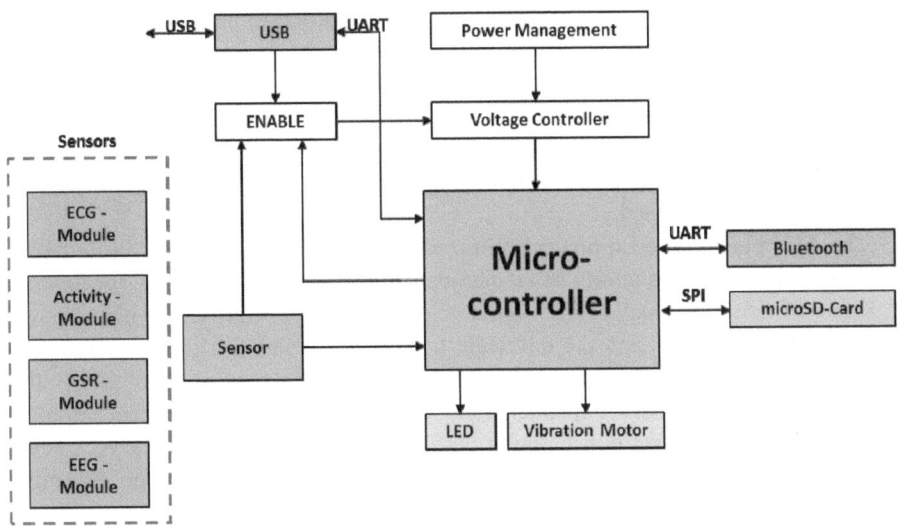

Fig. 2. Architecture of the sensor platform

The ECG module is a single channel ECG recorder with a 12 bit resolution and a sampling rate from 256 Hz to 1024 Hz. The electrodes are integrated into a wearable chest strap, which is light, small and comfortable. The electrodes are dry, allowing the everyday use of the chest strap.

The activity monitoring module consists of a triaxial acceleration sensor (adxl345, Analog Devices Inc.) with a range of ± 8 g and a sampling frequency of 64 Hz. The measuring unit has an additional air pressure sensor (BMP085, Bosch GmbH) with a sampling frequency of 8 Hz and a resolution of 0.03hPa (corresponding to 15 cm).

The galvanic skin response (GSR) module measures the skin conductance with a sampling rate of 32Hz. The measurement range of the GSR module is 2µS to 100µS and its resolution is 14 bit.

Beside the above mentioned modules, the sensor platform will include an additional EEG module, which will record the brain activity.

To assess additional context parameters like sound, light or geographic position, a smartphone is used. Connection between Smartphone, Sensor and Aggregator is also realized by Bluetooth interface.

2.2   Data Encryption Unit

In wirelessly transmitting medical and highly sensitive data, security support is a prerequisite of primary importance. Respective support pertains to data privacy, data integrity and authentication of communication parties. However, provision of security features pose significant challenges in sensor network due to extremely limited resources in critical areas such as processing power, available memory and available energy. Furthermore, although Bluetooth Technology offers security features with respect to both authentication and privacy, at the same time respective weaknesses and vulnerabilities are quite well-known [10]. Additionally, significant overhead imposed by software security implementations as opposed to hardware implemented counterparts must be taken into consideration [11].

Based on these considerations, an FPGA based hardware implementation solution has been selected, aiming to provide high level security services while minimizing respective performance overhead. An ultra-low power dissipation 128bit block AES encryption cipher comprises the core encryption algorithm upon which data privacy and authentication is based.

The AES block has been power optimized by using advanced power-aware design techniques coupled with a fully serial data-path architecture. Indicatively, for Spartan-6 Xilinx FPGA technology (45 nm process, core voltage 1 Volt), the dynamic power dissipation is 6 mWatts and the quiescent power dissipation is 11 mWatts assuming 10 MHz operating frequency and a worst case I/Os & FFs toggle rate of 100%. It is also noted that the FPGA implementation is used as a proof of concept approach concerning mainly power consumption performance while other approaches such as ASIC implementation can be considered at second phase in order to satisfy unobtrusiveness requirements.

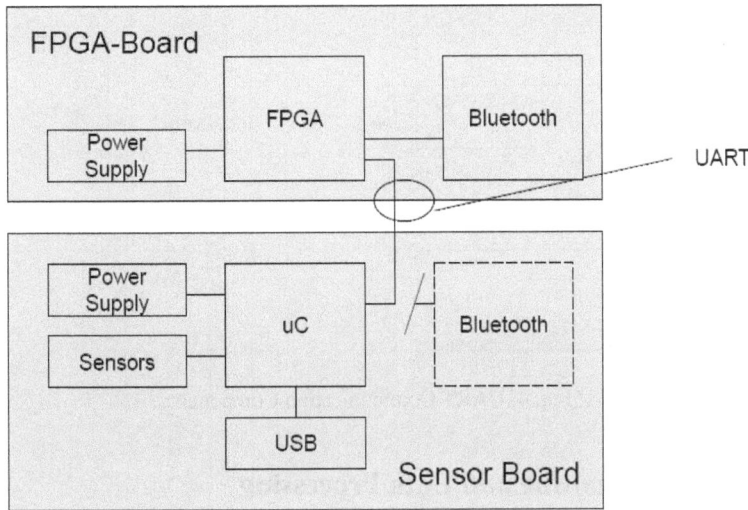

Fig. 3. Encryption and Data Acquisition Units Interconnection Design

A critical issue requiring careful consideration is the communication between the encryption unit and data acquisition unit; an abstract design of the proposed architecture is depicted in Fig. 3.

As indicated by the presented approach, the microcontroller - Bluetooth module connection is essentially interrupted and data is conveyed directly to the encryption unit. Following adequate data processing data is again directed to the Bluetooth unit to be wirelessly transmitted. An important advantage offered by this scheme is the opportunity to directly compare metrics of performance and power dissipation. This metrics consider all possible functional combinations between the hardware implemented AES cipher and Bluetooth provided security features.

Focusing on the interconnection implementation, the microcontroller unit provides the data blocks for encryption towards the FPGA platform via RS232 serial link. Therefore an adequate communication protocol is specified in order to enable a prompt implementation. Fig. 4 shows the components of the FPGA module and the communication among them.

As depicted, the data transferred over the UART link is stored in the register file. When a block of data is completed a respective status register indicates that a new data block is ready to be encrypted by the AES module.

Finally, as AES comprises one of the most prominent symmetric ciphers, appropriate encryption keys must be agreed between communicating parties. In that respect various scenarios in sensor network will be evaluated ranging from network wide keys, to pair-wise predefined keys [12]. Predefined keys appear as an appropriate approach since due to the nature of medical applications, nodes comprising a relative medical kit are expected to be also predefined. Provision of such kits are normally controlled and monitored by adequate medical facilities and personnel in order to adhere to the required privacy and ethical requirements [13].

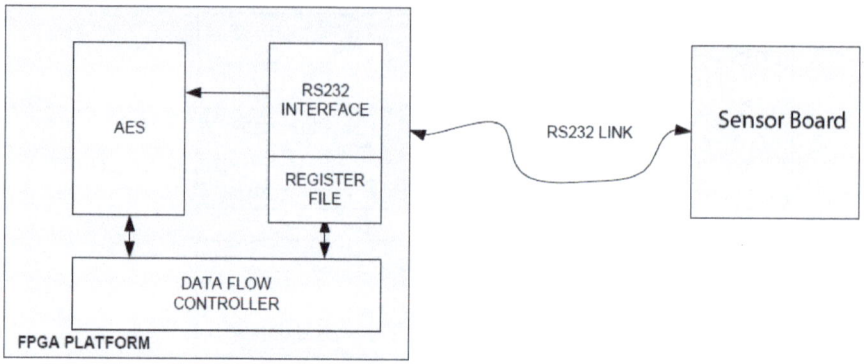

Fig. 4. UART Communication Components

3   Data Formatting and Data Processing

The data format which is being used is the unisens-format [5]. This is a universal and generic format suitable for recording and archiving sensor data from various recording systems and with various sampling frequencies.

The data acquisition on the aggregator side is performed by using xAffect [9]. xAffect is an open source software framework for online recording, processing and storage of multi sensor data. It was developed at FZI Research Center for Information Technology, Karlsruhe, Germany and can be used as a standalone application for data acquisition and visualization.

In the following significant types of measurements are presented and their role in epilepsy monitoring is depicted.

EEG monitoring is the state of the art while monitoring epileptic patients. It allows early detection of changes in the neurological status by providing dynamic information about brain function. In a clinical setting, a common practice involves examining short recordings of interictal periods. During this period, individual or isolated spikes, a sharp wave or a spike-and-wave complex are most commonly seen in epileptic patients [4].

ECG monitoring is one of the most crucial elements of monitoring in almost every disease. The ECG raw signal can be used to assess many parameters including Heart Rate (HR), Heart Rate Variability (HRV) parameters, heart rate changes and breathing rates when at rest. The above mentioned parameters have been proven useful for the measurement of autonomic functions and the automatic detection of seizures in patients with epilepsy [1, 2].

Activity sensors are useful, as they allow for the possibility to assess all the main motoric parameters. One can detect different activities (e.g. walking, jogging) or inactivity, different postures (e.g. lying left, lying prone), changes of body positions or estimate the consumed energy expenditure. Other than that, acceleration sensors also allow the detection of abnormal movements during myoclonic seizures [7] or possible falls [3] that can occur before, during or after seizures.

GSR monitoring measures the electrical conductance of the skin as it varies with moisture levels. This is a sensitive measurement of autonomic arousal and physiological state which reflects one's behavior. Studies have found that GSR biofeedback has the potential of being a potent adjunctive non-pharmacological means of reducing seizure frequency in epilepsy [6], and that seizure-induced EDA elevation is a possible sign of autonomic instability [8].

4   Results

In a first step we examined the life-time performance of the mobile sensor platform for different conditions of operation. For this, we varied the sampling frequency of different sensors, the number of online analysis performed on the mobile platform and transmission of data via Bluetooth interface. The data acquired are based on real and not simulated measurements.

On the acquisition side of the sensor module, the sampling rate for acceleration signals was varied between 32 Hz and 64 Hz, the sampling rate for ECG signal between 256 Hz and 1024 Hz. In addition to this, we added online analysis of pulse rate (bpmList) and the detection of normal R-peaks (nnList) in some cases. On the storage and transmission side of the module we changed between simple raw data acquisition and storage and additional data transmission via Bluetooth interface with different parameters. The results are presented in Table 1.

As we can see, the life time of the mobile platform depends essentially on wireless connection. The difference between wireless transmissions of different amount of data can be neglected. The use of this platform in monitoring of epileptic patients is possible regarding the results shown in this table. For all cases in which wireless connection is necessary, the future use of Bluetooth Low Energy module will provide adequate results.

Table 1. Life time performance of mobile sensor platform

Acquisition	Storage	Transmission	Life-time
acc 64 Hz, ecg 256 Hz, bpmList, nnList, press 8 Hz, temp 1 Hz	Raw data	-	2d 7h 33m
acc 32 Hz, activity, ecg 512 Hz, press 8 Hz, temp 1 Hz	Raw data	-	3d 6h 20
acc 64 Hz, ecg 1024 Hz, press 8 Hz, temp 1 Hz	Raw data	-	2d 14h 31m
acc 64 Hz, ecg 256 Hz, bpmList, nnList, press 8 Hz, temp 1 Hz	Raw data	256 Hz ECG-raw data	3h 10m
acc 64 Hz, ecg 256 Hz, bpmList, nnList, press 8 Hz, temp 1 Hz	Raw data	1 Hz HR	3h 15m
acc 64 Hz, ecg 256 Hz, bpmList, nnList, press 8 Hz, temp 1 Hz	Raw data	BT connection	3h 20m

5   Conclusion

The presented system is a complete monitoring system able to accurately acquire and assess multiple body and brain parameters. The goal of this paper was to provide a complete, secure and reliable solution for the monitoring of patients with epilepsy. The novelty of the system lies in the aspects taken into account for its realization (biomedical context, unobtrusiveness, security, software and hardware design) and its' special design to address the needs of epileptic patients.

The implementation of this solution presented here is still ongoing work.

Acknowledgements. This work has been co-funded by the European Commission within the European Union's Seventh Framework Programme ([FP7/2007-2013]) in the ARMOR project (http://www.armor-project.eu).

References

1. Ponnusamy, A., Marques, J.L., Reuber, M.: Comparison of heart rate variability parameters during complex partial seizures and psychogenic nonepileptic seizures. Epilepsia (2012)
2. Massé, F., Penders, J., Serteyn, A., van Bussel, M., Arends, J.: Miniaturized Wireless ECG-Monitor for Real-Time Detection of Epileptic Seizures. In: Wireless Health 2010, San Diego, USA (2010)
3. Bianchi, F., Redmond, S.J., Narayanan, M.R., Cerutti, S., Celler, B.G., Lovell, N.H.: Falls Event Detection Using Triaxial Accelerometry and Barometric Pressure Measurement. In: 31st Annual International Conference of the IEEE EMBS Minneapolis, Minnesota, USA (2009)
4. Gotman, J.: Automatic Detection of Seizures and Spikes. Journal of Clinical Neurophysiology 16(2), 130–140 (1999)
5. Krist, M., Ottenbacher, J.: http://www.unisens.org
6. Nagai, Y., Goldstein, L.H., Fenwick, P.B., Trimble, M.R.: Clinical efficacy of galvanic skin response biofeedback training in reducing seizures in adult epilepsy: a preliminary randomized controlled study. Epilepsy & Behavior 5(2), 216–223 (2004)
7. Nijsen, T.M., Arends, J.B., Griep, P.A., Cluitmans, P.J.: The potential value of three-dimensional accelerometry for detection of motor seizures in severe epilepsy. Epilepsy & Behavior 7(1), 74–84 (2005)
8. Poh, M.-Z., Loddenkemper, T., Swenson, N., Goyal, S., Madsen, J., Picard, R.: Continuous Monitoring of Electrodermal Activity During Epileptic Seizures Using a Wearable Sensor. In: 32nd Annual International Conference of the IEEE EMBS Buenos Aires, Argentina (2010)
9. Schaaff, K., Mueller, L., Kirst, M.: http://www.xaffect.org/
10. Hall, J.B.: Brush up on Bluetooth. GSEC Practical Assignment Version 1.4b, SANS Institute (2008)
11. Lee, J., Kapitanova, K., Son, S.H.: The Price of Security in Wireless Sensor Networks Computer Networks. The International Journal of Computer and Telecommunications Networking 54(17) (2010)
12. Bojkovic, Z.S., Bakmaz, B.M., Bakmaz, M.R.: Security Issues in Wireless Sensor Networks. International Journal of Communications 2(1) (2008)
13. Data Protection Directive (Directive 95/46/EC), http://eur-lex.europa.eu/ LexUriServ/LexUriServ.do?uri=CELEX:31995L0046:en:NOT

Sensor-Based Mobile Functional Movement Screening

Ulf Jensen[1], Fabian Weilbrenner[1], Franz Rott[2], and Bjoern Eskofier[1]

[1] Pattern Recognition Lab, University of Erlangen-Nuremberg, Germany
{ulf.jensen,bjoern.eskofier}@cs.fau.de,
fabian.weilbrenner@informatik.stud.uni-erlangen.de
[2] Adidas innovation team ait, adidas Group, Herzogenaurach, Germany
franz.rott@adidas.com

Abstract. The Functional Movement Screen[TM] (FMS) is a useful tool to assess functional abilities in a pre-participation screening. Its seven dynamic movement tests reveal shortcomings in stability and mobility and screen the whole body. However, the current test protocol delivers results that are subjective, qualitative and have to be manually processed. This article presents a semi-automatic system to overcome these limitations for the Deep Squat test. The system consists of four wireless inertial sensors and a central Android[TM]-based processing node for data analysis and result storage. We developed our system based on data from ten subjects and evaluated the results with the FMS scoring guidelines. The sensor-based scoring system completely agreed with the manual scoring in eight out of ten subjects. In addition, quantitative information in case of compensation movements was logged. Thus, our system is capable of simplifying the FMS test and enhances the score with objective, quantitive and automatic results.

Keywords: Functional Movement Screen[TM], Body Sensor Network, intertial sensors, semi-automatic screening, Android[TM] app.

1 Motivation

Functional movement assessment is established as a valuable procedure to test the preparedness of an individual for activity. It is combined with a prior medical examination and a following performance test for a comprehensive pre-participation screening. Thereby, functional examination reveals shortcomings in mobility and stability during basic functional movements. Seven of these movements have been defined as a standard full-body functional athlete assessment procedure, the Functional Movement Screen[TM] (FMS) [1,2]. The FMS comprises of predefined tests (e.g. special squats and push-ups) and rates individuals according to the quality and efficiency of their execution. Thus, it identifies movement inabilities and is a valuable tool for sports medicine as injuries and irritations can be proactively avoided. Currently, the seven FMS tests are scored by an experienced rater and manually entered into a result sheet. Additional

B. Godara and K.S. Nikita (Eds.): MobiHealth 2012, LNICST 61, pp. 215–223, 2013.
© Institute for Computer Sciences, Social Informatics and Telecommunications Engineering 2013

qualitative information that further specifies the score is optional and can be added in textual form. This procedure is rater-dependent, based on personal visual assessment and not automated in result processing.

The FMS is widely used in training science and sports medicine and established as a standard tool to assess functional movement abilities. A study that investigated the correlation between core stability, functional movement and performance concluded that the FMS scores quality and efficiency of movement [3]. They further conclude that the FMS is a suitable indicator for risk of injury and is not appropriate to predict performance. The performance has to be assessed in other parts of the pre-participation screening. These findings have been confirmed for sport-specific movements and the authors of [4] proposed to investigate athlete strength instead.

Peate et al. used the FMS to determine the risk of injury for professional firefighters [5]. The authors proved that the number of injuries can be decreased for individuals with a low FMS score with an adequate training program. Thus, they further support the findings that individuals with a lower FMS score are more likely to sustain an injury. The influence of specific training on the results of the FMS test with special emphasis on symmetry were investigated in [6]. The authors proved that the prescribed training helped to reach a FMS score above a predefined threshold score. Asymmetries detected during functional movement assessment were reduced with the training program.

The problem of interrater variability was addressed in [7] and the authors found a good agreement of expert raters and trained novices on videotaped tests. Nevertheless, some FMS tests revealed differences in the scoring and prove the limitations of human assessment. In addition, only a small group of raters was investigated, the intrarater and intrasession variability was not considered and the scoring was made on videotaped tests. Some of these limitations were addressed in [8] that investigated intersession and interrater reliability in real-time testing with the same number of raters. Again, the results proved that novice raters perform also well in real-time FMS scoring. However, the results from the intersession tests revealed a need for reliable scoring of the same person in different sessions as some tests showed only moderate or good reliability.

Body Sensor Networks (BSN) are used for different health and sports applications and are capable of collecting mobile physiological and kinematic data [9]. Software frameworks for the mobile sensor data collection for specific BSN components exist [10]. From an application perspective, BSN are e.g. applied in gait analysis for Parkinson's disease early detection and therapy monitoring [11] and in fatigue classification during activity [12]. Due to their miniaturization and low cost, inertial sensors gain more and more popularity and are applied for numerous purposes in medical engineering, movement science and consumer electronics.

This paper presents a system to address the limitations of the FMS which is a well-established screening test for injury prediction and training control. We propose a semi-automatic system that uses data from inertial body-worn sensors to determine more objective results, to enhance the score with quantitative results and to enable easier result processing.

2 Methods

2.1 Functional Movement Screen

The FMS consists of seven dynamic movement patterns to screen the whole body functional movement abilities [1,2]. The collected results can be further interpreted by medical or coaching experts for corresponding clinical implications. Thus, scoring results directly pinpoint affected muscle groups or joints that are prone to injury.

Each of the seven tests is scored on a 0-3 ordinal scale. The highest score of 3 is reached if the movement pattern is completed as described in the test specification. If the test is completed with compensational movements a score of 2 is given. Incomplete movement execution results in a score of 1 and the test is scored with 0 if any pain is involved during movement. Specific error patterns and scoring aspects have been defined for each test. Tests are repeated three times and, if the test is of asymmetrical nature, repeated for each side. The lowest score of all repetition of a single test is considered and summed up for an overall score that ranges between 0 and 21.

Beside the score, the rater can add textual comments that further specify the error pattern, level of compensation or affected side. This information pinpoints shortcomings and is a of great value for therapy planning and monitoring.

2.2 Overhead Squat

In our study, we focused on the Deep Squat test [1] that challenges the mechanics of the whole body. In this test (fig. 1), the individual performs a deep squat with an overhead dowel. The Deep Squat is a symmetric test and therefore repeated three times. If the tested individual does not reach the perfect score, the test is repeated with a heel-supporting block. From a functional perspective, the scoring is based on the deepness of the squat, the torso position and knee alignment during testing and the heel movement. We derived four typical error patterns that our systems addressed:

1. The heel is lifted during testing.
2. The femur is not below horizontal in end position.
3. The torso performs a compensational movement in the frontal plane.
4. The torso performs a compensational movement in the sagittal plane.

In addition, it is required that our system automatically detects one repetition of the test to enable the precise error detection and assign detailed information to specific repetitions.

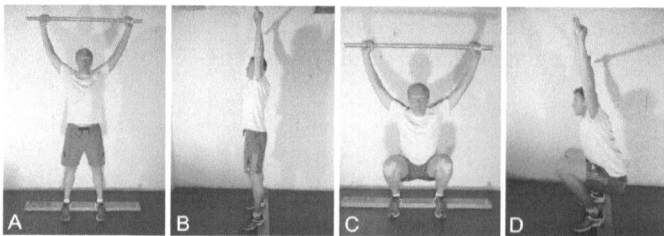

Fig. 1. Overview of the Deep Squat test. Initial positions in frontal view (A) and sagittal view (B) are shown on the left. End positions in frontal view (C) and sagittal view (D) are shown on the right. Positions are shown with the supporting heel block.

2.3   Body Sensor Network

Our BSN data collection system consisted of four SHIMMER^{TM} sensors [13] and a recording laptop. We positioned the sensor nodes on the dowel, the heel, the shank and the femur as displayed in figure 2. We chose to place the sensors on the right leg and heel. The internal three-axis accelerometer was set to a range of 2 g and was sampled with a frequency of 100 Hz. Data were wirelessly transmitted to the recording laptop and stored for further processing. The sensor data were calibrated with the standard procedure specified in the manufacturers user manual.

2.4   Data Collection

We collected Deep Squat test data from ten (1 female, 9 male) volunteers and videotaped the experiments for algorithm development and scoring. We used two videocameras for a frontal and a sagittal view of each repetition. As we did not live score the test during data collection, the test was always repeated with a heel-supporting block.

We followed a simple protocol in the test execution. First, the test was explained to the subjects and the sensors were placed. Second, the subjects were put in correct initial position. This position was recorded with the sensors and the videotaping was started. Third, the volunteers were asked to perform three squats. Fourth, the test was repeated with a heel-supporting block.

2.5   Repetition Detection

The automatic detection of error patterns required information about the beginning and the end of a repetition during testing. We therefore tracked the subjects' knee angle with data from the sensors on the femur and the shank. It was assumed that the knee behaved like a hinge joint during test execution so that the sensors were only rotated in the sagittal plane.

The knee angle calculation required the initial position r_i before the test was started and the current position x_i during repetitions for each sensor $i \in \{1, 2\}$

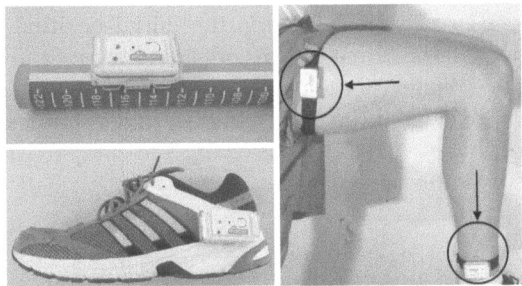

Fig. 2. Overview of sensor placement on the dowel (top left), the heel (bottom left) and the leg (right)

during testing. We calculated the current deviation angle α_i with regard to the starting position for each sensor i with eq. 1.

$$\alpha_i = \arccos\left(\frac{r_i \cdot x_i}{\|r_i\| \cdot \|x_i\|}\right) \tag{1}$$

The resulting knee angle α_{knee} was calculated with eq. 2.

$$\alpha_{knee} = \alpha_1 + \alpha_2 \tag{2}$$

These computations resulted in the knee angle for each sampled sensor value. We averaged the angle results of ten measurements to eliminate outliers and reduce noise. This averaging step was performed for all angle computations.
The knee angle was initialized during the idle phase in correct initial position. We set the value to zero in initial position with extended legs, thus the angle increased with knee flexion.

2.6 Error Pattern Determination

Heel Lift. According to test specification, the heel has to remain on the floor during test execution. We tracked the heel sensor to detect this error pattern and used eq. 1 for the computation.

Final Femur Position. Concerning the final position of the femur we used the same principle. The deviation angle of the femur sensor was calculated with eq. 1. In addition the maximum femur angle was recorded.

Torso Compensation. A compensational movement during a deep squat is composed of the compensation in sagittal plane and in frontal plane. In the Deep Squat scoring scheme, both aspects are regarded as one. As the sensor's coordinate system planes roughly coincided with the subjects plane, we were able to discriminate between the frontal and the sagittal plane and quantified the compensation angles with data from the dowel sensor. The difference in the planes were compensated with data from the initial position before test start. Thereby, we projected the three-dimensional vectors r_i and x_i in either the frontal or the sagittal plane. As the planes were defined by the axes of the sensor coordinate system, we deleted the corresponding dimension resulting in the two-dimensional projections $\hat{r}_i$ and $\hat{x}_i$. We used eq. 3 to compute the deviation angle for each plane in two-dimensional space.

$$\alpha_i = \arccos \left(\frac{\hat{r}_i \cdot \hat{x}_i}{\|\hat{r}_i\| \cdot \|\hat{x}_i\|} \right) \tag{3}$$

Only compensation movements during repetition were considered. We registered the error if a compensation was detected in at least one of the planes.

2.7   Implementation

The algorithms for repetition detection and error pattern determination were implemented in an Android^{TM} app running on Android-based devices like smart phones or tablets. The app built upon the software framework introduced in [10] which manages the connection between the sensors and the analysis device. We set up a user interaction with detailed descriptions of the FMS tests, user and test management and an automatic sensor calibration. The app included a database into which the results were automatically entered after three detected repetitions. Detailed quantified information like the knee angle and the compensation in frontal and sagittal plane were added accordingly.

2.8   Evaluation

The videotaped tests were scored and commented by a sport scientist according to the scoring guidelines in [1]. The automatic system scored accordingly and the score was decremented if at least one error pattern was registered. Thus, if one of the error patterns occurred in the first trial without heel-supporting block, the score was decremented. Subsequently, the second trial with heel support was considered and scored in the same way. Finally, the subject was asked if any pain occurred during testing.

   To evaluate our sensor-based semi-automatic system, we compared the results from the manual scoring (MANUAL) and our system (SENSOR). For this, we reran the recorded experiments with the Android implementation in simulation mode.

3   Results

To determine the beginning and the end of a repetition, we used a threshold value of 20 degrees from the knee angle computation. With this setting, our algorithms was able to correctly detect all squats performed during data collection.

   The thresholds for the detection of the error patterns were chosen according to the manual scoring. The final scoring results are compiled in tab. 1.

Table 1. Overview of the results of the manual (MANUAL) and sensor-based (SEN-SOR) scoring of the Deep Squat test. Results are given for subjects S1 - S10.

	S1	S2	S3	S4	S5	S6	S7	S8	S9	S10
MANUAL	2	2	1	1	2	1	2	2	2	2
SENSOR	2	2	1	1	2	2	2	1	2	2

4   Discussion

The results revealed that our system was capable of adequately scoring the Deep Squat test of the FMS. However, the algorithms are based on manually defined thresholds. In future research, these thresholds have to be defined by experienced raters or identified in a larger data collection study. In addition, some error patterns described in the FMS scoring scheme were not covered by the sensor-based system. In the Deep Squat test, this was the case for the alignment of the knee and the foot which has to be addressed in future research.

The Deep Squat test was chosen to provide a proof of concept of a sensor-based FMS scoring system and we are planning to integrate the missing six tests in future research. Some of the algorithms like the torso compensation are reusable for other tests with only little modification. However, the use of inertial sensors is not straightforward for tests like the Active Straight Leg Raise test or the Shoulder Mobility test. Nevertheless, a semi-automatic system will be capable of supporting these tests in result entry and storage.

We analyzed the subjects for which the scoring results did not agree in detail. In the test of subject S6, we detected a sagittal compensation movement in the video. However, this compensation was not detected by the sensor system. For subject S8, in contrast, a compensation movement was detected in the sensor result but not visible in the video data. This discrepancy was due to the threshold value we manually set. As mentioned before, the thresholds have to be confirmed by experts or quantitatively computed on a large database. We propose a training phase for our system where error patterns of different severity are scored by FMS experts to set the threshold angles adequately. However, one has to keep in mind that the scoring is subjective and that different raters will use different scales in their personal rating. Thus, this rating has to be repeated and averaged with different raters. The advantage of the resulting averaged automatic system is that it will always compute the same score for one single data set. A human rater, in contrast, might score different results on the same experiment if the scoring is repeated.

Furthermore, the sensor results need to be validated to prove the correctness of the measurement. This is particular important in the case for the final femur position error pattern where a specific angle was defined in the scoring manual. It has to be proven that the sensor systems is capable of computing the correct value. If this is the case, the quantitative sensor output can be interpreted from a biomechanical perspective and enhances the FMS score. We also experienced a couple of factors that interfere in the sensor measurements. These were the initial position of the sensor straps and the movement of sensor during testing due to muscle activity. We are planning to address these issues with the aid of a 3-D motion tracking system to validate the sensor data and quantify the influence of sensor position and movement.

We speculate that quantitative results are helpful for a rater and deduct two application scenarios. First, the support of an unexperienced rater that mainly relies on the automatic scoring and only changes the results if needed. Second, the support of an experienced rater with figures to tackle unclear cases. Beside the scoring aspect, these quantitative results can be used in therapy monitoring to identify improvements that are not reflected in an improvement of the score. An athlete might for example reduce its sagittal compensation by five degrees but still be scored with 1. Further research has to be conducted to prove the value of quantitative results. It can either be used for assisting the scoring or for a more detailed result than the 0-3 ordinal scale.

5   Summary and Outlook

We presented a sensor-based system to simplify the FMS scoring and to produce more objective and quantitative results. It consisted of four body-worn accelerometer sensors and a mobile Android device for data analysis. The comparison of manual and automatic scoring confirmed the applicability of our system to accomplish the scoring of the Deep Squat test.

However, challenges for training the system and sensor placement were identified to further improve our system. In addition, the system needs to be expanded to cover the complete FMS test. We are also planning to enhance our system with data mining functionality to facilitate therapy monitoring and team statistics.

Acknowledgments. The authors would like to thank all volunteers who participated in the study. This work was funded by the Bavarian Ministry for Economic Affairs, Infrastructure, Transport and Technology and the European Fund for Regional Development.

References

1. Cook, G., et al.: Pre-Participation Screening: The Use of Fundamental Movements as an Assessment of Function - Part 1. North American Journal of Sports Physical Therapy 1(2), 62–72 (2006)
2. Cook, G., et al.: Pre-Participation Screening: The Use of Fundamental Movements as an Assessment of Function - Part 2. North American Journal of Sports Physical Therapy 1(3), 132–139 (2006)
3. Okada, T., et al.: Relationship between Core Stability, Functional Movement, and Performance. Journal of Strength and Conditioning Research 25(1), 252–261 (2011)
4. Parchmann, C., et al.: Relationship between Functional Movement Screen and Athletic Performance. Journal of Strength and Conditioning Research 25(12), 3378–3384 (2011)
5. Peate, W., et al.: Core strength: A new model for injury prediction and prevention. Journal of Occupational Medicine and Toxicology 2(1), Art. Nr. 3 (2007)
6. Kiesel, K., et al.: Functional Movement Test Scores Improve Following a Standardized Off-season Intervention Program in Professional Football Players. Scand. J. Med. Sci. Sports 21(2), 287–292 (2011)

7. Minick, K., et al.: Interrater Reliability of the Functional Movement Screen. Journal of Strength and Conditioning Research 24(2), 479–486 (2010)
8. Onate, J., et al.: Real-time Intersession and Interrater Reliability of the Functional Movement Screen. Journal of Strength and Conditioning Research 26(2), 408–415 (2012)
9. Chen, M., et al.: Body Area Networks: A Survey. Mobile Networks and Applications 2(16), 171–193 (2011)
10. Kugler, P., et al.: Mobile Recording System for Sport Applications. In: Proc. of the 8th International Symposium on Computer Science in Sport (IACSS 2011), Shanghai, pp. 67–70 (2011)
11. Barth, J., et al.: Biometric and Mobile Gait Analysis for Early Detection and Therapy Monitoring in Parkinson's Disease. In: Proc. of the Annual International Conference of the IEEE Engineering in Medicine and Biology Society (EMBC 2011), Boston, pp. 868–871 (2011)
12. Eskofier, B., et al.: Embedded Classification of the Perceived Fatigue State of Runners: Towards a Body Sensor Network for Assessing the Fatigue State during Running. In: Proc. of the 9th International Conference on Wearable and Implantable Body Sensor Networks (BSN 2012), London, pp. 113–117 (2012)
13. McGrath, M., Dishongh, T.: A Common Personal Health Research Platform SHIMMER^{TM} and BioMOBIUS^{TM}. Intel Technology Journal 13(3), 122–147 (2009)

Depth Limited Treatment Planning and Scheduling for Electronic Triage System in MCI

Ayaka Kashiyama, Akira Uchiyama, and Teruo Higashino

Graduate School of Information Science and Technology, Osaka University,
1-5 Yamadaoka, Suita, Osaka 5650871, Japan
{a-kasiym,utiyama,higashino}@ist.osaka-u.ac.jp

Abstract. For supporting rescue operations in disasters, vital data collections in wireless sensor networks have been proposed so far. In such systems, we can expect to predict each patient's probability of survival based on real-time vital data. In this paper, we focus on prehospital care and propose a method to determine treatment plans and schedules of patients. The proposed method maximizes the number of expected saved patients under limited medical resources. This optimization problem is called Treatment Planning and Scheduling, which is NP-hard. Therefore, we propose a heuristic algorithm based on depth-limited search. We have compared the proposed method with greedy methods. The results show the proposed method can derive solutions in practical time and the average number of saved patients is 10% larger compared to the greedy methods.

Keywords: Mass Casualty Incident, Disaster Medical Care, Treatment Planning and Scheduling, NP-hard, Depth Limited Search.

1 Introduction

Triage is a process of prioritizing patients based on vital signs in Mass Casualty Incidents (MCIs) such as earthquakes and terrorism. The purpose of triage is to save as many patients as possible under limited medical resources, e.g. medical supplies and physicians. Our research group has been developing an electronic triage system called eTriage which uses wireless networks for supporting rescue and medical operations in disasters[1]. We have developed an electronic triage tag to measure a heart rate and a blood oxygen level of a patient. The electronic triage tag is capable of ZigBee communication, and wireless sensor networks are built over the tags attached to patients. Through monitoring patients' vital signs, a sudden change of each patient's condition is notified to healthcare workers. Similarly, AIDN(Advanced Health and Disaster Aid Network)[2] and WIISARD (Wireless Internet Information System for Medical Response in Disasters)[3] also investigate an advanced medical support system by using wireless networks.

Moreover, some medical research works have proposed methods for predicting patient survivability. For example, TRISS method[4] predicts the probability of

B. Godara and K.S. Nikita (Eds.): MobiHealth 2012, LNICST 61, pp. 224–233, 2013.

survival of a patient from the ISS (Injury Severity Score) and the RTS (Revised Trauma Score) calculated from anatomic, physiologic, and age characteristics. Such survivability prediction is expected to become more accurate and sophisticated in the future by collecting a large amount of vital data with the aid of ICT (Information and Computer Technology). Then, precise triage based on real-time vital data of patients will be possible.

There are some methods using ICT for supporting rescue operations in MCIs. Ref.[5] proposes a transportation scheduling algorithm from a disaster site to multiple hospitals to maximize total survivability of patients assuming future advanced survivability prediction. Ref.[6] presents an agent-based scheduling algorithm for patients in a hospital. However, in order to maximize the number of saved patients in MCIs, we need consider a large variety of operations including transportation and medical treatments in both a disaster site and a hospital.

In this paper, we focus on prehospital care in MCIs and propose a method to derive treatment plans and schedules of patients that maximize the number of saved patients under the assumption that accurate prediction of survivability is possible. For this purpose, we model prehospital care in MCIs as shown in Fig. 1 based on the Emergo Train System (ETS)[7], which is a widely used on-the-desk simulation toolkit for disaster medical care exercises in hospitals. Given conditions of each patient, we need decide treatment plans and schedules under limited medical resources. Deadlines and essential treatments for each patient are also given, and if essential treatments of a patient do not finish before the deadline, the patient is considered to die.

Our goal is to maximize the number of saved patients in this ETS-based disaster medical care model. We call this maximization problem as a Treatment Planning and Scheduling (TPS) problem, of which a sub-problem is equivalent to an Integrated Process Planning and Scheduling (IPPS) problem, known as NP-hard[8]. To solve TPS problem, we need choose treatment plans for each patient. For example, some patients may be treated completely in the disaster site and some others may be transported to the hospital without treatment. It may also increase the number of saved patients to treat some patients partly in the disaster site, which results in extensions of the patients' deadlines. Furthermore, after determining treatment plans, we need decide the treatment order of patients who use the same medical resources such as ambulances and physicians. As we mentioned above, deadlines of patients change if such treatment plans are chosen. On the other hand, deadlines are fixed and do not change depending on chosen plans in IPPS problems. For this reason, TPS problems are more complicated than IPPS problems and we cannot directly apply methods for IPPS[9,10] to TPS. Ref. [11] considers penalty functions over time to consider degradation of condition and proposes an algorithm for optimizing medical supply in disaster scenarios to minimize the total penalty. Our approach aims to treat as many patients as possible before deadlines and does not consider waiting time for treatment. In this sense, Ref. [11] is different from our approach.

Since TPS is difficult than NP-hard problem, we propose a heuristic algorithm using depth limited search to solve TPS problems in practical time. To the best of

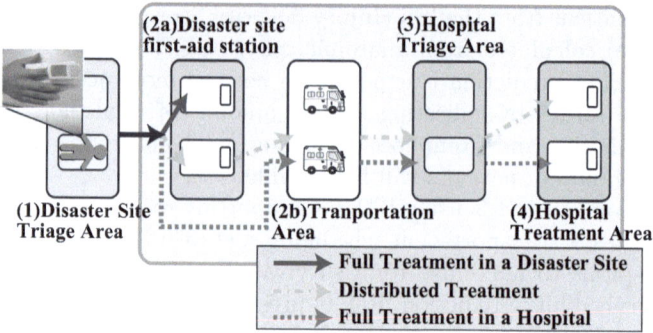

Fig. 1. Overview of Disaster Medical Care

our knowledge, there is no research on determining treatment plans and schedules of patients in MCIs focusing on the early stage of disaster medical care.

We have compared the proposed method with two deadline-based greedy methods for evaluation. The results show that the proposed method derives solutions that save approximately 10% more patients than the greedy methods in a few seconds.

2   Treatment Planning and Scheduling Problem

2.1   Assumptions and Disaster Medical Care Model

We assume our electronic triage tags are attached to all patients in a disaster site, and vital signs of the patients are transmitted to a server via wireless ad hoc networks. The changes of patient's survivability over time are predicted based on the collected vital data at the server. We also assume the server knows the numbers of patients that each area can treat/transport in parallel based on medical resource information such as the numbers of physicians, nurses, and ambulances. Then, our method determines how and in which order the patients should be treated.

Figure 1 shows the overview of the modeled disaster medical care. Hereafter, we target a case of a single hospital for simplicity of discussion. However, note that modeling of a case of multiple hospitals is also possible in the same manner. In this model, we assume that we cannot interrupt a treatment once it starts, and that multiple patients are not allowed to be treated by using the same medical resource simultaneously. We assume there are five areas as follows, and patients are treated at each area and transported to the next area as necessary.

1. Disaster site triage area: Firstly, every patient is moved from a disaster site to this area. In this area, electronic triage tags are attached to each patient on a First-Come, First-Served (FCFS) basis to monitor their vital signs.
2a. Disaster site first-aid station: Physicians and nurses treat patients in the disaster site.

Table 1. Notations Used for Formulation

Symbol	Explanation
P	A set of patients
M	A set of medical resources
R	A set of treatment plans
c_h^r	The hth operation in process plan r
$t_i[c_h^r, m]$	Required time for patient i's operation c_h^r using medical resource m
$T_i[c_h^r, m]$	Completion time of patient i's operation c_h^r using medical resource m
$d_i[c_h^r, m]$	Deadline of patient i's operation c_h^r using medical resource m
X_i^r	$\begin{cases} 1, \text{if treatment plan } r \text{ is selected for patient } i \\ 0, \text{otherwise} \end{cases}$
$Y_m[i, j, c_h^r, c_g^s]$	$\begin{cases} 1, \text{ if patient } i\text{'s operation } c_h^r \text{ precedes patient } j\text{'s operation } c_g^s \text{ on} \\ \quad \text{medical resource } m \\ 0, \text{ otherwise} \end{cases}$
$Z_i[c_h^r, m]$	$\begin{cases} 1, \text{ if medical resource } m \text{ is selected for patient } i\text{'s operation } c_h^r \\ 0, \text{ otherwise} \end{cases}$

2b. Transportation area: Patients are transported from the disaster site to a hospital by ambulances.

3. Hospital triage area: Conditions of patients are checked again. After that they are transported to a treatment area in the hospital.

4. Hospital treatment area: Physicians and nurses treat patients in the hospital. Usually, medical resources in the hospital are much more than those in the disaster site.

At first, an electronic triage tag is attached to a patient at (1) a disaster site triage area. Then, the patient is transported to the next area, which is either (2a) the disaster site first-aid station or (2b) a transportation area, depending on each patient's treatment plan. We can treat the patient by using medical resources in (2a) a disaster site first-aid station and (4) a hospital treatment area. After transportation by an ambulance, the patient has to be checked his condition at (3) the hospital triage area before transportation to (4) the hospital treatment area.

We assume there are two types of treatments: full treatment and distributed treatment. For each case, time required to finish treatment and deadlines for these treatments are given, and we need finish either of the treatment by the given deadline in order for saving the patient. Full treatment finishes patient's treatment at either the disaster site first-aid station or the hospital treatment area. On the other hand, in distributed treatment, we firstly treat a patient at the disaster site to prolong the deadline, transport the patient to the hospital, and then finish the remaining treatment in the hospital. Therefore, there are three treatment plans as shown by the arrows in Fig. 1.

2.2   Problem Formulation

We formulate TPS problem based on Ref.[11] which formulates Integrated Process Planning and Scheduling (IPPS) problem. Table 1 shows notations used in the formulation. There are $|R|$ treatment plans, and the sequence of operations for selected treatment plan $r \in R$ is denoted as $c_1^r, c_2^r, \ldots, c_{|r|}^r$. These operations include medical treatments such as full treatment and distributed treatment, and we regard transportation by an ambulance as one of the operations as well. For each patient i, time required to complete operation c_h^r by using medical resource $m \in M$ is given and denoted by $t_i[c_h^r, m]$ where M is a set of medical resources.

There are three constraints, that are (i) a treatment plan selection constraint, (ii) an operation sequence constraint, and (iii) an interruption constraint. Firstly, the equation (1) shows the treatment plan selection constraint which indicates each patient must select exactly one treatment plan.

$$\sum_{r=1}^{R} X_i^r = 1 \qquad \forall i \in P \qquad (1)$$

where P is a set of patients and X_i^r represents the selection state of treatment plan r for patient i.

Secondly, the operation sequence constraint is described as shown in the expression (2). This constraint means the sequence of operations must follow the sequence of operations $c_1^r, \ldots, c_{|r|}^r$ in treatment plan r if treatment plan r is selected for patient i.

$$X_i^r \times (Z_i[c_h^r, m_1] \times T_i[c_h^r, m_1] - Z_i[c_{h-1}^r, m_2] \times T_i[c_{h-1}^r, m_2])$$
$$\geq X_i^r \times t_i[c_h^r, m_1] \times Z_i[c_h^r, m_1]$$
$$\forall i \in P, \quad \forall r \in R, \quad \forall m_1, m_2 \in M, \quad \forall h \in [2, |r|] \quad (2)$$

Here, $T_i[c_h^r, m]$ is completion time of operation c_h^r for patient i by using medical resource m. $Z_i[c_h^r, m]$ indicates the selection state of medical resource m for operation c_h^r of patient i.

Finally, the interruption constraint is represented by the expression (3). This constraint indicates medical resources cannot handle two or more operations simultaneously and no operation is interrupted by other operations once it starts. A state binary $Y_m[i, j, c_h^r, c_g^s]$ represents the sequence of patient i's operation c_h^r and patient j's operation c_g^s that use the same machine m.

$$Y_m[i, j, c_h^r, c_g^s] \times (T_j[c_g^s, m] - T_i[c_h^r, m]) \geq Y_m[i, j, c_h^r, c_g^s] \times t_i[c_h^r, m]$$
$$\forall i, j \in P, \quad \forall r, s \in R, \quad \forall h \in [1, |r|], \quad \forall g \in [1, |s|], \quad \forall m \in M \quad (3)$$

For simplicity, we introduce another state binary D_i^r as follows, which indicates whether all operations of patient i finish before the deadlines on treatment plan r or not.

$$D_i^r = \begin{cases} 1, \text{ if } Z_i[c_h^r, m] \times (d_i[c_h^r, m] - T_i[c_h^r, m]) < 0 \\ \qquad\qquad\qquad\qquad \forall h \in [1, |r|], \quad \forall m \in M \qquad (4) \\ 0, \text{ otherwise} \end{cases}$$

Then, the objective function is defined as the following expression (5) that minimizes the number of deaths, which is equivalent to maximizing the number of saved patients.

$$\text{minimize} \sum_{i \in P} D_i^r \times X_i^r \quad \forall r \in R \tag{5}$$

Subject to: (1), (2), and (3).

3 Depth Limited Treatment Planning and Scheduling

3.1 Overview

In TPS problem, we need determine both treatment plans X_i^r and schedules $Y_m[i, j, c_h^r, c_g^s]$ for all patients. Schedules are determined for each area while treatment plans are selected right before the disaster site first-aid station because treatment plans branch after a patient is rescued from the disaster site.

For scheduling at each area, we apply deadline-based greedy scheduling because the more serious condition a patient is, the higher the patient's treatment priority is. However, there is possibility that we can save two or more patients by abandoning one patient. For example, a seriously injured patient may take long time for treatment, and if we treat the patient, other patients may die. Therefore, we explore such possibilities in addition to distributing medical workloads over the disaster site and the hospital. This means the number of treatment plans is four: (i) full treatment in the disaster site, (ii) distributed treatment in both the disaster site and the hospital, (iii) full treatment in the hospital, and (iv) abandonment.

3.2 Depth Limited Treatment Planning

We cannot solve TPS problem in practical time if we explore all combinations of treatment plans for all patients because it requires exponential time with respect to the number of patients. For this reason, we limit the number of patients to explore treatment plans. It is natural that exploring other plans of a seriously injured patient is more likely to improve the result. Hence we explore all plans of the k most serious patients with respect to deadlines, and choose such treatment plans for those k patients that maximize the number of saved patients. Hereafter, we describe a set of those k most serious patients with respect to deadlines in a set of patients P as P_k.

Given a candidate of treatment plans of k patients, we need assign treatment plans of the other patients in $P - P_k$ to compute the number of saved patients. We select treatment plans of the other patients in a greedy manner where full treatment in a disaster site is assigned. In this manner, we need not consider distributed treatment and abandonment for the patients in $P - P_k$, thus the computation time is reduced. Firstly, the proposed method sorts $|P|$ patients in ascending order right after the triage area. Secondly, it explores and determines top k patients' treatment plans. Then, we repeat the same process for the set of $P - P_k$ until the treatment plans of all patients are determined.

An example of the depth limited planning is shown in Fig. 2. Suppose there are 6 patients $A, B, \ldots, F$ in ascending order with respect to their deadlines. In this

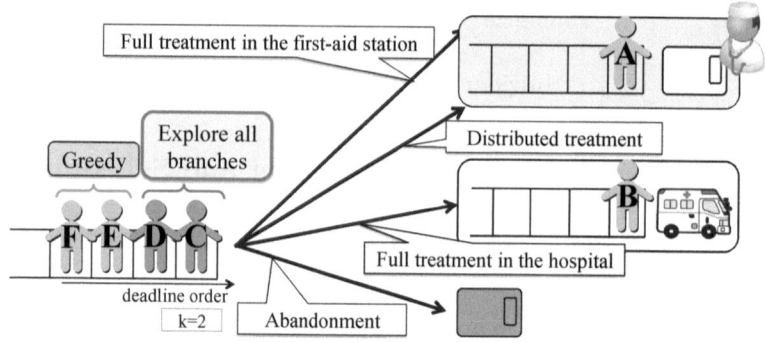

Fig. 2. Example of Depth Limited Treatment Planning

Table 2. Treatment Time and Deadlines Used in Simulation (sec.)

	Urgent	Priority	Delayed	Minimal
Treatment time t_f	[4000,5000]	[300,450]	[120,400]	[100,300]
Treatment time t_h	-	[300,450]	[200,400]	[300,500]
Deadline d	[100,900]	[780,1680]	[1700,3300]	[3300,6300]
Ext. deadline d'	-	[1000,1500]	[1000,2000]	[1000,2000]

example, we assume $k = 2$, and let treatment plans of A and B be determined as full treatment in the first-aid station and full treatment in the hospital, respectively. Then, the next k patients are C and D. We explore all treatment plans for C and D while treatment plans of E and F are selected greedily.

We also consider other criteria to derive a better solution. This is because it is likely to happen that the numbers of saved patients for different candidates are equal. In such cases, it is desirable to select the candidate which does not occupy medical resources in the disaster site as much as possible to keep medical resources available for the following patients. This means the proposed method prioritizes candidates with the maximum number of saved patients according to the following criteria: the number of abandoned patients, full treatment plans in the hospital, and distributed treatment plans. For example, suppose there are two candidates c_1 and c_2 with the maximum number of saved patients. If the number of abandoned patients in c_1 is larger than c_2, we select c_1 as the best treatment planning. If the numbers of abandoned patients are equal, the numbers of full treatment in a hospital are compared to determine the best planning.

4 Performance Evaluation

4.1 Settings

We have evaluated the performance of the proposed method through simulation. In the evaluation, we assume four categories: urgent, priority, delayed, and minimal. Particularly, deadlines of urgent patients are short while it takes long time to finish treatment. We have assigned patients one of the categories, and the treatment time and deadlines of the patients are randomly selected from the ranges shown in Table 2 according to their categories. Time required for distributed treatment is t_f in the first-aid station and t_h in the hospital. For treatment plans of full treatment, the time to complete the treatment operation is $t_f + t_h$ independently of treatment areas. Deadline d is extended by d' when distributed treatment is selected and the treatment operation in the first-aid station finished. We set the total number of patients to 100. We also set the numbers of patients that each area can handle simultaneously in the first-aid station, the transportation area, the hospital triage area, and the hospital treatment area to 6, 5, 7, and 21, respectively. We used a workstation with Intel Xeon 2.66 GHz and 23.6 GB memory for evaluation. The results are averages of 100 random cases.

We used two types of scenarios. The first one is a scenario with urgent patients, where there are 15 urgent, 40 priority, 35 delayed, 10 minimal patients, respectively. The second one is a scenario without urgent patients. For the scenario without urgent patients, we used 45 priority, 35 delayed, 20 minimal patients.

For comparison, we introduce two greedy approaches to determine treatment plans: a Disaster Site weighted greedy approach (DS-greedy) and a Hospital weighted greedy approach (H-greedy). The decision of DS greedy and H-greedy is different when (i) medical resources in the disaster site and the transportation area are available and (ii) medical resources in both areas are occupied. In the above two cases, DS-greedy selects full treatment in the disaster site while H-greedy selects full treatment in the hospital. In both greedy approaches, schedules are determined based on a FCFS basis. We have selected the above two approaches for comparison since we believe they are close to doctors' decision: doctors try to prioritize patients according to their conditions and treat them greedily with respect to the priorities.

4.2 Effect of Limited Depth k

To see the effect of depth k for limited search, we have measured computation time for different depth k in the scenario with urgent patients. The result is shown in Fig. 3. We can see the number of saved patients increases with the increase of k although computation time increases exponentially. This is because the number of combinations is $O(|R|^k)$ and in this case $|R| = 4$. It is obvious that there is a trade-off between computation time and the number of saved patients. From the result, $k = 4$ is the most balanced since the computation time is about 5 seconds and the result is comparable to that of $k = 5$. Therefore, we use $k = 4$ in the following evaluation.

4.3 Comparison with Greedy Methods

We have compared the proposed method with DS-greedy and H-greedy approaches in two simulation scenarios. Table 3 describes the results of the

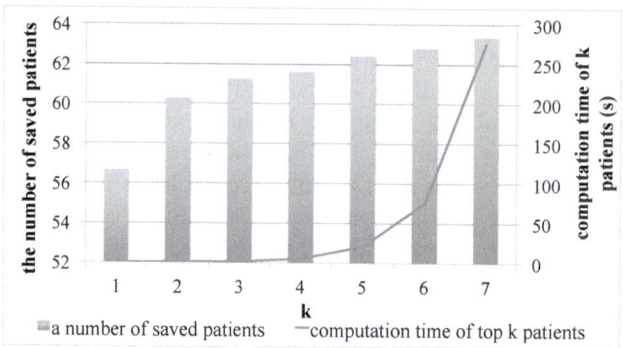

Fig. 3. Depth k vs. # of Saved Patients and Computation Time

Table 3. Comparison on the Number of Saved Patients with Greedy Methods

	DS-greedy	H-greedy	Proposed
Scenario w/ urgent patients	17.70	16.81	61.59
Scenario w/o urgent patients	65.82	65.89	74.93

comparison. The results show there is not much difference between two greedy methods. This is because there is not much difference between the amount of medical resources available in the first-aid station and the transportation area.

In the scenario with urgent patients, the number of the saved patients in the proposed method is more than three times of those in the greedy methods. The reason is that medical resources are occupied by urgent patients in the greedy methods since they do not abandon urgent patients those require long time for treatment. In contrast, the proposed method can derive better solutions because the proposed method explores possibilities of abandonment. Even in the scenario without urgent patients, the proposed method has achieved approximately 10% better result than the compared greedy approaches. This result indicates the effectiveness of distributing workload of the first-aid station and the hospital, which is explored by the proposed method. From the results, we have confirmed the proposed method can derive better solutions than the greedy methods by exploring all treatment plans for k patients.

5   Conclusion

In this paper, we modeled prehospital care and proposed a method to derive treatment plans and schedules of patients that maximize the number of saved patients in practical time under the assumption that accurate prediction of future probability of survival is possible. The proposed method uses depth-limited search to explore possibilities of improvement. We evaluated the proposed method through simulation and confirmed we could derive solutions that achieve better results than the compared greedy methods. Our future work includes considering arrival of new patients. For this purpose, we may apply a policy to keep some amount of medical resources depending on the estimated number of potential patients.

Acknowledgement. This research was supported by Japan Science and Technology Agency, Core Research for Evolutional Science and Technology(CREST).

References

1. Higashino, T., Uchiyama, A., Yasumoto, K.: eTriage: A wireless communication service platform for advanced rescue operations. In: Proceedings of ACM Workshop on Internet of Things and Service Patforms (IoTSP) (2011) (Invited talk)
2. Gao, T., Pesto, C., Selavo, L., Chen, Y., Ko, J.G., Lim, J.H., Terzis, A., Watt, A., Jeng, J., Chen, B.R., Lorincz, K., Welsh, M.: Wireless medical sensor networks in emergency response: Implementation and pilot results. In: Proceedings of 2008 IEEE Conference on Technologies for Homeland Security, pp. 187–192 (2008)
3. Lenert, L.A., Palmer, D.A., Chan, T.C., Rao, R.: An intelligent 802.11 triage tag for medical response to disasters. In: Proceedings of American Medical Informatics Association 2005 Symposium, pp. 440–444 (2005)
4. Champion, H.R., Copes, W.S., Sacco, W.J.: The major trauma outcome study: Establishing national norms for trauma care. Journal of Trauma 30, 1356–1365 (1990)
5. Mizumoto, T., Sun, W., Yasumoto, K., Ito, M.: Transportation scheduling method for patients in mci using electronic triage tag. In: Proceedings of International Conference on eHealth, Telemedicine, and Social Medicine (eTELEMED), pp. 156–163 (2011)
6. Amani, D., Hayfa, Z., Slim, H., Herve, H.: A dynamic patient scheduling at the emergency department in hospitals. In: Proceedings of IEEE Workshop on Health Care Management (WHCM), pp. 1–6 (2010)
7. Emergo Train System, http://www.emergotrain.com/
8. Khoshnevis, B., Chen, Q.: Integration of Process Planning and Scheduling Funtcions. Journal of Intelligent Manufacturing 2(3), 165–176 (1991)
9. Weintraub, A.J., Cormier, D., Hodgson, T.J., King, R.E., Wilson, J., Zozom Jr., A.: Hybrid Genetic Algorithm and Simulated Annealing Approach for the Optimisation of Process Plans for Prismatic Parts. International Journal of Production Research 40(8), 1899–1922 (2002)
10. Guo, Y.W., Li, W.D., Mileham, A.R., Owen, G.W.: Optimisation of Integrated Process Planning and Scheduling Using a Particle Swarm Optimisation Approach. International Journal of Production Research 47(14), 3775–3796 (2009)
11. Xinyu, L., Chaoyong, Z., Liang, G., Weidong, L., Xinyu, S.: An agent-based approach for integrated process planning and scheduling. Expert Systems with Applications 37(2), 1256–1264 (2010)

An Integrated Broker Platform
for Open eHealth Domain

Foteini Gr. Andriopoulou, Lamprini T. Kolovou, and Dimitrios K. Lymberopoulos

Wire Communications Laboratory, Electrical and Computer Engineering Department,
University of Patras,
University Campus, 265 04 Rio Patras, Greece
fandriop@upcatras.gr, lamprinik14@gmail.com,
dlympero@upatras.gr

Abstract. The adoption of personalized context aware services in healthcare domain has imposed new demands on IT providers and motivates integration and interoperability between heterogeneous healthcare systems. In this paper, we propose an Integrated Broker Platform – IBP that incorporates the benefits of the advanced technologies of Enterprise Service Bus (ESB) and Service Broker (SB) allowing the efficient provision of secure, interoperable, reliable and cost-efficient message and service delivery by dynamical and intelligent selection of services. IBP provides mediation functionalities that TSB supports but is enhanced with business logic from the SB. An architecture pattern for both TSB and SB is proposed, analyzed and prototyped.

Keywords: integrated broker platform (IBP), ESB, TSB, Service Broker-SB, healthcare.

1   Introduction

Nowadays, healthcare systems rapidly moved from treating isolated episodes towards a continuous treatment process involving multiple healthcare professionals and various healthcare infrastructures (e.g. hospitals, clinics, institutes). This rapid change in the healthcare domain imposes new demands on IT providers and motivates integration and interoperability among heterogeneous software components within the health information systems [1]. Integration and interoperability of different, heterogeneous software components, however, is a difficult task, as applications usually are vendor proprietary and not designed to cooperate with other vendor applications. Today powerful integration tools (e.g. application servers, object brokers, different kinds of message-oriented middleware, integrated platforms, Enterprise Service Bus (ESBs), Service Delivery Platforms (SDPs), etc) are available to overcome the heterogeneity of system components [2].

ESB is an evolution in the integrated middleware software architecture that has gained the attention of architects and developers, as it provides interoperability, integration, mediation, security and reliability. The main role of the ESB is to serve as a communication bus accepting a variety of input message formats and transforming them to different output formats and thus providing a transparent communication

B. Godara and K.S. Nikita (Eds.): MobiHealth 2012, LNICST 61, pp. 234–246, 2013.

interface. Nevertheless, ESB implementation itself is not standardized but offers a messaging infrastructure based on standardized protocols. As a result, there are major differences in the feature sets of available ESBs (e.g. Oracle, IBM, Microsoft, Nokia, Siemens, etc) as vendors try to differentiate from each other.

In the eHealth domain, some enterprises have proposed and implement healthcare integration solutions such as IBM, Microsoft that are fully vendor proprietary and based on web service technologies. Moreover, some research efforts are trying on to create open ESBs for healthcare purposes but all of them focus on web services technologies. In [3] L.Gonzalez et al have proposed an e-health integration platform that is based on semantic and web service technologies for social security services. In addition, S. Van Hoecke et al in [4] have proposed a user- friendly and secure broker platform for e-homecare services that was designed using web service technology. It provided a well established mechanism for authenticating user once and being always connected, also for the implementation used an open ESB for the integration between requestors (users) and providers. Nevertheless, in the Hoecke proposal the syntactic, semantic and ontology integration is still a complex and complicated issue. Moreover, the Open eHealth Foundation [5] has already proposed and implemented an Open eHealth Integration Platform (IPF) that is based on open standards and Apache Camel [6]. Since IPF is licensed by Apache Software Foundation [6] the whole implementation is based on Apache software products and tends to be vendor proprietary even if Apache supports open source projects.

In this paper, we propose an Integrated Broker Platform (IBP) for open eHealth domain that supports the mobility of citizens and caregivers by providing the integration of various services through a unique framework. We propose the IBP architecture pattern and the functionalities that an open platform should have so as to let any developer and enterprise to create their own or use proprietary and legacy technologies. IBP provides syntactic and semantic interoperability by performing related transformations and is based on open standards in order to achieve the interoperable cooperation of different communication protocols and interfaces. IBP is a combination of cooperating but autonomous brokers. Each broker has its own functionalities and mechanisms so as to be completely autonomous and independent of the others in order to support a scalable and horizontal architecture. The autonomy and independency of each single broker provides the openness of IBP. Moreover, IBP is characterized as intelligent since it routes intelligently the messages to the appropriate brokers and provides an intelligent way to find/ bind and invoke services. In this paper, we demonstrate a fundamental IBP structure with a message and a service broker. The proposed architecture tends to bring interoperability both in personalized and mobile services [1].

2   Functionality of the Proposed

2.1   An overview of the IBP

The IBP for eHealth domain enables integration of services and data, and ensures interoperability between different proprietary devices, software systems, operating systems and implementation languages. IBP aims to simplify user interactions, provide security and guarantee quality requirements (e.g. QoS, QoE, etc).

The proposed IBP, as presented in Figure 1, is composed of: (a) a Telemedicine Service Bus (TSB) that is used as a backbone broker providing efficient message transformation and intelligent message routing [2] and (b) a Service Broker (SB) acting as the integration engine for finding/ binding and invoking of the requested service.

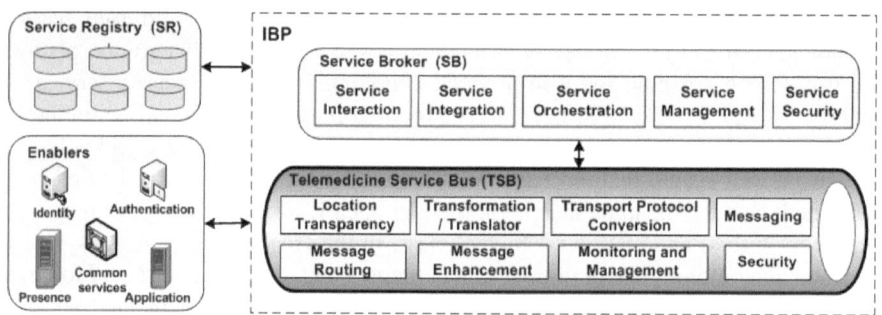

Fig. 1. An overview of the IBP

IBP is activated by event messages from various Enablers [2, 7] that acquire context aware data and provide operational events of any personalized healthcare case (e.g. elderly and disable people). Internal mechanisms of Enablers (e.g. control, administration mechanisms, etc) create standardized messages for the communication of these data and events with IBP through standardized APIs [Parlay/ETSI [8]]. These messages contain a Header and a Content (Body) part; however this message structure is out of the scope of this paper.

TSB is the receiver of the incoming message forwarded by the Enablers. Actually, TSB is a message channel, constructed as a common open source ESB based on Service Oriented Architecture (SOA) and enhanced with protocols for healthcare domain (e.g. DICOM, HL7, CDA, etc). The basic functionality of TSB is to mediate the messages from the Enablers to the SB [2, and 7]. The SB receives the transformed messages from TSB and provides mechanisms for processing the content of the messages in order to find/ bind and invoke the requested service from a Service Registry (SR). The SB is enhanced with open standard interfaces for sending and receiving messages from TSB to 3rd party providers and applications. These interfaces are combined with a set of strong rules in order to guarantee message delivery and processing [2, 7]. Finally, one or more SRs contain the lists of the services and URLs provided by 3rd party providers so as their services and resources to be accessible and discoverable from the SB [2, 7].

2.2   IBP Fundamentals

The proposed IBP is a brokering platform that provides end-to-end communication service through independent and operating autonomous brokers (TSB and SB).

In order to provide the full functionality character of the brokering platform, both the TSB and SB support the basic functionalities of message transferring, storing and verification.

- *Message Transferring*: The service components (TSB, SB) are responsible for transferring, handling, addressing, identifying and converting messages from the Enablers or from the Service Registry. For the efficient and secure transferring of these messages it is essential to manage and negotiate user's capabilities and relevant security issues.
- *Message Storing* is provided by service components such as data stores that handle the transmission and receipt of messages from or to the message storing entities.
- *Resource Verification* is essential in a brokering system in order to prevent malicious use for both the service components of the IBP and the end users.

2.3   TSB Messages

There are two discrete categories of messages in the proposed IBP architecture (Figure 1). The incoming messages created from Enablers that mentioned in section 2.1 and are out of the scope of this paper and the messages constructed by the TSB for internal message exchanging and routing. The messages constructed by the TSB have a common structure and consist of two parts, (a) the envelope that is constituted of four segments of fields and (b) the content that includes the initial incoming message from Enablers (section 2.1). The envelope includes the minimal information to support the required functionality so as not to increase significantly the size of the message and ensure the optimal use of the available resources. Moreover, it provides consistently the operation of TSB and its structure is presented in Figure 2.

```
<envelope>
        <originator></originator>
        <recipients>
                <recipient></recipient>
                ...
                <recipient></recipient>
                </recipients>
        <session_ID></session_ID>
        <message_ID></message_ID>
</envelope>
```

Fig. 2. The structure of envelope constructed by TSB

2.4   TSB Functionality

According to the functionalities that a brokering system has in the IBP (section 2.2), TSB is designed to be a lightweight, personalized integration solution with guaranteed reliability, which provides transparency from the application layer. In order to provide openness and flexibility, TSB should be designed following an abstract pattern and typical features [9]. Openness and flexibility allow 3rd party software developers to integrate their services, frameworks or enablers with no or minimal code modification to the system. To meet these major challenges the TSB includes the following key functions:

- **Location Transparency**: TSB contains and configures message endpoints so that to provide message transportation. These message's endpoints are a set of interfaces (APIs [8]), that contain information about the operating capabilities both of the applications and the messaging systems, bridging them transparently and knowledge independently from the location that the requestors and the receivers have.
- **Transformation/Translation**: TSB converts messages from one format to another based on open standards (e.g. XSLT, XPath, etc) and translates them according to syntactic and semantic rules.
- **Protocol Conversion**: TSB accepts messages sent with a variety of different application layer protocols (e.g. SOAP) and converts them to a format required by the Enablers, the SR and the SB.
- **Messaging**: TSB supports synchronous, asynchronous, point-to-point, and publish-subscribe operational modes for sending and receiving messages either from the Enablers or from the SB and SR.
- **Message Routing**: TSB provides flexible and intelligent routing by the means of a dynamic router, which allows the routing logic to be modified by sending control messages. Routing is an essential feature because allows to decouple the source of the message from the ultimate destination providing transparency between message requestor and receiver.
- **Message Enhancement**: TSB checks and compares the messages before delivering them to the SB. If there is an error in the transformation phase, then retrieves the missing data based on the existing message.
- **Monitoring and Management** are mechanisms for easy monitoring the performance and controlling the runtime execution of the message flows. Moreover, provides auditing mechanisms so as to be high performing and reliable [9].
- **Security** in TSB involves authentication, authorization and encryption or decryption functionality both into incoming and outgoing messages so as to prevent malicious use and handles messages in a fully secure manner [9].

2.5   SB Functionality

The key functionality of the SB is to process a received message from TSB and interact with SR so as to find, bind and invoke services and finally integrate, orchestrate the response of the message and forward it to the TSB. SB includes the following key functions similarly to the functionalities mentioned in section 2.3:

- **Service Interaction:** SB contains interfaces (APIs) to enable interaction and communication directly with the applications and services from 3rd party providers and supports standards for web service communication (e.g. SOAP, WSDL, etc). Moreover, Java Message Service (JMS) API and the J2EE Connector Architecture (JCA) are implemented for integration between application servers and message oriented middleware (MOM) [9]. Finally, are supported underlying protocols and communication mechanisms such as TCP, HTTP, SMTP, FTP, JBI, POP3, etc.

• **Service Integration:** The SB negotiates and enforces policies among service providers to guarantee secure service invocation.

• **Service Orchestration:** The received responses from the providers are processed using Business Process Execution Language (BPEL) and then integrated into a unified message with a common format so as to be invoked by the end user of the service.

• **Service Security:** Handles access control and authentication for messaging TSB and services provided by 3rd party providers. Moreover, encrypts and decrypts the content of messages preventing malicious interventions.

• **Service Management:** SB provides auditing facilities for monitoring the process execution and integration scenario.

3   Architecture of the Proposed IBP

In this section, according to the IBP functionality mentioned above, we analyze the architecture and Functional Entities (FEs) of the TSB and SB that compose IBP. It should be mentioned that all the Enablers and 3rd party providers are registered to the IBP so as to be widely accessible. Moreover, we consider that the monitoring, auditing and administrating mechanisms operate parallel with the TSB and SB FEs.

3.1   TSB Architectures and FEs

TSB roots the messages "onward towards to the intended recipients" by the means of the functional entities of the architecture that is presented in Figure 3.

TSB contains unique endpoints for the inbound and the outbound messages. Whenever messages either from Enablers or message responses from SB and SR trigger the TSB, the Inbound endpoint activates the Listener (step 1). Listener is permanently 'alive' and ready to accept messages. As soon as it receives a message it checks: (a) the validity of the message and the users' capabilities and (b) the available resources of TSB by the means of a filter and the central data store. If the incoming message is not certified as valid, the sender of the message is properly informed about the cause of failure and the actions to be performed to restart the session.

Listener automatically forwards the message to the TSB central data store (step 2). TSB central data store contains: (a) temporarily the incoming message for security and recovery purposes until the session is released/completed, (b)temporarily information about the users' capabilities and provide a Single-Sign-On ticket [2, 7] to be always connected, (c) rules for message translation and conversion and (d) 'traces' from the originated and delivered messages. The available resources of all FEs of TSB architecture are also registered in this data store. Moreover, Listener forwards the incoming message to a filter for validation (step 3). Since the message is validated and certificated, then the Message Creator (step 4) constructs the envelope for the message transition using identifying and structuring mechanisms. The enhanced message is composed of the envelope and the originated message. This enhanced message is forwarded into a message queue (step 5). The Message Processor gets the messages from the message queue (step 6), analyzes their envelope to identify the transition / transformation / conversion conditions and implements the necessary reformatting (syntactic level) and translation (semantic level) to the payload of the message using the information that is provided by the central data store. After structuring the new message it puts it to the queue of one of the available message stores of TSB (step 7). If the structuring of the new message cannot be completed due to the lack of some information into the payload of the message, then the 'trace' and the prior registered information from the TSB central data store are used to re-process the message (error handling) (step 8). Additionally, the Message Allocator interacts with a filter to certify the validity of the message derived from the message stores using the information that is provided by the central data store (step 9). In the case of a failure the TSB central data store is properly updated and a new session is started by the Listener (step 10). Finally, the Outbound message is delivered to the final recipient(s) by the Router that 'reads' the envelope to define the end-destination(s) and if necessary, it divides or multiply the payload of the message based on the conditions of transition (step 11).

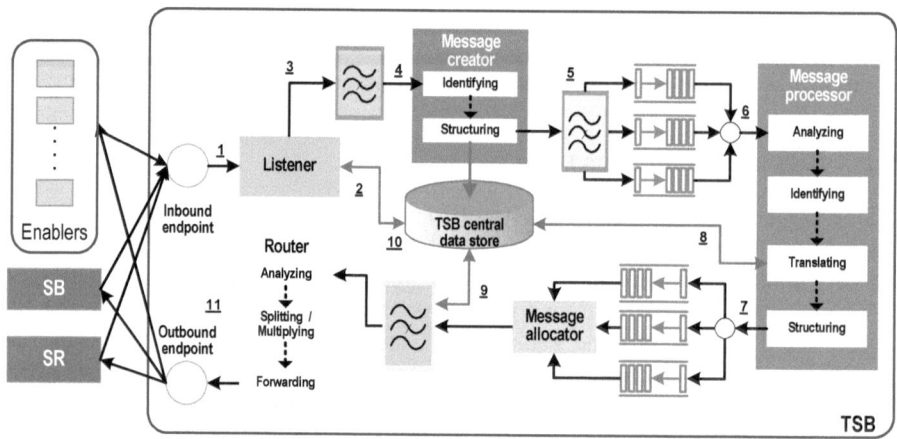

Fig. 3. TSB architecture

During the entire communication an auditing mechanism is enabled. For each process the exact time details (timestamps), successful and failed attempts are marked to monitor the performance, the effectiveness and the quality of the provided service.

3.2   SB Architectures and FEs

The architecture of SB follows the design of TSB architecture, since both of them are brokers and there are similar requirements for message administration (Figure 4). Respectively to TSB architecture, SB architecture contains a SB data store that keeps information about the APIs that are used for the interaction with the 3rd party providers and some policy aspects so as to provide an effective communication and ensure a secure invocation of the services provided by 3rd party providers.

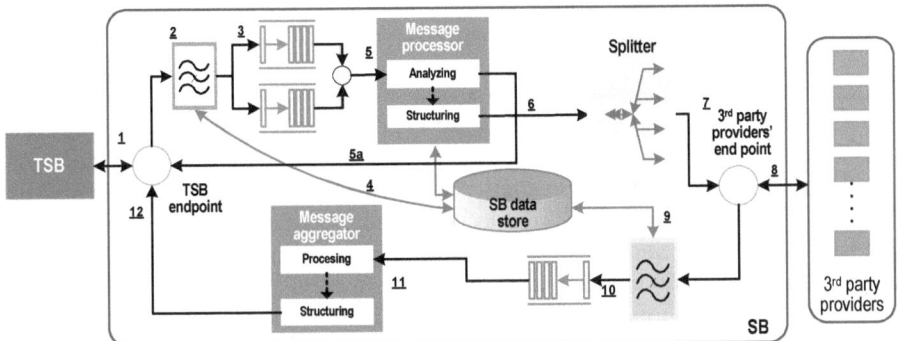

Fig. 4. SB architecture

Whenever a message triggers the TSB endpoint of SB, a session between the TSB and SB is activated (step 1). The inbound message from TSB endpoint is validated through a filter (step 2). The filter enforces some authentication and message validity control mechanisms using the information that is registered to the SB data store and puts the message to the queue of a message store (step 3). For the supervision of the entire communication a copy of the originated message is filed also to the SB data store (step 4). Then, the Message Processor gets the stored message from the queue and reads its content. The content of the message provides information about the required service of the end- user. For the efficient routing of the message into the appropriate service providers, the SB must communicate with the SR so as to find the most appropriate service for the end-user's request. For this reason, Message Processor sends back to TSB a request in order to activate/ trigger SR. SR is activated by the TSB, finds the appropriate service(s) and sends a response back to the TSB that gathers the message from SR with the service's URL and API(s). TSB forwards this message to the Message Processor following the above analyzed steps 1-5. Since Message Processor has successfully analyzed the content of the initial message, then through a structuring mechanism enhances the analyzed content with API information and the enhanced messages will continue to be delivered to the 3rd party providers (step 5). These messages are forwarded to the Splitter (step 6). In the real world, a received message is most of the times a complex process which is composed of many sub-processes for finding and binding more than one service from different service providers. The Splitter shares these messages simultaneously to the appropriate service providers so as to bind the appropriate service for the end-user (step 7). interaction with the 3rd party providers is provided through a unique 3rd party provider's endpoint (step 8). The inbound responses are filtered and checked for the validity of the messages retrieving the necessary information from the SB data store (step 9). The valid messages are put to the queue of a message store (step 10).

Moreover, The Message Aggregator processes the received messages using the BPEL and then it integrates them to a unified message (step 11), which is forwarded to TSB endpoint and finally to the TSB for continuing the session with the service applicant (step 12).

4   Implementation of the Proposed IBP

Today, in the market field there is available a variety of different ESB products such as Oracle ESB, JBOSS, OpenESB, MuleSoft ESB- MuleESB, and other [10, 11, 12, 13,]. Our IBP architecture is based on open standards and provides integration independent from the software products what will be used for implementing either the TSB or the SB. For this reason, we selected from a list of open source ESB software products [12, 13], the MuleESB [14] for a prototype implementation. The MuleESB is a very famous and not commercial product that supports a wide variety of transport protocols, data transformation, data formats, programming languages, web services, cloud connectors and security mechanisms. Moreover, according to Z. Siddiqui et al [15] analysis based on Analytical Hierarchy Process (AHP), MuleESB is more preferable, information secure, high available and interoperable in contrast to FuseESB. In contrast with the JBoss [16], MuleESB's performance in a typical message routing without business logic was 3 times faster.

The proposed IBP has been implemented as prototype to provide medical personalized services and its pilot operation performed into the laboratory. For the exchanged messages the HL7 v2.x and HL7 v3 standards were applied and for the implementation of them the NeoTool Library was used. The engines of IBP that provide the messaging, the routing and the translation / conversion mechanisms were implemented as independent Java modules using the Eclipse IDE that is a platform compatible with the MuleESB.

For evaluating the prototype implementation a simple communication scenario was built utilizing already developed Medical Information Systems (MISs). In this scenario, we consider that the tele-healthcare service used by the physician is authorized to receive data from a MIS provided that the two systems ought to satisfy and fulfill the appropriate policy agreements and Service Level Agreements (SLAs). In this case study, we also consider that the doctor's application is a telemedicine service using the HL7 v.2.0 for the message administration and transformation. In the same time the MIS is an EHR system that applies the HL7 v.3.0 standard for the organization, administration and transmission of messages.

In the pilot operation, the IBP platform is triggered by the physician's application/ enabler to retrieve data (e.g. user's profile and laboratory exams) stored in an EHR (of the 'healthcare center' where the patient has been hospitalized). The IBP receives a message/ request for data retrieval, the Listener of TSB is automatically activated and the whole service recovery process in collaboration to the SB (analyzed in section 3) takes place. The SB authorizes, authenticates and validates doctor's access for this request. Since SB identifies the physician's privileges, then sends via the IBP a request to trigger the appropriate EHR's units, retrieves, collects and sends the requested on demand data to the physician.

To monitor the whole process and evaluate the response time of the IBP, a logging service (auditing service) was implemented, which is activated during the entire communication and messages transformation / exchange creating log files with all the necessary information regarding: successful or non - execution of the message processing and transmission from one system to the other, the response times of IBP and the overall time of the session (from receiving the original message to return the requested data).

These parameters were the base for the extraction of statistical and evaluation of quality factors for the developed IBP, according to the ISO 9126 model's characteristics [17] that regard the Functionality, the Reliability and the Efficiency. The results for these three factors are presented in the following diagrams and the Table includes the relative logged measures.

Table 1. Logged evaluation parameters of IBP

Evaluation parameters	Measurements	Statistical	
Set 1: Number of transgerred messages	*(messages)*		
Messages originally sent	616	-	-
Delivered & acknowledged messages	606	98.38%	1.62%
Rejected by filters	7	1.14%	98.86%
Resent (delivered / not)	134	99.26%	0.74%
Set 2: Times and delays	*(sec)*		
Memory queuing time	1.7	-	-
Resending delay	2.1	-	-
Total transferring time	24	-	-
Total completing session time	48	-	-
Set 3: Sessions through IBP	*(sessions)*		
Attempted sessions	388	-	-
Complete TSB-SB sessions	383	98.71%	1.29%
Complete MIS-IBP sessions	381	98.20%	1.80%
Complete transfers of messages	380	97.94%	2.06%

By analyzing the results of this process, it came out that the IBP achieves to satisfy this specific and simple communication by finalizing successfully all the processes for message transformation and elaboration, even though the response times remain in tolerated, but not in satisfactory levels. This arises the need for optimization the modules of IBP that implement the message processing concerning the algorithms that they use and the lack of parallel processors that share the message traffic.

From the whole process of implementation and the pilot operation of the IBP, it was validated that for the communication of the external systems no alteration is needed as regards the end-user services that these provide.

Meaning that, the architecture and the communication models provided and supported by the IBP do not interfere at all to the harmonious operation of the existing systems and no effort is needed for the integration of IBP to already applied business models into a healthcare organization.

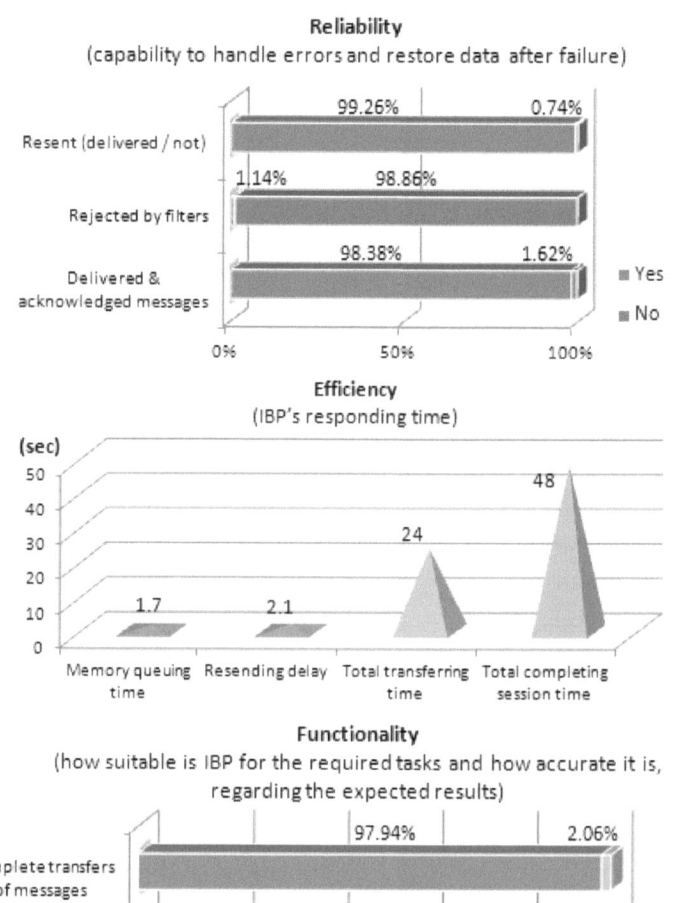

Fig. 5. IBP quality factors

5   Conclusion

This paper proposes an open IBP architecture for the eHealth domain. We analyzed thoroughly the architecture and the functionality of each of the core brokering components (TSB and SB) for message and service delivery purposes. In order to clarify the potential role of the IBP architecture in the real world for personalized and mobile services, we described analytically the message and service delivery processes that provide location transparency and are aware of contexts. Finally a prototype was implemented using an open source, non commercial software product, the MuleESB.

For future work, we plan to study the performance of the IBP, evaluating the IBP's behavior in real world. This real world IBP environment will be consisted of more than four autonomous and independent brokers such as context broker that will enhance the functionality of IBP with advanced personalized features.

References

1. Continua Health Alliance, http://www.continuaalliance.org/index.html
2. Andriopoulou, F., Lymberopoulos, D.: A new platform for delivery interoperable Telemedicine services. In: Proc. Second Int. ICST Conf on Wireless Mobile Communication and Healthcare, Kos Island, October 5-7, pp. 181–188 (2011)
3. Gonzalez, L., Llambias, G., Pazos, P.: Towards an e-health integration platform to support social security services. In: Proc. 6th International Policy and Research Conference on Social Security, Luxembourg, September 29-October 1(2010)
4. Van Hoecke, S., Steurbaut, K., Taveirne, K., De Turck, F., Dhoedt, B.: Design and implementation of a secure and user-friendly broker platform supporting the end –to-end provisioning of e-homecare services. Journal of Telemedicine and Telecare 16, 42–47 (2010)
5. Open eHealth Foundation,
   http://www.openehealth.org/display/OEHF/Foundation
6. The Apache Software Foundation, http://www.apache.org/
7. Andriopoulou, F., Lazarou, N., Lymperopoulos, D.: A proposed Next Generation Service Delivery Platform (NG-SDP) for eHealth domain. In: Proc. of 34th Annual Intern. Conf. of the IEEE Engineering in Medicine and Biology Society, San Diego, August 28-September 1 (2012)
8. ETSI ES 203 915-3 V1.2.1, Open Service Access (OSA); Application Programming Interface (API); Part 3, Framework, Parlay 5 (2007)
9. Menge, F.: Enterprise Service Bus. In: Proc. of Free and Open Source Software Conference (2007)
10. Woolley, R.: Enterprise Service Bus (ESB) Product Evaluation Comparisons. UTAH Department of Technology Services (October 18, 2006)
11. Mr. Gupta, Enterprise Service Bus Capabilities Comparison, in Project Performance Corporation Part of AEA Group (April 2008), http://www.ppc.com/documents/enterprisebus.pdf
12. Pronschinske, M.: Top Open Source ESB Projects (October 2009), http://architects.dzone.com/news/top-open-source-esbs
13. Cope, R.: Comparison of Open Source ESB Solutions (August 2010), http://www.openlogic.com/

14. MuleSoft [TM], http://www.mulesoft.com/company
15. Siddiqui, Z., Abdullah, A.H., Khan, M.K., Alghathbar, K.: Analysis of enterprise service buses based on information security, interoperability and high availability using Analytical Hierarchy Process (AHP) method. Inter. Journal of Physical Sciences 6(1), 35–42 (2011)
16. Tiwari, N.: JBOSS ESB vs Mule Performance (August 2008),
    https://community.jboss.org/message/506587
17. ISO/IEC 9126, International Standard, Information Technology – Software Product Evaluation – Quality characteristics and guidelines for their use (1991),
    http://www.usabilitynet.org/tools/r_international.htm

Group Profile Creation in Ubiquitous Healthcare Environment Applying the Analytic Hierarchy Process

Maria-Anna Fengou, Georgia Athanasiou,
Georgios Mantas, and Dimitrios Lymberopoulos

Wire Communications Laboratory, Electrical and Computer Engineering Department,
University of Patras
University Campus, 265 04 Rio Patras, Greece
{afengoum,gman,dlympero}@upatras.gr, gathana@ece.upatras.gr

Abstract. Nowadays, the personalization in ubiquitous healthcare is of utmost importance for enabling the provision of services tailored to the patient's needs and interests. The personalization of the ubiquitous healthcare services is based on the profiles of the entities participating in these services. Such an application is the dynamic creation of the group of the entities that is formed to deliver the healthcare service to the patient. In this paper, we propose an approach for achieving creation of group profiles in a ubiquitous healthcare environment applying the Analytic Hierarchy Process.

Keywords: ubiquitous healthcare, group profile management, analytic hierarchy process.

1 Introduction

Nowadays, ubiquitous healthcare (UH) plays a major role in the patient-centric model since it requires the provision of healthcare to anyone, anytime and anywhere without limitations on time and location. Thus, UH services are designed having the patient as the core entity. The patient not anymore passively receives the healthcare service, but participates dynamically in service deployment and provision. The different states of the patient's health condition lead to different treatment schemes. The entities that are involved in these schemes should be dynamically organized per case in order to form the group that will deliver the UH service. To achieve such personalization in UH services, the existence of the profile for all the participating entities is required as well as the creation of a group profile.

In this paper, we carry on our work from [1], in which a group profile management system for UH environment is presented. In particular, we propose an approach for achieving creation of group profiles in a UH environment applying the Analytic Hierarchy Process (AHP) [2].

Following the introduction, this paper is organized as follows. In Section 2, related work to the group profile management in UH as well as to applications of AHP in UH is presented. In Section 3, the proposed approach for implementation of the group profile creation mechanism is presented. In section 4, a scenario of the implementation of the

B. Godara and K.S. Nikita (Eds.): MobiHealth 2012, LNICST 61, pp. 247–254, 2013.

analytic hierarchy process in the group profile creation in UH environment is deployed and then the scenario is evaluated. Finally, Section 5 concludes the paper and discusses the future work.

2   Related Work

2.1   Group Profile Management in Ubiquitous Healthcare

The work in [1] introduces a Group Profile Management System in a UH environment. The proposed system integrates the following four mechanisms: the Event Handler, the Role Assignment, the Group Profile Creation and the Group Profile Update that are responsible for the dynamic creation of the group profile and its management. It is considered that a UH environment is composed by UH entities with the patient being in the center.

Each of the participating entities in the UH environment has a profile. The state of the patient's health condition is the inception for a UH service to be delivered. At a time, the patient's healthcare condition can be in only one state. At each state, certain UH services are provided to the patient by certain entities. For the provision of such services, the determination of the entities that will participate to form dynamically the group is of great importance. For that reason, the group profile integrates two main types of information; the roles and the rules. The roles correspond to the participating entities that are essential for each group in order to accomplish the overall tasks. The group consists of entities with discrete roles in the provision of the UH service. The rules are statements required for the selection of the appropriate entities.

2.2   Analytic Hierarchy Process in Healthcare

AHP, proposed by Saaty [2], is a structured technique for organizing and analyzing complex decisions. It is used with success in a wide variety of decision situations, in many different fields such as everyday life issues [3], socio-economic planning sciences [4], military [5] and resource allocation and management [6]. AHP has also been applied in healthcare for solving multi-attribute decision making problems.

The work [7] deals with strategic enterprise resource planning (ERP) in a health-care system using a multi-criteria decision-making (MCDM) model. The model is developed and analyzed on the basis of the data obtained from a leading patient-oriented provider of health-care services in Korea. Goal criteria and priorities are identified and established via the AHP.

DIABRA (DIABetes Risk Assessment) [8] is a knowledge-based expert system developed to aid individuals to assess their chance for getting Type 2 diabetes. The system core is a quantitative model, implemented by AHP mechanism, to evaluate the developed scenarios. The acquired knowledge as scenarios are scored by AHP mechanism and represented in the DIABRA. The validation results show the expert system gives a highly satisfactory performance when compared to human experts.

This work [9] showed how the AHP decision support technique can be applied to clinical engineering health technology assessment projects. AHP provides a structured method of organizing and documenting the decision process and takes into consideration the many tradeoffs that exist between alternate choices. When an AHP model is properly designed and implemented, it facilitates interdepartmental and interdisciplinary communication and results in a decision support tool that represents a consensus model. The AHP model can then be used to compare health technology alternatives and delivers a composite score for each alternative that identifies the best choice. AHP produces a clinical engineering decision support tool for the hospital that identifies the best technology alternative for their specific need.

The work [10] examines clinical laboratory and pharmacy deliveries in middle to large size hospitals, in order to evaluate whether or not a fleet of mobile robots can replace a traditional human-based delivery system. The complexity of the problem derives from its multi-objective character, since several, often contrasting factors must be taken under consideration. The Analytic Hierarchy Process was used to build a decision problem that synthesized economic and technical performance as well as social, human and environmental factors. This research provides a methodology to approach automation introduction evaluation in a hospital environment.

The objective of the work [11] is to introduce the AHP as a preference elicitation method in health technology assessment (HTA). Patient involvement is widely acknowledged to be a valuable component in HTA and healthcare decision making. However, quantitative approaches to ascertain patients' preferences for treatment endpoints are not yet established. It is concluded that AHP can be used in HTA to give a quantitative dimension to patients' preferences for treatment endpoints.

The objective of the work [12] is to illustrate how the AHP can be used to promote shared decision-making and enhance clinician–patient communication. The AHP promotes shared decision-making by creating a framework that is used to define the decision, summarize the information available, prioritize information needs, elicit preferences and values, and foster meaningful communication among decision stakeholders. AHP is a well-developed method that provides a practical approach for improving patient–provider communication, clinical decision-making, and the quality of patient care in these situations.

3   Proposed Approach for Implementation of the Group Profile Creation Mechanism

As we proposed in [1], the group profile creation mechanism is used for the creation of the required group profile based on the current patient's health condition. To determine each of the participating entities of the group profile, we propose the use of the AHP.

To select the appropriate entity is a complex decision since many criteria should be taken into consideration. These criteria are related to the participating entities in the group profile with the patient being the center of the provisioned UH services. For instance, two criteria may be the availability of the potential participating entities and the patient's preference on the potential participating entities.

The potential participating entities that can be assigned to a role are called alternatives. Based on the criteria, the alternatives will be ranked in order to be selected the alternative with the highest priority. AHP is used to determine the entity that will eventually participate in the group profile. The AHP is a method consisting of the following four concrete steps.

In the first step, to select the participating entity that will participate in the group profile, we define the goal, the criteria and the alternatives which are structured in a hierarchy as depicted in Fig. 1. The goal which is the selection of the appropriate entity is in the top level of the hierarchy. The criteria which contribute to the goal are in the middle level, and the alternative participating entities, who are to be evaluated in terms of the criteria, are in the bottom level of the hierarchy.

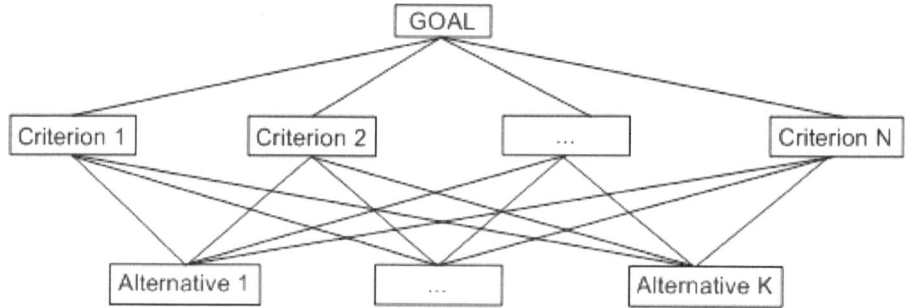

Fig. 1. Principal hierarchical structure

In the second step, according to the AHP process the criteria are constructed as a set of pairwise comparison judgments in a reciprocal matrix i.e. $a_{ji}=1/a_{ij}$, $a_{ii}=a_{jj}=1$. For this comparison, a scale of numbers (1-9), which is validated for effectiveness, is used. That scale indicates how many times more important or dominant one criterion is over another criterion with respect to the criterion to which is compared. The result of this process is the Relative Value Vector (RVV) which is the principal eigenvector of the matrix. The RVV gives the relative priority of the criteria measured on a ratio scale i.e. which criteria have the highest priority with a ratio of influence.

In the third step, the alternatives (bottom level of the hierarchy) are compared in pairwise with respect to how much better one is than the other for the satisfaction of each criterion defined in the middle level. The judgments of the matrices depend on the characteristics of the alternatives with regard to each of the criteria. The process results to the Local Value Vector (LVV) that gives the local priorities of the alternatives on a ratio scale.

To deduce the objectiveness of the judgments in the above matrices, the consistency ratio (CR) is checked when each matrix is constructed. The CR should range between 0 and 0.1 in order the matrix to be consistent. To have a final selection of a participating entity that has not been determined randomly, the CR should not exceed the upper limit in all matrices.

The result of the fourth step is the desired vector of the alternatives from which it is deduced the participating entity that will be eventually chosen. This vector is called Global Value Vector (GVV).and is calculated by the following process: a) the LVV of all the alternatives with respect to each of the criteria is laid out in a matrix, b) each column of these vectors is multiplied by the RVV that shows the priority of the corresponding criterion and c) each row is added across. This process is given by the following formula:

$$GVV = RVV \times LVV \tag{1}$$

4 Implementation and Evaluation

4.1 Scenario

We consider that the current patient's health condition is the emergency state and the patient requires a specific healthcare service. For the provision of this service, the roles that are essential for the group creation are the role of a doctor and the role of a relative. Thus, two different decisions should be made for the group creation. The first one is related to the selection of the most suitable doctor and the second one is associated with the selection of the appropriate relative. In our scenario, the selection of the doctor is analyzed in details below.

Initially, the criteria that will determine this decision are defined. From the patient's perspective, it is important to be treated by a preferred doctor. For that reason, as we presented in [1], the patient has already defined in his profile a catalogue with the potential participating entities for each role of the group profile that he would prefer to participate in his treatment. In this catalogue, the preferred doctors for his treatment are also defined. In this scenario, in the patient's profile there are five potential doctors ranked according to his preferences. Another criterion is the location of the potential participating entity (e.g. doctor). When the doctor is closer to him, the patient may feel safer. From the doctor's perspective, an important criterion is his availability as well as the capabilities of his devices that determine the quality of the provided healthcare service.

In Fig. 2, it is depicted the scenario structured in a hierarchy. The selection of the appropriate doctor is the goal, the five doctors are the alternatives, and the criteria for evaluating these alternatives are four.

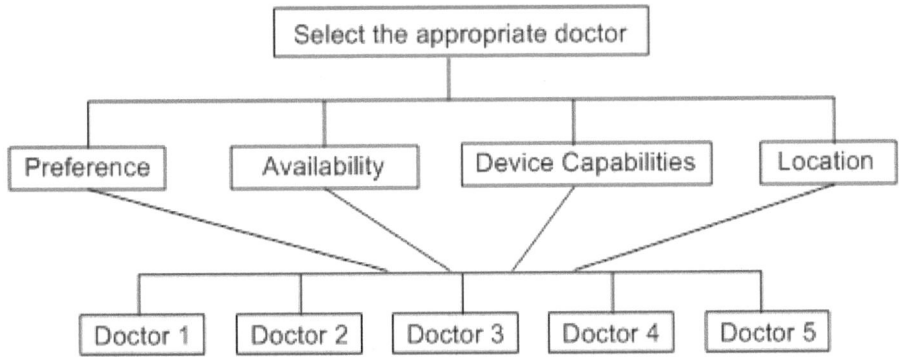

Fig. 2. Scenario analyzed in a hierarchical structure

To apply the AHP in group profile creation we consider that the five potential doctors that exist in the patient's profile have the following characteristics at the time of the decision.

Doctor 1 is on a private examination far from the patient, carrying only his mobile phone of poor capabilities. In the patient's profile, Doctor 1 is designated as the first choice because he is the doctor that formally treats him.

Doctor 2 is at his house which is in the same neighborhood with the patient. However, he has set himself available for offering healthcare service only if needed. He is carrying a mobile phone of new generation. In the patient's profile, Doctor 2 is designated as the second choice for being selected.

Doctor 3 has just walked away from a private examination carrying with him the PDA. He is located close to the patient's house. Therefore, he is totally available for offering his healthcare services, if needed. Moreover, he is ranked as the third preferred selection in the patient's profile.

Doctor 4 is at his office which is very close to patient's house. Non-having examinations and sitting in front of his desktop, he can offer his healthcare services. However, he is set nearly on the bottom of the patient's preferences, as he is non-aware of patient's medical history but he had examined the patient in the past.

Doctor 5 is on duty at the hospital far from the patient's location carrying his PDA. He is designated as the last preferred option in the patient's profile.

4.2   Evaluation

Based on the above scenario, we run the decision making algorithm to select the appropriate participating entity in the UH group profile. Inspired by AHP method, we applied this algorithm for the selection of the one of the five doctors that will participate in the group profile. The results from the simulation are presented in this section.

The pairwise comparison matrix for the criteria with respect to the goal is depicted in Fig. 3. Comparing the criteria on the left with the criteria on the top as to their importance, it emerges that the patient's preference has the highest priority with 55,34% of the influence. The CR is 0.071.

	Preference	Availability	Device	Location	Relative Value Vector
Preference	1	3	6	8	0.5534
Availability	1/3	1	5	7	0.3023
Device	1/6	1/5	1	3	0.0969
Location	1/8	1/7	1/3	1	0.0474

Fig. 3. Pairwise comparison matrix of the criteria

There are four 5 X 5 matrices of judgments since there are four criteria in the second level, and 5 doctors to be pairwise compared for each criterion. These pairwise comparison matrices for the alternatives with respect to each one of the criteria are depicted in Fig. 4.

CRITERIA		Doctor 1	Doctor 2	Doctor 3	Doctor 4	Doctor 5	Local Value Vector
PREFERENCE	Doctor 1	1	3	5	7	9	0.5028
	Doctor 2	1/3	1	3	5	7	0.2602
	Doctor 3	1/5	1/3	1	3	5	0.1344
	Doctor 4	1/7	1/5	1/3	1	3	0.0678
	Doctor 5	1/9	1/7	1/5	1/3	1	0.0348
							CR=0.053
AVAILABILITY	Doctor 1	1	6	1/5	1/2	7	0.1728
	Doctor 2	1/6	1	1/8	1/7	2	0.0478
	Doctor 3	5	8	1	3	9	0.4970
	Doctor 4	2	7	1/3	1	8	0.2492
	Doctor 5	1/7	1/2	1/9	1/8	1	0.0331
							CR=0.065
DEVICE	Doctor 1	1	1/3	1/5	1/9	1/5	0.0400
	Doctor 2	3	1	1/3	1/7	1/3	0.0805
	Doctor 3	5	3	1	1/3	1	0.1975
	Doctor 4	9	7	3	1	2	0.4684
	Doctor 5	5	3	1	1/2	1	0.2135
							CR=0.017
DISTANCE	Doctor 1	1	1/7	1/3	1/4	3	0.0702
	Doctor 2	7	1	5	3	9	0.5127
	Doctor 3	3	1/5	1	1/2	6	0.1516
	Doctor 4	4	1/3	2	1	7	0.2313
	Doctor 5	1/3	1/9	1/6	1/7	1	0.0342
							CR=0.043

Fig. 4. Pairwise comparison matrix for the alternatives with respect to each of the criteria

The desired Global Value Vector of the alternatives is depicted in Fig. 5.

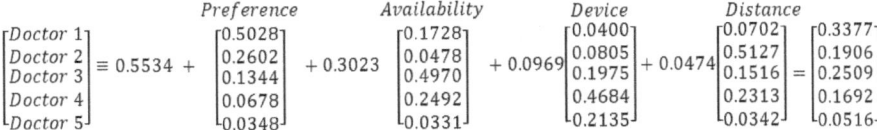

Fig. 5. Priority ranking of the alternatives

Observing the resulted GVV, Doctor 1 has the largest priority to be selected to participate in the group. This selection is also the most desirable with respect to the patient's preferences (the highest priority criterion). Doctor 3 is the second choice to participate in the group even if he was not declared as the second choice in the profile.

5   Conclusion and Future Work

In this paper, we have proposed an approach for achieving the creation of group profiles in a UH environment applying the AHP. The results indicate that AHP leads to an optimal selection of the participating entity taking into account all the required criteria. As future work, we intend to customize the AHP in order to optimize its performance for group profile creation in a UH environment. The integration of the customized AHP in the group profile creation process will lead to a more efficient health delivery process.

References

1. Fengou, M.-A., Mantas, G., Lymberopoulos, D.: Group Profile Management in Ubiquitous Healthcare Environment. In: 34th Annual International Conference of the IEEE Engineering in Medicine and Biology Society, EMBC (2012)
2. Saaty, T.L.: Decision making with the analytic hierarchy process. Int. J. Services Sciences 1(1), 83–98 (2008)
3. Chou, W.-H.: Using AHP to Assess a Plan of Training the Adolescent Golf Player. In: 5th IEEE International Conference on Fuzzy Systems and Knowledge Discovery, pp. 575–579 (2008)
4. Srdjevic, B.: Linking analytic hierarchy process and social choice methods to support group decision-making in water management. Decision Support Systems in Emerging Economies 42(4), 2261–2273 (2007)
5. Yao, Y., Zhao, J., Sun, J., Wang, Y.: The MADM-AHP method on estimating attempt of target in air defense. In: IEEE Conference on Intelligent Computing and Intelligent Systems, pp. 526–529 (2010)
6. Min, W., Shining, L.: An energy-efficient load-balanceable multipath routing algorithm based on AHP for wireless sensor networks. In: IEEE Conference on Intelligent Computing and Intelligent Systems, pp. 251–256 (2010)
7. Lee, C.W., Kwak, N.K.: Strategic Enterprise Resource Planning in a Health-Care System Using a Multicriteria Decision-Making Model. J. Med. Syst., 265–275 (2011)
8. Amin-Naseri, M.R., Neshat, N.: An Expert System Based on Analytical Hierarchy Process for Diabetes Risk Assessment (DIABRA). In: Tan, Y., Shi, Y., Chai, Y., Wang, G. (eds.) ICSI 2011, Part II. LNCS, vol. 6729, pp. 252–259. Springer, Heidelberg (2011)
9. Sloane, E.B.: Clinical engineering technology assessment decision support: a case study using the analytic hierarchy process (AHP). In: 24th Conference of the Biomedical Engineering Society, vol. 3, pp. 1950–1951. Springer, Heidelberg (2002)
10. Rossetti, M.D.: Multi-objective analysis of hospital delivery systems. Computers and Industrial Engineering 41(3), 309–333 (2001)
11. Danner, M., et al.: Integrating patient's views into health technology assessment: Analytic hierarchy process (AHP) as a method to elicit patient preferences. Int. J. Technol. Assess. Health Care, 369–375 (2011)
12. Dolan, J.G.: Shared decision-making – transferring research into practice: The Analytic Hierarchy Process (AHP). In: 4th Conference on Shared Decision Making, vol. 73(3), pp. 418–425 (2008)

Data Processing from mHealth Patient Data Acquisition Related to Extracting Structured Data from EH Records

Stefan Balogh, Fedor Lehocki, Daniel Ivaniš, Erik Kučera,
Miloš Lajtman, and Igor Miňo

Slovak University of Technology, Faculty of Electrical Engineering and Information
Technology, Institute of Computer Science and Mathematics, Ilkovicova 3,
812 19 Bratislava, Slovakia
{stefan.balogh,fedor.lehocki,daniel.ivanis,erik.kucera,
milos.lajtman,igor.mino}@stuba.sk

Abstract. Application of mobile devices in healthcare is a pervasive way how to asses patient health status. Adding just another data source to overwhelmed physician requires technologies for their effective processing. Despite the fact that the problem of extracting clinical information from free-text health reports for computerized applications or for decision support systems is a lot discussed issue, it is still complicated and unresolved question. In general Natural language processing (NLP) systems are implemented to solve the task. However NLP system works only for relatively narrow clinical domains because the format of the language used in the reports is not standardized and the reports vary depending on the domain. We describe methodology suggested for extracting structured data from EHR focusing especially on EHR in Slovak language. Further, we discuss problems concerning a task of extracting required data from free-text health reports. In the conclusion we present test results and possible implementations.

Keywords: Natural language processing, NLP, health reports, structured data, telemedicine.

1 Introduction

Increasing healthcare costs and shortage of physicians pave the road for new technologies to enter the healthcare sector. Although mHealth is around for some time, wide spread of mobile WWAN/ WLAN networks and cost effective wireless sensor equipment enable real pervasiveness of mobile health. This provides reliable and cost effective access for patients and physicians to health monitoring, data collection, delivery and support of health information, diagnosis and treatments, research and education. In this paper we would like to emphasize more on what happens "behind the curtain" i.e. when data are collected and stored. We believe that adding another data source to fill up data storage will not improve the quality of information or bring knowledge to support physician in his daily routine. Not all data collected by mHealth solution are structured. For example in case of self-management of diabetes [1], besides creating the structured data related to glycemia measurements and other relevant data,

B. Godara and K.S. Nikita (Eds.): MobiHealth 2012, LNICST 61, pp. 255–262, 2013.
© Institute for Computer Sciences, Social Informatics and Telecommunications Engineering 2013

patient can also create custom notes of unstructured text. These notes include observations about patient's general health with specific symptoms (in case of infection) or comments related to diabetes (hypoglycemia during the night). It would be interesting to incorporate methods for analyses of free-text in electronic health records (EHR) as part of mHealth solution related to data processing [2]. Data from EHR can be used also for provision of clinical decision support services. The unstructured content of patient's reports stored in EHR represents a rich source of data. Therefore it becomes a major bottleneck hindering widespread deployment of effective clinical applications because it is difficult, if not impossible, to access the textual information reliably by computerized processes [3]. For solving this problem different Natural language processing (NLP) systems were developed. A NLP-based approach has been applied for a variety of problems. These include identifying patient cohorts, reporting of diseases, syndrome surveillance, diagnostic classification, identifying co-morbidities, medication event extraction, adverse event detection, identification of postoperative complications, and disease management [8].

The paper focuses on describing the problems that are related to the processing of unstructured text contained in medical records taking into account various possible forms of the records defined for example by particular writing style of a physician. Aim of the presented work is to highlight design of the whole process of obtaining structured information from unstructured documents. Being aware of the particularities of Slovak language, we tried to describe all particular phases of the whole extracting process in detail. Sections 1.1 and 1.2 describe the existing work and specific problems, in section 2 we focus on suggested methodology, and in the section 3 related to conclusion we discuss the advances and shortcomings of the presented methodology.

1.1   Related Works

The related works can be divided into those where the text parser for concrete task in clinical area is described and those which deal with the text parser for general solution searching approaches. Friedman [3] analyzes semantic methods that map narrative patient information to a structured coded form. In [4] challenges are discussed related to processing of clinical reports like performance, availability and confidentiality of clinical texts, intra- and inter-operability. Other works concentrate more on development of accurate decision support system and free-text processor for extracting required information from reports. For example Aronsky *et al* [5] has demonstrated the development of accurate clinical decision support system (CDSS) for diagnosing pneumonia that utilized a free-text processor for pneumonia reports. Demner-Fushman *et al* [6] have discussed the potential of NLP to enhance CDSS. Dupuis *et al* [7] recently constructed a free-text parser to identify abnormal Pap reports. In [8] authors claim that the application of NLP for clinical decision support has been deferred, possibly because of the requirement for a high accuracy.

1.2   Specific Problems in NLP Systems

The main known problems which occur during application of NLP systems for extracting structures and codification of clinical information from the health reports are already described in [3]. It includes expressiveness, heterogeneous formats, abbreviated text, interpreting of clinical information, rare events. Also, physicians use their own special terms and abbreviations, so each report can have different terms, depending on an author (physician). Taking into account these problems we would like to present a design of a theoretical model for extraction of clinical structured information for medical application. Our target is to map the extracted information for a controlled vocabulary and for a standard domain representational model. The representational model of medical language is essential for interpreting the underlying meaning of clinical information in the reports and relations among the information. Creating such model is a demanding task already. Moreover, mapping of extracted terms from the health reports for that model is even more challenging.

2   Methodology

Core NLP system usually uses syntax and semantics analysis for achieving the correct result. Syntactic analysis determines the structure of a sentence and the relationships among the words in the sentence. Semantic analysis is a process that determines what words and phrases in the text are clinically relevant, and determines their semantic relations. An important requirement of semantic analysis is a semantic model of the domain or ontology [3]. The NLP system usually has components for morphological analysis, lexical look up, syntactic analysis, semantic analysis and encoding, still many variations are possible. More about these components can be found in [9]. For our purpose of extracting clinical information from various kinds of reports we have created our own methodology which deals with problems mentioned in previous section. The methodology consists of two phases, the preparation phase and the processing phase.

The preparation phase has the following activities: 1. Morphological analysis – (lematization); 2. Creating a list of words used in reports; 3. Lematizator completion; 4. Manual division of reports into logical sections; 5. Training the machine learning algorithm; 6. Obtaining required information from logical section into defined structure.

The processing phase consists of the following activities: 1. Lemmatization of a report; 2. Division of report into sections; 3. Encoding the required information to defined structure.

Further we describe all the activities in more detail for better understanding.

2.1   Preparation Phase

Preparation phase is necessary to avoid the previously mentioned problems for NLP systems and to adapt the system to real situation. It can be achieved by text normalization in reports. The medical reports are frequently written in technical language using loan words and their derivations, even in neologisms. Some physicians use their own special terms or abbreviations. Therefore, it is required to figure out a way to include these words in the process of lemmatization or, in case of abbreviations, to translate the words into their original form. To break up the original words in a text to their canonical forms in Slovak language we used lematizator called Morphonary [12]. Morphonary works with three dictionaries - Dictionary of Foreign/Derived Words (Slovník cudzích slov- SCS), Dictionary of the Slovak Language (Slovník slovenského jazyka- SSJ) and the Declined Words Dictionary. SCS contains about 60,000 words in the base form, SSJ two times more. The key vocabulary in this methodology is the Declined Words (DW) Dictionary. This dictionary contains 1730 words in the base form, as well as their all declined (inflected) forms. This dictionary is composed from a selection of such terms and words that make the best representation within variability of declined forms of words. In this dictionary there are pairs of words "basic form - declined form". During preparation phase we configured all components for reports from department of internal medicine taking into account text formats, sections format and specific words.

In the preparation phase we make **lemmatization** [12] of chosen number of reports using Morphonary and DW dictionary with default words. It is required in the process of examination of the list of the most common words in the reports. In the list we can find special medical terms or physicians own custom expressions, abbreviated text and words not included in our dictionary and therefore not corrected during lemmatization. In cooperation with medical staff we tried to find the real meaning of the words or abbreviated text. Then, during the lemmatization completion activity, we created a new pair in the Declined Words Dictionary. For example, if doctors used the abbreviation "pcnt" rather than the "patient", we have added to the DW dictionary pair "pcnt - patient". Then during lemmatization process this atypical shortcut is replaced with usual word "patient". Also we divided the report into logical sections manually in a chosen number of reports to enable training of the machine learning algorithm. As a last activity in this phase we choose an algorithm for obtaining required information from report into defined structure.

Creating a list of words used in reports - We examined the lemmatized texts using the application RapidMiner [1] and have created a list of the most common words. To obtain a list of words (wordlist) of selected documents we have used procedure including pre-processing, text tokenization and removing stop-words. Wordlist conveys the desired list of words. Therefore we removed the common words with the aid of dictionary of stop words. This provides the list of words and abbreviations that are specific to the reports and they should be identified and included into the DW dictionary.

Manual division of reports into logical sections - Logical section can be understood as part of a report describing the relevant topic, e.g. anamnesis, medications, laboratory results, diagnosis, etc. It can consist of several paragraphs (or vice versa).

Division of a report to its logical sections is necessary to provide correct data for machine learning algorithm. Usually logical section of a report can be generally

---

[1] http://rapid-i.com/content/view/181/190/

recognized but sometimes it must be discussed with the specialist who created the report. The first step is to split the text into paragraphs according to the written arrangement (usually defined by the writing style of a physician) of a document. It is based on the assumption that physician is also dividing text into paragraphs during creation of the patient's report.

During analysis of the available documents (approximately 3000 reports), in many cases text was structured into different paragraphs, although the unit has the same semantic part (logical section). To structure the parts of the texts in such documents doctor leaves out a line for each paragraph. Based on these findings, we implemented in the application the possibility of dividing a document according to paragraphs or left out lines. For the case of our reports we have divided paragraphs into nine sections: 1. Doctors' names, outpatient facilities; 2. Objective examinations and laboratory testing; 3. Medications, therapy; 4. Recommendations, conclusions; 5. Epicrisis; 6. ID code of physician and specialization; 7. Subjective problems; 8. Meaningless characters; 9. mixture of various categories.

Training the machine learning algorithm - This training is essential for the algorithm in categorization while performing supervised learning. The task is to train the algorithm for each kind of reports for its specific logical sections. Therefore, for the purposes of training data, only manually divided logical sections from the previous activity were used. For logical structure of our reports (divided into 9 sections as mentioned above), the most suitable was naive Bayes classifier.

Obtaining required information from logical section into defined structure - This part of the process requires defining the information and terms from the logical sections of the individual medical records and finding suitable methods for their accurate identification. It is usually not easy to decide on the right approach for solving this type of task. As we mentioned above we can use syntax tools or tools based on semantic analysis. But semantic approaches, while more precise, are subject to poorer coverage than syntax approaches [10]. Therefore in many cases the balanced approaches are used. Balanced approaches utilize more equal amounts of syntax and semantic processing. First comes the syntax processing and then the semantic analysis is applied to eliminate incorrect syntactic parse trees and to further identify domain words. Despite measures such as dividing into section it is necessary to use more advanced methods for correct identification of expression. The rule base may vary for each term and it is not possible to establish a general procedure. Therefore solutions need to be found for each term individually. The next necessary step is setting up the system that receives and manages to save those terms. In some cases, to correctly recognize them it is essential to use semantic analysis and create ontology. For example, in our case we configured the system for identification of drugs, blood pressure, and diagnosis. More complex structures for drugs were created that contained the name, dosage and prescribed quantity. Our rule base for obtaining structured information was developed and tested using the corpus of 3 000 test reports from department of internal medicine. We can see the example of identified structure related to drug data in report (Fig. 1) and the identified and filled structure of blood pressure on Fig. 2.

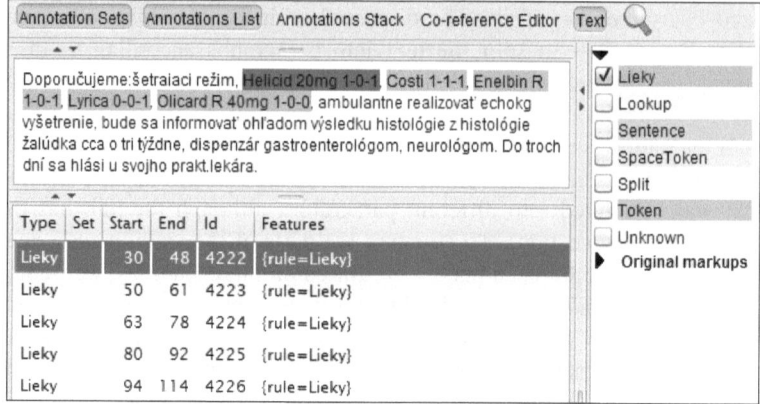

Fig. 1. Identified the structure of drugs

2.2   The Processing Phase

The processing phase has following activities: lemmatization of report, division of report into sections and encoding a particular phrase to relevant structure.

Lemmatization of report - For lemmatization we have used the DW dictionary prepared in preparation phase, so we can eliminate the problem of ambiguous abbreviations and specific medical terms in the given type of reports.

Division of the report into sections - For division we have used the chosen machine learning algorithm from preparation phase. The output is stored in text files which are systematically labeled by index number of the paragraphs in the original document. This ensures the possibility to re-stack the original document. Thanks to this extension we have solved the problem of heterogeneous report format and also this helps us to deal better with expressiveness-and interpreting clinical information.

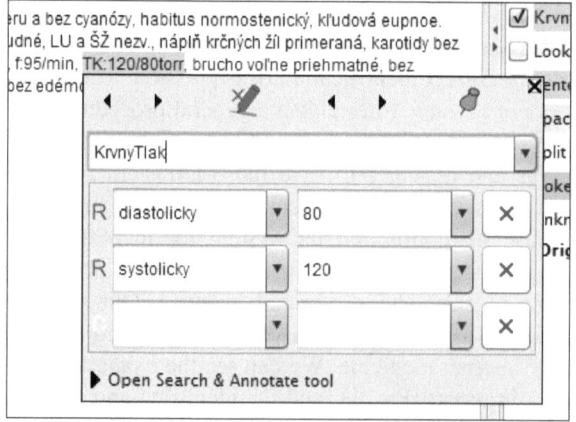

Fig. 2. Filled structure for blood pressure

Encoding the required information to defined structure - This was the last activity, where we have searched for specified information and filled them into desired structure for each logical section separately. We have used rule bases created in the preparation phase for processing of each logical section. Example of encoded particular phrase to a relevant structure is shown on Fig. 2.

3   Conclusion

The whole process is more complex in the final realization and it depends on many conditions. The main distinguishing factor is the purpose for which the information is gained, whether it is a single-purposed application based on a decision support system or whether the information must be available for different applications. In the latter case it is important to achieve the maximal re usability of data with respect to existing standards (e.g. archetypes). Importance of the whole methodology does not lie in the design of the process phase, but in the design of methodology of the preparation phase. The process stage is very simple. Lematize report and divide it into sections using selected and pre-configured techniques to store information to designated structures which can be used by other applications and systems. In the preparation phase the primary task is the setting up of lematizator. The new idea is using lemmatization process and Morphonary DW dictionary for Slovak language to translate and map the unknown words and the clinically relevant terms to well defined concepts in a controlled vocabulary (such as the known clinical healthcare terminology vocabularies like UMLS, ICD-9 or SNOMED) and to the original form of words. Also, new approach is represented in use of wordlist and stop words dictionary to filter familiar words which support easier identification of special unknown terms, completion of abbreviations and terms unknown to lematizator. The setting of the method for dividing paragraphs into given optional sections will extend to exploration and testing of different methods for text categorization and testing their effectiveness for the type of records. For finding and correct recognition of clinical information and inserting a particular phrase to a relevant structure (e.g. standard archetypes), syntactic and semantic analysis is used. The creation of such systems is also not a trivial problem. At the same time the tools that use syntax parsing seek to relate semantically relevant phrases via the syntactic structure of the sentence. In this sense, syntax serves as a "bridge" to semantics [11]. So we must find combination of syntax tool with suitable semantic one to achieve the goal. Cooperation with medical personnel is critical in achieving this goal. Without their support it would not be possible to configure the system or to create the ontology correctly (not mentioning the identification of abbreviation or special words). The methodology we have created had some shortcomings related to elegance in its application in different phases and activities (e.g. lematization, search and encoding information to relevant structures, splitting the unstructured text into logical sections, etc.). This also includes selection of a suitable machine learning algorithm for division report into logical sections. Overall, presented methodology provides complete and complex solution with explicitly defined phases and activities. Each activity can be implemented with different approach than described above. This is determined by the logical structure of the unstructured patient report and type of information that we search for in the text, i.e. position of desired information in the text like drugs, diagnosis, lab results etc.

Acknowledgments. The authors would like to acknowledge the support for research under following projects: Measuring, Communication and Information Systems for Monitoring of Cardiovascular Risk in Hypertension Patients (APVV-0513-10); Analytics Services for SMARTer Healthcare (IBM SUR project); Research & Development Operational Programme for the project Support of Center of Excellence for Smart Technologies, Systems and Services I and II (ITMS 26240120005, ITMS 26240120029), Competence Centre of Intelligent Technologies for Electronisation and Informatisation of Systems and Services (ITMS 26240220072), Knowledge discovery (ITMS 26240220063) co-funded by the ERDF.

References

1. Tatara, N., Arsand, E., Nilsen, H., Hartvigsen, G.: A review of mobile terminal-based applications for self-management of patients with diabetes. In: Intl. Confernce on eHealth, Telemedicine, and Social Medicine, Mexico, pp. 166–175 (2009)
2. NHS Choices UK's health website, http://www.nhs.uk
3. Friedman, C.: Semantic Text Parsing for Patient Records. Published in Medical Informatics: Knowledge Management and Data Mining in Biomedicine. Springer (2005)
4. Friedman, C., Johnson, S.B.: Natural Language and Text in Processing in Biomedicine. In: Biomedical Informatics: Computer Applications in Health Care and Medicine. Springer (2005)
5. Aronsky, D., Fiszman, M., Chapman, W.W., et al.: Combining decision support methodologies to diagnose pneumonia. In: Proc. AMIA Symp., pp. 12–16 (2001)
6. Demner-Fushman, D., Chapman, W.W., McDonald, C.J.: What can natural language processing do for clinical decision support? J. Biomed. Inform. 42, 760–772 (2009)
7. Dupuis, E.A., White, H.F., Newman, D., et al.: Tracking abnormal cervical cancer screening: evaluation of an EMR-based intervention. J. Gen. Intern. Med. 25, 575–580 (2010)
8. Wagholikar, K.B., MacLaughlin, K.L., Henry, M.R., Greenes, R.A., Hankey, R.A., Liu, H., Chaudhry, R.: Clinical decision support with automated text processing for cervical cancer screening. J. Am. Med. Inform. Assoc. (Published Online First April 29, 2012)
9. Chen, H., Fuller, S.S., Friedman, C., Hersh, W.: Medical Informatics: Knowledge Management and Data Mining in Biomedicine. Integrated Series in Information Systems, vol. 8. Springer (2005)
10. McDonal, D.M., Su, H., Xu, J., Tseng, C.-J., Chen, H.: Gene Pathway Text Mining and Visualization published in Medical Informatics: Knowledge Management and Data Mining in Biomedicine. Springer (2005)
11. Buchholz, S.N.: Memory-Based Grammatical Relation Finding. Computer Science 2, 17 (2002)
12. Krajči, S., Novotný, R.: Lemmatization of Slovak words by a tool Morphonary, Tools for Acquisition, Organisation and Presenting of Information and Knowledge (2). In: Proceedings in Informatics and Information Technologies, Vydavateľstvo STU, pp. 115–118 (2007) ISBN 978-80-227-2716-7

A Fuzzy Decision Support Language for Building Mobile DSSs for Healthcare Applications

Aniello Minutolo, Massimo Esposito, and Giuseppe De Pietro

Institute for High Performance Computing and Networking, ICAR-CNR
Via P. Castellino, 111-80131, Napoli, Italy
{minutolo.a,esposito.m,depietro.g}@na.icar.cnr.it

Abstract. Recently, Fuzzy Logic has been proposed as the most suitable approach for profitably tackling uncertainty and vagueness in clinical guidelines, and providing a new mobile generation of Decision Support Systems. This paper presents an intuitive XML-based language, named Fuzzy Decision Support Language, for both configuring a fuzzy inference system and encoding fuzzy medical knowledge to be embedded into a mobile DSS. Such a language enables the encoding of: i) fuzzy medical knowledge, in terms of groups of positive evidence rules and fuzzy ELSE rules assembling all the negative evidence for a specific situation; ii) input and output data, respectively elaborated or produced by the fuzzy DSS, in order to provide meaningful and semantically well-defined advices. As a proof of concept, the proposed language has been applied to encode, into a mobile DSS, the medical knowledge required to remotely detect suspicious situations of sleep apnea or heart failure in patients affected by cardiovascular diseases.

Keywords: Decision Support Systems, Fuzzy Logic, Clinical Guidelines, Mobile Computing, XML technologies.

1 Introduction

In the last decade, a new mobile generation of Decision Support Systems (DSSs) for healthcare applications is increasingly appearing on smart phones, aimed at locally reasoning about patient data and providing case-specific advices to health professionals, patients themselves or other concerned about them [1-2]. In particular, recent implementations of DSSs in medicine [3-5] rely on clinical practice guidelines encoded into crisp-based logical formalisms for simulating the process followed by the physicians and improving the efficiency of medical practices. However, they are not able to reproduce the real physician's decision-making process, since clinical practice guidelines are often pervaded by uncertainty and vagueness in both their recommendations and the clinical signs triggering them.

In this respect, Fuzzy Logic [6] has been proposed as the most suitable approach for profitably tackling uncertainty and vagueness in natural (textual) clinical guidelines, and providing enhanced DSSs [7-8]. One prerequisite for the broad usage of fuzzy DSSs in mobile applications and their efficient application to medical

B. Godara and K.S. Nikita (Eds.): MobiHealth 2012, LNICST 61, pp. 263–270, 2013.

settings is the guarantee of a high level of upgradability and maintainability in order to: i) change clinical rules according to their evolution in terms of medical progresses in the treatment of individual diseases; ii) adapt generic, site-independent clinical rules to the specific patient to be treated. These issues point out two main needs: first, fuzzy medical knowledge to be embedded in a DSS should be represented by means of a well-defined and machine-readable language to enable both easy of formalization and management; the mobile scenario demands for a technology to share fuzzy data and structure by granting portability, extensibility and re-use.

Several studies [9-11] have analyzed and proposed XML-based solutions to represent the knowledge base embedded into a fuzzy intelligent system in a common and human comprehensible manner, with the aim of supporting the seamless collaboration between developers and final users. Anyway, the existing solutions provide many general-purpose facilities for modeling fuzzy knowledge, without any form of vertical arrangement for the particular domain of interest. Specifically, to the best of our knowledge, so far, none of the existing approaches is specifically tailored to face two main issues regarding the encoding of fuzzy knowledge underpinning clinical practice guidelines: i) each guideline is made of a group of recommendations which contribute as a whole to detect the positive evidence of a single abnormal situation; ii) no recommendation is formulated to encode the negative medical evidence, i.e. when no abnormal situation is happened, and, thus, physicians are forced to write ad-hoc recommendations also for this case.

In this respect, an intuitive XML-based language, named Fuzzy Decision Support Language (in the following, FdsL), has been proposed and implemented for both configuring a Fuzzy Inference System (in the following, FIS) and encoding fuzzy medical knowledge to be embedded into a mobile DSS. In detail, two types of knowledge can be modeled: i) fuzzy terminological knowledge, in terms of both groups of positive evidence rules, which can be customized by means of a peculiar configuration for the inference, and fuzzy ELSE rules assembling all the negative evidence for a specific situation; ii) fuzzy assertional knowledge in terms of input and output data, respectively elaborated or produced by the fuzzy DSS, in order to provide meaningful and semantically well-defined advices and significantly increase the users' confidence in the final system.

The rest of the paper is organized as follows. Section 2 describes the proposed markup language, whereas, Section 3 depicts a proof of concept regarding a mobile DSS for detecting sleep apnea or heart failure. Finally, Section 4 concludes the work.

2   Fuzzy Decision Support Language

The approach, presented here, is to create the domain-specific language FdsL that unambiguously specifies all the parameters needed to build the FIS underpinning a DSS for mobile healthcare scenarios without enforcing a particular software framework. In addition, FdsL also enables the encoding of both the input and output data, respectively elaborated or produced by the fuzzy DSS, with the aim of encouraging the rapid development of DSSs for mobile healthcare applications and, contextually, to allow medical experts both i) to communicate domain-specific knowledge clearly when describing their decision-making procedures and ii) to simply understand the DSS's outcome, so that the learning curve is diminished or removed. Therefore, FdsL has been devised as simple as possible, yet as comprehensive as needed to provide general utility in fuzzy modeling with respect to mobile healthcare scenarios. As fundamental step necessary to achieve this objective, XML-derived technologies have been chosen since they allow to create data-oriented markup languages able to describe information in a designed working context. In particular, FdsL has been designed as an XML language in order to exploit its capability of defining a rudimentary syntax for specifying hierarchical data. Indeed, on the one hand, all the parameters needed to build a FIS, and, on the other hand, the input and output data elaborated or produced by the fuzzy DSS, have been arranged in accordance with a tree structure, whose FdsL formalizations is provided hereafter.

FIS. It can be modeled by means of a tag named <fuzzyInferenceSystem>, which represents the root node opening a FdsL markup program. Such a tag has two attributes: *name* and *note*. The *name* attribute permits to specify the name of the FIS, whereas *note* is used to provide a textual description about the final DSS based on it.

Concerning the definition of structural and logical parameters of the FIS, first of all, the set of fuzzy variables composing the knowledge base can be encoded by means of a set of nested tags, namely <fuzzyVariable>, to describe a linguistic concept, and <fuzzySet> to define a linguistic term associated to the concept.

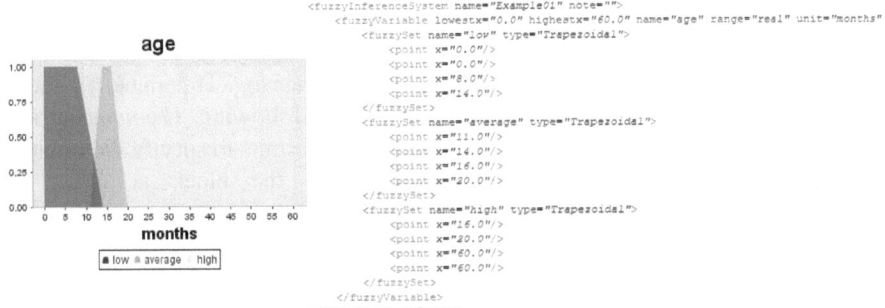

Fig. 1. A FdsL fragment modeling a linguistic variable "age"

More in detail, the attributes of the tag <fuzzyVariable > are: *name, range, unit, lowestx, highestx*. The *name* attribute defines the name of linguistic fuzzy concept; *range* and *unit* are used to define how it is measured; *lowestx, highestx* are used to model its universe of discourse. The tag <fuzzySet>uses two attributes, describing its *name* and the *type* of membership function used. A variety of shapes is supported for the membership functions, each of them customizable via a set of nested tags specifying its operational parameters. In detail, *Trapezoidal, Triangular, Singleton*, and *Piecewise* are describable by indicating their most significant points of their geometric shape by using the tag <point>. This tag uses one or two attributes, namely *x* and *y,* for defining the coordinates of the single points. In detail, if the attributes *y* are not expressed, the corresponding fuzzy sets are supposed as normal (i.e. for trapezoidal and triangular shapes, if the ordinates of their points are not expressed, they are automatically fixed as [0, 1, 1, 0], and [0, 1, 0], respectively). Other supported membership functions, which are *Bellcurve, Cosine, Gaussian,* and *Sigmoidal*, are not describable point by point but the tag <parameter> and its attributes *name* and *value* are used to define the parameters characterizing a specific function (i.e. for Gaussian shapes, parameters to be specified are mean and variance).

Considering as example, Figure 1 shows the FdsL fragment modeling the fuzzy variable "age" of a monitored patient, in terms of three trapezoidal fuzzy sets.

After defining the knowledge base of the FIS, the rule base can be modeled through a set of nodes named <rulesBlock>, placed under the root note through a father-child relation. This tag has been devised to group a set of fuzzy if-then rules depending on a same linguistic variable used in their consequent parts. Such a way, clinical guidelines, typically composed of isolated care recommendations linked to the same final action [12], can be encoded into the FIS. In this respect, Figure 2 shows an example of clinical guideline made of three recommendations linked to the same action, i.e. the lumbar puncture (LP) in children aged up to 60 months.

> IF the child age is low,
>   then LP is *strongly considered*
>
> IF the child age is average,
>   then LP is *considered*
>
> IF the child age is high,
>   then LP is *not routinely warranted*

Fig. 2. Clinical guidelines involved in the decision to perform the lumbar puncture

Since each rule block can be characterized by peculiar logical parameters, the tag <rulesBlock> uses the set of attributes described in the following. The *name* attribute uniquely identifies the rule block, *outputVar* attribute permits to specify the linguistic variable common to all the rules belonging to the block at issue. The *implicationMethod, aggregationMethod* and *defuzzificationMethod* attributes define the methods used to implication, aggregation ant defuzzification processes, respectively. The *andMethod* and *orMethod* attributes define, respectively, the fuzzy *And* and *Or* operators to connect the different clauses in antecedent parts of the rules belonging to the block. Such a way, the fuzzy inference is configurable with respect the single block of rules to best fit the peculiarities of the guideline evaluated.

In order to define the single implication rule within a block, the tag <rule> is used, which contemplates two attributes, namely *name,* to identify the rule, and *weight,* to encode the rule relevance to be considered during the inference process.

Each implication rule is characterized by two nodes, the <if> node containing the antecedent part of the rule, and the <then> node containing the consequent part of the rule. They can be used to model pieces of positive evidence, i.e. looking for those manifestations sufficient to establish a positive conclusion.

For what concerns the <if> node, rule antecedents can assume the form of: (i) a simple expression of only one clause (e.g., A is large); (ii) two clauses (e.g., A is large AND B is small), or (iii) composite expressions (e.g., A is large AND (B is small OR C is high)), where priorities have to be also managed. A simple expression of only one clause can be modeled by means of the <ruleClause> tag, directly nested under the <if> node. This tag uses four attributes, namely *variable* and *set* to indicate the fuzzy linguistic concept and term involved, *connector,* which can be either *is* or *isNot,* to relate the variable to a set or its complement, and *modifier* to associate a modification to the fuzzy set.

A rule antecedent of two clauses can be modeled by using the <ruleExpression> tag, directly nested under the <if> node, and a couple of <ruleClause> tags to express the clauses involved. The <ruleExpression> tag uses two attributes, namely *connection,* to express the logical connection between the clauses involved, and *isnegated,* to model the logical complement of the whole expression. Finally, composite expressions can be encoded by means of a set of nested <ruleExpression> tags, where the order of evaluation goes from the most internal rule expression to the most external one. As a result, a <ruleExpression> tag can contain two or more nested nodes, where each node can be either a <ruleClause> term or a <ruleExpression> one.

For what concerns the <then> node, the <ruleClause> tag is used to define the rule's conclusion about the linguistic variable associated to the rule block.

Finally, a <rulesBlock> can also contain one <elseRule> tag to model a rule for the negative evidence that is activated when the other rules of the block are weakly satisfied or not satisfied at all. Similarly to the <then> node, <ruleClause> tag is admitted to formalize the conclusion of the ELSE rule [13] about the linguistic variable associated to the rule block and, thus, to face the lack of exclusionary clinical recommendations in clinical guidelines. Figure 3 depicts the detailed structure of the whole FdsL model, designed for representing the FIS underpinning a DSS.

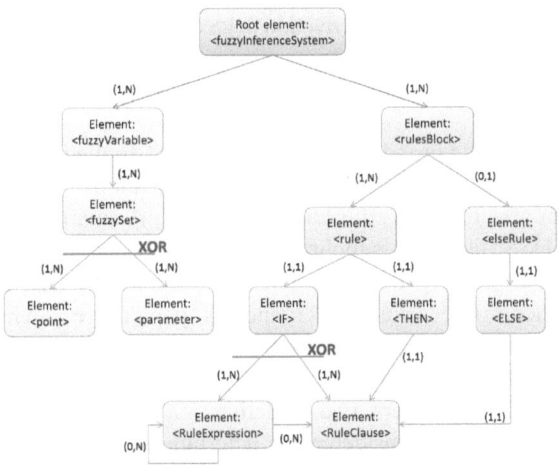

Fig. 3. The FdsL model for representing a FIS

Input and output data. The input and output data, respectively elaborated or produced by the fuzzy DSS, can be codified through two different FdsL descriptions, starting with the root tags named <reasoningInput> and <reasoningOutput>, respectively. Such tags have an attribute *name* which permits to specify the name of the input/output dataset. They admit the nested tags <fuzzyInferenceSystem>, to specify the system to be referred to, and <dataset>, which defines the collection of input data to be evaluated or output data inferred. Each element in this collection is referred by means of the <item>

tag. This tag uses the attribute *id* to specify a univocal identification number with respect to the dataset. Each <item> tag can contain two child tags, namely <input> and <output>, where the latter one is always omitted in the FdsL description of an input dataset.

The <input> tag contains one or more nested <fuzzyVariable> tags which specify the linguistic variables involved. Each <fuzzyVariable> tag can contain either a <fuzzySet> tag or a <crispValue> tag to express respectively its fuzzy or crisp input value. The attributes of the <fuzzySet> tag have been already described above, whereas <crispValue> tag uses the attribute *value* to indicate its input value.

The <output> tag contains one or more nested <fuzzyVariable> tags which specify the inferred fuzzy values for each linguistic variable involved in every single rule block of the FIS. In this context, the <fuzzyVariable> tag includes a nested <fuzzySet> tag to specify the inferred fuzzy value, a nested <defuzzifiedValue> tag to indicate the corresponding crisp value defuzzified according to the method set in the rule block, and, finally a set of <rulesActivationDegrees> tags to report the activation degree of each rule contained into the block. The attributes of the <fuzzySet> tag have been already described above, even if it is important to note that, in this situation, the only value admitted for the attribute *type* is Piecewise, since the shape of the inferred fuzzy set does not match with one of the predefined ones but it has to be specified point by point. The <defuzzifiedValue > tag uses the attribute *value* to indicate its output value. The <rulesActivationDegrees> tag uses the attribute <rulesBlock> to specify the block to be referred to, and includes a set of nested tags, namely <rule> and <else>. Both these tags use the attributes *name* and *degree* to describe the name of the rule and its activation degree, respectively.

3   A Mobile DSS for Detecting Sleep Apnea or Heart Failure

As a proof of concept, the proposed language has been applied to encode the medical knowledge required to remotely detect suspicious situations of sleep apnea or heart failure in patients affected by cardiovascular diseases. A smart phone, equipped with a mobile fuzzy DSS, has been supplied to the patient and wirelessly connected to some wearable sensors for gathering significant parameters, such as the respiratory rate (RR), the heart rate value (HR) and its percentage deviation (HR_Δ), the percentage deviation of the heart rate from respiratory rate ($RRHR_\Delta$), the hemoglobin oxygen saturation (SpO_2), and an estimation of the current physical activity.

Starting from such parameters, two guidelines, each of them made of four clinical recommendations, has been considered for determining situations of sleep apnea or heart failure, as shown in Figure 4. Each guideline has been modeled as a block of rules, where the first three ones enable to identify the positive evidence of the suspicious situations, whereas the last ones are ELSE rules, used when the other ones are weakly satisfied or not satisfied at all, to model the negative evidence.

Afterwards, the knowledge base of fuzzy linguistic variables has been constructed based on the ranges of the measured parameters. Finally, the rule base, the knowledge base and the whole set of parameters needed to configure the fuzzy inference engine underpinning the mobile DSS have been codified in FdsL as reported in the Figure 5. Such a FdsL program has been used to configure the fuzzy DSS deployed on the smart phone of the patient. Considering as a proof of the effectiveness of the proposed

r1: IF |RRHR$_\Delta$| is Negligible, THEN Apnea is Present	r5: IF HR is High AND Activity is Resting, THEN Heart-Failure is Present
r2: IF |HR$_\Delta$| is Great, THEN Apnea is Present	r6: IF HR is Low AND (Activity is Walking OR Activity is Running), THEN Heart-Failure is Present
r3: IF SpO$_2$ is Low, THEN Apnea is Present	r7: IF HR is VeryHigh OR HR is VeryLow, THEN Heart-Failure is Present
r4: ELSE Apnea is Absent	r8: ELSE Heart-Failure is Absent

Fig. 4. The fuzzy clinical guidelines of the considered case of study

```xml
<?xml version="1.0" encoding="UTF-8"?>
<fuzzyInferenceSystem name="FIS" note="">
  <fuzzyVariable lowestx="0.0" highestx="10.0" name="abs(RR_HR_delta)" range="real" unit="%">
    <fuzzySet name="Negligible" type="Triangular">
      <point x="0.0"/> <point x="0.0"/> <point x="10.0"/> </fuzzySet>
  </fuzzyVariable>
  <fuzzyVariable lowestx="10.0" highestx="30.0" name="abs(HR_delta)" range="real" unit="%">
    <fuzzySet name="Great" type="Trapezoidal">
      <point x="10.0"/> <point x="20.0"/> <point x="30.0"/> <point x="30.0"/> </fuzzySet>
  </fuzzyVariable>
  ...
  <rulesBlock aggregationMethod="max" andMethod="min" defuzzificationMethod="centerOfGravity"
        implicationMethod="min" name="Apnea" orMethod="max" outputVar="Apnea">
    <rule name="Rule1" note="" weight="1.0">
      <if> <ruleClause connector="is" set="Negligible" variable="abs(RR_HR_delta)"/> </if>
      <then> <ruleClause connector="is" set="Present" variable="Apnea"/> </then> </rule>
      ...
    <elseRule name="Rule4" weight="1.0" note="otherwise Apnea is Absent">
      <else> <ruleClause connector="is" set="Absent" variable="Apnea"/> </else> </elseRule>
  </rulesBlock>
  ...
</fuzzyInferenceSystem>
```

Fig. 5. The medical knowledge of the considered case of study codified in FdsL language

approach, some experimental tests have been produced and the corresponding outputs have been formalized according to the FdsL language. Figure 6 depicts a FdsL fragment of the encoded outcome for a single item of the input dataset used.

```xml
<?xml version="1.0" encoding="UTF-8"?>
<reasoningOutput name="FIS_reasoningOutput_test">
  <fuzzyInferenceSystem name="FIS"/>
  <dataset>
    <item id="1">
      <input>
        <fuzzyVariable name="abs(RR_HR_delta)"> <crispValue value="20.0"/> </fuzzyVariable>
        <fuzzyVariable name="abs(HR_delta)"> <crispValue value="5.0"/> </fuzzyVariable>
        <fuzzyVariable name="SpO2"> <crispValue value="98.0"/> </fuzzyVariable>
        <fuzzyVariable name="Activity"> <crispValue value="30.0"/> </fuzzyVariable>
        <fuzzyVariable name="HR"> <crispValue value="100.0"/> </fuzzyVariable> </input>
      <output>
        <fuzzyVariable highestx="100.0" lowestx="0.0" name="Apnea" range="real" unit="%">
          <fuzzySet name="Apnea" type="Piecewise">
            <point x="0.0" y="1.0"/> <point x="15.0" y="1.0"/> <point x="60.0" y="0.0"/> </fuzzySet>
          <defuzzifiedValue value="20.972"/>
          <rulesActivationDegrees rulesBlock="Apnea">
            <rule degree="0.0" name="Rule1"/>
            <rule degree="0.0" name="Rule2"/>
            <rule degree="0.0" name="Rule3"/>
            <else degree="1.0" name="Rule4"/> </rulesActivationDegrees> </fuzzyVariable>
        <fuzzyVariable highestx="100.0" lowestx="0.0" name="HFailure" range="real" unit="%">
          <fuzzySet name="HFailure" type="Piecewise">
            <point x="0.0" y="1.0"/> <point x="15.0" y="1.0"/> <point x="60.0" y="0.0"/> </fuzzySet>
          <defuzzifiedValue value="20.972"/>
          <rulesActivationDegrees rulesBlock="HFailure">
            <rule degree="0.0" name="Rule5"/>
            <rule degree="0.0" name="Rule6"/>
            <rule degree="0.0" name="Rule7"/>
            <else degree="1.0" name="Rule8"/> </rulesActivationDegrees> </fuzzyVariable> </output>
    </item>
    ...
  </dataset>
</reasoningOutput>
```

Fig. 6. FdsL fragment of the encoded outcome for a single item of the input dataset used

4   Conclusions

In this paper, the XML-based FdsL language has been proposed for defining all the parameters needed to build a FIS underpinning a DSS for mobile healthcare scenarios.

Differently from existing solutions, which provide general-purpose facilities for modeling fuzzy knowledge, without any form of vertical arrangement for the particular domain of interest, the FdsL language enables the encoding of: i) fuzzy medical knowledge, in terms of both groups of positive evidence rules and fuzzy ELSE rules assembling all the negative evidence for a specific situation; ii) input and output data, respectively elaborated or produced by the fuzzy DSS, in order to provide meaningful and semantically well-defined advices and significantly increase the users' confidence in the final system. As a proof of concept, a case study has been arranged, where the proposed language has been applied to encode into a mobile DSS the medical knowledge required to remotely detect suspicious situations of sleep apnea or heart failure in patients affected by cardiovascular diseases. Next step of the research activities will regard the design and development of an editing and visualization framework supporting the proposed knowledge formalization language, for enabling physicians to update and handle the fuzzy medical knowledge embedded into the clinical decision support components deployed on mobile devices while they are running by avoiding any service interrupt.

References

1. Li, K.F.: Smart Home Technology for Telemedicine and Emergency Management. Journal of Ambient Intelligence and Humanized Computing (2012)
2. Eren, A., Subasi, A., Coskun, O.: A Decision Support System for Telemedicine Through the Mobile Telecommunications Platform. J. Med. Syst. 32(1), 31–35 (2008)
3. Lv, Z., Xia, F., Wu, G., Yao, L., Chen, Z.: Icare: A mobile health monitoring system for the elderly. In: IEEE-ACM Int'l Conf. Green Computing and Communications and Int'l Conf. Cyber, Physical and Social Computing, Los Alamitos, CA, USA, pp. 699–705 (2010)
4. Minutolo, A., Esposito, M., De Pietro, G.: A Mobile Reasoning System for Supporting the Monitoring of Chronic Diseases. In: Nikita, K.S., Lin, J.C., Fotiadis, D.I., Arredondo Waldmeyer, M.-T. (eds.) MobiHealth 2011. LNICST, vol. 83, pp. 225–232. Springer, Heidelberg (2012)
5. Lasierra, N., Alesanco, A., Garcia, J.: Home-based telemonitoring architecture to manage health information based on ontology solutions. In: The IEEE International Conference on Information Technology and Applications in Biomedicine (ITAB), November 3-5, pp. 1–4 (2010)
6. Zadeh, L.: FuzzySets. Inform. Control. 8, 338–353 (1965)
7. Warren, J., Beliakov, G., Zwaag, B.: Fuzzy logic in clinical practice decision support system. In: Proceedings of the 33rd Hawaii Inter. Conference on System Sciences (2000)
8. Alayón, S., Robertson, R., Warfield, S.K., Ruiz-Alzola, J.: A fuzzy system for helping medical diagnosis of malformations of cortical development. J. B. Inf. 40, 221–235 (2007)
9. Thomas, O., Dollmann, T.: Fuzzy-EPC markup language: XML based interchange formats for fuzzy process models. Soft Computing in XML Data Management 255, 227–257 (2010)
10. Tseng, C., Khamisy, W., Vu, T.: Universal fuzzy system representation with XML. Computer Standards & Interfaces 28, 218–230 (2005)
11. Acampora, G., Loia, V.: Fuzzy Markup Language: A new solution for transparent intelligent agents. In: IEEE Symposium on Intelligent Agent, April 11-15, pp. 1–6 (2011)
12. Shiffman, R.: Representation of clinical practice guidelines in conventional and augmented decision tables. J. of the American Medical Informatics Association 4(5), 382–393 (1997)
13. Esposito, M., De Falco, I., De Pietro, G.: An evolutionary-fuzzy DSS for assessing health status in multiple sclerosis disease. Int. J. of Med. Inf. 80(12), e245–e254 (2011)

Performance Evaluation of EC-ElGamal Encryption Algorithm for Wireless Sensor Networks

Soufiene Ben Othman[1], Abdelbasset Trad[1], Hani Alzaid[2], and Habib Youssef[1]

[1] UR PRINCE, ISITcom, Hammam Sousse University of Sousse, Tunisia
[2] Computer Research Institute, King Abdulaziz City for Science and Technology, Riyadh, Saudi Arabia
ben_oth_soufiene@yahoo.fr, abdelbasset.trad@isigk.rnu.tn, hmalzaid@kacst.edu.sa

Abstract. The rapid development in the Wireless Sensor Networks (WSNs) filed has allowed this technology to be used in many applications. In some of these applications, wireless sensor devices must be secured, especially when the captured information is valuable, sensitive, or for military usage. However, the implementation of security mechanisms on WSNs is a non-trivial task. Limitations in processing speed, battery power, bandwidth and memory constrain the applicability of existing cryptography algorithms for WSNs. The security of WSNs poses challenges because of the criticality of the data sensed by a node and in turn the node meets severe constraints like minimal energy, computational and communicational capabilities. Taking all the above said challenges energy efficiency or battery life time plays a major role in network lifetime. Providing security consumes some energy used by a node, so there is a need to minimize the energy consumption of any security algorithm that will be implemented in WSNs. As a solution, we apply an additive homomorphic encryption scheme, namely the elliptic curve ElGamal (EC-ElGamal) cryptosystem, and present the performance results of our implementation for the prominent sensor platform MicaZ mote.

Keywords: Wireless sensor network, security, elliptic curve ElGamal, Energy consumption analysis.

1   Introduction

Wireless Sensor Networks (WSNs) **have** emerged as an important new area in wireless technology. A wireless sensor network [1] is a distributed system interacting with physical environment. It consists of motes equipped with task-specific sensors to measure the surrounding environment, e.g., temperature, movement, etc. It provides solutions to many challenging problems such as wildlife, battlefield, wildfire, or building safety monitoring. A key component in a WSN is the sensor mote, which contains (a) a simple microprocessor, (b) application-specific sensors, and (c) a wireless transceiver. Each sensor mote is typically powered by batteries, making energy consumption an issue. Security is vital aspect in WSN applications.

B. Godara and K.S. Nikita (Eds.): MobiHealth 2012, LNICST 61, pp. 271–285, 2013.
© Institute for Computer Sciences, Social Informatics and Telecommunications Engineering 2013

The implementation of security policies is a complex and challenging issue because of resource constrained nodes. Short transmission distances reduce some of the security threats, but there are risks, for example, related to spoofing, message altering and replaying, and flooding and wormhole attacks [2]. It is important therefore to consider security solutions that guarantee data authenticity, freshness, replay protection, **integrity and confidentiality.** For secure communication in WSNs, efficient cryptographic algorithm suitable for WSNs environment is required. It is ideal to choose the most efficient cryptographic algorithm in all aspects; operation speed, storage and power consumption. However, since each cryptographic algorithm applied in WSNs has distinguished advantages, it is important to choose a cryptographic algorithm suitable for each environment WSNs are exploited.

The data encryption algorithms used in WSNs **are** generally divided into three major categories: symmetric-key algorithms, asymmetric-key algorithms, and hash algorithms. A number of papers, [1–2], have investigated using asymmetric-key algorithms in WSNs. However, the results they present reveal that despite the use of energy efficient techniques, such as elliptic curve cryptography or dedicated cryptography coprocessors, asymmetric-key algorithms consume more energy than symmetric-key algorithms. Hash functions, on the other hand, are typically used for verifying the integrity of the exchanged messages and may increase the transmission cost [3,4]. To prevent information and communication systems from illegal delivery and modification, message authentication and identification need to be examined through certificated mechanisms. Therefore, the receiver has to authenticate messages transmitted from the sensor nodes over a wireless sensor network. This is done through cryptography. It is a challenge to find out suitable cryptography for wireless sensor network due to limitations with respect to power, computational efficiency, and enough storage capabilities [2].

In this paper, an efficient implementation of EC-ElGamal scheme on MicaZ is presented in order to get better understanding of the usage of public encryption in WSNs. It is important to consider minimizing the code size of the implementation of ECC since sensor nodes keep in its memory other information required to make these sensors alive and functioning. For the data memory usage a similar motivation holds. In comparison to code and memory size, the execution time is not as critical as them. Therefore, this work focuses respectively on the optimization of code size, memory usage, and computation time. In comparison with similar implementations from the literature, the proposed implementation requires less storage for code, consumes less memory, and offers faster operation. Note that the EC-ElGamal scheme shares many properties with other standard EC algorithm. Thus, the major parts from this proposed work are also applicable to other EC implementations on small general purpose processors. The rest of the paper is structured as follows: Wireless Sensor Networks are discussed in Section 2. Then, the related work is highlighted in Section 3. Moreover, elliptic curve ElGamal cryptosystem is illustrated in Section 4. Performance results and evaluation of cryptographic algorithms are presented in Section 5. Finally, Section 6 concludes the paper and then final considerations and future works are given.

2   Wireless Sensor Network

A wireless sensor network (WSN) consists of a large number of tiny sensor nodes deployed over a geographical area also referred as sensing field. Each node is a low-power device that integrates computing, wireless communication and sensing capabilities [8] [9]. Nodes organize themselves in clusters and networks and then they cooperate to perform an assigned monitoring (and/or control) task without any human intervention. Sensor nodes are able to sense physical environmental information such as temperature, humidity, vibration, acceleration and then process locally the acquired data both at sensors and cluster level. The proposed information is then sent to the cluster (or the sink) as in Figure 1.

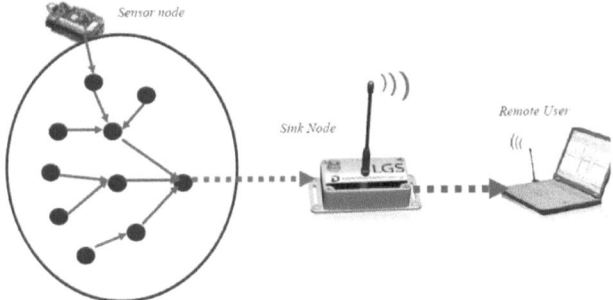

Fig. 1. A typical sensor network architecture

A WSN can thus be viewed as an intelligent distributed measurement technology adequate for many different monitoring and control contexts. In recent years, the number of sensor network deployments for real-life applications has rapidly increased [15]. Examples of WSNs applications in different domains are as follows: environmental monitoring [10], agriculture [11], production and delivery [12], military [10], structure monitoring [13] and medical applications [14]. However, energy consumption still remains one of the main obstacles to the diffusion of this technology, especially in application scenarios where a long network lifetime and a high quality of service are required. In fact, nodes are generally powered by batteries which have limited capacity and often can neither be replaced nor recharged due to environmental constraints. Despite the fact that energy scavenging mechanisms can be adopted to recharge batteries such as through solar panels, piezoelectric or acoustic transducers, energy is a limited resource and must be used judiciously. Interested reader can refer to [16] for more information on scavenging mechanisms. Hence, efficient energy management strategies must be devised at both sensor nodes level and cluster level to prolong the network lifetime as much as possible.

2.1   Security Goals and Challenges

Achieved security goals vary from one security mechanism to another due to the adversarial model considered at the design time. In other words, depending on the attacks that need to be mitigated, the provided security goals may vary. These security goals are discussed as follows [18]:

- **Data Confidentiality:** Confidentiality means keeping information secret from unauthorized parties. A sensor network should not leak sensor readings to neighboring networks. In many applications (e.g. key distribution) nodes exchange highly sensitive data. The standard approach for keeping sensitive data secret is to encrypt the data with a secret key that only intended receivers can possess, hence achieving confidentiality. Since public-key cryptography is too expensive to be used in the resource constrained sensor networks, most of the proposed protocols use symmetric key encryption methods. The authors of TinySec [18] argue that cipher block chaining (CBC) is the most appropriate encryption scheme for sensor networks. They found RC5 and Skipjack to be most appropriate for software implementation on embedded microcontrollers. The default block cipher in TinySec is Skipjack. SPINS uses RC6 as its cipher.

- **Data Authenticity:** In a wireless medium, an adversary can easily inject messages, if no mechanism to prevent unpermitted parties from participating in the network is in place. Thus, the receiver needs to make sure that the data used in any decision making process originates from the correct source. Data authentication prevents unauthorized parties from participating in the network and legitimate nodes should be able to detect messages from unauthorized nodes and reject them. In the two party communication case, data authentication can be achieved through a purely symmetric mechanism. The sender and the receiver share a secret key to compute a message authentication code (MAC) of all exchanged data. When a message with a correct MAC arrives, the receiver knows that it must have been sent by the sender. However, authentication for broadcast messages requires stronger trust assumptions on the network nodes. The authors of SPINS [19] contend that it is insecure to send authenticated data to mutually untrusted receivers, using a symmetric MAC is insecure since any one of the receivers know the MAC key, and hence could impersonate the sender and forge messages to other parties. SPINS constructs authenticated broadcast from symmetric primitives, but introduces asymmetry with delayed key disclosure and one-way function key chains. LEAP [20] uses a globally shared symmetric key for broadcast messages to the whole group. However, since the group key is shared among all the nodes in the network, an efficient rekeying mechanism is defined for updating this key after a compromised node is revoked. This means that LEAP has also defined an efficient mechanism to verify whether a node has been compromised.

- **Data Integrity:** Data integrity ensures the receiver that the received data is not altered in transit either maliciously or accidentally. This property can help to filter out incorrect/altered data and save the processing energy if the data travelled all the way to the base station.

- **Data Freshness:** Data freshness implies that the data is recent, and no old messages have been replayed. A common defense (used by SNEP [19]) is to include a monotonically increasing counter with every message and reject messages with old counter values. With this policy, every recipient must maintain a table of the last value from every sender it receives. However, for RAM constrained sensor nodes, this defense becomes problematic for even modestly sized networks. Assuming nodes devote only a small fraction of their RAM for this neighbor table, an adversary replaying broadcast messages from many different senders can fill up the table. At this point, the recipient has one of two options: ignore any messages from senders not in its neighbor table, or purge entries from the table. Neither is acceptable; the first creates a DoS attack and the second permits replay attacks. In [21], the authors contend that protection against the replay of data packets should be provided at the application layer and not by a secure routing protocol as only the application can fully and accurately detect the replay of data packets (as opposed to retransmissions ,for example). In [18], the authors reason that by using information about the network's topology and communication patterns, the application and routing layers can properly and efficiently manage a limited amount of memory devoted to replay detection. In [19], the authors have identified two types of freshness: weak freshness, and strong freshness. On one hand, the weak freshness provides partial message ordering, but carries no delay information. This type of freshness is suitable sensor measurements. On the other hand, the strong freshness provides a total order on a request response pair, and allows for delay estimation. This type is useful for time synchronization within the network.

2.2   Types of Attacks on WSNs

Wireless networks are vulnerable to security attacks due to the broadcast nature of the transmission medium. Furthermore, wireless sensor networks have an additional vulnerability because nodes are often placed in a hostile or dangerous environment where they are not physically protected. This section summaries types of attacks may be launched in WSNs. These attacks are as follows:

- **Passive Information Gathering:** An intruder with an appropriately powerful receiver and well-designed antenna can easily pick off the data stream. Interception of the messages containing the physical locations of sensor nodes allows an attacker to locate the nodes and destroy them. Besides the locations of sensor nodes, an adversary can observe the application specific content of messages including message IDs, timestamps and other fields. To minimize the threats of passive information gathering, strong encryption techniques needs to be used.

- **Subversion of a Node:** A particular sensor might be captured, and information stored on it (such as the key) might then be obtained by an adversary. If a node has been compromised then how to exclude that node, and that node only, from the sensor network is at issue (LEAP [22] suggests an efficient way to do so).

- **False Node and malicious data:** An intruder might add a node to the system that feeds false data or prevents the exchange of true data. Such messages also consume the scarce energy resources of the nodes. This type of attack is called "sleep deprivation torture" in [23]. Insertion of malicious code is one of the most dangerous attacks that can occur. Malicious code injected in the network could spread to all nodes, potentially destroying the whole network, or even worse, taking over the network on behalf of an adversary. A seized sensor network can either send false observations about the environment to a legitimate user or send observations about the monitored area to a malicious user. By spoofing, altering, or replaying routing information, adversaries may be able to create routing loops, attract or repel network traffic, extend or shorten source routes, generate false error messages, partition the network, increase end-to-end latency, etc. Strong authentication techniques can prevent an adversary from impersonating as a valid node in the sensor network.

- **The Sybil attack**: In a Sybil attack [24], a single node presents multiple identities to other nodes in the network. They pose a significant threat to geographic routing protocols, where location aware routing requires nodes to exchange coordinate information with their neighbors to efficiently route geographically addressed packets. Authentication and encryption techniques can prevent an outsider from launching a Sybil attack on the sensor network. However, an insider cannot be prevented from participating in the network, but (s)he should only be able to do so using the identities of the nodes (s)he has compromised. Using globally shared key allows an insider to masquerade as any (possibly even nonexistent) node. Public key cryptography can prevent such an insider attack, but it is too expensive to be used in the resource constrained sensor networks. One solution is to have a shared unique symmetric key between each node and a trusted base station. Two nodes can then use a Needham- Schroeder like protocol to verify each other's identity and establish a shared key. A pair of neighboring nodes can use the resulting key to implement an authenticated, encrypted link between them. An example of a protocol which uses such a scheme is LEAP [22], which supports the establishment of four types of keys.

- **Sinkhole attacks:** In a sinkhole attack, the adversary's goal is to lure nearly all the traffic from a particular area through a compromised node, creating a metaphorical sinkhole with the adversary at the center. Sinkhole attacks typically work by making a compromised node look especially attractive to surrounding nodes with respect to the routing algorithm. For instance, an adversary could spoof or replay an advertisement for an extremely high quality route to a base station. Due to either the real or imagined high quality route through the compromised node, it is likely each neighboring node of the adversary will forward packets destined for a base station through the adversary, and also propagate the attractiveness of the route to its neighbors. Effectively, the adversary creates a large *"sphere of influence"* [25], attracting all traffic destined for a base station from nodes several hops away from the compromised node.

- **Wormholes:** In the wormhole attack [26], an adversary records a packet at one location in the network, tunnels the packet to another location over a low latency link, and replays it at another part of the network. The simplest instance of this attack is a single node situated between two other nodes forwarding messages between the two of them. However, wormhole attacks more commonly involve two distant malicious nodes colluding to understate their distance from each other by relaying packets along an out-of-bound channel available only to the attacker. An adversary situated close to a base station may be able to completely disrupt routing by creating a well-placed wormhole. An adversary could convince nodes that would normally be multiple hops from a base station that they are only one or two hops away via the wormhole. This can create a sinkhole, since the adversary on the other side of the wormhole can artificially provide a high quality route to the base station, potentially all traffic in the surrounding area will be drawn through the adversary if alternate routes are significantly less attractive.

3   Related Works

One of the first requirements for providing a security mechanism is establishing the cryptographic keys to be used by the encryption algorithms. Due to the limited resources and the need for scalability in WSNs, the key establishment protocols used in other fields are not suitable for WSN environments. To address this problem, a lot of work has been done to develop and evaluate specialized key establishment protocols [7], [6], [27]. Publications like [17] mimic asymmetric signatures schemes by a relatively complex scheme of two party hash chains, so do [5] and [6]. Other work like [7] try to establish pairwise secret keys to avoid public and private key schemes or Diffie-Hellman like key exchanges.

In [27] and [28] the authors implement elliptic curve cryptography for sensor networks. However the underlying hardware is quite sophisticated consisting of 16 Bit microcontrollers with 16 MHz clock frequency. Therefore the results are only of limited value as typical sensor hardware does not dispose of such powerful computing resource. As mentioned before sensor networks can in general not afford high clock frequencies and potent CPUs, because of cost and energy saving issues associated.

In [29] a high-performance microcontroller offerings 24 MIPS, i.e. 3 times more than the usual ATMEGA 128, is utilized. The work is based on special Galois fields called *optimal extension fields* where field multiplication can be done quite efficiently. However, the security of this fields is unclear because of the Weil descent attack [28]. The proposals trying to implement elliptic curves on 8Bit ATMEGA128 chips like in [30] and [31] reach extremely poor performance. For example, a signature generation over 1:08 min of expensive computing and battery time has to be spent, which surely is not affordable. In addition the cost for necessary field operations are not mentioned at all.

4   Elliptic Curve El-Gamal Encryption Scheme

The original ElGamal encryption scheme, see [32], is not additive homomorphic. However, the elliptic curve group is an additive group, which can be used to get an additive homomorphic scheme. Algorithm 1 and Algorithm 2 show the methods for EC-ElGamal encryption and decryption, respectively. Therein, E is an elliptic curve over the finite field $GF(p)$. The order of the curve E is denoted $n = \#E$ and G is the generator point of the curve E. The secret key is defined as integer number x 2 GF(p), while the public key is determined as Y = xG.

The function map () is a deterministic mapping function used to map values mi 2 GF(p) into plaintext curve points Mi 2 E such that

$$Map\ (m1 + m2 +. .) = map\ (m_1) + map\ (m_2) + ...map\ (m_n) \qquad (1)$$
$$\underbrace{\qquad}_{M_1} \quad \underbrace{\qquad}_{M_2} \quad \underbrace{\qquad}_{M_N}$$

holds, whereby m_1, $m_2 \in GF(p)$. Since the addition operation over an elliptic curve requires both operands to be on that curve, prior to performing an addition of two integers, they should be mapped to the corresponding elliptic curve points. This explains why the mapping function is necessary. As proposed in [32] the homomorphic mapping function used in TinyPEDS is based on using multiples of the generator point G of the elliptic curve. This means that the mapping function converts a plaintext m to the point mG. The reverse mapping function *rmap* ( ) then extracts m from a given point mG. The mapping function, namely holds with m_1, m_2, ... $m_n \in GF(p)$, the generator point G, and the modulus p.

$$map: m \longrightarrow mG \text{ with } m \in GF\ (p) \qquad (2)$$

fulfills the required homomorphic property due to the fact that the equation

$$M_1 + M_2 + ... + M_n = map\ (m_1 + m_2 + ... + m_n) \qquad (3)$$
$$= (m_1 + m_2 + ... + m_n)\ G$$
$$= m_1G + m_2G + ... + m_nG$$

The mapping function is not security relevant, since it only converts an integer to an elliptic curve point. This means, it neither increases nor decreases the security of the EC-ElGamal encryption scheme. Note that the reverse mapping function is the same as solving the *discrete logarithm problem* over an elliptic curve and, therefore, a weakness of this scheme. However, since the mapping function is only performed on the reader device, which is assumed to have unlimited resources, this disadvantage does not affect the performance and resource consumption within the network.

In conclusion, according to the analysis made in [32], the EC-ElGamal scheme becomes the most promising candidate for using in TinyPEDS, because of its efficiency both in computation and bandwidth. However, the main disadvantage of this scheme is that the reverse mapping function required during decryption may be in some cases too costly. However, since the number of the aggregated values is limited and the maximum length of the final aggregation is assumed to be at most three bytes, see [46], the reverse mapping of the point mG with 24-bit m can be calculated fast enough on the reader device.

Algorithm 1: EC-ElGamal encryption

Require: public key Y, plaintext m
Ensure: ciphertext (R, S)
1: choose random $k \, 2 \, [1, n - 1]$
2: $M := map(m)$
3: $R := kG$
4: $S := M + kY$ (4)
5: return (R, S)

Algorithm 2: EC-ElGamal decryption

Require: secret key x, ciphertext (R, S)
Ensure: plaintext m
1: $M := -xR + S$
2: $m := rmap(M)$
3: return m

---

5   Implementation

The implementation was done on the Mica-Z mote, the operating system employed in the implementation is TinyOS-2.0 [33], an open-source operating system designed for wireless embedded sensor networks. In TinyOS there are two kinds of components, namely configurations and modules. Configurations connect modules, while the required functionality, e.g. arithmetic operations, is implemented in modules [33]. Figure 2 depicts a graphical representation of the EC-ElGamal configuration.

5.1   ECElGamalM

The module ECElGamalM implements the EC ElGamal encryption scheme and the arithmetic operations such as homomorphic addition operation.

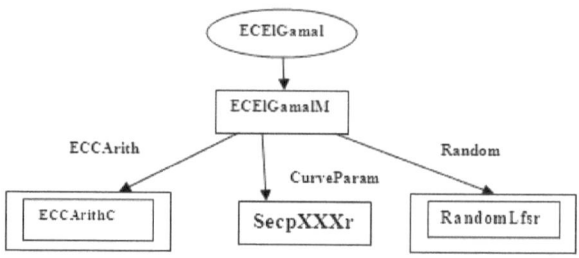

Fig. 2. Graphical representation of elliptic curve ElGamal implementation

Thus, in ECElGamalM following functions are implemented.

- **Void init ():** Initializes the parameters, e.g. G, Y and the pre-computed points, required by the mapping and the encryption function.
- **Void generateRandomNum (FF_DIGIT *k):** This function generates the random k required in the EC-ElGamal encryption. Note that the random number generation is based on the method rand16() from the module RandomLfsrC which is contained in TinyOS. Therefore, ECElGamalM calls the external method rand16() and this method call is represented as arrow in figure 2.
- **Void map(Point *M, FF_DIGIT *m, FF_DIGIT lengthOfm):** Software implementation of the mapping function shown in equation 2, m is mapped to a elliptic curve point M, whereby $M = mG$.
- **Void enc (ECElGamalCipher *cipher, FF_DIGIT *m, FF_DIGIT lengthOfm):** Software implementation of the EC-ElGamal encryption scheme as described in algorithm 1, whereby $cipher = enc(m)$.
- **Void homAdd(ECElGamalCipher *cipher, ECElGamalCipher *cipher1, ECElGamalCipher *cipher2):** Software implementation of the homomorphic addition operation $\otimes$, see equation 3, with $cipher = cipher1 \otimes cipher2$.

5.2 ECCArithC

As depicted in Figure 2, the component **ECCArithC** consists of two modules, namely **ECCArithM** and **FFArithM**, which implement the arithmetic operations at elliptic curve and finite field level, respectively.

- **ECCArithM :** The module **ECCArithM** implements the following operations from the elliptic curve level.
- **FFArithM :** The module **FFArithM** implements the following finite field arithmetic operations.

5.3   SecpXXXr1

Elliptic curve parameters such as the base point **G** and the point **Y** and pre-computed points are set in this module.

5.4   RandomLfsrC

This module is already implemented in TinyOS and part of the operating system. The following method is employed from this module. Note that the **RandomLfsrC** does not generate good pseudo-random numbers, which may lead to security problems. However, as they are not within the scope of this paper, the security analysis of weak pseudo-random numbers is not covered in this work.

6   Performance Evaluations

This section presents a comparative performance and energy consumption analysis of this algorithm. We have selected three crucial parameters; memory efficiency, execution time (operation speed), and energy efficiency.

6.1   Memory Efficiency

Memory usually includes flash memory (ROM) and RAM. Flash memory is classified into programming flash memory and data flash memory. Programming flash memory is used to store downloaded application programming code. Data flash memory stores temporary or sensing data. RAM is used for program execution. Because memory in a sensor node is not only limited but also require energy to retain or store data, efficient usage of memory is important.

Besides computing time memory consumption is an important criteria for the use in sensor networks. Figure 3 gives an overview over the memory use of our implementation.

6.2   Operation Time

Operation speed is also an important factor when evaluating performance. After estimating operation time by repeatedly executing encryption and decryption process, we calculate the average of estimated value.

Table 1 shows the performance of the different realizations of the EC-ElGamal, which contains two point multiplications with n-bit scalar k and one short point multiplication with the sensed data m, see Algorithm 1. Note that for testing purposes m was chosen to be 8-bit.

6.3   Energy Efficiency

The energy consumed by a processor during the execution of a piece of software, such as a block cipher, corresponds to the product of the average power dissipation and the

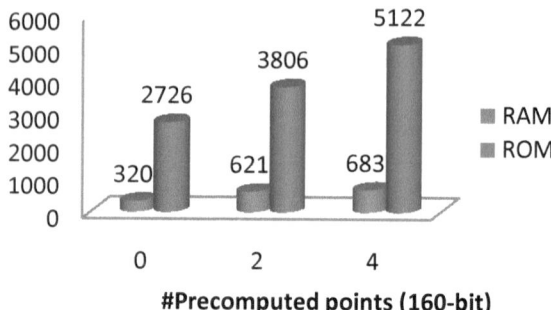

Fig. 3. Memory requirements of each algorithm

Table 1. Operation time requirements of each algorithm

# Recomputed points (160-bit)	Execution time [s]
0	2.14
2	1.22
4	0.97

total running time. The former depends on a number of factors including supply voltage, clock frequency, and the average current drawn by the processor while executing individual instructions of the program code. The computational complexity of an algorithm translates directly to its energy consumption. Assuming the energy per CPU cycle is fixed, by measuring the number of CPU cycle executed per byte of plaintext processed, we get the amount of energy consumed per byte.

We estimate CPU cycle by using Power TOSSIM, which is extension of TOSSIM, an event driven simulation environment for TinyOS applications. Power TOSSIM provides accurate estimation of power consumption for a range of applications and scales to support very large simulation. The energy consumed by a processor during the execution of a piece of software, such as a block cipher, corresponds to the product of the average power dissipation and the total running time.

Table 2 represents the power consumption of the implementations from this work, when those operations are performed.

Table 2. Energy Efficiency requirements of each algorithm

# Recomputed points (160-bit)	Execution time [s]
0	10.556
2	5.560
4	5.918

7   Conclusion

The performance evaluation of cryptographic algorithms is vital for the safe and efficient development of cryptosystem in devices with low computational power.
Due to the resource restrictions of sensor nodes, several algorithms required for implementing the EC-ElGamal cryptosystem are analyzed. Thus, the time efficiency, code size, and memory consumption of each candidate algorithm were compared and the most promising algorithms were selected and implemented.

Moreover, the programming style was selected such that unnecessary overhead in terms of code performance, code size, and memory usage were reduced to minimum.
One future research direction is to explore adaptive cryptographic mechanisms to optimize energy consumption by varying cipher parameters with timely acquisition of resource-context in WSN environment. The adaptability of the security system will improve sensor nodes battery's lifetime.

References

1. Bertoni, G., Breveglieri, L., Venturi, M.: Power aware design of an elliptic curve coprocessor for 8 bit platforms. In: PERCOMW 2006, p. 337 (2006)
2. Wander, A.S., Gura, N., Eberle, H., Gupta, V., Shantz, S.C.: Energy analysis of public-key cryptography for wireless sensor networks. In: PERCOM 2005, pp. 324–328 (2005)
3. Potlapally, N.R., Ravi, S., Raghunathan, A., Jha, N.K.: A study of the energy consumption characteristics of cryptographic algorithms and security protocols. In: IEEE TMC 2005, pp. 128–143 (2005)
4. Chang, C.-C., Muftic, S., Nagel, D.J.: Measurement of energy costs of security in wireless sensor nodes. In: ICCCN 2007, pp. 95–102 (2007)
5. Weimerskirch, A., Westhoff, D.: Zero Common-Knowledge Authentication for Pervasive Networks. In: Matsui, M., Zuccherato, R.J. (eds.) SAC 2003. LNCS, vol. 3006, pp. 73–87. Springer, Heidelberg (2004)
6. Weimerskirch, A., Westhoff, D.: Identity Certified Authentication for Ad-hoc Networks. In: 10th Workshop on Security of Ad Hoc and Sensor Networks (2003)
7. Balfanz, D., Smetters, D., Stewart, P., Wong, H.: Talking to strangers: Authentication in adhoc wireless networks. In: Symposium on Network and Distributed Systems Security (2002)
8. Akyildiz, I.F., Su, W., Sankarasubramaniam, Y., Capirci, E.: Wireless Sensor Networks: a Survey. Computer Networks 38(4) (March 2002)
9. Romer, K., Mattern, F.: The design space of wireless sensor networks. IEEE Wireless Communications 11(6), 54–61 (2004)
10. Mainwaring, A., Culler, D., Polastre, J., Szewczyk, R., Anderson, J.: Wireless sensor networks for habitat monitoring. In: Proc. ACM International Workshop on Wireless Sensor Networks and Applications, pp. 88–97 (2002)
11. Werner-Allen, G., Johnson, J., Ruiz, M., Lees, J., Welsh, M.: Monitoring volcanic eruptions with a wireless sensor network. In: Proceeedings of the Wireless Sensor Networks, pp. 108–120 (2005)
12. Lee, K.B., Reichardt, M.E.: Open standards for homeland security sensor networks. IEEE Magazine on Instrumentation & Measurement 8(5), 14–21 (2005)

13. Baldus, H., Klabunde, K., Müsch, G.: Reliable Set-Up of Medical Body-Sensor Networks. In: Karl, H., Wolisz, A., Willig, A. (eds.) EWSN 2004. LNCS, vol. 2920, pp. 353–363. Springer, Heidelberg (2004)

14. Alippi, C., Galperti, C.: An Adaptive System for Optimal Solar Energy Harvesting in Wireless Sensor Network Nodes. IEEE Transactions on Circuits and Systems I: Regular Papers 55(6), 1742–1750 (2008)

15. Slijepcevic, S., Potkonjak, M., Tsiatsis, V., Zimbeck, S., Srivastava, M.B.: On communication security in wireless ad-hoc sensor networks. In: Proceedings of 11th IEEE International Workshop on Enabling Technologies: Infrastructure for Collaborative Enterprises (WETICE 2002), pp. 139–144 (2002)

16. Carman, D.W., Krus, P.S., Matt, B.J.: Constraints and approaches for distributed sensor network security., Technical Report 00-010, NAI Labs, Network Associates Inc., Glenwood, MD (2009)

17. Anderson, R., Bergadano, F., Crispo, B., Lee, J., Manifavas, C., Needham, R.: A New Family of Authentication Protocols. ACMOSR: ACM Operating Systems Review (1998)

18. Karlof, C., Sastry, N., Wagner, D.: TinySec: A Link Layer Security Architecture for Wireless Sensor Networks. In: ACM SenSys 2004, November 3-5 (2004)

19. Xiao, Y. (ed.): Wireless Sensor Network Security: A Survey. Security in Distributed, Grid, and Pervasive Computing. Auerbach Publications, CRC Press (2006)

20. Estrin, D., Govindan, R., Heidemann, J.S., Kumar, S.: Next century challenges: Scalable coordination in sensor networks. In: Mobile Computing and Networking, pp. 263–270 (1999)

21. Karp, B., Kung, H.T.: GPSR: greedy perimeter stateless routing for wireless networks. In: Proceedings of the 6th Annual International Conference on Mobile Computing and Networking, pp. 243–254. ACM Press (2000)

22. Zhu, S., Setia, S., Jajodia, S.: LEAP: Efficient Security Mechanisms for Large-Scale Distributed Sensor Networks. In: The Proceedings of the 10th ACM Conference on Computer and Communications Security (2003)

23. Stajano, F., Anderson, R.: The Resurrecting Duckling: Security Issues for Ad-hoc Wireless Networks. In: 3rd AT&T Software Symposium, Middletown, NJ (October 1999)

24. Madden, S.R., Franklin, M.J., Hellerstein, J.M., Hong, W.: TAG: A tiny aggregation service for ad-hoc sensor networks. In: The Fifth Symposium on Operating Systems Design and Implementation, OSDI 2002 (2002)

25. Wagner, C.K.D. Secure Routing in Wireless Sensor Networks: Attacks and Countermeasures

26. Hu, Y.C., Perrig, A., Johnson, D.B.: Wormhole detection in wireless ad hoc networks. Department of Computer Science, Rice University, Tech. Rep. TR01-384 (June 2002)

27. Huang, Q., Cukier, J., Kobayashi, H., Liu, B., Zhang, J.: Fast Authenticated Key Establishment Protocols for Self-Organizing Sensor Networks. In: International Conference on Wireless Sensor Networks and Applications (2003)

28. Huang, Q., Kobayashi, H.: Energy/security scalable mobile cryptosystem. IEEE Personal, Indoor and Mobile Radio Communications (2003)

29. Kumar, S., Girimondo, M., Weimerskirch, A., Paar, C., Patel, A., Wander, S.: Embedded End-to-End Wireless Security with ECDH Key Exchange. In: The 46th IEEE Midwest Symposium on Circuits and Systems (2003)

30. Malan, D.J., Welsh, M., Smith, M.D.: A Public-Key Infrastructure for Key Distribution in TinyOS Based on Elliptic Curve Cryptography. In: First IEEE International Conference on Sensor and Ad Hoc Communications and Networks (2004)

31. Lorincz, K., Malan, D.J., Fulford-Jones, T.R.F., Nawoj, A., Clavel, A., Shnayder, V., Mainland, G., Moulton, S., Welsh, M.: Sensor Networks for Emergency Response: Challenges and Opportunities. IEEE Pervasive Computing (2004)

32. El Gamal, T.: A Public Key Cryptosystem and a Signature Scheme Based on Discrete Logarithms. In: Blakely, G.R., Chaum, D. (eds.) CRYPTO 1984. LNCS, vol. 196, pp. 10–18. Springer, Heidelberg (1985)

33. http://www.tinyos.net

Endocom and Cyclope – Two Smart Biomedical Sensors for Cardio-Vascular Surgery and Gastro-Enterology

Patrick Garda[1], Olivier Romain[2], Aymeric Histace[2], Bertrand Granado[1], Andrea Pinna[1], and Xavier Dray[3]

[1] UPMC, Université Pierre et Marie Curie; LIP6, CNRS UMR 7606; Paris, France
[2] UCP, Université de Cergy Pontoise; ETIS, CNRS UMR 8051; Cergy Pontoise, France
[3] Hôpital Lariboisière; AP-HP ; Paris, France
{Patrick.Garda,Bertrand.Granado,Andrea.Pinna}@upmc.fr,
{Olivier.Romain,Aymeric.Histace}@u-cergy.fr,
Xavier.Dray@lrb.aphp.fr

Abstract. In this paper we present two case studies of electronic embedded systems for biomedical applications: ENDOCOM and CYCLOPE. In the former, we designed and realized the prototype of an implantable pressure sensor for the follow-up of the abdominal aortic aneurysm treated by a stent. Numerical modeling, in vitro experiments and in vivo tests on large animal model demonstrated the successful real-time follow-up of the pressure in the aneurysm sac. In the latter, we designed an embedded active multispectral vision system for the real time detection of polyps based both on the classification of the 3D reconstruction of the polyps by SVM and the classification of the texture by boosting methods. An FPGA-based demonstrator of the system was realized. Experiments in laboratory, in vitro and in vivo on a pig were performed to obtain its performances. This system could be integrated into a wireless capsule for colorectal endoscopy.

Keywords: Smart sensors, implants, biomedical systems, embedded systems, mems, wireless communications, cardio-vascular surgery, abdominal aortic aneurysm, pressure sensor, 3d imaging, polyps, gastro-enterology, wireless capsule endoscopy.

1 Introduction

In this paper we present two case studies of implantable electronic embedded systems for biomedical applications: ENDOCOM and CYCLOPE. They were designed and studied in collaboration between the LIP6 and ETIS laboratories in the Paris area.

2 ENDOCOM: Smart Biomedical Sensor for the Follow Up of Abdominal Aortic Aneurysm

An Abdominal Aortic Aneurysm (AAA) is a localized and permanent dilatation of the aorta. It affects 6 to 7% of the population over 65 years [1] and the mortality rate of

B. Godara and K.S. Nikita (Eds.): MobiHealth 2012, LNICST 61, pp. 286–294, 2013.

ruptured aneurysms is currently of 80% [2]. Several surgical procedures are available for the treatment of AAAs. The conventional surgical treatment is well established and results in a low mortality, below 3-5% [3] and a post-surgery morbidity rate between 15 to 35% [4]. In the endovascular treatment, a covered stent is introduced via the femoral aorta (see Figure 1). The aortic blood flow is then guided through the stent and the pressure on the aneurysm wall is stabilized [5]. Unfortunately, in some cases the rupture risk persists [6]. In order to prevent the rupture, the patient is subjected to many imaging examinations after the endovascular treatment [7]. The objective of the ENDOCOM was to investigate the possibility to replace this monitoring of the geometry of the aneurysmal sac, by a monitoring of the pressure in the sac.

2.1   ENDOCOM Overview

For several years, biomedical research and industrial laboratories have been developing new generic pressure sensors and transducer systems for cardiovascular applications [8] [9] [10] [11] [12]. Two of the most accomplished and relevant projects related to the problem of AAA leaks following an endovascular treatment are CardioMEMS [13] [14] and Remon Medical Technologies [15]. Both methods use analogue signal transmissions. Therefore, no wireless sensor network configuration can be used.

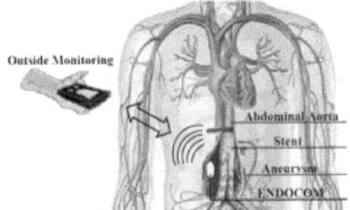

Fig. 1. ENDOCOM system

The changing properties (geometry, elasticity) of the aneurysm, the changing nature of the blood clot, and the distribution of hypothetical leaks lead us to assume that the pressure field inside an excluded aneurysmal sac is non-uniform. As a consequence, we expect that a randomly placed sensor could be inefficient at detecting a highly localized leak. Moreover, due to the aneurysm location deep inside the abdomen, several layers (skin, fat, muscle, thrombus) may perturb the transmission signal.

Placing itself within this context, the ENDOCOM project aims [16] to develop a communicating endo-prosthesis (fig. 1) based on a wireless sensor network. This prosthesis will include integrated sensors, made of a pressure transducer and a

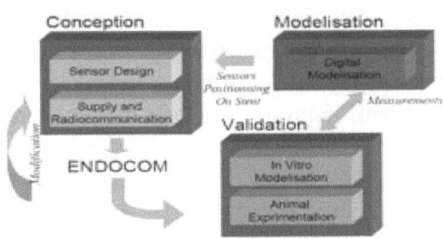

Fig. 2. Conception Flow

wireless processing architecture. The electronic system will be remotely powered during radio transmission. Regular recordings of the pressure in the aneurysmal sac during post-surgical consultations will provide a means to monitor the evolution of the AAA's condition after the intervention. This represents a reliable and cheaper alternative to current medical imaging options. The full development of the system required a specific workflow (Fig 2) that integrated three main parts: the design of the implantable wireless pressure sensor, the *in vitro* and *in vivo* test bench, and, finally numerical modeling. The latter aimed to determine the optimum position of the sensor in the aneurysmal sac depending on the geometrical characteristics of the patient's aneurysm.

2.2   Architecture of the Implantable Wireless Sensor

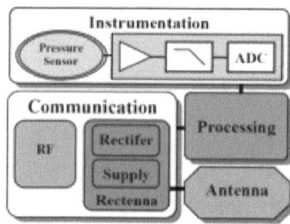

Fig. 3. ENDOCOM system

The architecture of the wireless pressure sensor is based on a RFID tag at 13.56MHz with an instrumentation block (Fig. 3). The wireless sensor uses both the 15693 RFID standard and I2C for the communication. The instrumentation block provides a measurement of the absolute pressure, which is adapted for numerical treatment. The treatment block makes sure that the sensor tasks are operating correctly (acquisition, energy management, emission/reception) and are in accordance with its internal state and its supply level. The communication block contains, in addition to the telecommunication part, a ted coil and a rectifier for the circuit supply management in respect to the antenna's output signal.

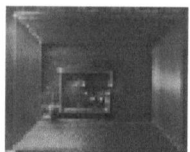 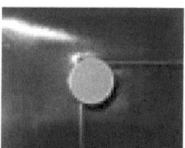

Fig. 4. RFID tag planar coil with the pressure sensor chip embedded in the middle

An integrated prototype was realized with a biocompatible titanium package (fig 4.). The transponder was composed of a 1.5cm × 1.85 cm planar rectangular coil.

2.3   In Vivo Experiments

The objective was to create a porcine model of AAA similar to the human pathology in order to finally perform in vivo implantation of the pressure sensor fixed on an endograft. For that purpose, after several trials, an original AAA model was created, it presents 3 main characteristics: it is compliant, reproducible and its diameter represents 3 to 4 fold the native aortic diameter.

2.4   In Vitro Test Bench

An experimental device dedicated to the ENDOCOM project was sized and designed to mimic the blood flows in a model of abdominal aortic aneurysm of a pig (AAA).

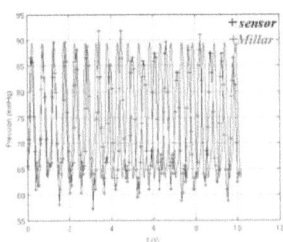

Fig. 5. Comparison between Endocom's sensor and Millar

Given the variability of geometric models of AAAs of animals, an average and axisymmetric geometry was first chosen. Given the variability of flow curves and pressure recorded during animal protocols, mean values of flow rates and pressures are taken to model these quantities in the in vitro experiments.

Pressure measurements were performed in the non-excluded AAA and in the aneurysm sac excluded by a stent similar to that used in vivo. These measurements are obtained using Millar pressure sensors and wired pressure sensor designed during the ENDOCOM project. Comparisons between the different signals obtained in the non-excluded AAA showed a good quantitative agreement (Figure 5).

2.5   3D Reconstruction and Numerical Modeling

In some animal trials, the vessel anatomy was obtained from 2 incidences of 2D angiography performed on pigs. The 3-D reconstruction was achieved using a specific algorithm developed under Solidworks®, previously described in [17] and adapted from coronary vessel to the specificity of AAA.

Then, a numerical model involving a compliant stent immersed in a compliant aneurysm was developed. A special effort was dedicated to devise a robust fluid-solid coupling algorithm adapted to this configuration. The incompressibility of the blood in a confined elastic region was indeed responsible for numerical instabilities with standard algorithms [18]. The simulations run with realistic physiological pressures and flow rates, provided by the data acquisitions in the in vitro or in vivo experiments. In the considered configurations, it was observed that the pressure is essentially homogeneous in the sac. The pressure sensor could therefore be safely located anywhere within the aneurysm. Future works will address other situations, including for example collateral vessels.

2.6   Discussion

This section proposed an overview of the ENDOCOM project. This project aimed to develop an implantable pressure sensor based on the RFID standard at 13.56MHz. A specific workflow was developed in order to design this sensor and to elaborate the *in vitro* and *in vivo* test benches for the interpretation of the measurements. In parallel, numerical modelling was also investigated in order to determine the optimal position of the sensor in the aneurysmal sac depending on the geometrical characteristics of the patient's aneurysm. Some preliminary results were presented. The implantable pressure sensor measures 5mm x 2mm and its flexible antenna 1.5cm x 1.85cm. In a near future, the wireless sensor will be tested in a pig and *in vitro*. These experiments will provide some data about the distribution of pressure in the excluded AAA.

3   CYCLOPE: Smart Biomedical Sensor for Colonoscopic Applications

The colonoscopic polypectomy consists of removing malignant colon polyps [19]. Therefore, an accurate and reliable 3D colon polyp classification is critical. We chose active stereovision methods as they offer an alternative approach to the classical use of two cameras. They are based on the projection of a set of structured rays on the studied object. In this case, only one image is necessary. In our research work, we focused on an integrated 3D active vision sensor: "Cyclope" [20]. This prototype sensor allows making real time 3D objects reconstruction and continues to be optimized technically to improve the consistency of differentiation between captured objects, while respecting the size and power consumption constraints of embedded systems [21].

A range of different materials and techniques were investigated to correctly realize the whole system. Among them, we focus in this section on the implementation of the support vector machines (SVM) in order to classify objects captured by our active stereovision system. The choice of support vector machines is motivated by the fact that they proved powerful classifiers in various pattern recognition applications [22].

To demonstrate the performance of the proposed technique, we applied it to the detection of polyps in the colon wall. Since, there are two different types of colon polyps, namely hyperplasias and adenomas [23]. Hyperplasias are benign polyps and do not have chance to evolve into cancer and, therefore, do not need to be removed. By contrast, adenomas have a strong tendency to become malignant. Therefore, they have to be removed immediately via polypectomy.

Our contributions are first, to extract the most suitable features describing the polyp models; second to choose an appropriate structure of the classification model to accurately discriminate between different 3D polyps respecting computation time and hardware requirements for our embedded sensor.

3.1   The Architecture of *Cyclope*

The "Cyclope" system (figure 6) is composed of three essential parts [20] [21]:

Instrumentation block. It contains a CMOS camera and a structured light projection system. The laser projector illuminates the studied scene with an array of 361 (19x19) laser beams.

Processing block. It integrates a microprocessor core and a reconfigurable array, the microprocessor is used for sequential processing and the reconfigurable array is used to implement

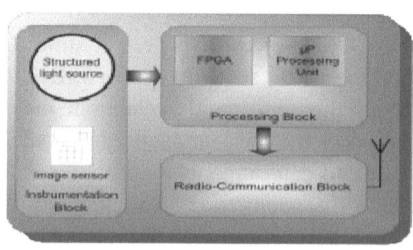

Fig. 6. Block diagram of CYCLOPE

time consuming algorithms needed for image processing and objects recognition task. The images captured by the active stereovision system are preprocessed to handle 3D information for extracted interest points. A small set of suitable features will be computed later from these points to be used as inputs to the SVM classifier.

Wireless communication block. This part is dedicated to the OTA (Over the Air) communication to have a wireless sensor.

3.2   Processing

As in traditional pattern recognition systems, discriminating between different shapes during endoscopic imaging is divided into three phases: data acquisition, feature extraction, and decision classification.

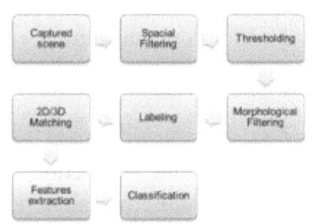

Fig. 7. CYCLOPE algorithmic chain

Data acquisition. This phase uses our stereovision system as input sensor by applying several processing techniques to the captured image in order to improve its quality and prepare it for the reconstruction stage. At the end of this phase a cloud of 3D points is obtained after stereo-matching operation.

Feature extraction. Given a cloud of points from the surface of studied objects (polyp models in this demo) defined by their 3D coordinates. We might wish to favor a small number of suitable characteristic features in order to discriminate as well as possible between different studied objects. These extracted features will be fed to the SVM classifier (third phase) in order to recognize the studied object.

Classification. We used an SVM classifier to make the final decision and classify the captured 3D objects. In this study, we tested the performance of our system for the colonoscopy, to make decision whether the captured image belongs to a benign or malignant polyp.

The input of SVM is a set of suitable features extracted from the surface of each object under study, and the output is a soft label denoting the class this object belongs to (Adenoma or Hyperplasia).

The recognition system involves several stages of operation to be performed beforehand during an off-line analysis. These activities include the calibration of the stereovision system, the feature selection process to reduce the dimensionality of the feature space, the training of the SVM classifier, the model selection and the cross-validation to find out the best parameters of the classifier.

3.3 Large Scale Demonstrator

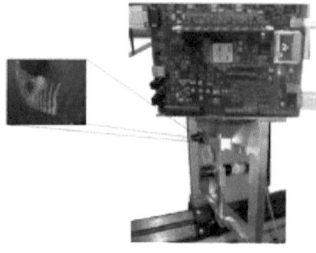

Fig.8. Large scale demonstrator

To test and validate our system, a large scale demonstrator was realized: several 3D models were created to generate a dataset consisting of 111 polyps (40 adenomas and 81 hyperplasias). These polyps were built in silicone with a scale factor of 2. Polyps are fixed on the internal wall of the intestine. The intestine was simulated by a tube in silicone with a scale factor of 2 compared to the human size. Their image sequences were captured by an active stereovision sensor (see figure 10) created by an original ¼" color CMOS imager with digital output (356×292 array size), and a structured light generator constituted by an array of 361 laser beams [24]. The Processing block was constituted by a XUP Virtex-II Pro Development System Board, and a Zigbee module was used for communication.

3.4 Discussion

We described a multi-stage system for the automatic feature extraction and classification of colon polyps using 3D data obtained from active stereovision system. On our own polyp database, we achieved a correct classification rate of approximately 96.9%, obtained by combining RBF kernel function and SVM models.

Note that this was an ideal example, because the scene was very simple and the size of the training set iwa small. Further work is clearly required to investigate different feature areas, like second order statistics features (co-occurrence matrices), and to evaluate system performance for multi-classification.

4 Conclusion

We presented two case studies of implantable electronic embedded systems for biomedical applications: ENDOCOM and CYCLOPE. Both led to prototype realizations and in vivo measurements.

Acknowledgments. The ENDOCOM project was supported by the French ANR TECSAN 2007 Program. We thank the teams from IJLRA, INRA, INRIA, IRPHE, L2E, Orange Labs and UTC for their collaborations.

References

1. Laheij, R.J.F., Buth, J., Harris, P.L., Moll, F.L., Stelter, W.J., Verhoeven, E.L.G.: Need for secondary interventions after endovascular repair of abdominal aortic aneurysms. Intermediate-term follow-up results of a European collaborative registry (EUROSTAR). Br. J. Surg. 87, 1666–1673 (2000)

2. Bhuyan, R.R., et al.: Outcomes of surgical management of ruptured abdominal aortic aneurysm. Indian Journal of Thoracic and Cardiovascular Surger 22, 132–136 (2006)
3. de Carvalho, A.T.Y., et al.: Morbidity and mortality factors in the elective surgery of infrarenal abdominal aortic aneurysm: a case study with 134 patients. J. Vasc. Bras. 7(3) (2008) ISSN 1677-5449
4. Lederle, F.A., et al.: Risk of rupture for large infrarenal abdominal aortic aneurysm. Journal of American Medical Association 287, 2968–2972 (2002)
5. Elkouri, S., et al.: Most patients with abdominal aortic aneurysm are suitable for endovascular repair using currently approved bifurcated stent-grafts. Proc. XVI on Endovascular Interventions. Vascular and Endovascular Surgery 38(5), 401–412 (2004)
6. Veith, F.J.: Nature and significance of endoleaks and endotension. Journal of Vascular Surgery 35, 1029–1035 (2002)
7. Elkouri, S., Panneton, J.M., Andrews, J.C., Lewis, B.D., et al.: Computed tomography and ultrasound in follow-up of patients after endovascular repair of abdominal aortic aneurysm. Ann Vascular Surgery 18(3), 271–279 (2004)
8. Schnakenberg, U., Kruger, C., Pfeffer, J., Mokwa, W., Bogel, G., Gunther, R., Schmitz-Rode, T.: Intravascular pressure monitoring system. Sensors and Actuators 110(1-3), 61–67 (2004)
9. Huang, Q., Oberle, M.: A 0.5-mW Passive Telemetry IC for Biomedical Applications. IEEE Journal of Solid-State Circuits 33(7), 937–941 (1998)
10. Eggers, T., Marschner, C., Marchner, U., Clasbrummel, B., Laur, R., Binder, J.: Advanced hybrid integrated low-power telemetric pressure monitoring system for biomedical applications. In: The Thirteenth Annual International Conference on Micro Electro Mechanical Systems, MEMS 2000, pp. 329–334. IEEE Press (2000)
11. Hierold, C., Clasbrummel, B., Behrend, D.: Low power integrated pressure sensor system for biomedical application. Sensors and Actuators 73(9), 58–67 (1999)
12. Kovacs, G., Knapp, T.: Implantable biosensing transponder. WO patent no 5 833 603 (1998)
13. Allen, M., Fonseca, M., White, J.: Implantable wireless sensor for blood pressure measurement within an artery. WO Patent no 2004014456 (2004)
14. Allen, M.: Micromachined endovascularly-implatable wireless aneurysm pressure sensors: from concept to clinic. In: Proceeding of Transducteur Conference, pp. 275–279 (2005)
15. Portat, Y., Penner, A.: Implantable acoustic bio-sensing system and method. WO Patent no US6432050 B1 (2002)
16. Mazeyrat, J., Romain, O., Garda, P., Lagree, P.Y., Leprince, P., Karouia, M.: Wireless communicative stent for follow-up of abdominal aortic aneurysm. In: IEEE Biomedical Circuits and Systems Conference, pp. 237–240. IEEE Press (2006)
17. Berthier, B., Bouzerar, B., Legallais, C.: Blood flow patterns in an anatomically realistic coronary vessel: Influence of 3 different reconstruction methods. J. Biomech. 35, 1347–1356 (2002)
18. Mura, J., Fernandez, M.A., Gerbeau, J.-F.: Numerical simulation of the fluid-structure interaction in stented aneurysm. In: 5th European Conference on Computational Fluid Dynamics ECCOMAS CFD (2010)
19. Rex, D.K., Petrini, J.L., Baron, T.H., Chak, A., Cohen, J., Deal, S.E., Hoffman, B., Jacobson, B.C., Mergener, K., Petersen, B.T., Safdi, M.A., Faigel, D.O., Pike, I.M.: Quality indicators for colonoscopy. American Journal of Gastroenterol 101, 873–885 (2006)
20. Graba, T., Granado, B., Romain, O., Ea, T., Pinna, A., Garda, P.: Cyclope: an integrated real-time 3d image sensor. In: XIX Conference on Design of Circuits and Integrated Systems (2004)

21. Kolar, A., Graba, T., Pinna, A., Romain, O., Granado, B., Belhaire, E.: Smart Bi-Spectral Image Sensor for 3D Vision. IEEE Sensors, 577–580 (2007)
22. Tchangani, P.: Support Vector Machines: A Tool for Pattern Recognition and Classification. Studies in Informatics & Control Journal 14(2), 99–109, 1220-1766
23. Stehle, T., Auer, R., et al.: Classification of Colon Polyps in NBI Endoscopy Using Vascularization Features. In: Proc. SPIE 7260, Medical Imaging 2009: Computer-Aided Diagnosis. SPIE Press (2009)
24. Kolar, A., Romain, O., Ayoub, J., Faura, D., Viateur, S., Granado, B., Graba, T.: A system for an accurate 3D reconstruction in Video Endoscopy Capsule. EURASIP Journal on Embedded Systems (2009)

An Analog Front-End and ADC Integrated Circuit for Implantable Force and Orientation Measurements in Joint Prosthesis

Steve Tanner[1], Shafqat Ali[1], Mirjana Banjevic[1], Arash Arami[2], Kamiar Aminian[2], Willyan Hasenkamp[2], Arnaud Bertsch[2], Philippe Renaud[2], and Pierre-André Farine[1]

[1] Ecole Polytechnique Fédérale de Lausanne, Rue Breguet 2, CH2000 Neuchâtel, Switzerland
[2] Ecole Polytechnique Fédérale de Lausanne, Station 11, CH1015 Lausanne, Switzerland
{steve.tanner,shafqat.ali,pierre-andre.farine}@epfl.ch

Abstract. The paper presents an analogue front-end and ADC integrated circuit for processing signals of sensors implanted into joint prosthesis. The circuit is designed to be operated with Wheatstone bridge sensors, such as strain gauges, pressure, Hall Effect, magneto-resistive sensors, etc. It performs sensor supply multiplexing, sensor signal amplification with chopper modulation, offset compensation and 14-bit analog to digital conversion in a single chip. It can operate simultaneously up to eight sensors at an overall bandwidth of 8 kHz, and can be directly interfaced to a remotely powered RFID system in order to constitute a complete multi-sensor, low-power, small size and externally powered micro-system. Integrated into a 180 nm CMOS process, it measures 5 mm^2, is supplied with 1.8 Volt and consumes 1.8 mW.

Keywords: kinematics, prosthesis, strain gauge, telemetry, front-end, integrated circuit, ADC, monitoring, implantable, electronic.

1 Introduction

In vivo biomechanical monitoring of joint prosthesis and orthopedic implants has gained interest in the last years [1], [2] as a mean to detect premature implant failure, which could avoid harmful and costly revision surgery. It is also of interest during implantation operation, for improving the insertion accuracy, and in the long-term for monitoring the aging of the prosthesis and its impact on the surrounding tissues. The parameters of interest to be measured are the forces applied to the joint, the kinematics of the prosthesis (relative orientation and movements), and its micro-motions and vibrations, which can give indication on the interface between the prosthesis and the surrounding tissues. The first difficulty in the design of such an implant is to find an adequate set of sensors and their efficient placement in the insert to get good sensing accuracy without changing the mechanical and biocompatible properties of the prosthesis, submitted to strict regulations. The second difficulty is to design a compact electronics that does not change significantly the prosthesis properties, and that can be powered and monitored remotely so as to avoid batteries.

B. Godara and K.S. Nikita (Eds.): MobiHealth 2012, LNICST 61, pp. 295–302, 2013.

This implies to use a high level of integration, and to minimize the power consumption for allowing small antennas for inductive powering of the system. Finally, the kinematics measurement of the prosthesis from the inside of the body is a challenge; while forces can be measured using strain gauges positioned on the joint interface, and vibrations are detected with accelerometers, the prosthesis kinematics cannot be sensed with traditional methods, due to the impossibility of electrical or optical communication between the two joint parts of the implant. A solution is to use a local magnetic field generated by a permanent magnet located in one part of the prosthesis, and to measure its field intensity by multiple magnetic sensors located in the other part and sensitive to different directions [3]. The 3D relative orientation of the two prosthesis parts can then be computed by merging the different sensor signals.

This paper presents an integrated circuit designed to operate force and magnetic sensors for a microsystem inserted into a joint knee prosthesis. The circuit can power and operate up to eight sensors arranged in a Wheatstone bridge configuration, such as strain gauges, anisotropic magneto-resistive (AMR), and Hall-effect. It embeds a low-noise, high-gain amplification chain, and a 14-bit ADC. It has also a 12-bit DAC for sensor offset compensation. It is powered at 1.8 Volt and consumes 1.8 mW. It can be directly interfaced to an RF communication and power supply system (RFID).

2   Sensors Configuration

The considered prosthesis is a total knee prosthesis, made of a femoral and a tibial part, separated by a polyethylene bearing plate. This plate, of a thickness of 8 to 10 mm, is the ideal location for sensors and electronics. Metallic film strain gauges placed in a Wheatstone bridge were selected for force sensing, and placed at the contact points of the femoral part on the plate (Fig. 1). Depending on the bridge connection, the force difference between the two bridge branches, or the total force, can be measured. This is especially useful for the knee, to measure either force unbalance between two joint sides, or the total force on the joint. The strain gauge signals are weak (in the order of 50 μV) and need amplification by a factor of >1000 to get useful signal for ADC conversion.

There exist several magnetic sensors. The two considered for miniaturization and power consumption reasons are the magneto-resistive and the Hall-effect sensors. Although they use different physical principles, they are relatively similar in terms of input and output impedance (typically 1 to 3 kΩ), and output signal amplitude (a few tenths of mV), considering the targeted magnetic intensity to be measured (10^{-3} to 10^{-2} gauss). Therefore, they do not require high amplification. Regarding their number, like in all triangulation measurements, a higher number of sensed directions and channels increase the accuracy. In the present case, six channels were selected to be a good compromise between accuracy and hardware complexity. Experimental measurements were carried out with a knee simulator and six AMR sensors to validate the accuracy of the proposed orientation sensing principle [3]. A difference of 0.6° RMS was obtained in the dynamic angle estimation compared with an external optical measurement with vicon cameras (Fig. 1).

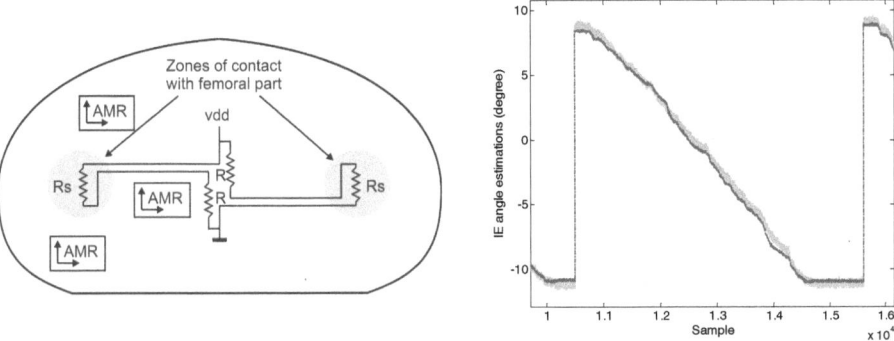

Fig. 1. Left: Location of strain gauge resistors Rs and typical location of three 2-axis AMR sensors in the insert. Right: comparison of two angle measurements of a knee prosthesis placed in a simulator; one with the AMR, and the other with external vision camera system. The RMS difference is 0.6°.

The use of strain gauges to sense efforts in the joint prosthesis determines the parameters for signal conditioning. First, the bandwidth is chosen to be 500 Hz per channel to allow sensing short shocks. Then, the SNR of strain gauge signals is set to 40 dB (100:1) to allow reasonable accuracy measurement at full bandwidth. This sets the input-referred noise density to about 22 nV/Hz$^{0.5}$. For magnetic sensors, an ADC of 14-bit of resolution is needed to fully exploit the sensor sensitivity.

3   Amplification Chain

The architecture of the amplification chain is show in Fig. 2. It includes three stages for high gain, high speed and low power consumption amplification, and input and output chopper switches for flicker noise cancellation.

The first stage is built around a Differential Difference Amplifier (DDA) [4] having a Miller two-stage structure with resistive feedback to provide a programmable voltage gain between 2 and 16. Since its noise is the dominant contribution in the chain, it is carefully designed to provide a low thermal input-referred noise density of 12 nV/Hz$^{0.5}$, and a flicker noise corner frequency at around 15 kHz. The unit capacitor R is 750 Ohm to provide low thermal noise contribution.

The second and third stages are built around a two-stage Miller Differential OTA with capacitive feedback C of 0.6 pF. The input capacitor is programmable from 1.2 to 9.6 pF to allow an overall voltage gain between 2 and 16. In order to set the input common-mode voltage of the amplifiers, a feedback resistor is implemented by means of a switched capacitor circuit with a small capacitor Cr of 10 fF and two switches clocked with non-overlapping phases 1 and 2 at twice the chopper frequency.

The chopper modulation is applied at the input with four switches controlled by signal m, and the demodulation is applied at the output by the same switch arrangement. A second-order passive low-pass filter with a cutoff frequency of 20 kHz (not shown) is present after demodulation to attenuate harmonics resulting from the modulation. The chopper frequency is programmable, from 25 to 35 kHz. Table 1 shows the key parameters of the amplification chain obtained from simulations.

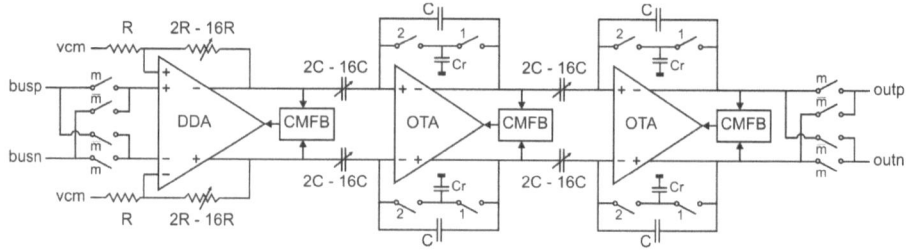

Fig. 2. Amplification chain schematic diagram

Table 1. Performance of amplification chain with chopper modulation

Parameter	Value	Unit
Voltage gain	8 to 4096	
Input bandwidth	10	kHz
Input-referred noise, 0 – 10 kHz	30	$nV/Hz^{0.5}$
Input impedance	>1	MOhm
Max. differential input swing	70	mV
Input common-mode range	0.8 – 1.2	V
Current consumption	600	μA

4   Analog to Digital Converter

To reach 14-bit of resolution, a Sigma-Delta Modulator structure was chosen, whose structure is shown in Fig. 3. It is a third-order modulator with a multi-bit resolution of 4 bit in the feedback path. A multi-bit implementation allows reaching a better SNR for the same oversampling ratio, therefore permits lower power consumption. The modulator includes feed-forward paths on all stages that reduce the signal dynamic, thus strongly relaxes the linearity requirements of the integrators. The 4-bit quantizer includes also passive feed-forward at its input stage. On the feedback path, the 4-bit DACs are implemented on each stage input with a capacitive network of 15 unit capacitors.

Normally, the SNR of a multi-bit Sigma-Delta modulator is limited to 10 bit by the linearity of the first stage DAC, if no linearization technique is used. In order to reach 14-bit, two techniques are implemented. The first uses dynamic element matching, and consists of a scrambling logic on the digital feedback path that selects different DAC unit elements at each conversion, in a way that their mismatch is averaged and the resulting non-linearity is strongly reduced. Data-Weighted Averaging [5] is the chosen algorithm as scrambling law.

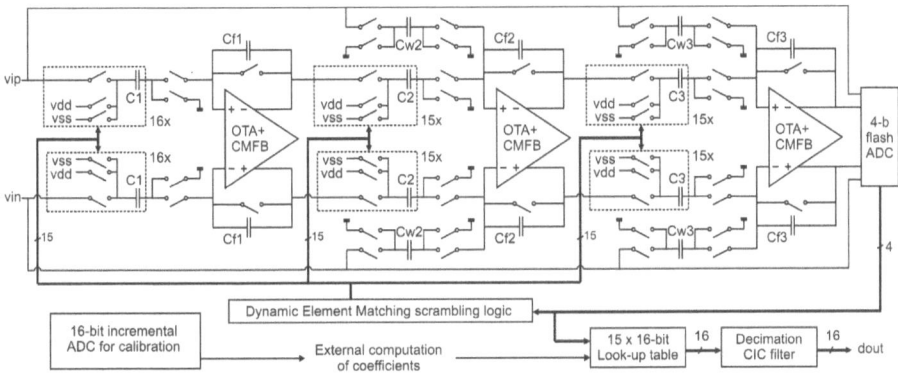

Fig. 3. Analog to Digital Converter schematic diagram

The second linearization technique is based on a background calibration that can be run continuously during circuit operation [6]. The 4-bit DAC of the first stage is made of an array of 16 elements. Each one of these elements can be disconnected from the bank and connected to an incremental 16-bit ADC that measures the capacitor value against a reference capacitor. The correction coefficients can then be computed by the host processor, and written back in a 15x 16-bit Look-Up Table placed before the ADC output decimation filter.

The ADC decimation filter is a standard Cascaded Integrator Comb structure with 5 stages, allowing attenuation of 85 dB before down-sampling by a factor of 32. The output sampling rate is 52 kHz, while the modulator is clocked at a frequency of 1.695 MHz. The ADC modulator consumes 160 μA, and the DEM logic and CIC filter consume together 60 μA. The SNDR of the modulator was simulated at 87 dB.

5   DAC for Sensor Offset Calibration

Since their resistors are subject to mismatch, Wheatstone bridge sensors are affected by offset, which needs to be compensated before amplification. For this, a simple offset compensation scheme is used, consisting of biasing one of the two bridge branches with a resistor and a voltage from a DAC. Choosing an appropriate DAC output voltage allows to modify the DC voltage of the branch and to compensate for sensor offset. The on-chip implementation relies on a programmable resistor whose value can be tuned between 10 and 160 kOhm by steps of 10 kOhm to accommodate for various sensor impedances and offset variations, and on a 12-bit DAC for having a small quantization error. The schematic diagram of the DAC with programmable bias resistor is shown in Fig. 4. Since the DAC is used in a calibration procedure, its integral non-linearity is not critical but the differential non-linearity must remain below 1 LSB. A sub-ranging structure is proposed, made of a first resistive voltage divider with 64 resistors of 3.4 kOhm (6 most significant bits). A 6-bit decoder and a double switch array allow to select the upper and lower point of a given resistor, and to pass the corresponding voltages to voltage buffers. These buffers power a second resistive divider, with 64 resistors of 3.4 kOhm. A second 6-bit decoder and switch array permit the selection of the final output voltage, which is buffered before being applied to the programmable bias resistor. The DAC has a DNL level of 12-bit, consumes 140 µA and has a bandwidth of 20 kHz.

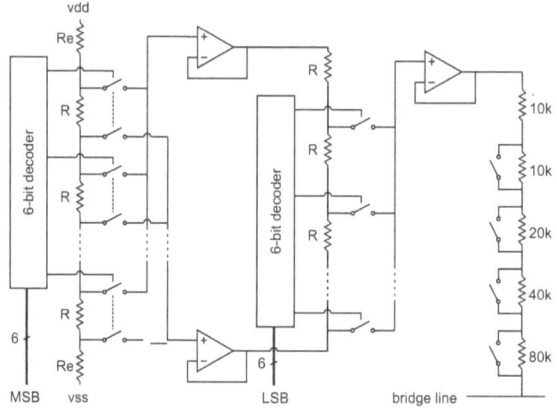

Fig. 4. Offset compensation DAC with programmable bias resistor

6   Chip Architecture

6.1   Input Switches

Fig. 5 shows the internal switches performing multiplexing and powering for the eight sensor channels. To obtain low system power consumption, the sensors must be supplied only when they are read out. For this, the circuit includes one supply line for each sensor, active when the sensor is addressed (signal s active). Two channels are equipped with a 4-wire configuration allowing to swap the resistors of one half bridge to perform summing (signal a active) or differential (signal a inactive) readout modes.

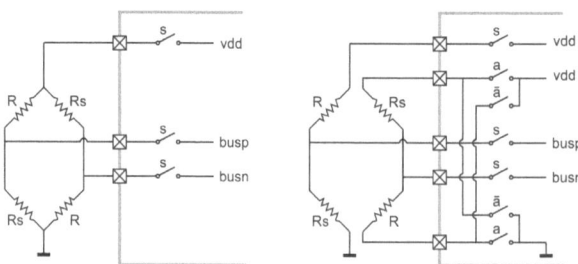

Fig. 5. Internal switches for sensor selection and powering. Left: 2-wire sensor, right: 4-wire sensor for summing or differential readout modes.

6.2   Top-Level

The circuit overall architecture is represented in Fig. 6. Up to 8 sensor bridges can be connected, two of them in a 4-wire configuration. After channel multiplexing, one of the signal bus lines is connected to the offset compensation DAC through the programmable bias resistor. The sensor signal is fed to the amplification chain, the low-pass filtering, and the Sigma-Delta modulator. An on-chip PTAT current reference provides the analog blocks with biasing. The circuit includes digital functions related to ADC (decimation filter, dynamic element matching logic), control logic and a bank of 64 x 8-bit registers which can be read through an SPI interface. The channel selection is controlled through the same SPI. The registers contain individual gain and offset settings for all channels, allowing fast channel switching.

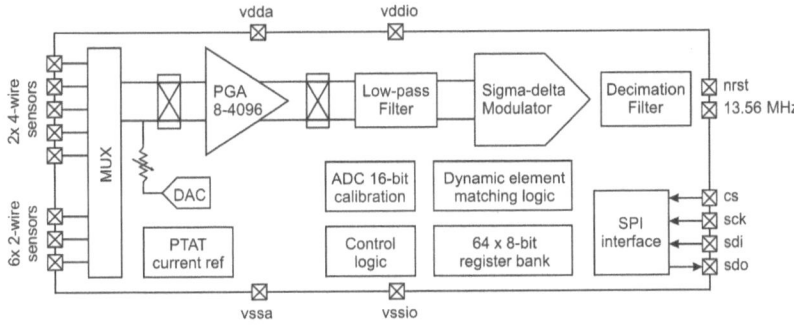

Fig. 6. Top-level circuit architecture

6.3   Layout and Performance Summary

The circuit was integrated into a CMOS 180 nm process technology. The layout is shown in Fig. 7. The circuit expected performances are summarized in Table 2.

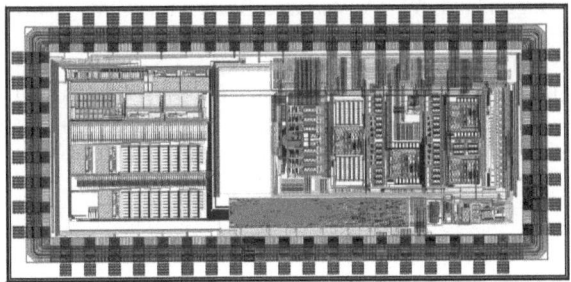

Fig. 7. Circuit layout. Dimensions are 3.2 x 1.6 mm

Table 2. Circuit main parameters and expected performances

Parameter	Value	Unit
Voltage supply	1.8	V
Input clock	13.56	MHz
Current consumption	1	mA
Max. bandwidth per channel	1	kHz
SNR, strain gauges, BW = 500 Hz	40	dB
SNR, magneto-resistors	80	dB

7   Conclusion

The paper presented an integrated circuit for operating 2 strain gauge and 6 magneto-resistive sensors in a knee prosthesis for in vivo force and orientation measurements. The circuit will contribute to high level of integration, small size and low power consumption of the implant.

Acknowledgements. This work was funded under Swiss Science National Foundation Grant SNF20NAN1_123630. The project partners are gratefully acknowledged.

References

1. Graichen, F., Arnold, R., Rohlmann, A., Bergmann, G.: Implantable 9-channel telemetry system for in vivo load measurements with orthopedic implants. IEEE Transactions on Biomedical Engineering 54, 253–261 (2007)
2. Liu, M., Hong, C., Zhang, X., Wang, Z.: Low-Power SoC Design for Ligament Balance Measuring System in Total Knee Arthroplasty. In: Proc. 33rd Annual Int. Conf. of the IEEE EMBS, pp. 5860–5863 (2011)
3. Arami, A., Miehlbradt, J., Aminian, K.: Accurate internal–external rotation measurement in total knee prostheses: A magnetic solution. Journal of Biomechanics 45, 2023–2027 (2012)
4. Säckinger, E., Guggenbühl, W.: A Versatile Block: The CMOS Differential Difference Amplifier. IEEE J. Solid-State Circuits sc-22(2), 287–294 (1987)
5. Baird, R., Fiez, T.: Linearity enhancement of multibit delta–sigma A/D and D/A converters using data weighted averaging. IEEE Trans. Circuits Syst. II 42, 753–762 (1995)
6. Ali, S., Tanner, S., Farine, P.-A.: A Background Calibration Method for DAC Mismatch Correction in Multibit Sigma-Delta Modulators. In: Proc. Int. Soc. Design Conf. (2012)

Improving Power Efficiency in WBAN Communication Using Wake Up Methods

Stevan Marinkovic[1], Emanuel Popovici[2], and Emil Jovanov[3]

[1] ABB Corporate Research, Baden-Dättwil, Switzerland
stevan.marinkovic@ch.abb.com
[2] University College Cork, Cork, Ireland
e.popovici@ucc.ie
[3] The University of Alabama, Huntsville, USA
emil.jovanov@uah.edu

Abstract. Power efficient communication in a Wireless Body Area Network (WBAN) is critical for successful system deployment. Stringent constraints of size and weight of sensors significantly limit available sensor power, particularly in the case of implantable sensors. This paper discusses and analyses methods that could be used to improve power efficiency of implantable WBAN systems, with focus on the Wake Up Radio (WUR), which allows power efficient listening of wireless channel. The paper presents analysis of existing hardware and design trade offs in WUR implementation.

Keywords: Wireless Body Area Networks, Wake-up Radio, Ultra Low Power.

1 Introduction

Wireless Body Area Networks (WBAN) have witnessed a surge of resurgence in research and applications in recent years [1, 2, 3, 4]. This trend is facilitated by advances in sensing, processing and communication algorithms and technologies. WBANs integrate a number of wearable or implanted sensors and may integrate environmental sensors in the vicinity of the user. Environmental sensors typically provide context of physiological or activity records. User convenience and ubiquitous connectivity, among other advantages, make WBANs the most promising application of wireless sensor networks. WBAN applications have the potential to dramatically change the field of monitoring, telemedicine, drug delivery and compliance monitoring, as well as computer assisted rehabilitation.

WBAN based systems introduce a very specific design space with stringent constraints of weight and size, resulting in significant resource constraints. The most limiting factor is power source, which determines maximum power consumption of the system. This is particularly important for implanted sensors, such as pacemakers, where battery life is expected to exceed 10 years [5]. Wireless communication is typically dominant component in the power budget, with several times higher power consumption than processing in the active mode. This

B. Godara and K.S. Nikita (Eds.): MobiHealth 2012, LNICST 61, pp. 303–317, 2013.

paper presents a survey of power efficient WBAN protocols and architectures, with emphasis on benefits of integration of Wake Up Radio as resource that facilitates power efficient WBAN communication.

2   Communication in WBAN

Due to the power constraints, a typical WBAN implements a simple network topology, while supporting sophisticated protocols and signal processing algorithms as well as high quality of service required by health monitoring systems. This section presents commonly used wireless communication standards and system support for power efficient wireless communication.

2.1   Standard Wireless Communication

Choice of wireless standard is mostly driven by requirements for power efficiency and system support. Consequently, most research projects employ IEEE 802.15.1 (Bluetooth [6]) or IEEE 802.15.4 (ZigBee [7]) protocols. These wireless standards are well researched, documented and tested, but are not an optimal technologies for the wireless BAN, since they target a large application space, more flexible networks than WBAN and are used for longer transmission ranges [8]. This makes them less energy efficient than the protocols specifically targeting WBANs such as [9]. A comparison and optimization of two popular WBAN technologies, Bluetooth and ZigBee, is given in the comparative study [10], in terms of design, cost, performance and energy efficiency. Demand for low power consumption, essential for WBAN applications led to the modification of the original Bluetooth standard and introduction of Bluetooth Low Energy (LE). Figure 1 shows the typical WBAN implementation. Smartphone serves as a master node controlling the WBAN and gateway for integration of data from wearable or implanted sensors

The long term health monitoring of patients requires low power techniques [11]. Medium Access Control (MAC) protocols play a significant role in determining the energy consumption in wireless communication. Traditional MAC protocols mainly focus on improving bandwidth utilization, throughput, and latency. However, they lack energy conserving mechanisms, which is one of the most important constraints of a WBAN. The main sources of energy waste are *collision, idle listening, overhearing, and control packet overhead*. MAC protocols maximize the network lifetime by controlling the aforementioned sources of energy waste. Some contention based protocols such as WiseMAC [12], BMAC [13] and [14] use low power listening and preamble sampling techniques to reduce idle listening. Other protocols such as SMAC [15], TMAC [16] and PMAC [17] reduce idle listening by applying a synchronized schedule between the nodes. Contention-based solutions are not suitable for WBAN since most of the traffic is correlated.

Some research groups used TDMA-based MAC protocols for wireless sensor networks [18, 19, 20] and protocols especially for WBAN [21, 22, 23, 24]. Some protocols are designed to support application specific transceivers [21, 22].

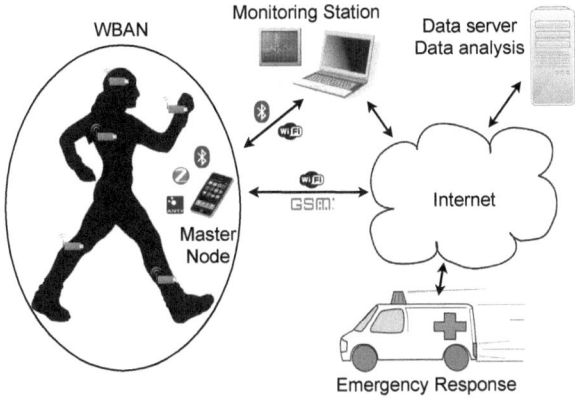

Fig. 1. Wireless Body Area Network example

The main schemes for MAC protocols for sensor networks are CSMA/CA (Carrier Sense Multiple Access / Collision Avoidance) and TDMA (Time Division Multiple Access). FDMA (Frequency Division Multiple Access) requires complex hardware and CDMA (Code Division Multiple Access) has high computational demands. A comparison between TDMA and CSMA protocols is given in Table 1, as reported in [25], where is shown that the TDMA method is more suitable for static types of networks. It is presumed that a BAN is not a dynamic network structure.

Table 1. Comparison of TDMA and CSMA/CA

Communication Strategy	TDMA	CSMA/CA
Power Consumption	Low	High
Bandwidth Utilisation	Maximum	Low
Preferred Traffic Level	High	Low
Dynamic (Network Change)	Poor	Good
Effect of Packet Failure	Latency	Low
Synchronisation	Essential	-

TDMA based protocols outperform CSMA based protocols in all areas except the protocol adaptability to changes in network topology. On the other hand TDMA based protocols need a good synchronization scheme. Such schemes are not easy to implement in a dynamic network, but since BAN has relatively constant network structure and fixed sensor functions synchronization can be simplified.

Additionally, most of the contention-based protocols use Clear Channel Assessment (CCA) to determine the status of the channel. However, this is not always guaranteed in WBAN due to the high path loss inside or outside the human body. Schedule-based protocols such as Time Division Multiple Access (TDMA) provide good solutions to the traffic correlation and CCA problems. These protocols are energy conserving protocols because the duty cycle is reduced and there is no contention, idle listening, and overhearing problem. However, common TDMA needs extra energy for periodic time synchronization. All the sensors (with and without data) are required to receive periodic control packets in order to synchronize their clocks.

2.2   Preamble Sampling

Another method for reducing time spent on idle listening is called preamble sampling method. This method is based on the principle of short duration of radio activity, to determine if there is activity on the channel, in order to wake up. Sensor node wakes up periodically, and if the channel is busy the node remains awake; if not, the node returns to sleep. Time between two channel samples is fixed and known by the network. Therefore, in order to wake up the nodes, before transmission one must ensure that the preamble before the transmission is long enough (at least as long as this time between the channel sampling).

Table 2. Summary of preamble sampling methods [26]

Category	Energy	Sync. Requirements	Implementation	Adaptability
Basic preamble sampling	Average	None	Simple	Bad
Short preamble burst	Good	None	Simple	Bad
Sync. info. advantage	Very good	Sync. needed	Average	Bad
Adaptive duty cycle	Good	None	Not simple	Good

As summarised in Cano et.al. [26], Preamble sampling techniques can be split into the following four 4 categories:

1. **Basic preamble sampling.** - This technique is first presented in 2002 [27], where it was implemented in Aloha and called "preamble sampling". Around same time it was presented in [28], where it was combined with CSMA and called "low power listening". Later, Berkeley MAC was presented [13], which had clear channel assessment (CSA) strategy, where noise floor was measured in the period where it was known that there is no communication on the channel.

2. **Short preamble burst.** - This method is a bit different from the previous in a sense that long preamble is split into a series of short packets. In such way, preamble sampling can detect channel activity and read a short packet of data that will most commonly be a short address (destination identifier), allowing to target specific node. In this way, unnecessary listening is avoided. Example of these are Enhanced B-MAC [29]. Also, one can include information when will the data transmission start, allowing the node to return to sleep mode for a while [13, 30, 31, 32, 33]. Further improvements of this method can be: The transmission of early acknowledgement, to stop the transmission of the burst if the node has nothing to transmit, as presented in [34, 35, 36, 31, 37] and others; Repetitions of data packet, where full data message is repeated [30]; or packet dependent behaviour, that depends on the type of the packet being sent [38, 31, 39].

3. **Taking advantage of synchronisation information.** - This preamble sampling category is a combination of preamble sampling and synchronisation mechanism, with the goal of reducing the length of the preamble. There are two methods of achieving this, either the network coordinator memorises the wake-up time of each receiver, and positions its preamble at that time [12, 35, 32, 40]; or wake up schedules of sensors are synchronised [41, 39].

4. **Adaptive duty cycle.** - This technique is based on changing of the duty cycle of the preamble sampling, channel listening, to adapt to the network traffic change. This makes the protocol to be better adaptive to the network changes, and traffic intensity change, without much idle listening but requires a more complicated algorithm to run. This duty cycle change can be either request based, where duty cycle is adapted on the requests in transmission [12, 42, 43, 44], or traffic load based, where the duty cycle is changed with the observed traffic load [45, 46, 47, 41, 36]. A survey and comparison of WUR methods is presented in [26] and outlined in Table 2.

2.3   Wake Up Radio

The problem of idle listening for events can be solved using the separate hardware that is continuously listening for a certain wake up signal. Typical application will be in a WBAN network with ranges less than 2m. There will be a dedicated device acting as a Master Node that will act as a network coordinator. This device would send wake up signals, and receive data packets from sensors. In 2001, [48] presented the advantages of wake up radio and estimated that a specialised radio interface could consume as little energy as $1\mu W$.

The wake up receiver intended for WBAN is expected to operate in the dense network environment. At any given moment some nodes will be communicating within a WBAN, while some may stay in a sleep mode, monitoring the channel for communication requests. Also, we can expect numerous high power transceivers and noise in the vicinity of a network. The optimal WUR must be immune to to this ambient traffic and should avoid waking up the sensor on signals intended for the neighbouring nodes, as well as on the ambient noise.

From a functional perspective, WUR is not as restricted regarding bit error rate and data rate as the standard receiver. The metric of interest is probability of detection of wake up signals and probability of false alarms. Retransmissions increase power consumption for the transmitter as well as the latency. False alarms are costly from a power perspective because of the needless sensor activations.

There are two functional groups of WUR: *wake up circuits* and *wake up receivers*.

Wake up circuits can have very low power consumption (even zero power), but these only detect the activity on a channel, and cannot distinguish a wake up signal from other RF activity of sufficient power. They are mostly realised using a charge pump. This concept was first presented and simulated in [49]. The circuit is zero power, and it is realised using the Schottky diodes. A similar solution using MOSFET is presented in [50]. Also, battery assisted (semi passive) RFID tags demand similar solutions for their power-on sensing circuitry as explained in [51]. In 1998 an RF field detector was presented as a low power wake up method that could be used in semi passive RFID tags [52]. Another design, with a power-on circuit based on multi stage charge pump is presented in [53]. A complete micro-power sensor node with RF quasi-passive wake-up circuit is presented in [54].

Wake up receivers (WUR) have the ability to demodulate and decode some packet of information following the signal, which can be used for addressing to reduce the number of activations. A low power WUR that has addressing capabilities is presented by [55]. A solution with a Schottky voltage doubler followed by a programmable amplifier and integrator is developed in [56]. Alternative approach based on a zero-bias Schottky voltage doubler (charge pump, envelope detector), is simulated in [57]. A design based solely on amplifiers is presented in [58]. Another low voltage - low power ASIC solution is presented in [59]. This WUR has a very good sensitivity of -71dBm. [60] proposes a WUR that has a dedicated low power microcontroller for packet decoding. The solution published in [61] is a wake-up transceiver, meaning that a dedicated transmitter was developed with the WUR. [62] have developed a low-power, low-frequency WUR with an integrated correlator which compares the received signal to a byte pattern saved in a configuration register. Another integrated solution has been developed at Fraunhofer institute [63].

Currently, the lowest power WUR, specially designed for the WBAN and implant communication is presented in [64]. This receiver is a full WUR solution, working in 400MHz range, that continuously listens on a wireless channel for the Wake Up Packet - a packet of OOK data that contains the address of the targeted device. Any transmitter that can work in OOK mode can be used for the transmission of the wake up packet. Ideally, one would use a transmitter that has a OOK and FSK mode, where OOK would be used for the wake up, and FSK for the regular communication. Example can be Texas Instruments CC430, which can provide a full solution with the processor for protocol and wake-up handling, and transceiver for the communication that can be used for wake up

Table 3. Wake-up receiver prototypes

Authors	Year	f [MHz]	Rate [kb/s]	S [dBm]	P [μW]
Pletcher [58]	2009	2000	100	-72	52
Fraunhofer [63]	2010	868	1	-60	33
Le-Huy [57]	2008	2400	50	-50	20
Durante [56]	2009	2400	100	-53	12.5
Gamm [62]	2010	868	NA	-52	2.78
Doorn [60]	2009	868	0.862	-51	2.6
Ansari [55]	2009	868	0.75	N/A	2.6
Hambeck [59]	2011	868	100	-71	2.4
Marinkovic [64]	2011	434	5.5	-51	0.270

packet transmission in OOK mode. It is currently the WUR prototype with the lowest power consumption and very low latency that was achieved at the cost of somewhat reduced sensitivity optimized for typical WBAN ranges.

Finally, Zarlink [65] present and produce a full commercial solution of wake up receiver and a transceiver, intended for implant communication. This is not a continuous listening WUR, but separate low power 2.4GHz receiver that is duty cycled, acting as a WUR. Reason is that this band allows for higher output power than the MICS band [66] and somewhat longer range. Although this is in a sense a preamble sampling mechanism, it is a separate circuit with a very low power consumption, and can be considered as a Wake Up Receiver.

Jelicic et.al. [67] finely summarises the state of the art in WUR designs and prototypes (Table 3) for the last three years. The paper also contains more detailed analysis of the WUR implementation in communication protocols. For the implant communication, one should consider the lower power WUR solutions in the 1μW range. Two solutions, [65] and [64] have reduced the power consumption below 1μW, which makes them suitable for the implant communication. They both have advantages and disadvantages, which will be discussed in the next section.

3   Power Efficiency with WUR

The main issue in low power wireless networking is to keep the network functionality, but to lower the power consumption. This is achieved by deliberately increasing the communication latency, to reduce the communication duty cycle. Most of the proposed and cited protocols are based around a centralised network structure and beacon communication. This means that either the network coordinator sends beacons at regular time intervals, or the sensor scans the channel at regular time intervals, in order to keep the network alive, and to synchronise for data transfer. Since data transfer cannot happen in those protocols before the initial polling (reception of the beacon and request for data send/receive), the maximum latency is the time interval between two beacons.

Table 4. Comparison between communication methods

Communication method	Node responsiveness †	Range	Power consumption ‡
Standard Protocol	Slow	High	High
Preamble Sampling	Slow	High	Medium
Strobed WUR (Zarlink)	Fast	Medium	Low
WUR	Very fast	Low	Low

† - Comparison with given power consumption target
‡ - Comparison with given latency / response time target

When the communication is frequent, this is proper way to organise a network, since a timeslot can be given and data can be sent during regular time intervals, but when communication is scarce, or irregular, this regular awakening becomes the main communication power consumer, especially when desired latency is low. It is not mentioned in the literature, but in practice, this kind of operation requires an active timing and control circuit, which if not implemented within the transceiver, is usually a microcontroller that consumes current by staying in active mode or running the timers.

The WUR can be used on top of the existing protocols, as a method to control the power consumption, and solve the latency problem, by allowing the rest of the circuit to be in the low power "sleep" mode, while continuously listening to a wireless channel. The next sections discuss the usage of the proposed WUR, and its benefits in the standardised and frequently used WBAN protocols.

Introducing the wake up receiver as a component that can listen to a channel reduces the duty cycle (time spent on idle listening), but introduces new component with quiescent power consumption. Good power model must be derived to justify the introduction of this component and maximum power consumption it can have in order to be practical in applications.

Table 4 presents the functional comparison between communication methods in WBAN. The main point is that WUR enabled devices will have lower power consumption while maintaining the lower node response times (fast responsiveness). Of course this is achieved at the cost of the receiver sensitivity, and limitation of the effective communication range. Therefore, since the ranges in WBAN are not long and power consumption requirements are strict, one can conclude that WUR is the good approach in the implant communication, where responsiveness has to be relatively fast.

In order to determine the power consumption benefits, usage of WUR will be compared to three popular protocols. Zigbee and Bluetooth Low Power as the standard protocols, and Wise MAC as preamble sampling protocol.

ZigBee is a specification for a suite of high level communication protocols using small, low-power digital radios based on the IEEE 802.15.4-2003 standard for Low-Rate Wireless Personal Area Networks (LR-WPANs), such as wireless light switches with lamps, electrical meters with in-home-displays, consumer electronics equipment via short-range radio needing low rates of data transfer. The technology defined by the ZigBee specification is intended to be simpler and less expensive than other WPANs, such as Bluetooth. ZigBee is targeted at RF applications that require a low data rate, long battery life, and secure networking [7].

Bluetooth Low Energy (LE) is one of the most popular WBAN protocols, and it is used today for the variety of applications. It uses a TDMA based master-slave protocol, consisting of piconets with one master and up to 7 slaves [68]. Bluetooth channels use a Frequency-Hop/Time-Division-Duplex (FH/TDD) scheme in which the time is divided into $625\mu sec$ intervals called slots. The master-to-slave transmission starts in even numbered slots, while the slave-to-master transmission starts in odd-numbered slots.

The WiseMAC [12] is a popular low power MAC protocol, based on preamble sampling which is discussed for the next standard in the 802.15 CSEM FM-UWB Proposal [69] for wide band personal area networks. WiseMAC is based on the preamble sampling technique which consists in regularly sampling the medium to check for activity. All sensor nodes in a network sample the medium with the same constant period TW but their relative sampling schedule offsets are independent and constant. If the medium is found busy, a sensor node continues to listen until a data frame is received or until the medium becomes idle again. At the access point, a wake-up preamble of size equal to the sampling period is transmitted as a preamble of every data frame to ensure that the receiver will be awake when the data portion of the packet arrives. The access point (coordinator node) knows the sampling schedule of all sensor nodes, therefore it starts the transmission just at the right time with a wake-up preamble. This wake up preamble is received with the conventional receiver. The access point is the only initiator of the communications.

However losses in the body signal propagation are considerable despite the fact that WBAN implant communication ranges are low. Therefore one has to keep balance between power consumption, receiver sensitivity, and responsiveness. Depending on the application, one can choose *strobed WUR* (Higher range, slower response) or *continuous WUR* (Lower range, faster response). Both methods are much more power efficient than regular communication, or preamble sampling using the high sensitivity receiver.

Figure 2 compares the power consumption of three protocols, Zigbee, Bluetooth LE and WiseMAC, for connection events only - wireless overhead communication that is required just to keep the network alive and not to transmit or receive any data. Values for calculation was extracted from application note [70] for Bluetooth LE, application note [71] for Zigbee and [12] for WiseMAC. Data from these papers was used to calculate the energy needed for one connection event. The figure presents the average power consumption of these connection events, as a function of their frequency (time between them). In order to compare, the line "With WUR" shows the power consumption of a receiver and uC processor sleep mode plus the power consumption of WUR presented in [64]. This is not a function of connection events frequency, as the protocol implementing WUR would not use connection events.

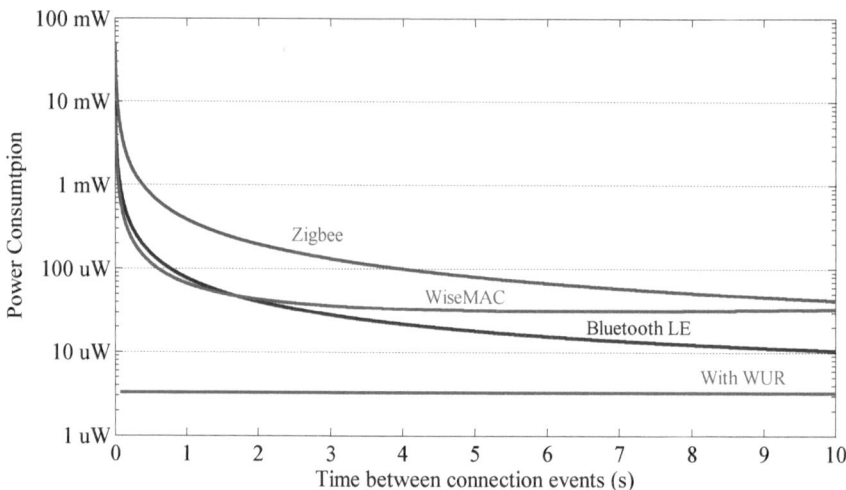

Fig. 2. Comparison between Zigbee, Bluetooth LE, WiseMAC and a protocol that would implement WUR

There are not many protocols that consider the WUR hardware in the MAC design, and this area is currently being researched. Examples are traffic-adaptive MAC protocol (TaMAC) for WBAN that improves energy efficiency by exploiting the traffic information (traffic-patterns) of the nodes is presented in [11]. Other solutions that incorporate WUR for energy efficiency is presented in [72, 55]. These solutions are based on a fictional (concept) WUR, but prove that if presented with a WUR device, the power consumption of any protocol can be significantly reduced. [73] proposes a communication method for medical oriented scenarios using the WUR [64].

4   Conclusion

Efficient integration of implanted sensors into WBANs must provide effective trade off between low power consumption and the responsiveness of the implanted node to external requests. Keeping responsiveness using traditional wireless method of connection events is relatively power consuming, even in the case of low power protocols. Therefore, one should consider the new technologies of wake up receivers used for channel monitoring. In this paper we presented alternative approaches, the preamble sampling WUR by Zarlink and continuous channel listening as state of the art in this area and as seen in Figure 2, this might be a possible and promising technology for future WBAN development.

References

[1] Istepanian, R., Jovanov, E., Zhang, Y.: Guest editorial introduction to the special section on M-Health: beyond seamless mobility and global wireless Health-Care connectivity. IEEE Transactions on Information Technology in Biomedicine 8(4), 405–414 (2004)

[2] Ullah, S., Higgins, H., Braem, B., Latre, B., Blondia, C., Moerman, I., Saleem, S., Rahman, Z., Kwak, K.: A comprehensive survey of wireless body area networks. Journal of Medical Systems, 1–30 (2010)

[3] Milosevic, M., Shrove, M., Jovanov, E.: Applications of smartphones for ubiquitous health monitoring and wellbeing management. JITA 1(1), 7–15 (2011)

[4] Jovanov, E., Milenkovic, A.: Body area networks for ubiquitous healthcare applications: Opportunities and challenges. J. Med. Syst. (2011)

[5] Shi, W.V., Zhou, M.: Body sensors applied in pacemakers: A survey. IEEE Sensors Journal 12(6), 1817–1827 (2012)

[6] Bluetooth SIG: Specification of the bluetooth system, version 4.0 (2010)

[7] ZigBee Alliance: Zigbee wireless standard (2003),
http://www.zigbee.org/Standards/Overview.aspx

[8] Drude, S.: Requirements and application scenarios for body area networks. In: Mobile and Wireless Communications Summit 16th IST pp. 1–5 (2007)

[9] Marinkovic, S.J., Popovici, E.M., Spagnol, C., Faul, S., Marnane, W.P.: Energy-efficient low duty cycle MAC protocol for wireless body area networks. IEEE Transactions on Information Technology in Biomedicine 13(6), 915–925 (2009)

[10] Yan, L., Zhong, L., Jha, N.: Energy comparison and optimization of wireless body-area network technologies. In: Proc. Int'l Conf. Body Area Networks, BodyNets, pp. 1–8 (2007)

[11] Ullah, S., Kwak, K.S.: An ultra low-power and traffic-adaptive medium access control protocol for wireless body area network. Journal of Medical Systems, 1–10 (2010)

[12] Hoiydi, E., Decotignie, J.: Wisemac: An ultra low power mac protocol for the downlink of infrastructure wsns. In: Ninth International Symposium on Computers and Communications (ISCC), pp. 244–251 (2004)

[13] Polastre, J., Hill, J., Culler, D.: Versatile low power media access for wireless sensor networks. In: 2nd International Conference on Embedded Networked Sensor Systems, pp. 95–107 (2004)

[14] Hauer, J.-H., Handziski, V., Köpke, A., Willig, A., Wolisz, A.: A component framework for content-based publish/subscribe in sensor networks. In: Verdone, R. (ed.) EWSN 2008. LNCS, vol. 4913, pp. 369–385. Springer, Heidelberg (2008)

[15] Wei, Y., Heidemann, J., Estrin, D.: An energy-efficient mac protocol for wireless sensor networks. In: IEEE Infocom Conference, pp. 1567–1576 (2002)

[16] van Dam, T., Langendoen, K.: An adaptive energy-efficient mac protocol for wsns. In: 1st ACM Conf. on Embedded Networked Sensor Systems (SenSys), pp. 171–180 (2003)

[17] Khan, N., Boncelet, C.: Pmac: Energy efficient medium access control protocol for wireless sensor networks. In: IEEE Military Communications Conference, pp. 1–5 (2006)

[18] Lee, W., Datta, A., Cardell-Oliver, R.: Fleximac: A flexible tdma-based mac protocol for fault-tolerant and energy-efficient wireless sensor networks. In: 14th IEEE Int'l Conf. Networks (ICON), pp. 1–6 (2006)

[19] Elsaify, A., Padhy, P., Martinez, K., Zou, G.: Gwmac- a tdma based mac protocol for a glacial sensor network. In: 4th ACM PE-WASUN, pp. 54–61 (2007)

[20] van Hoeselt, L., Niebergt, T., Kipt, H.J., Havingar, P.: Advantages of a tdma based, energy-efficient, self-organizing mac protocol for wsns. In: IEEE 59th Vehicular Technology Conference, vol. 3, pp. 1598–1602 (2004)

[21] Chen, Z., Khokhar, A.: Self organization and energy efficient TDMA MAC protocol by wake up for wireless sensor networks. In: First Annual IEEE Communications Society Conference on Sensor and Ad Hoc Communications and Networks, pp. 335–341 (2004)

[22] Omeni, O., Wong, A., Burdett, A., Toumazou, C.: Energy efficient medium access protocol for wireless medical body area sensor networks. IEEE Transactions on Biomedical Circuits and Systems 2, 251–259 (2007)

[23] Milenkovic, A., Otto, C., Jovanov, E.: Wireless sensor network for personal health monitoring: issues and an implementation. Computer Communications 29, 2521–2533 (2006)

[24] Latre, B., Braem, B., Moerman, I., Blondia, C., Reusens, E., Joseph, W., Demeester, P.: A low-delay protocol for multi-hop wireless body area networks. In: 4th Int'l Conference, MobiQuitous, pp. 1–8 (2007)

[25] Cionca, V., Newe, T., Dadarlat, V.: Tdma protocol requirements for wireless sensor networks. In: 2nd Int'l Conf., Sensorcomm, pp. 30–35 (2008)

[26] Cano, C., Bellalta, B., Sfairopoulou, A., Oliver, M.: Low energy operation in wsns: A survey of preamble sampling mac protocols. Computer Networks 55(15), 3351–3363 (2011)

[27] El-Hoiydi, A.: Aloha with preamble sampling for sporadic traffic in ad hoc wireless sensor networks. In: IEEE International Conference on Communications, ICC 2002, vol. 5, pp. 3418–3423. IEEE (2002)

[28] Hill, J., Culler, D.: Mica: A wireless platform for deeply embedded networks. IEEE Micro 22(6), 12–24 (2002)

[29] Lim, S., Kim, S.-H., Cho, J., An, S.-S.: Medium access control with an energy-efficient algorithm for wireless sensor networks. In: Cuenca, P., Orozco-Barbosa, L. (eds.) PWC 2006. LNCS, vol. 4217, pp. 334–343. Springer, Heidelberg (2006)

[30] Wong, K., Arvind, D.: Speckmac: low-power decentralised mac protocols for low data rate transmissions in specknets. In: Proceedings of the 2nd International Workshop on Multi-Hop ad Hoc Networks: from Theory to Reality, pp. 71–78. ACM (2006)

[31] Lim, S., Ji, Y., Cho, J., An, S.-S.: An ultra low power medium access control protocol with the divided preamble sampling. In: Youn, H.Y., Kim, M., Morikawa, H. (eds.) UCS 2006. LNCS, vol. 4239, pp. 210–224. Springer, Heidelberg (2006)

[32] Shi, X., Stromberg, G.: Syncwuf: An ultra low-power mac protocol for wireless sensor networks. IEEE Transactions on Mobile Computing 6(1), 115–125 (2007)

[33] Han, K., Lim, S., Lee, S., Lee, J., An, S.: Signaling-embedded short preamble mac for multihop wireless sensor networks. In: Information Networking. Towards Ubiquitous Networking and Services, pp. 1–10 (2008)

[34] Lin, E., Rabaey, J., Wolisz, A.: Power-efficient rendez-vous schemes for dense wireless sensor networks. In: 2004 IEEE International Conference on Communications, vol. 7, pp. 3769–3776. IEEE (2004)

[35] Mahlknecht, S., Bock, M.: Csma-mps: A minimum preamble sampling mac protocol for low power wireless sensor networks. In: Proceedings of the 2004 IEEE International Workshop on Factory Communication Systems, pp. 73–80. IEEE (2004)

[36] Buettner, M., Yee, G., Anderson, E., Han, R.: X-mac: a short preamble mac protocol for duty-cycled wireless sensor networks. In: Proceedings of the 4th International Conference on Embedded Networked Sensor Systems, pp. 307–320. ACM (2006)

[37] Liu, S., Fan, K., Sinha, P.: Cmac: an energy-efficient mac layer protocol using convergent packet forwarding for wireless sensor networks. ACM Transactions on Sensor Networks (TOSN) 5(4), 29 (2009)

[38] Bernardo, L., Oliveira, R., Pereira, M., Macedo, M., Pinto, P.: A wireless sensor mac protocol for bursty data traffic. In: IEEE 18th International Symposium on Personal, Indoor and Mobile Radio Communications, PIMRC 2007, pp. 1–5. IEEE (2007)

[39] Merlin, C., Heinzelman, W.: Schedule adaptation of low-power-listening protocols for wireless sensor networks. IEEE Transactions on Mobile Computing 9(5), 672–685 (2010)

[40] Zhang, X., Ansari, J., Mähönen, P.: Traffic aware medium access control protocol for wireless sensor networks. In: Proceedings of the 7th ACM International Symposium on Mobility Management and Wireless Access, pp. 140–148. ACM (2009)

[41] Ye, W., Silva, F., Heidemann, J.: Ultra-low duty cycle mac with scheduled channel polling, pp. 321–334 (2006)

[42] Anwander, M., Wagenknecht, G., Braun, T., Dolfus, K.: Beam: A burst-aware energy-efficient adaptive mac protocol for wireless sensor networks. In: International Conference on Networked Sensing Systems, INSS (2010)

[43] Bing, L., Lin, Z., Huimin, Z.: An adaptive schedule medium access control for wireless sensor networks. In: Sixth International Conference on Networking, ICN 2007, p. 12. IEEE (2007)

[44] Kumar, P., Gunes, M., Mushtaq, Q., Blywis, B.: A real-time and energy-efficient mac protocol for wireless sensor networks. International Journal of Ultra Wideband Communications and Systems 1(2), 128–142 (2009)

[45] Avvenuti, M., Vecchio, A.: Adaptability in the b-mac+ protocol. In: International Symposium on Parallel and Distributed Processing with Applications, ISPA 2008, pp. 946–951. IEEE (2008)

[46] Hurni, P., Braun, T.: MaxMAC: A maximally traffic-adaptive MAC protocol for wireless sensor networks. In: Silva, J.S., Krishnamachari, B., Boavida, F. (eds.) EWSN 2010. LNCS, vol. 5970, pp. 289–305. Springer, Heidelberg (2010)

[47] Cano, C., Bellalta, B., Sfairopoulou, A., Barceló, J.: A low power listening mac with scheduled wake up after transmissions for wsns. IEEE Communications Letters 13(4), 221–223 (2009)

[48] da Silva Jr., J.L., Shamberger, J., Ammer, M.J., Guo, C., Li, S., Shah, R., Tuan, T., Sheets, M., Rabaey, J.M., Nikolic, B.: et al.: Design methodology for PicoRadio networks. In: Proceedings of the Conference on Design, Automation and Test in Europe, pp. 314–325 (2001)

[49] Gu, L., Stankovic, J.A.: Radio-triggered wake-up for wireless sensor networks. Real-Time Systems 29(2), 157–182 (2005)

[50] Kim, H., Cho, H., Xi, Y., Kim, M., Kwon, S., Lim, J., Yang, Y.: CMOS passive wake-up circuit for sensor network applications. Microwave and Optical Technology Letters 52, 597–600 (2010)

[51] Protocols, E.R.F.I.: Uhf rfid protocol for communications at 860 mhz -960 mhz, version 1.0.9 (2005)

[52] Lee, M.: Zero-bias detector yields high sensitivity with nanopower consumption. Linear Technology Magazine 8(1), 28 (1998)

[53] Wenyi, C., Shuo, G., Xiao, W., Tingwen, X., Jingtian, X., Xi, T., Na, Y., Hao, M.: Analysis and design of power efficient semi-passive RFID tag. Journal of Semiconductors 31(7), 075013 (2010)

[54] Malinowski, M., Moskwa, M., Feldmeier, M., Laibowitz, M., Paradiso, J.A.: CargoNet: a low-cost micropower sensor node exploiting quasi-passive wakeup for adaptive asynchronous monitoring of exceptional events. In: Proceedings of the 5th International Conference on Embedded Networked Sensor Systems (SenSys), pp. 145–159 (2007)

[55] Ansari, J., Pankin, D., Mahonen, P.: Radio-triggered wake-ups with addressing capabilities for extremely low power sensor network applications. International Journal of Wireless Information Networks 16(3), 118–130 (2009)

[56] Durante, M.S., Mahlknecht, S.: An ultra low power wakeup receiver for wireless sensor nodes. In: Proceedings of the Third International Conference on Sensor Technologies and Applications (SENSORCOMM), pp. 167–170 (2009)

[57] Le-Huy, P., Roy, S.: Low-Power Wake-Up radio for wireless sensor networks. In: Mobile Networks and Applications, pp. 1–11 (2008)

[58] Pletcher, N., Gambini, S., Rabaey, J.: A 52 μW wake-up receiver with -72 dbm sensitivity using an uncertain-IF architecture. IEEE Journal of Solid-State Circuits 44(1), 269–280 (2009)

[59] Hambeck, C., Mahlknecht, S., Herndl, T.: A 2.4 μw wake-up receiver for wireless sensor nodes with- 71dbm sensitivity. In: 2011 IEEE International Symposium on Circuits and Systems (ISCAS), pp. 534–537. IEEE (2011)

[60] der Doorn, B.V., Kavelaars, W., Langendoen, K.: A prototype Low-Cost wakeup radio for the 868 MHz band. Int. Journal of Sensor Networks 5(1), 22–32 (2009)

[61] Van Langevelde, R., Van Elzakker, M., Van Goor, D., Termeer, H., Moss, J., Davie, A.: An ultra-low-power 868/915 mhz rf transceiver for wireless sensor network applications. In: IEEE Radio Frequency Integrated Circuits Symposium, RFIC 2009, pp. 113–116. IEEE (2009)

[62] Gamm, G., Sippel, M., Kostic, M., Reindl, L.: Low power wake-up receiver for wireless sensor nodes. In: 2010 Sixth International Conference on Intelligent Sensors, Sensor Networks and Information Processing (ISSNIP), pp. 121–126. IEEE (2010)

[63] Fraunhofer Institute: Wakeup receiver (2010),
http://www.iis.fraunhofer.de/en/bf/ic/komp/rf/hew.html

[64] Marinkovic, S.J., Popovici, E.M.: Nano-power wireless wake-up receiver with serial peripheral interface. IEEE Journal on Selected Areas in Communications 29, 1641–1647 (2011)

[65] Zarlink Semiconductor Inc.: Medical implantable rf transceiver mics rf telemetry (2010), http://www.zarlink.com/zarlink/zl70102-shortform-datasheet-jun10.pdf

[66] Rules, F.: Regulations: Mics band plan (2003)

[67] Jelicic, V., Magno, M., Brunelli, D., Bilas, V., Benini, L.: Analytic comparison of wake-up receivers for wsns and benefits over the wake-on radio scheme. In: Proceedings of the 7th ACM Workshop on Performance Monitoring and Measurement of Heterogeneous Wireless and Wired Networks, pp. 99–106. ACM (2012)

[68] Zussman, G., Segall, A.: Bluetooth time division duplex - analysis as a polling system, pp. 547–556. Columbia University (2004)

[69] Farserotu, J., Gerrits, J., van Veenendaal, G., Lobeira, M., Long, J.: Csem fm-uwb proposal. IEEE P802.15 Working Group for Wireless Personal Area Networks, WPANs (2009)

[70] Kamath, S.: Application note an092 - measuring bluetooth low energy power consumption. Texas Instruments (2010)

[71] Selvig, B.: Application note an053 - measuring power consumption with cc2430 & z-stack. Texas Instruments (2007)

[72] Miller, M., Vaidya, N.: A mac protocol to reduce sensor network energy consumption using a wakeup radio. IEEE Transactions on Mobile Computing, 228–242 (2005)

[73] Marinkovic, S., Popovici, E.: Ultra low power signal oriented approach for wireless health monitoring. Sensors 12(6), 7917–7937 (2012)

Active Textile Antennas as a Platform for More Energy-Efficient and Reliable Wireless Links in Healthcare

Hendrik Rogier[1,2], Frederick Declercq[1,2], Patrick Van Torre[1], and Luigi Vallozzi[1]

[1] Ghent University, Dept. of Information Technology
Sint-Pietersnieuwstraat 41, B-9000 Ghent, Belgium
`Hendrik.Rogier@intec.UGent.be`
[2] IMEC, INTEC Division, Ghent, Belgium

Abstract. New wireless wearable monitoring systems worn by patients and caregivers require a high degree of reliability and autonomy. We show that active textile antenna systems may serve as robust platforms to deploy such wireless links, in the meanwhile being comfortable and invisible to the wearer, thanks to recent developments in the design process combined with dedicated signal processing techniques. The key idea is to exploit the large amount of real estate available in patients' and caregivers' garments to deploy multiple textile antennas each with a size large enough to make them efficient radiators when deployed on the body. The antenna area is then reused by positioning active electronics directly underneath and energy harvesters directly on top of the antenna patch, ensuring the autonomy of the module. Combining different antenna signals by means of low-power multi-antenna processing techniques then ensures good signal quality at low transmit power in all situations.

Keywords: Smart Fabrics and Interactive Textiles, wearable electronics, active textile antennas, MIMO signal processing.

1 Introduction

The explosive developments in the field of smart fabrics and interactive textiles (SFIT) have opened a wide range of exciting possibilities in the field of healthcare. Remote monitoring of patients may be provided by wearable systems that are unobtrusively integrated into patient garments, in the meanwhile continuously monitoring life signs, activities and environmental conditions, and relaying these data wirelessly to a remote location for supervision by a caregiver. Such intelligent garments may be deployed both in the hospital and in the home environment of the wearer. Also caregivers may be equipped with wearable systems, either to collect and transmit their own parameters during interventions in hazardous situations, or as a personal wearable computer that receives, interprets and displays patient data to help a caregiver in making decisions.

B. Godara and K.S. Nikita (Eds.): MobiHealth 2012, LNICST 61, pp. 318–325, 2013.

As SFIT systems are to be deployed in critical applications such as patient monitoring and rescue missions, their reliability and autonomy are two key concerns of the designers. To ensure sufficient autonomy without the use of heavy batteries, we need to satisfy two requirements: First, the wireless communication module, and in particular the transceiver module responsible for setting up the wireless link is typically one of the largest energy consumers of the wearable system. Therefore, we need to design a highly energy-efficient communication system, in which textile antennas are critical components. Indeed, an efficient wearable antenna providing off-body communication with high gain and large radiation efficiency typically consumes quite a lot of space, as a large ground plane is required to avoid absorption of antenna radiation by the human body. Yet, this space is widely available in garments. However, the large flexible textile antenna [6, 4, 5, 3] will typically be subject to bending, wrinkling and crumpling as the wearer moves around. This should be taken into account during the design phase of these antennas. Second, to ensure sufficient autonomy to the SFIT system, energy harvesters should be added that make use of the large number of energy sources available in the neighbourhood of the body to scavenge energy.

In this contribution, we will review and evaluate a number of techniques that may be implemented on textile antennas to increase the energy-efficiency and autonomy of SFIT systems. The key idea is to increase performance and functionality by reusing surface area for multiple purposes. This is done at two levels: First, the garment, offering protection and comfort to the wearer, is reused as a platform for a wearable multi-antenna system. Second, the textile antenna itself, being the largest component of each wearable module, is reused as a platform for active electronic circuits implementing sensing and communication, and for energy-scavengers with energy-management circuits.

In Section 2 we show how active electronic circuits may be directly integrated underneath the wearable antenna, resulting in a compact communication module. Moreover, by adopting a full-wave/circuit co-design and co-optimizing strategy, optimal active antenna performance can be obtained, aiming either for optimal noise or impedance matching. Next, we show in Section 3 how one can integrate a set of solar cells on top of the antenna patch, without disturbing the radiation characteristics of the textile antennas. In Section 4 we show that by combining multiple wearable antennas, integrating them in the front and back sections of a garment and relying on diversity techniques at both ends of the link, the reliability of wireless communication links can be improved tremendously. Diversity techniques can easily be implemented at the receiver side, but the use of space-time codes can be quite energy-consuming as codes must be generated at the transmitting side, whereas accurate channel estimation is required at the receiver. Section 5 presents some energy-efficient alternatives, such as passive beamforming and channel state tracking. It is shown that these techniques provide an almost equal performance while relying on much simpler and less energy-consuming signal processing algorithms. Finally, we formulate some conclusions in Section 6.

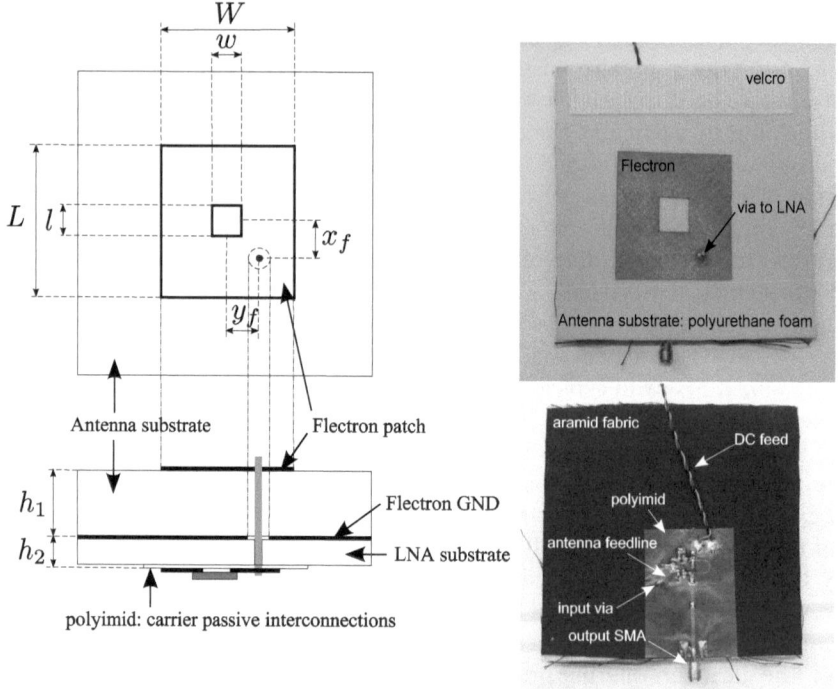

Fig. 1. Active wearable receive antenna operating in 2.45GHz ISM band

2   Full-Wave/Circuit Co-design of Active Wearable Antennas

Although the development of wearable electronics systems has boomed over the last decade, most of the research focused on converting conventional rigid electronic circuits into flexible wearable components that are compatible with integration into fabric. The complete wearable electronic system is then constructed by interconnecting the set of wearable components needed to implement the desired functionality. This approach, however, results in a fragile overall system, with many weak links that easily break. Moreover, as all components are designed separately, optimal performance of the overall system is not guaranteed. Therefore, we have adopted a new design strategy [2] where we aim to integrate as many components as possible on the textile antenna(s) of the wearable system, in the meanwhile reusing the large area that we need to ensure high gain and good radiation efficiency, and opening new opportunities to co-optimize the performance of the antenna together with the active circuits. At the same time, improving overall system performance also increases the autonomy of the wireless system and reduces the risk of interference with other systems. Both problems are highly relevant in healthcare applications.

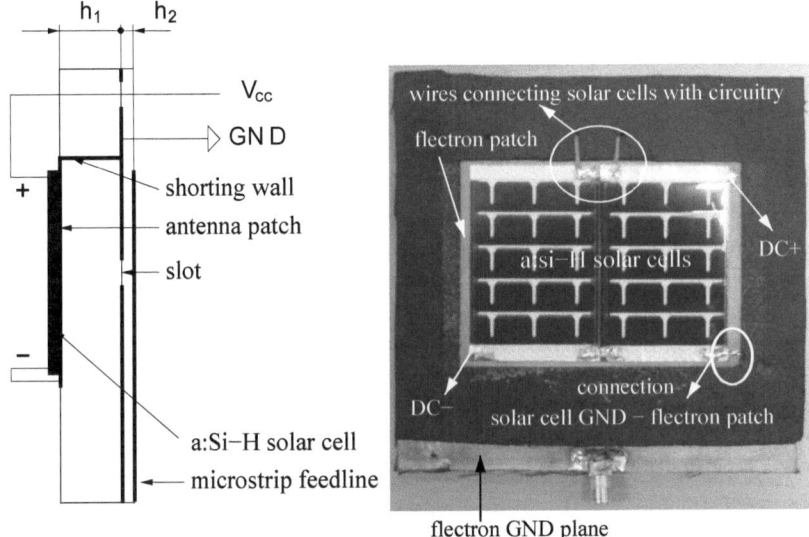

Fig. 2. Aperture-coupled shorted wearable solar patch antenna for 902–928 MHz UHF band

In Fig. 1 we present an active wearable antenna, for which the full-wave/circuit co-design approach was applied to integrate a low-noise amplifier (LNA) directly underneath a textile patch antenna. As the antenna feed is directly connected to the LNA input by means of a short via, RF connection losses are reduced. Moreover, careful co-optimization of the patch dimensions, the position of the antenna feed point and the elements composing the LNA circuit results in optimal noise performance, high gain and 50Ω matching at the output of the LNA, leading to a highly sensitive receive antenna that operates in the 2.45GHz ISM band.

3   Integration of a Solar Cell on a Wearable Antenna

Ensuring acceptable autonomy is of major concern for wearable systems, since batteries rapidly increase the weight and may reduce the flexibility. An exciting new area of the research focusses on harvesting energy from the body and its environment to power the system. In particular, solar energy and kinetic energy originating from body movement are important sources the wearable system may rely upon. In addition to placing active electronics below the antenna patch, we now also integrate energy harvesters directly on top of the wearable antenna module [1]. In Fig. 3 we present an aperture-coupled shorted wearable solar patch antenna for communication in the 902–928 MHz UHF band.

4   MIMO Techniques for Wearable Systems

In indoor environments, wireless communication systems suffer from multipath fading, which significantly reduces the reliability of the data link. In case of wearable SFIT units, their deployment in the direct neighborhood of the human body results in important additional shadowing effects. To overcome shadowing and fading, typically higher transmit powers are required to achieve acceptable Bit Error Rates (BERs), which seriously reduces the autonomy of the wearable system. However, by making use of a garment as a platform for the integration of multiple wearable transmit/receive units and by relying on MIMO diversity schemes [8], highly reliable links may be implemented using low transmit power. Fig. 3 demonstrates the improvement in terms of BER for different MIMO schemes that were implemented using a wearable system consisting of two dual-polarized textile antennas integrated in a professional garment. The link quality was studied for a person walking around in an indoor office environment in non-line-of-sight conditions. It is, however, important to approach BER results based on measured instantaneous signal levels like the ones obtained in Fig. 3 with care. In reality, the BER for the real data demodulation suffers from imperfect channel estimation in case of low signal levels. In case of erroneous channel estimation, the space-time codes will not offer the full diversity gain expected from theory. A transmission of 100 frames with channel estimation by 300 BPSK pilot symbols at an average SNR of 10dB resulted in a BER at the receiver of 1.7e-2 for a 4×1, 8e-3 for a 4×2 and 1.7e-3 for a 4×4 link. Clearly, the measured improvements in wireless link quality are found to be much lower than expected from theory. It was found that, by just increasing the average SNR from 10dB to 12dB, for the set of 100 transmitted frames the number of bit errors dropped to zero for the 4×4 communication link.

5   Energy-Efficient Multi-antenna Processing Techniques

Although space-time coding (STC) via multiple antenna offers large potential benefits in terms of link quality, it comes at a cost in terms of required processing power to manipulate the codes and to perform accurate channel estimates. Therefore, we have investigated an alternative approach where simple static beamforming is performed using a four-element textile antenna array that transmits a beam confined in the vertical direction [7], resulting in a larger received signal level and reducing the number of received multipath components. This in turn decreases the fluctuations in received signal level. In Fig. 4 we compare space-time coding and static beam forming in non-line-of-sight conditions in an indoor environment. Moreover, BER versus SNR curves are presented for two receiver configurations: a single-antenna receiver without diversity versus a four-antenna receiver implementing maximum ratio combining (MRC). The curves were normalized to include TX array gain, which corresponds to ensuring an equal total transmitted energy per information bit $E_{b,tr}$ at the transmitter. In absence of receiver diversity, the space-time code clearly outperforms beamforming

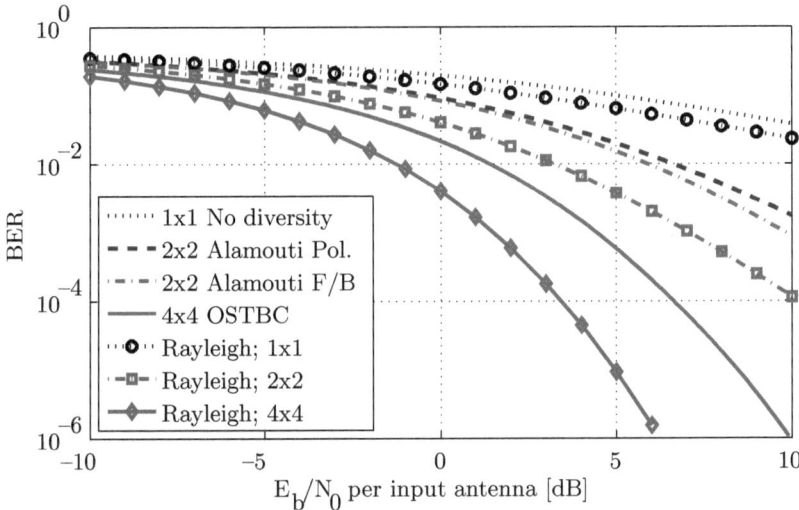

Fig. 3. Bit Error Rate versus Signal to Noise Ratio for various orders of MIMO systems implementing front/back (F/B) and/or polarization (Pol.) diversity by means of Orthogonal Space-Time Block Codes (OSTBCs). The curves derived from measured instantaneous signal levels for a person walking in an indoor environment are compared to the theoretically achievable gains in case of ideal Rayleigh fading.

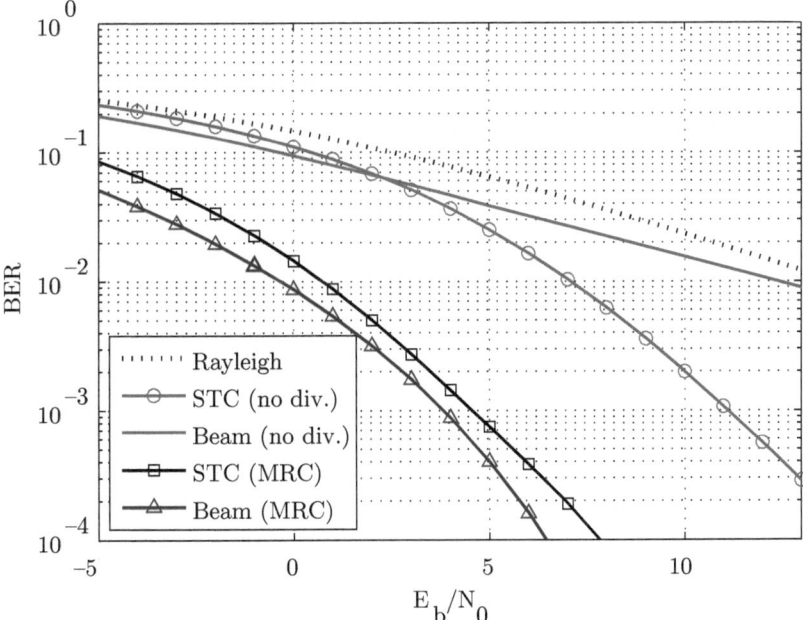

Fig. 4. Bit Error Rate versus Signal to Noise Ratio: comparison between Space-Time Coding (STC) and beam forming (Beam) with 4th order receive diversity (MRC combining) and in absence of diversity

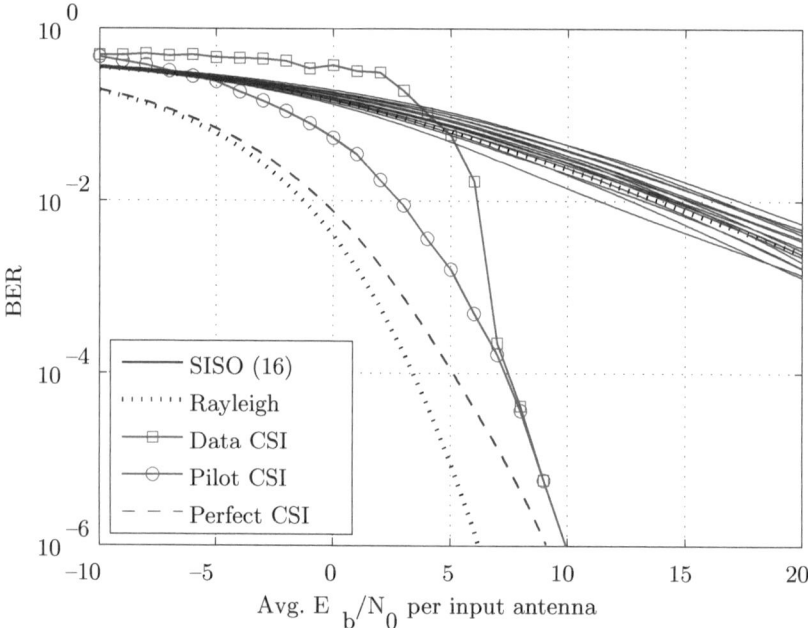

Fig. 5. Bit Error Rate versus Signal to Noise Ratio for the 4×4 MIMO channel: comparison between perfect channel knowledge, estimation based on pilot symbols and data driven channel tracking

as for the higher E_b/N_0 values, the transmit diversity gain rapidly exceeds the beamforming power gain. In case of receiver diversity, however, the beamforming BER is lower than the BER for space-time coding over the full range we considered.

If we prefer the benefits of additional diversity gain offered by the space-time codes, we need to implement techniques that alleviate the additional processing cost. One approach consists of reducing the overhead in terms of pilot symbols that are needed to make accurate channel estimates at the receiver. This is done by implementing data driven channel tracking [9], where we use the detected data symbols as substitutes for the pilot symbols to keep track in time of the correct channel state. Fig. 5 compares the performance in terms of BER of a 4x4 MIMO system that has perfect channel knowledge at the receiver with an implementation that makes abundant use of pilot symbols for channel estimation (300 pilot symbols transmitted in separate time-slots for each transmit channel in addition to 528 symbols of space-time coded data per frame) and a link for which data driven channel tracking is implemented at the receiver. We observe that, once the BER drops below 2e-4, the STBC-MIMO system with channel tracking offers a performance similar to that of the MIMO system using large amounts of pilot symbols for channel estimation.

6   Conclusion

It was shown that garments of patients and caregivers may be used as platforms to deploy wearable multi-antenna systems that sense the wearer and his/her surroundings. Direct integration of active electronics and energy scavengers onto the active textile antennas lead to compact and energy-efficient modules that are light-weight and comfortable to wear.

References

[1] Declercq, F., Georgiadis, A., Rogier, H.: Wearable Aperture-Coupled Shorted Solar-Patch Antenna for Remote Tracking and Monitoring Applications. In: Fifth European Conference on Antennas and Propagation - EuCAP 2011, Rome, Italy, pp. 2992–2996 (April 2011)

[2] Declercq, F., Rogier, H.: Active Integrated Wearable Textile Antenna With Optimized Noise Characteristics. IEEE Trans. on Antennas and Propagation 58(9), 3050–3054 (2010)

[3] Hertleer, C., Rogier, H., Vallozzi, L., Van Langenhove, L.: A textile antenna for off-body communication integrated into protective clothing for firefighters. IEEE Trans. on Antennas and Propagation 57(4), 919–925 (2009)

[4] Locher, I., Klemm, M., Kirstein, T., Troster, G.: Design and characterization of purely textile patch antennas. IEEE Transactions on Advanced Packaging 29(4), 777–788 (2006)

[5] Salonen, P., Rahmat-Samii, Y.: Textile antennas: Effects of antenna bending on input matching and impedance bandwidth. IEEE Aerospace and Electronic Systems Magazine 22(12), 18–22 (2007)

[6] Tronquo, A., Rogier, H., Hertleer, C., Van Langenhove, L.: Robust planar textile antenna for wireless body LANs operating in 2. 45 GHz ISM band. IEE Electronic Letters 42(3), 142–146 (2006)

[7] Van Torre, P., Scarpello, M.L., Vallozzi, L., Rogier, H., Moeneclaey, M., Vande Ginste, D., Verhaevert, J.: Indoor Off-Body Wireless Communication: Static Beamforming versus Space-Time Coding. Intern. Journal of Antennas and Propagation, Article ID 413683 (2012)

[8] Van Torre, P., Vallozzi, L., Hertleer, C., Rogier, H., Moeneclaey, M., Verhaevert, J.: Indoor Off-Body Wireless MIMO Communication With Dual Polarized Textile Antennas. IEEE Trans. on Antennas and Propagation 59(2), 631–642 (2011)

[9] Van Torre, P., Vallozzi, L., Rogier, H., Moeneclaey, M., Verhaevert, J.: Channel Characterization and Robust Tracking for Diversity Reception over Time-Variant Off-Body Wireless Communication Channels. EURASIP Journ. on Advances in Signal Processing, Article ID 978085 (2010)

An Antenna for Footwear

Max J. Ammann[1], Patrick McEvoy[1], Domenico Gaetano[1],
Louise Keating [2], and Frances Horgan [2]

[1] Antenna and High Frequency Research Centre
Dublin Institute of Technology
Kevin Street, Dublin 8, Ireland
Max.Ammann@dit.com
[2] School of Physiotherapy
Royal College of Surgeons in Ireland
St Stephen's Green, Dublin 2, Ireland

Abstract. Antenna design for footwear is an essential part of enabling reliable wireless links with lower-limb sensors used in body centric networks. Sensors can report biomechanical pressure data to analyse kinematic and posture parameters for a range of medical and sporting applications. Consideration is given to antenna shapes, the fit with shoe shapes, the positioning on the shoe and the radiation patterns suited to on body and off-body communications.

Keywords: Biomedical telemetry, body sensor networks, footwear industry, ultra wideband antennas.

1   Introduction

Intelligent footwear technologies that will report sensor information through radio links require suitable antennas to overcome adverse propagation influences near to ground level, variable tuning in close proximity to the human body and to ensure compatibility with various fabrics subject to scuffing, flexing and changing moisture conditions. Opportunities in various applications will present slightly differing antenna requirements but any approaches should take account of user influences on the designs and should avoid interfering with the user's typical stride or posture.

Around one in three older people fall each year [1] often with serious consequences including an increased likelihood of nursing home admission [2]. Every year, 10% of all older people need medical treatment following an injury and falls cause 75% of these injuries. Almost 7,000 older people were admitted to Irish hospitals with a fall in 2001 (ESRI 2001). Some recent Irish data profiled falls in an acute hospital over a one year period (Cotter et al 2006). There were 810 fall-related admissions, resulting in 8,300 acute bed days, and 6,220 rehabilitation bed days, costing €10.3 million. Fall-related readmissions resulted in 650 bed-days, bringing the total cost to €10.8 million. A typical hip fracture incident admission episode costs €14,300. The Royal College Surgeons in Ireland have shown that in frail older women, wearing their own footwear significantly improved balance compared to being barefoot with the greatest

B. Godara and K.S. Nikita (Eds.): MobiHealth 2012, LNICST 61, pp. 326–331, 2013.

benefit being seen in those with the poorest balance [3]. The cause of this benefit is unclear though it may be that patients with poorer balance have deficits in foot and ankle architecture that are compensated for by footwear. Understanding the features of footwear that benefit balance in at-risk elderly individuals could lead to practical and inexpensive ways of preventing falls. In order to advance this field of research, collaboration between clinicians and engineering professionals is essential.

Future communications using miniaturised radios will enable many aspects of body-centric sensors for medical, occupational and leisure applications. Published research on wireless systems is dominated by upper-body scenarios [4]-[8] and there are many opportunities associated with extending the technology downwards to footwear. Wirelessly connected pressure sensors would dramatically enhance the clinical analysis of dynamic activities, such as gait or running in patient and sporting groups. For example, older people at risk of falls could be monitored at home or in the wider community, with a truly wireless, mobile system. This would enable detailed analysis without encumbering elderly people with wires or significantly distracting them with large devise.

Linked with other compatible technologies, they could also be the basis of new sporting performance analysis and gaming applications. For example, increased participation in endurance type activities such as marathon running, have been associated with a shift in musculoskeletal injury patterns from acute (sprains, strains, contusions, etc.) to overuse injury types. Biomechanical factors are thought to have a role in the development of these types of injuries. Antenna functionality in this particularly adverse environment for radiowave propagation has been substantially published. An appropriate balance of several competing antenna parameters will be a key requirement for communications given the adverse propagation conditions in which the devices will be expected function reliably.

Electrically small antennas radiate as a function of their close proximity surroundings. Design and performance considerations should include, inter alia, the different materials and shapes of footwear, the movement of the subject and the characteristic propagation environment. Selection of antenna positions on footwear relate to how the sensors are integrated, the resilience to material flexing and the line-of-sight visibility to the upper body or to off-body data stations. The close and varying proximity of the antenna to the ground surface beneath a foot is expected to present conditions of propagation fading. Ultra wideband (UWB) offers a suitable propagation range for body area networks and the spectrum bandwidth can offset the impact of fading loss.

2   Methodology

Computer based simulations and anechoic chamber measurements were used to evaluate how antennas would perform on the footwear. Antenna types were selected based on suitable radiation patterns at various positions on the footwear. Predictive simulations using CST Microwave Studio on a 2.40 GHz quad-core processor PC with 12 Gbytes of memory allowed researchers to evaluate performance stability. Two NVIDIA® Tesla C1026 accelerator cards were used to reduce the experimental time to around 9 hours of computational time.

A lower limb and shoe model was developed in tandem with a phantom model for measurements. The geometric features and dielectric properties were derived from the sample shoe and the homogeneous foot phantom which was constructed for the experiment.

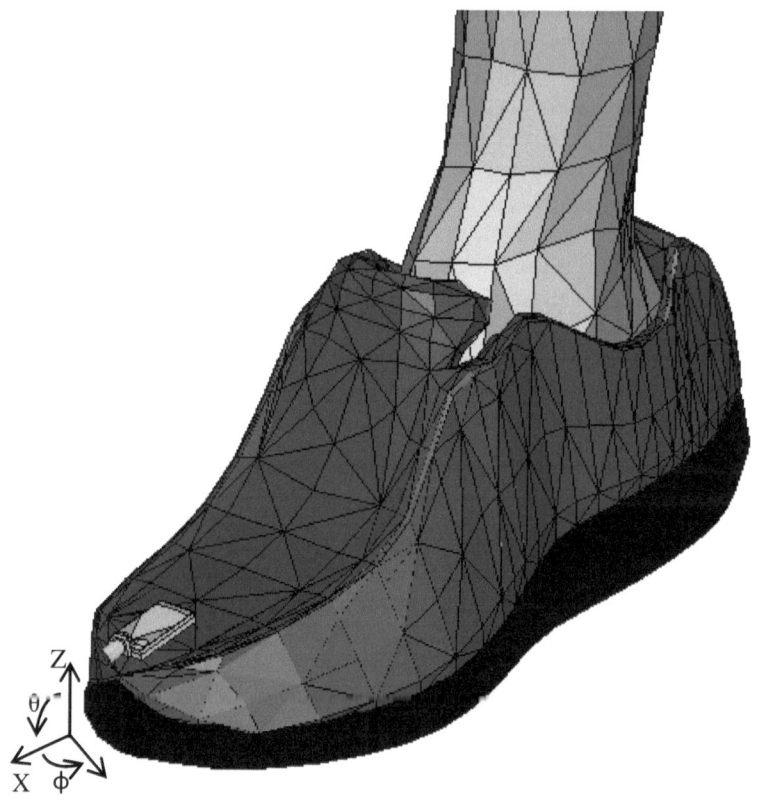

Fig. 1. CST model of foot-phantom and shoe with antenna on toe area

3   Monopole Antenna Design

A monopole antenna, in Fig. 2 comprises single-sided FR-4 dielectric with 0.2 mm thickness with an SMA feed connector. The parameters dimensions were refined for the footwear using a multi-objective algorithm to enhance a quasi-omnidirectional pattern in the 6 - 8.5 GHz band. The overall dimensions were limited $W = 15.7$ mm, $L = 25.63$ mm to minimize the overlay area on the shoe. The optimised parameters are $W_f = 1$ mm, $S_f = 0.56$ mm, $L_g = 2.4$ mm, $H_g = 3.6$ mm, $L_{a1} = 6.17$ mm, $L_{a2} = 2.96$ mm, $L_{a3} = 2$ mm, $D = 1.47$ mm, $D_g = 3.2$ mm. The CPW groundplane profile was refined to manage the surface currents that would otherwise impact the radiation patterns at upper frequencies.

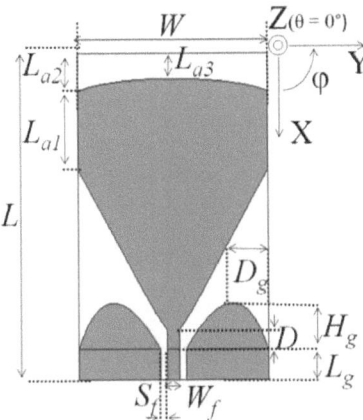

Fig. 2. Monopole Antenna

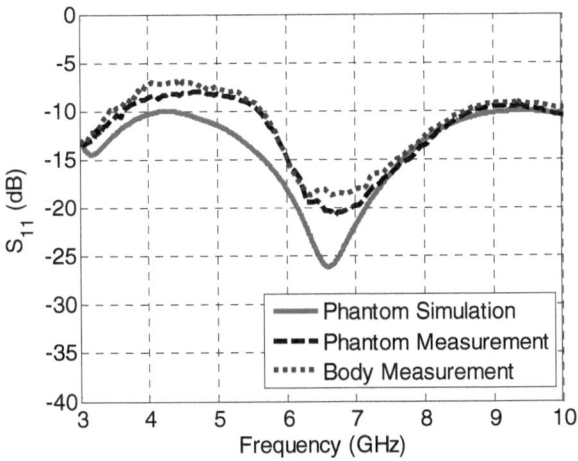

Fig. 3. S11 comparison for the material loaded monopole antenna

Fig. 3 shows the S_{11} achieved -10 dB match across 6 - 8.5 GHz for simulation and measurement. Comparing simulated and measured materially-loaded radiation patterns shown in Fig. 4 for the 7.5 GHz frequency indicates that the design produced a quasi-omnidirectional pattern in the $\varphi = 0°$ plane. Considering the 6 - 8.5 GHz bandwidth, the mean value of the simulated realized gain in the $\varphi = 90°$ plane $(-180° < \theta < 180°)$ is greater than 1 dBi. Discrepancies in the patterns are attributed to interaction of surface currents on the measurement cable with the small ground plane.

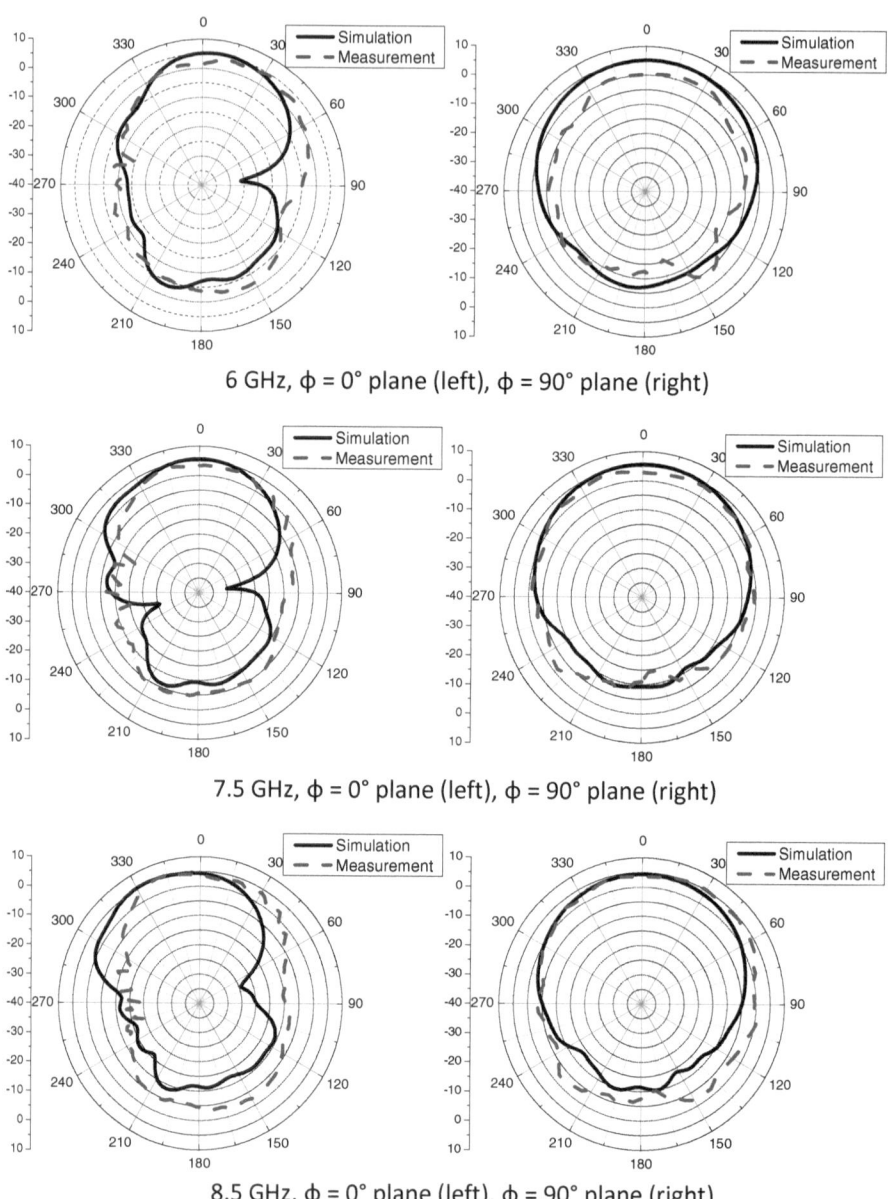

Fig. 4. Realized gain patterns (dBi) for the materially-loaded monopole antenna

The omni-directional characteristic that is characteristically exhibited in free-space changes predominantly in the back-lobe due to the presence of the shoe and the human body. While there is an approximate 3 dB reduction in the frequency-averaged realized gain in the $-180° < \theta < 180°$ plane respect to the empty shoe case, in the $90° < \theta < 90°$ the average simulated realized gain is greater than 1 dB for all the UWB frequencies.

4   Conclusion

Robust antenna performance designs are essential for sensors within wireless body area networks. Footwear mounted systems will enable real-time reporting of biomechanical parameters from ground level for sporting and medical purposes. Such short range on-body and off-body radio links can enable high-speed analysis of gait, stride and kinetic function, in addition to environmental sensing for occupational purposes.

The antenna design reported here is for the UWB 6 – 8.5 GHz frequencies on the toe area of a sports shoe. The design incorporates the influence of the footwear material properties and dielectric loading of a homogenous foot-shaped phantom. The simulation and measurement results indicate that a monopole antenna solution can provide stable performances in the UWB frequencies.

References

1. Tinetti, M.E., Williams, C.S.: Falls, injuries due to falls, and the risk of admission to a nursing home. N. Engl. J. Med. 337(18), 1279–1284 (1997)
2. Menz, H.B., Morris, M.E., Lord, S.R.: Footwear characteristics and risk of indoor and outdoor falls in older people. Gerontology 52(3), 174–180 (2006)
3. Cotter, P.E., Timmons, S., O'Connor, M., Twomey, C., O'Mahony, D.: The financial implications of falls in older people for an acute hospital. Ir. J. Med. Sci. 175(2), 11–13 (2006), PMID: 16872021 [PubMed - indexed for MEDLINE]
4. Conway, G.A., Scanlon, W.G.: Low-Profile Patch Antennas for Over-Body-Surface Communication at 2.45 GHz. In: International Workshop on Antenna Technology: Small and Smart Antennas Metamaterials and Applications, IWAT 2007 (2007)
5. See, T.S., Chen, Z.N.: Experimental Characterization of UWB Antennas for On-Body Communications. IEEE Transactions on Antennas and Propag. 57, 866–874
6. Alomainy, A., Sani, A., Rahman, A., Santas, J.G., Hao, Y.: Transient Characteristics of Wearable Antennas and Radio Propagation Channels for Ultrawideband Body-Centric Wireless Communications. IEEE Transactions on Antennas and Propagation 57, 875–884 (2009)
7. Chahat, N., Zhadobov, M., Sauleau, R., Ito, K.: A Compact UWB Antenna for On-Body Applications. IEEE Transactions on Antennas and Propagation 59, 1123–1131 (2011)
8. Duan, Z., Linton, D., Scanlon, W., Conway, G.: Improving wearable slot antenna performance with EBG structures. In: Antennas and Propag. Conference, LAPC 2008, Loughborough (2008)

RF Sensor for Non-invasive Cardiopulmonary Monitoring

Andrea Serra[1], Ruggero Reggiannini[1], Riccardo Massini[2], and Paolo Nepa[1]

[1] Dept. of Information Engineering, University of Pisa,
Via G. Caruso 16, 56122, Pisa, Italy
{andrea.serra,r.reggiannini,p.nepa}@iet.unipi.it
[2] CUBIT scarl
Via Giuntini 13, 56023 - Navacchio di Cascina, Pisa, Italy
riccardo.massini@cubitlab.com

Abstract. Cardiopulmonary information can be extracted from the temporal variations of the input reflection coefficient of a single wearable antenna placed in close proximity of the human thorax. In a previous paper, the authors have shown the potentials of such non-invasive measurement technique through experimental results; as a proof of concept, phase samples were collected by using a Vector Network Analyzer, and conventional non-linear filtering techniques were used to isolate the spectral components related to heartbeat and respiration rate. To get more realistic measurement data, a first prototype of a low-cost RF sensor has been implemented, and improved algorithms have been developed to estimate both heartbeat and breathing rate. Preliminary measurement results are shown to validate the approach, and the effects of the human body movements are discussed.

Keywords: beat rate measurements, non-invasive cardiopulmonary RF sensor.

1 Introduction

Microwave Doppler radars have been suggested as non-contact devices for non-invasive vital signs sensing since 1970s [1]-[4]. The quasi-periodic chest movements induced by the cardiopulmonary activity determine a phase modulation of an electro-magnetic wave reflected by (or transmitted through) the human thorax; then through optimized signal processing techniques applied to the demodulated signal, heartbeat and breathing rates, as well as heart rate variability, can be extracted.

A novel non-invasive RF measurement approach has been proposed in [5]-[6] for non-contact measuring of both heartbeat and breathing rate, which makes use of a single wearable antenna close to the body surface. Basically, it has been demonstrated that quasi-periodic movements induced by the cardiopulmonary activities affect the input impedance of the antenna, when the human thorax occupies most of the antenna near field region. To validate the methodology, a preliminary measurement campaign using a Vector Network Analyzer (VNA) was set up; measurements were taken at different frequencies in the UHF band, during regular breathing activity. The col-

B. Godara and K.S. Nikita (Eds.): MobiHealth 2012, LNICST 61, pp. 332–340, 2013.
© Institute for Computer Sciences, Social Informatics and Telecommunications Engineering 2013

lected signal (namely samples of the phase of the antenna reflection coefficient recorded in a temporal interval of some tens of seconds) was analyzed in the frequency domain in order to extract the desired spectral components. The respiration information was clearly and promptly detectable as breathing variations affect appreciably the collected signal, while the heartbeat frequency component was not so perceptible. Therefore a deeper analysis was necessary to isolate the heartbeat-induced spectral component; as a first attempt, two conventional non-linear filtering techniques have been checked. Although the proposed method employs an RF transmitting antenna, the authors believe that the physical principle used to achieve vital signs sensing is different from the Doppler effect [1]-[4]. The effectiveness of this novel approach has been confirmed by recent results in [7]-[10].

In this context, the primary goal of this paper is to demonstrate the feasibility of a simple low-cost hardware solution for the RF sensor based on the approach outlined in [5]-[6], for detection and monitoring of both heartbeat and respiration rate. As far as signal processing is concerned, the main enhancement proposed here with respect to the technique in [5]-[6] is the application of a recursive minimum mean square error (Kalman) tracker for estimation of the signal low-frequency (pulmonary) component. It is shown that this technique permits a more reliable extraction and elaboration of the weaker cardiac spectral component.

2   Measurement Set-Up and Phase-Detector Implementation

This section describes the device used for the acquisition of the samples of the reflection coefficient phase of an antenna in close proximity of the human thorax. In the proposed method the antenna must be located as close as possible to the human body (a direct contact is not required, and the antenna can operate through clothing), while Doppler radar prototypes have been always tested with the antenna at a distance of around 0.5-1m from the body. The RF sensor has been designed and built at CUBIT laboratories (Consortium UBIquitous Technologies, Pisa, Italy). Basically, the device is a reflectometer that measures the magnitude ratio and phase difference of signals that are incident on and reflected from a load (in this case the load is represented by the antenna placed in the chest proximity). The analog voltage outputs, representing the two above quantities, are sampled and stored with a sample rate less than 100 Hz (high enough, however, in view of the speed of typical person movements). Processing of the collected data allows to measure the time-varying phase of the antenna reflection coefficient, from which it is possible to extract information about the heartbeat and respiratory rates. Since above phase variations are of the order of tenths of a degree, the measurement device must be capable to detect variations at least one order of magnitude lower. Fig. 1 shows the block diagram of the device that has been prototyped. Preliminary measurements in different frequency bands (400 MHz, 800 MHz, 1500 MHz) showed that lower frequencies can provide larger phase variations (i.e., a higher system sensitivity) [6]; this is in contrast with Doppler-based sensor technology where instead high frequencies are preferred. The realized prototype operates in the ISM band at 433 MHz. Fig. 2 shows a photo of the device. The device uses an oscillator with an output level of about 6 dBm, which feeds the antenna. A pair of directional couplers test the incident and reflected signals and send them to the inputs of a Gain and Phase Detector (GPD), which produces two analog voltages proportional to the magnitude ratio and phase difference of the incident and reflected signals.

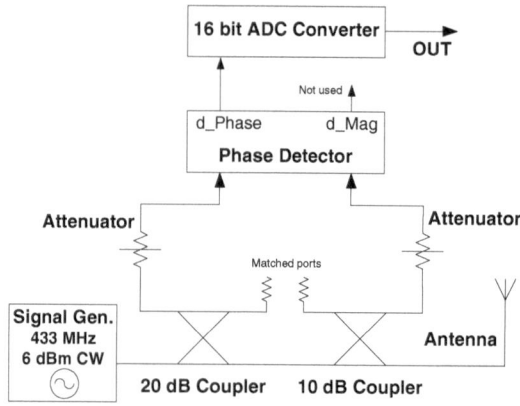

Fig. 1. Block diagram of the device used to get samples of the phase of the reflection coefficient of a wearable antenna

The estimated amplitude of the reflection coefficient is less than -10 dB since the antenna is matched at the working frequency; to approximately balance the level of the two signals at the GPD input, the two directional couplers have different coupling coefficients (20 dB for the incident signal and only 10 dB for the reflected one). Furthermore, the two attenuators set the signal levels around the middle of the GPD dynamic range.

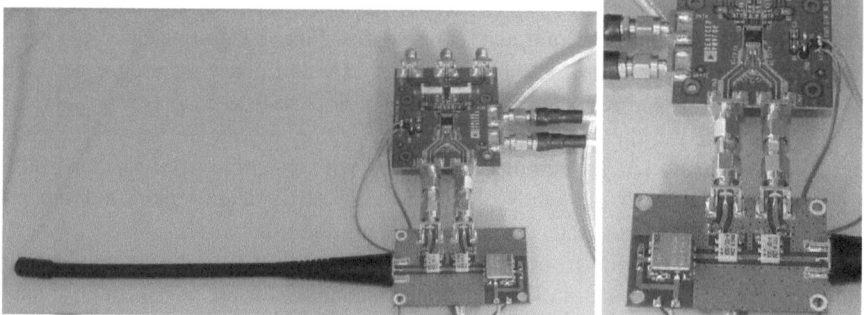

Fig. 2. The RF sensor prototype: the signal generator and the two directional couplers are clearly visible within the PCB (4cmx6cm) at the bottom side of both photos. The Gain and Phase Detector (GPD) based on the AD8302 log detector from Analog Devices is at the top side of the photos.

The GPD is based on the AD8302 log detector from Analog Devices, which produces output voltages in the range 0-1.8 V, with a slope of 10mV/deg. Since it is required to resolve a hundredth of degree of phase change, a voltage resolution of at least one tenth of mV is needed, which can be obtained by a 16-bit A/D converter with +/-2V input range. To increase the signal-to-noise ratio, the output signal is low-pass filtered. Since in this application only the phase variations must be monitored, it is not necessary to perform a calibration usually required to exclude a measurement setup bias. The only care to be taken is to avoid having a starting value of the phase difference in the proximity of 0 ° or 180 ° values, where the phase detector exhibits a dead zone. It is worth noting that a standard monopole has been used as an antenna. This is possible since the performance of the proposed method does not depend significantly by the antenna shape and technology [6]. This means that an ordinary wearable antenna can be used (in a practical implementation, this latter could be the antenna of a communication device already worn by the user!).

3   Algorithm Description and Performance Analysis

As mentioned earlier, the adoption of a low-cost wearable sensor prompted us to seek and test powerful algorithms capable of a more accurate separation of the pulmonary and cardiac components of the input signal, as compared to those utilized in the previous related literature [6]. Specifically, here we focus on recursive minimum mean square error (MMSE) estimation, or Kalman filtering, for accurate extraction of the signal components slower than the cardiac waveform. The idea behind this approach is similar to that already pursued in [6], i.e., we first try to get as accurate an estimate as possible of the slower-than-cardiac signal fluctuations (dominated by the pulmonary track) and then, as a next step, we proceed removing the cited slow components from the observed data so as to improve the visibility of the (tiny) cardiac waveform over the remaining disturbance, represented by low-frequency residual components, wideband noise and interference. We show that the above MMSE-track-and-subtract approach permits to significantly improve the detectability of the cardiac waveform over previously proposed techniques, such as those in [6].

The MMSE filter was implemented assuming the signal component to be tracked is generated by a linear stationary system described by two state variables, namely, the parameter to be tracked $x(t)$ and its derivative, governed by the same state equations as a simple one-dimensional mechanical system represented by a point mass of position $x(t)$ subject to a random acceleration. Using discrete-time representation with sample spacing T_s, the system inherent state evolution is assumed of the type

$$\mathbf{x}_k = \mathbf{F}\mathbf{x}_{k-1} + \mathbf{w}_k, \quad k = 1, 2, \cdots, N , \tag{1}$$

N being the observation length and $\mathbf{F} = \begin{bmatrix} 1 & T_s; 1 & 1 \end{bmatrix}$ the state transition matrix, while $\mathbf{w}_k$ indicates the vector noise process, generated assuming that the second derivative of $x(t)$ is zero-mean white Gaussian noise (WGN) with variance σ_p^2.

As for the observations, we assume the following linear time-invariant model:

$$\mathbf{z}_k = \mathbf{H}\mathbf{x}_k + \mathbf{v}_k, \quad k = 1, 2, \cdots, N , \tag{2}$$

where $\mathbf{H} = [1 \quad 0]$ and the single real-valued component $\mathbf{v}_k$ is the observation noise, modeled as zero-mean WGN with variance σ_n^2. We observe that parameters σ_n^2 and σ_p^2 have to be jointly calibrated on a trial-and-error basis so as to have the above models fit the level and quality of disturbance affecting the experimental data. The Kalman filter was implemented in Matlab$^{©}$ environment using a conventional formulation [11] and applied to experimental data blocks collected either in the presence or in the absence of respiratory activity as well as body motion of the cooperating subject. The results presented here are only relevant to the subject breathing normally, as the apnea condition was deemed to be unrealistic in an operating scenario. The sampling frequency used to collect the phase of the reflection coefficient is $f_s = 1/T_s = 50$ Hz. The data block size is around 10000 samples, corresponding to a length of 3-4 minutes. Prior to being fed to the Kalman filter, the arithmetic mean of the block is calculated and removed from the data set. Next, the sequence produced by the filter is subtracted from the input block, so as to attempt canceling the slowly-varying components from the input signal. The sequence emerging from the above cancellation procedure eventually undergoes spectral analysis aimed at revealing the most significant residual narrowband components. The analysis software allows to select the segment of time in the input data block to be processed. This can either coincide with the whole block length except for an initial interval (of arbitrary length) containing the filter transient response, or any fragment of the record whatever, presenting features of interest. Spectral analysis is carried out by estimating the signal power spectrum via the periodogram method. The block of experimental data to be analyzed is subdivided into segments ("windows") of equal length, then for each segment the squared modulus of the discrete Fourier transform (DFT) is calculated via the Fast Fourier transform (FFT) algorithm and finally the resulting sequences are averaged. This approach offers a twofold advantage: on one side, it permits to control the spectral analysis resolution, that for the application at hand does not need to be extremely narrow, but compatible with the bandwidth occupancy of the cardiac signal, that is nonzero because of the physiological fluctuations of the heartbeat period. Moreover, to relieve complexity it seems reasonable that the above resolution is chosen not to be far smaller than the maximum tolerable error in the measurement of the cardiac rate. Assuming that the latter is estimated by simply reading the position on the frequency axis of the bin where the periodogram peaks, it turns out that the maximum absolute estimation error is equal to half the spectral resolution. Collecting the above criteria, the resolution should be chosen so as to neither exceed twice the tolerable error in the cardiac rate, nor to be smaller than the cardiac rate instability. The curves presented in this section were produced using 512-point windows, corresponding to a frequency spacing between DFT samples of around 0.1 Hz, i.e. a maximum absolute frequency error of 0.05 Hz, or plus or minus three beats per minute. If this inherent uncertainty seems excessive, it can be considerably reduced by resorting to some form of interpolation on the DFT samples. However the above choice for the resolution allows to safely separate the cardiac from the respiratory components, since these are considerably spaced apart. The second advantage implicit in the above mentioned segmentation of the experimental data blocks stands in the possibility of averaging the partial spectral estimates originating from the single segments, thus obtaining a significant reduction of the fluctuations due to the random disturbance affecting the signal. Using 512-point windows and data block lengths in the order of 10,000 samples permits to average over some twenty spectral estimates, with a reduction of 4-5 times of the RMS disturbance. The figures presented below were obtained after a calibration of the parameters σ_p^2 and σ_n^2 involved in the dynamic models implicit in the Kalman tracker. A combination that proved to be nearly optimal for most of the available experimental data is $\sigma_p = 0.004 \div 0.006$ and $\sigma_n = 0.1 \div 0.2$. The actual selection for these parameters is specified in the figure captions below. In Figs. 3-4, we present numerical results for two blocks of data (identified as Block #i, i=1, 2), the first relevant to the cooperating subject standing still and normally breathing, the second with the addition of wide movements of both chest and arms in the first half of the record, followed by stillness in the second half. For each of the mentioned cases we present a

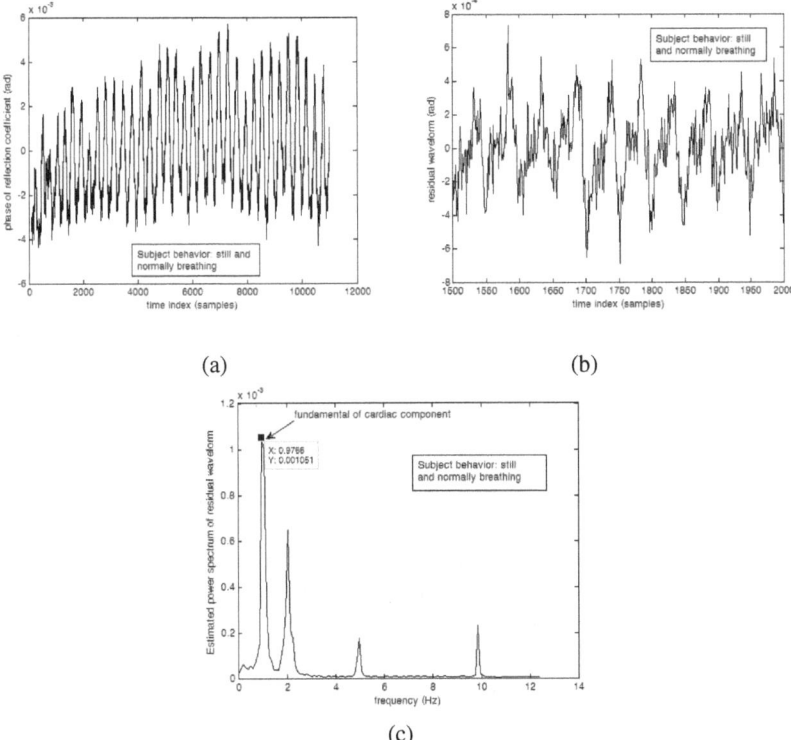

(a)   (b)

(c)

Fig. 3. Block #1: (a) diagram of the observed raw phase of the reflection coefficient; (b) diagram of the residual waveform (difference between the observed phase of the reflection coefficient and the output of the Kalman tracker); (c) Estimated power spectrum of residual waveform. $\sigma_p = 0.005$, $\sigma_n = 0.2$.

set of three figures: *a*) raw data vs. time for the whole block length, *b*) a fragment of the residual signal after cancellation of the slowly-varying component (i.e. the difference between the raw data and the Kalman filter output), *c*) finally, the averaged power spectrum estimate of the cited residual waveform. As for Block #2, a fourth figure is added (Fig. 4.d) showing the estimated spectrum of the residual signal in the second half of Block #2 where the subject is again still.

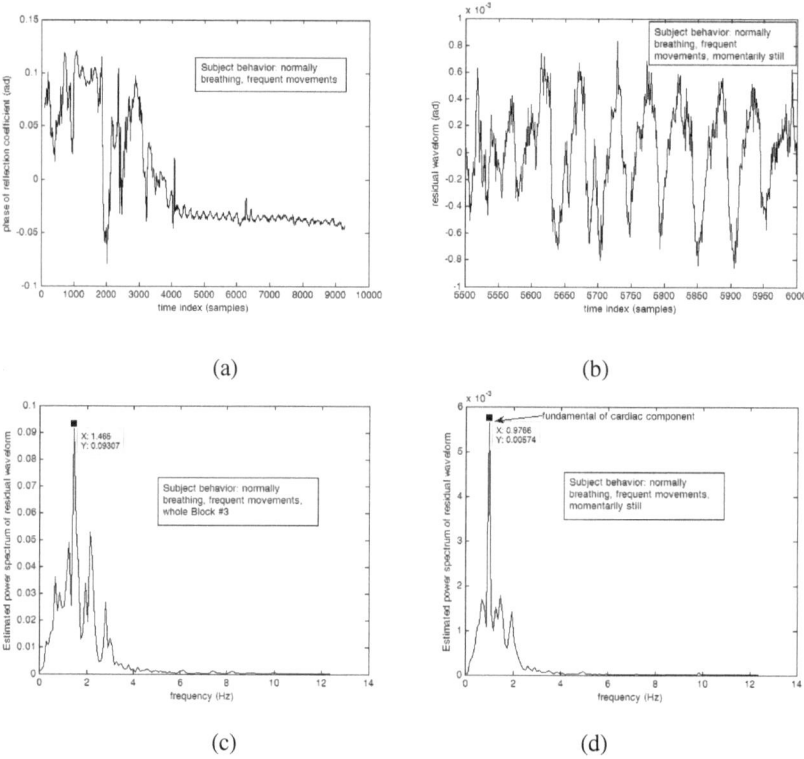

(a)   (b)

(c)   (d)

Fig. 4. Block #2: (a) diagram of the observed raw phase of the reflection coefficient (the impact of subject motion is visible in the first half of record); (b) diagram of the residual waveform in a segment where the subject is still; (c) estimated power spectrum of residual waveform (whole block); (d) estimated power spectrum of residual waveform starting from the sample with index 4300. $\sigma_p = 0.005$, $\sigma_n = 0.2$.

Inspection of the figures reveals that for Blocks #1 it is possible to neatly detect a narrowband spectral component centered on the cardiac rate, slightly less than 1 Hz (Figs. 3.c). Conversely, the same tone is not clearly visible in the spectrum obtained from the residual signal relative to the whole Block #2 (Fig. 4.c), while it pops up again if the elaboration is limited to the second part of the same record (Fig. 4.d). We also observe from Figs. 3.c and 4.d that the respiratory component is almost absent in the residual waveform, thus confirming the good accuracy in tracking and cancellation allowed by the Kalman filter. Other spectral components are visible in the figures, notably the one falling in the vicinity of 2 Hz, most likely the first harmonic of the cardiac signal, whereas the peaks around 5 Hz and 10 Hz could not be unequivocally ascribed to a specific source. As for the curve in Fig. 4.c, produced from the entire Block #2, it is worth observing that it exhibits a main spectral peak around 1.5 Hz, that is not correlated to the cardiac component, its position on the frequency axis being too high. This peak is presumably to be ascribed to the random fluctuations of the residual waveform and also to the possible presence of other pseudo-periodic signal components in the first part of the record, affected by movements of the cooperating subject. A possible criterion to distinguish between a situation of this type with respect to the one in which the peak is actually produced by the cardiac activity could be based on the calculation of the mean squared value of the residual signal: this in fact appears to be far larger (around two orders of magnitude for the data processed in the examples, see Figs. 4.c-d) when the cooperating subject makes movements leading to large errors in the Kalman tracker. This seems one of the topics worth investigating further, in the search of safe criteria for automatic recognition of the signal segments where the above procedure is more likely to be successful.

4   Conclusions

Non-invasive sensing of cardiopulmonary activity is feasible by deploying an RF antenna close to the human thorax. Encouraging preliminary results have been obtained by applying Kalman filtering techniques to real data acquired through a low-cost RF device. Work is in progress to get a smaller device through integrated circuit technology, which can be integrated in a commercial communication device or a radio beacon, such as those carried on by rescue operators and miners [12].

References

1. Lin, J.C., Kiernicki, J., Kiernicki, M., Wollschlaeger, P.B.: Microwave apexcardiography. IEEE Trans. Microwaves Theory and Techniques 27, 618–620 (1979)
2. Lin, J.C.: Microwave sensing of physiological movement and volume change: a review. Bioelectromagnetics 13, 567–575 (1992)
3. Obeid, D., Sadek, S., Zaharia, G., El Zein, G.: Multitunable microwave system for touchless heartbeat detection and heart rate variability extraction. Microwave and Optical Technology Letters 52(1), 192–198 (2010)
4. Obeid, D., Sadek, S., Zaharia, G., El Zein, G.: Microwave doppler radar for heartbeat detec-tion vs electrocardiogram. Microwave and Optical Tech. Lett. 54(11), 2610–2617 (2012)
5. Serra, A.A., Nepa, P., Manara, G.: On-body antenna input-impedance phase-modulation induced by breathing and heart activity. In: URSI Intern. Symposium. IEEE Press (2008)
6. Serra, A.A., Nepa, P., Manara, G., Corsini, G., Volakis, J.L.: A single on-body antenna as a sensor for cardiopulmonary monitoring. IEEE Antenna and Wireless Propagation Letters 9, 930–933 (2010)

7. Fletcher, R.R., Kulkarni, S.: Clip-on Wireless Wearable Microwave Sensor for Ambulatory Cardiac Monitoring. In: 32nd International Conference of the IEEE EMBS, pp. 365–369 (2010)
8. Gagarin, R., Celik, N., Youn, H.S., Iskander, M.F.: Microwave Stethoscope: a new method for measuring human vital signs. In: IEEE International Symposium on Antennas and Propagation, pp. 404–407. IEEE Press (2011)
9. Celik, N., Gagarin, R., Youn, H.S., Iskander, M.F.: A Noninvasive Microwave Sensor and Signal Processing Technique for Continuous Monitoring of Vital Signs. IEEE Antenna and Wireless Propagation Letters 9, 930–933 (2011)
10. Tariq, A., Ghafouri-Shiraz, H.: On-body antenna for vital signs and hearth rate vari-ability monitoring. In: 2011 Loughborough Antenna & Propagation Conference, pp. 1–4 (2011)
11. Wikipedia, http://en.wikipedia.org/wiki/Kalman_filter
12. Dubrovka, R.F., Shirokov, I.B.: On-body antenna for the miners cardiac rhythm sensor. In: Antennas & Propagation Conference, Loughborough, pp. 581–584 (2009)

Identifying Physiological Features from the Radio Propagation Signal of Low-Power Wireless Sensors

Max Munoz Torrico, Robert Foster, and Yang Hao

School of Electronic Engineering and Computer Science
Queen Mary, University of London
Mile End Road, London, E1 4NS, United Kingdom
{max.munoz,robert.foster,yang.hao}@eecs.qmul.ac.uk

Abstract. The radio propagation signal between a pair of low-power wireless sensor nodes is analysed with the aim to identify and retrieve embedded physiological features. The latter is post-processed using popular time-frequency analyses, such as such as the Fast Fourier transform (FFT). The results show initial evidence that the electromagnetic wave propagation contains bio-mechanical markers, such as gait pattern and thoracic displacements.

Keywords: physiological features, wireless sensors, low power, radio propagation, on-body communications, bio-mechanical markers.

1   Introduction

Compact and low-power devices interacting seamlessly through wireless connections are now integral parts of our daily lifestyle. The ubiquitous wireless connectivity between different devices has enabled the real-time transmission of sensed information (i.e., wireless pervasive sensing). Wirelessly connected miniaturized sensors and actuators placed in, on, and around the body define a Wireless Body Area Network (WBAN) [1, 2], which combines the continuous, automated, and unobtrusive monitoring of physiological signs to support medical, lifestyle and entertainment applications. The continuous monitoring of patients recovering from surgery, without constraining their normal recovery activities, in hospitals and home environments are active research topics.

It is evident that different areas of the body have unique characteristics; hence, the travelling electromagnetic wave behaves differently (e.g., absorption and exposure level). Additionally, external perturbations, such as human mobility and operation in cluttered environments, define a complex environment for the propagation characteristics of wearable devices [3, 4].

The interest in biomedical research is especially directed at continuous monitoring and quantification of physiological body signals, as well as at the development of personalized healthcare devices. Tele-monitoring and tele-diagnostics systems in smart home environments provide large amounts of health-related information from

B. Godara and K.S. Nikita (Eds.): MobiHealth 2012, LNICST 61, pp. 341–350, 2013.
© Institute for Computer Sciences, Social Informatics and Telecommunications Engineering 2013

strategically-placed body-worn sensors which sample, process, and transmit vital signs (e.g., heart-rate, blood pressure, skin temperature, pH, respiration, oxygen saturation).

Many studies have shown the potential of contactless sensors for the retrieval of physiological signals (e.g., breathing, heartbeat, gait pattern). Biomechanical features are embedded in the reflected waves which present shifts on frequency and phase when compared to the transmitted signal [5-8] (i.e., the Doppler Effect). The results presented in [8] indicate that heartbeat and respiration rates are clearly detectable at lower frequencies (i.e., 370 MHz) in the reflection coefficient of a single antenna. The physiological information was extracted using well-known non-linear filtering techniques. Other studies showed limb movement classification using the received signal values of multiple body-worn wireless modules. Different activities were recognized implementing supervised learning models such as support vector machine (SVM) and K-nearest neighbour (K-NN) methods [9]. The microwave sensors literature contains different contactless sensor prototypes. Different electromagnetic sources propagate within outdoor and indoor environments (e.g., Wi-Fi, GSM, GPS, Bluetooth, and ZigBee), to which human bodies are greatly exposed. Therefore, the radio propagation signal from each source could be used as a potential contactless sensing technology.

The current work investigates this possibility and the use of an alternative sensing method, by means of the received signal strength (RSS) of low-power wireless sensors operating in the 2.45 GHz ISM band. RSS is a commonly available parameter in commercially-available wireless transceivers, requiring no additional hardware. The received signal for a waist-to-chest channel is recorded in two different scenarios (i.e., motionless and jogging). The stored data is later extracted and characterized using well known time-frequency domain techniques, where the components of each signal is analysed and quantified at different scales.

The rest of the paper is organized as follows: Section 2 describes the in-house wireless sensors and the measurement procedure. In Section 3, the time domain signal acquired by the electrocardiograph is transformed to the frequency domain where main harmonic components are classified. Similar process is applied to the data recorded by wireless sensor nodes which is described in section 4. Additionally, the obtained results are compared with the spectral response of ECG signals. The conclusions are drawn in Section 5.

2   Measurement Procedure

The measurements were taken in Queen Mary's Human Performance Laboratory (i.e., indoor laboratory environment). The experimental research was carried out by a male subject of 168 cm height and 80 kg weight. The transmitter node (Tx node) was fixed on the right waist and the receiver node (Rx node) was fixed on the upper middle section of the thoracic wall (i.e., waist-to-chest channel). Fig. 1a shows Queen Mary's Human Performance Laboratory and Fig. 1b depicts the on-body locations for the on-body Rx and Tx nodes.

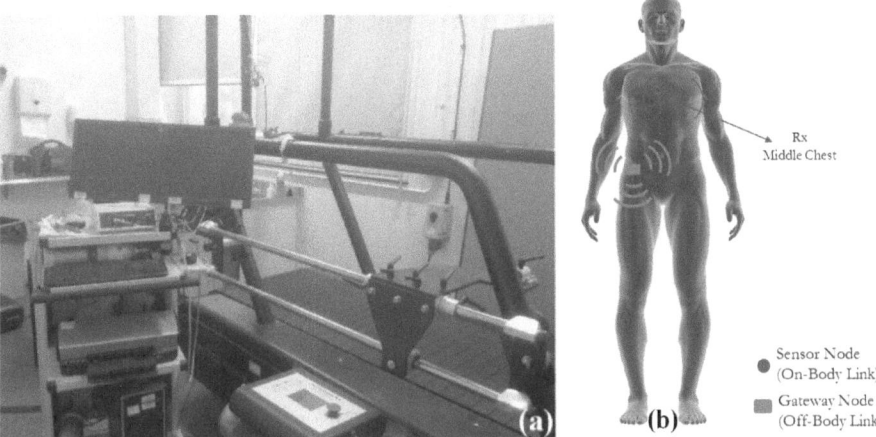

Fig. 1. Queen Mary's Human Performance Laboratory: (a) treadmill machine used for the experiments; (b) on-body location of custom-built wireless sensor nodes used for the radio propagation recording.

Each wireless sensor node is assembled using a Texas Instruments transceiver, the CC2420 [10], and an ultra-low power microcontroller, the PIC18F2620 [11]. The latter not only configures and controls the transceiver chip, but also records the radio propagation signal based on RSS characteristics in the internal flash memory. The acquired data was later extracted and analysed. The Tx and Rx nodes communicated using the IEEE 802.15.4 standard [12].

The radiating element of each wireless sensor node was a microstrip patch antenna printed on top of a FR-4 substrate material of 1.6 mm thickness. The simulated results of the microstrip patch antenna (i.e., 3D radiation pattern) and the custom-built wireless sensor node used for this study are shown in Fig. 2a and Fig. 2b, respectively. A summary of the performance of each antenna (i.e., Tx and Rx antennas) and additional information of the antenna design, radiation performance and the spectrum response of each low power wireless sensor can be found in [4, 13].

The acquisition of the data was taken in two different scenarios:

(a) Motionless test subject (i.e., standing on the treadmill machine),
(b) Jogging test subject at a constant speed of 5 km per hour (5km/h).

The jogging exercise was performed on a motorized treadmill machine equipped with a digital display and an electronic control console (see Fig. 1a). The tilt of the conveyor belt was set flat (no tilt), in order to simulate normal outdoor jogging.

In both scenarios, electrocardiogram (ECG) recordings were taken by a certified 12-Lead electrocardiograph, the Cardio Collect 12, with a sampling rate of 500 Hz. The ECG is a popular method to record the electrical impulses that the heart produces every time it beats. In this study, the ECG data provided additional information which helped with the data classification and interpretation.

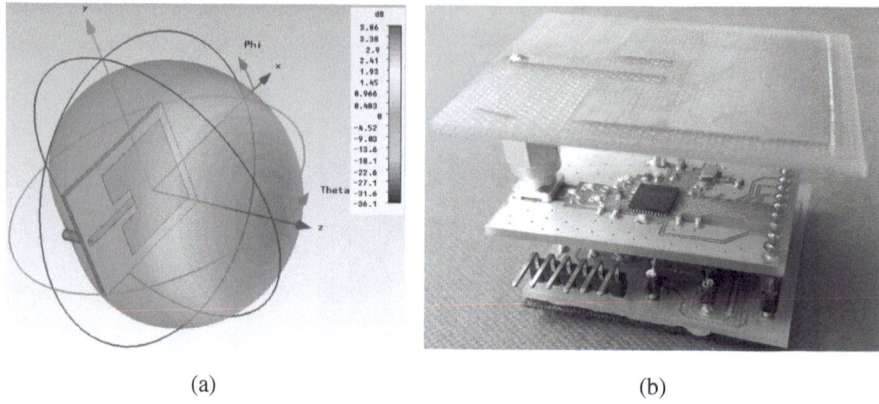

(a)   (b)

Fig. 2. Antenna used for on-body measurements: (a) simulated free-space radiation pattern for the microstrip patch antenna using CST Microwave Studio; (b) implemented wireless sensor node

VELCRO tape was fitted on each wireless sensor; thus, the location displacement due to the constant movement was significantly reduced. For each activity, the receiver node records an average of 6000 samples of the RSS at a rate of 14 ms per sample. For a jogging scenario, the receiver node started recording data only when the user had a constant speed. Both ECG recording and treadmill operation were controlled by a computer, thus avoiding synchronization errors.

3   Analysis of the Recorded Electrocardiogram Signals

The Cardio Collect ECG report gives average heart rates of 85 BPM and 108 BPM for a motionless and jogging activity, respectively. The ECG plots for each scenario are shown in Fig. 3a and Fig. 4a. The ECG recordings were extracted from the report for frequency analysis.

In order to recognize the main frequency components, a Fast Fourier Transform was applied to each recorded ECG signal. The time-sampled sequence, $x(n)$, is multiplied by a window function, $w(n)$, which limits the extent of the sequence and provides a more stationary spectral characteristic. The current study made use of a Hanning window. In our analysis, the length of the window $N = 4096$.

The resulting plots for a motionless and jogging activity are illustrated in Fig. 3b and Fig. 4b, respectively. The spectral plots identify main harmonics of 1.46 Hz for a motionless test subject (see Fig. 3b) and 1.77 Hz for a jogging test subject (see Fig. 4b).

A summary of the results is listed in Table 1. It is important to highlight that the transformation from time to frequency domain (the FFT process) has introduced a deviation of ≈3.4% from the average values given in the ECG report. The difference is mainly attributed to the truncation limits of the FFT summation, the FFT coefficient rounding errors and floating point arithmetic quantization errors. These results indicate the expected frequencies that should be observed based on thoracic wall movements for the two activities.

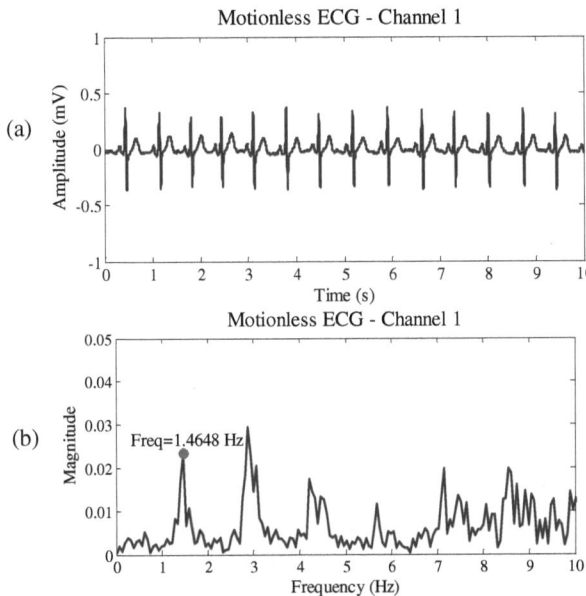

Fig. 3. Resulting plots while the test subject is standing on the treadmill machine (motionless scenario): (a) ECG signal acquired with the Cardio Collect 12. Average heartbeat is 85 BPM; (b) Spectral response of the recorded ECG signal.

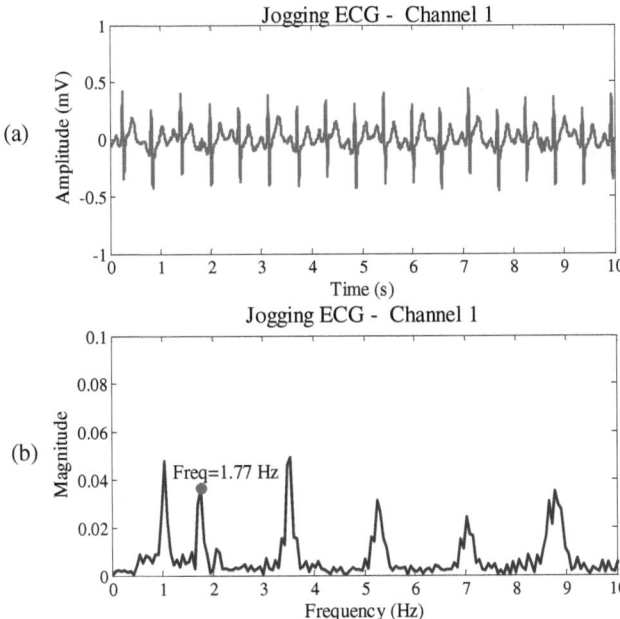

Fig. 4. Resulting plots while the test subject is jogging at a constant speed of 5 km/h (jogging scenario): (a) ECG signal acquired with the Cardio Collect 12. Average heartbeat is 108 BPM; (b) Spectral response of the recorded ECG signal.

Table 1. Comparison of estimated harmonics derived from ECG recordings acquired by the Cardio Collect 12, to the average heart rate provided by the Cardio Collect 12. Two different scenarios are considered: a motionless test subject and jogging at a constant speed of 5 km/h.

ECG Description	Average Heart Beat BPM	Spectral Harmonic Hz	Estimated Heart Beat BPM	Deviation %
Motionless	85	1.46	87.88	3.39
Jogging at 5 km/h	108	1.77	106.2	1.66

4   On-body Radio Propagation Analysis

It is evident that the practice of any sport activity will produce a high level of fluctuations on the received signal, which are the consequence of the continuous movement of the human body. In the case of jogging activity, our results show variations of ±15 dB from the average received signal; this is significantly greater than received signals of a motionless user, where the variations are ±3 dB. Fig. 5 depicts the received signal for both scenarios, jogging and motionless. The graph plots a 45 s window length of a waist-to-chest channel.

The data acquired by the on-body wireless sensors are rich in detail, but they are also highly non-stationary signals (i.e., frequencies, amplitudes and phases change with time). The transmitting node antenna radiates electromagnetic waves that propagate through both free space and human body. The main radiation beam of the

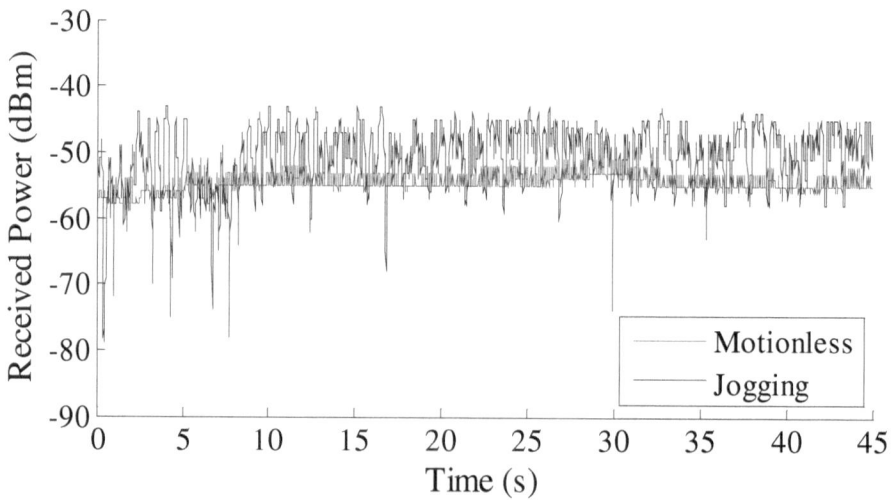

Fig. 5. Comparison of received signal, for a waist-to-chest channel, when the test subject is jogging and motionless in Queen Mary's Human Performance Laboratory

patch antenna is normal to the body; however, there are also electromagnetic waves travelling along the body's surface which are mainly triggered by the fringing fields and backscattering energy.

The spectral content for a motionless scenario (test subject standing on the treadmill machine) is shown in Fig. 6a. The latter takes into consideration the coherence gain factor (i.e., loss introduced due to the Hanning window). The search of the local maximum within expected frequencies (i.e., 1-2 Hz) shows 1.24 Hz as the local maximum. The small magnitude may indicate a sensitivity issue.

Fig. 6b plots the spectral components of the recorded RSS for a jogging scenario. Two main harmonics are clearly identified: the first at 0.9 Hz and the second at 1.79 Hz. It is known that human locomotion depends on two main factors, stride length and stride frequency, both of which contribute to a jogging activity [14].

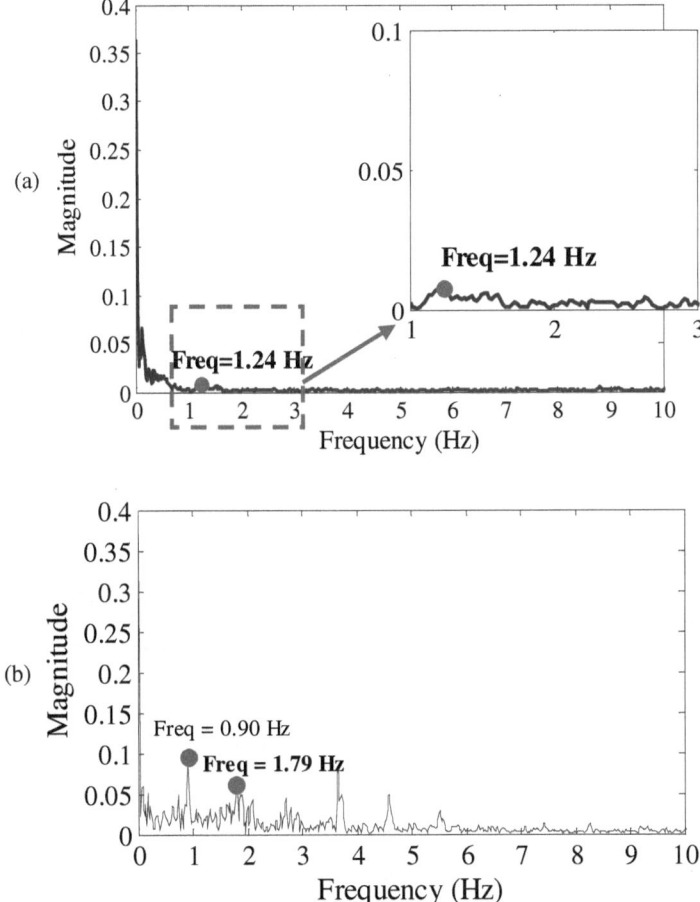

Fig. 6. Radio channel signal acquired by custom-built wireless sensor nodes: (a) spectral response while the subject is standing on the treadmill machine (i.e., motionless scenario), (b) spectral response of the received signal while jogging at a constant speed of 5 km/h.

The constant speed of 1.38 m/s (i.e., 5 km/h) and the average stride length of 1.5 m give rise to the first harmonic, 0.9 Hz. This is product of the periodic kinematic of the human body, which is mainly dominated by the head and the thoracic wall.

The second component is characterized by the quasi-synchronous movement of the arms and legs. The cyclic movement of the extremities, which is repeated during the entire jogging process, creates angular variations on the radiation of the patch antenna (i.e., normal to the body) and changes in the multipath propagation (i.e., multipath fading channel), and thus producing a harmonic at 1.79 Hz, almost twice that of the main frequency component. Although this harmonic is mainly dominated by small scale fading introduced by the upper extremities motion, it is also expected to embed the relative movement of the thoracic wall (due to the limbs movement), which not only contains comparative contributions of the limb motion, but also human breathing process and heart palpitation. The relative magnitudes of these aspects are much smaller than the fading observed due to motion. It may be that the coincidence of heart rate and motion harmonics can be avoided with different stride rates, allowing the thoracic wall movements to be detected; this is an objective of our future work.

The spectral content of the electrocardiogram maintains a high level of detail, unlike the spectral plot of the signal recorded by the wireless sensor nodes. This is likely the result of the sensing methods acquiring different aspects of the heart. The ECG mainly records electrical variation of the heart over a period of time across the electrodes, whereas the wireless nodes are affected by the mechanical movement of the heart over a period of time, thus recording the thoracic movement produced by each palpitation on the propagation of the electromagnetic wave.

Additionally, the spectral plot of a jogging scenario (see Fig. 6b) presents main harmonic components that can be classified as gait pattern descriptors of the test subject (i.e., human motion and limb movement). A summary of the obtained results is presented in Table 2. The results are compared with those obtained by the electrocardiograph.

The computed deviation of a resting scenario, shown in Table 1 and Table 2, is higher than of a jogging scenario. In both cases, the deviation is highly affected by three factors: (1) the heart rate variability (HRV) over a period of time (i.e., R-wave to R-wave interval fluctuations); (2) the angular variation of the radiating beam due to motion; and (3) the truncation limits of the FFT. For example, if the RR interval variance is 2000 ms^2, the acquired heartbeat data will fluctuate between 79.93 BPM and 90.74 BPM and the deviation would change accordingly (between 6.91% and 18%, respectively). Moreover, the radiating beam of the current antenna is normal to the body which makes it more sensitive to multipath fading. Future work will enclose wireless sensor nodes housing antennas that radiate tangentially to the human body thus the main propagation path is alongside the thoracic wall; therefore, changes produced by the respiration process and heartbeat are maximized. Although the initial results are only compared with ECG recordings, further studies will use a cardiopulmonary kit which can measure and monitor ECG and respiratory signals while synchronized to the treadmill machine. It will also consider different stride lengths in order to distinguish the harmonics from the human kinematics and those produced by the heartbeat and breathing process.

Table 2. Comparison of estimated harmonics derived from RSS recordings acquired by the custom-built wireless sensor nodes. Two different scenarios are considered: a motionless test subject and jogging test subject at a constant speed of 5 km/h.

Wireless sensor nodes	Average Heart Beat BPM	Spectral Harmonic Hz	Estimated Heart Beat BPM	Deviation %
Motionless	85	1.24	74.4	12.47
Jogging at 5 km/h	108	1.79	107.4	0.55

5   Conclusions and Future Work

The paper presented the radio-channel characterization of a particular on-body radio link (waist-to-chest channel). It was shown that the continuous movement of the human body, trunk and the limbs, for non-stationary scenarios (e.g., jogging exercise) produces cyclic changes in the multipath propagation, thus producing signal fluctuations of ±15 dB (maximum level from the average received signal).

Comparison of the on-body radio channel (which not only include radio propagation characteristics, but also embed biomechanical information, such as the gait pattern and thoracic wall movement) for a motionless and jogging activity showed noticeable differences in channel parameters. Moreover, the analysis of the signal spectra identified distinct frequency components for each recorded scenario. The analysis and quantification of the spectral components in the context of the activities and physiological signals provide a potential model for activity recognition and bio-mechanical feature extraction. The work proposed in this paper may open up a new possibility of non-invasive physiological monitoring based on EM sensing from on-body wireless sensor nodes.

References

1. Hall, P.S., Hao, Y.: Antennas and propagation for body-centric wireless communications. Artech House, Boston (2006)
2. Hao, Y., Foster, R.: Wireless body sensor networks for health-monitoring applications. Physiological Measurement 29, R27 (2008)
3. Gallo, M., Hall, P.S., Bozzetti, M.: Simulation And Measurement of Body Dynamics For On-Body Channel Characterisation. In: 2007 IET Seminar on Antennas and Propagation for Body-Centric Wireless Communications, pp. 71–74 (2007)
4. Munoz, M.O., Foster, R., Yang, H.: On-Body Channel Measurement Using Wireless Sensors. IEEE Transactions on Antennas and Propagation 60, 3397–3406 (2012)
5. Obeid, D., Issa, G., Sadek, S., Zaharia, G., El Zein, G.: Low power microwave systems for heartbeat rate detection at 2.4, 5.8, 10 and 16 GHz. In: First International Symposium on Applied Sciences on Biomedical and Communication Technologies, ISABEL 2008, pp. 1–5 (2008)

6. Lin, J.C., Kiernicki, J., Kiernicki, M., Wollschlaeger, P.B.: Microwave Apexcardiography. IEEE Transactions on Microwave Theory and Techniques 27, 618–620 (1979)
7. Lin, J.C.: Microwave sensing of physiological movement and volume change: a review. Bioelectromagnetics 13, 557–565 (1992)
8. Serra, A.A., Nepa, P., Manara, G., Corsini, G., Volakis, J.L.: A Single On-Body Antenna as a Sensor for Cardiopulmonary Monitoring. IEEE Antennas and Wireless Propagation Letters 9, 930–933 (2010)
9. Guraliuc, A.R., Barsocchi, P., Potortí, F., Nepa, P.: Limb Movements Classification Using Wearable Wireless Transceivers. IEEE Transactions on Information Technology in Biomedicine 15, 474–480 (2011)
10. Texas Instruments, 2.4 GHz IEEE 802.15.4 / ZigBee-ready RF Transceiver (2007), http://focus.ti.com/lit/ds/symlink/cc2420.pdf
11. Microchip, PIC18F2620 28-Pin Enhanced Flash Microcontrollers with 10-Bit A/D and NanoWatt Technology (2008), http://ww1.microchip.com/downloads/en/DeviceDoc/39626e.pdf
12. IEEE 802.15.4 Standard, Wireless Medium Access Control (MAC) and Physical Layer (PHY) Specifications for Low Rate Wireless Personal Area Networks, LR-WPANs (2006), http://standards.ieee.org/getieee802/download/802.15.4-2006.pdf
13. Munoz, M., Foster, R., Hao, Y.: On-body performance of wireless sensor nodes using IEEE 802.15.4. In: Proceedings of the 5th European Conference on Antennas and Propagation (EUCAP), pp. 3783–3786 (2011)
14. Maud, P.J., Foster, C.: Physiological assessment of human fitness. Human Kinetics Publishers (2006)

Cooperative and Low-Power Wireless Sensor Network for Efficient Body-Centric Communications in Healthcare Applications

Raffaele Di Bari, Akram Alomainy, and Yang Hao

Antennas and Electromagnetics Research Group
School of Electronic Engineering and Computer Science
Queen Mary, University of London
Mile End Road, London E1 4NS, UK
akram.alomainy@eecs.qmul.ac.uk

Abstract. Body Sensor Networks are an interesting emerging application to improve healthcare and the quality of life monitoring. In this paper, we compare the performances of multi-hop cooperative and single-hop networks with real-world sensor networks based on Zigbee technology. The network reliability, the data flow rate, the packet delivery ratio and the energy consumption are included as performances criteria. It is shown experimentally that the cooperative approach can provide a network more robust to link losses at the expenses of a lower bit rate and higher energy consumption. Specifically, for a packet delivery ratio >0.9, the cooperative scheme can provide the network with a link gain up to 14 dB traded off with an energy demand up to 30.7% higher and a data flow rate about 20% lower than a single-hop system. This work is a first exercise step in assessing reliability and life time trade-off with real-world platforms for body area sensor networks. Follow-up studies will address wireless ECG emulators with higher number of sensors (e.g. up to 10 for a typical 12-leads ECG system) employing ultra-low power chipsets in different specific health monitoring environments.

Keywords: Body-centric wireless communication, co-operative networks, energy efficiency, healthcare monitoring.

1 Introduction

Research on sensor network has been carried out using small, low-power digital radios based on an IEEE 802.15 standard [1], a high-level communication protocols suitable for WBANs [2-3]. The most straightforward approach to deploy a WBAN is considering single-hop (SH) communications between sensors and the sink. However, the body impact on the signal can result in severe path losses, even larger than 50dB [4]. Due to these high losses, direct communication between the sensors and the sink will not always be convenient (or even possible), especially when extended sensor lifetime is targeted deploying ultra-low range transceivers [5].

B. Godara and K.S. Nikita (Eds.): MobiHealth 2012, LNICST 61, pp. 351–360, 2013.
© Institute for Computer Sciences, Social Informatics and Telecommunications Engineering 2013

In a relay MH network, each sensor is dedicated to transmit or relay information packets, while in cooperative MH network each sensor can performs both operations. An example of MH WBAN benefits is introduced in [10], where spatial diversity gain is analyzed for a two-relay assisted transmission link, while a tree cross-layer protocols such CICADA [11] and WASP scheme [12] aimed to achieve WBANs reliability and low delay, although no considerable attention is focused on balancing the power consumption between the interconnected sensors [13]. Several researchers also attempted to design energy-aware MH protocols, considering also different metrics such as delay and reliability as Quality of Service requirements [14-17]. Although these studies shows that MH communications are suitable to overcome link blockage in sensor WBANs, the MH energy efficiency compared to the SH schemes is still an open issues and depends on several system parameters, including chipset implementation, sensors distance, and network topologies. A recent network design proposed in [18], shown a significant increase in battery life for relay MH scenarios considering only the transmit power.

The main objective of this paper is to compare experimentally the performances of MH cooperative and SH schemes for a WBAN. The power margins, the data flow rate, the sensor packet delivery ratio (PDR) and the average energy consumption are selected as a main performance criterion. The sensors generate and transmit data at regular intervals with a data flow rate suitable for ECG constant monitoring system.

2   Practical Considerations of the Body Sensor Network

A prototype synchronous sensor network at 2.4 GHz is set-up, where each sensor consists of a Sentilla Perk mote [22], standard compliant with the IEEE 802.15.4/Zigbee protocol. A total number of 4 sensors (with index i = 1, 2, 3 and 4) were placed on human volunteer (each attached on head, left leg, left wrist, and back) in sitting postural as shown in Fig. 1, while a sensor acting as sink is placed in the waist area. This is a representative scenario for patients who are resting for a major part of the day. The sensor 4 is placed on the volunteer's back diametrically opposite sensor 3. The sensors are placed such that batteries are closest to skin, with the antennas being further away. With respect to the sink, two sensors are in quasi-LOS (e.g. 1 and 2) while two others are in NLOS (e.g. 3 and 4). Experiments were run in office indoor scenario.

The sink collects raw data, and sends statistics to an off-body server using a wireless link. The network operations can ideally be cyclically repeated and they can be divided in 3 main phases: (1) setting-up of the routing tree topology, (2) time-slot transmission synchronization, and (3) data transmission. A time-synchronous architecture approach was selected as best suited to maximize the data delivery ratio. The first two phases can be ranked as start-up phases, the latter as steady-state phase. The sensors send routing messages in phase 1, dummy messages in phase 2 for synchronization purposes, and actual data messages during phase 3. The network performs cycles of the 3 phases with periodicity T_N to adapt its topology to the body movements and postural and environment changes.

2.1   Topology Update (Phase A)

The Minimum Cost Forwarding (MCF) network routing protocol [23] has been implemented on the top of the standard connection functionality provided by the Sentilla motes kit. The routing algorithm adopted seeks to achieve minimum cost from each sensor toward the sink, where costs are proportional to the RSSI. In SH case, each sensor transmits by default to the sink so no routing data is required, while in MH protocol case, each sensor retains the next hop target sensor address to build the tree topology. From previous published works [24, 28], the RSSI seems to provide a good estimation of packet loss rates; e.g. RSSI of −90 dBm or larger always corresponds to a PDR of 95% or more. The RSSI comes from the CC2420 built-in register, whose values are estimated in accordance to [1]. The RSSI register value $RSSI_{VAL}$ can be referred to the power P_{RF} at the RF pins by using the following equations:

$$P_{RF} = RSSI_{VAL} + RSSI_{OFFSET} \qquad (1)$$

where the $RSSI_{OFFSET}$ is approximately −45 (e.g. if reading a value of −20 from the $RSSI_{VAL}$ register, the P_{RF} is approximately −65 dBm). The $RSSI_{VAL}$ can directly be related to the path loss L_P and to the transmit power P_{TX} according

$$RSSI_{VAL} = P_{TX} - L_P - RSSI_{OFFSET} \qquad (2)$$

As transmit and receive antenna gain cannot be explicitly estimated because of the relative orientation and body impact, they are considered as embedded in the LP term. The PRF values are not numerically suitable as link costs for the routing algorithm. In fact, the sum of any MH links combination will not be lower than the SH links, even for MH power-wise convenient routes.

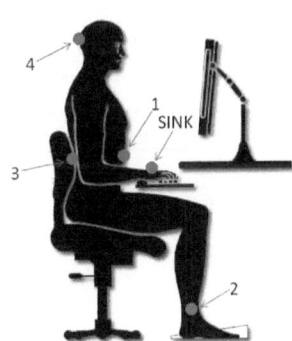

Fig. 1. Displacement map of 4 sensors and a sink network on volunteer body

2.2   Synchronisation (*Phase B*)

The transmit time slots are synchronised in Phase 2 using beacons with a unique sensor address periodically sent by the sink. In this phase, each sensor is constantly in receiving mode, listening for sink beacons and other sensor massages. If a beacon is received, the sensor set up a wake-up timer and send a packet to the next hop target sensor (or to the sink in case of SH scheme). If a sensor receives a message, it simply relays to the next hop. Thus, the sink and the sensors involved in relaying can synchronize their wake-up timers for receiving the messages from neighbourhood sensors. As the sink knows the total number of sensors (but not the network topology nor the latency *a priori*), it does not send a new beacon until a packet is received from the target sensor. As the massage delay depends of number of hops, R is expected to lower in MH scheme. After phase 2, the sink and the sensor have set a wake-up time, and no beacons are required anymore.

2.3   Transmission (*Phase C*)

At the end of phase 2, the communication between sensors is time-slotted according the wake up times to avoid idle listening and save energy. Each sensor regularly transmits data packets of 75 bytes of payload. In case of MH protocol, a sensor relays messages from neighbourhood sensors immediately after reception, with no data buffering. The sensor operation type (e.g. transmit or transmit and relay) depends on the network topology and it can dynamically change every cycle T_N. Considering a sensor in transmit operation type as shown in Fig. 2, the communication tasks are divided into 3 time slots: in T_P, the sensor generate data to transmit, in T_{TX} the sensor transmit the data packets, while in T_S the sensor is in sleeping mode. T_{TX} is fixed and empirically estimated to be ~108ms. This value includes value data serialization, a method of transforming Java objects into a byte stream (binary form), so they can be sent and received over the radio. Thus, the actual time required to transmit data itself is <100 ms. The sensor sleeping time is T_S and it varies according the synchronisations, while the active time is defined as $T_A = T_{TX} + T_P$, where T_P is ~72ms.

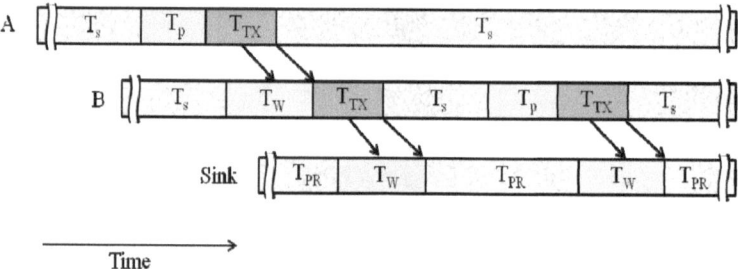

Fig. 2. Packet data communication tasks for a (A) transmit sensor, (B) relay sensor and Sink sensors operation modes (blocks are not in scale)

3   Experimental Investigations and Analyses

This section presents the results of the real-world tests. Considering a static posture of the patient, we assume a constant time average for RSSI is assumed per each link.

Each body link has been preliminary characterized in terms of measured average RSSI; data are stored in the devices memory and associated to each link before the experiments. As the links costs are now fixed, a single network cycle T_N is enough for each test. This approach has the benefits of comparing the SH and MH energy consumptions for the same network topology, enabling a separate study of the packet losses due to the synchronization drifts from those due to the P_{RF} dropping below the sensitivity threshold, and the repeatability of the results.

3.1   Network Topologies and Body Links Characterization

A preliminary characterization of the network topology in terms of link cost and time variability is performed. Per each link (e.g. γ_{13}), a data packet was sent every 1 second at 0 dBm of transmit power, for an observation time of 2 minutes. Each measurement was repeated 3 times and data were merged in a single history vector for each link. Per each packet, a RSSI measurement based on the Zigbee standard was stored and the path losses statistics are derived these values. While taking measurements, the volunteer was allowed to perform changes in the posture, as naturally happens in such scenario. Figure 3 shows the averaged RSSI and received power from measurements of the sitting postural set-up. Higher RSSI values correspond to a lower link costs. In case of SH scheme, the sensors 1, 2, 3, and 4 can only transmit directly to the sink.

In case of MH scheme, the routing protocol sets the sensor 1, 2 and 4 to communicate directly to the sink, as these links have a lower link cost if compared with any other MH link combination. The sensor 3 transmits to the sensor 4 and the latter acts as relay. In fact, considering the RSSI, the γ_{S3} link cost (where S stands for sink) is higher than the sum of γ_{13} and γ_{4S} link costs (e.g. (-16)+(-9)<-30). This can potentially results in transmit a power margin for the sensor 3 of 14 dB if compared to the SH case. The P_{RF} values are not numerically suitable as link costs for the routing algorithm. In fact, the sum of any MH links combination will not be lower than the SH links, even for MH power-wise convenient routes. As discussed before, only the 4 links relative to the sink are of interest for both SH and MH, while γ_{34} is of interest for MH only. The L_S time histories of these links are shown in Fig. 4, while Table 1 shows the statistical parameters. The standard variation σ spans from 5 dB to 8.1 dB, while the power range is up to 66 dB.

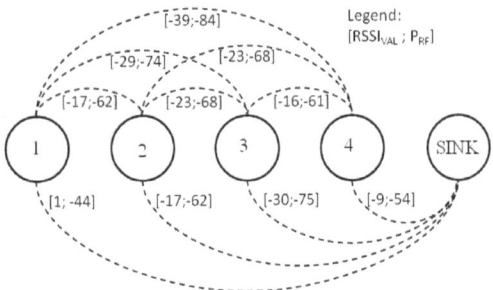

Fig. 3. Averaged RSSI and RF powers in dBm for sitting postural set-up

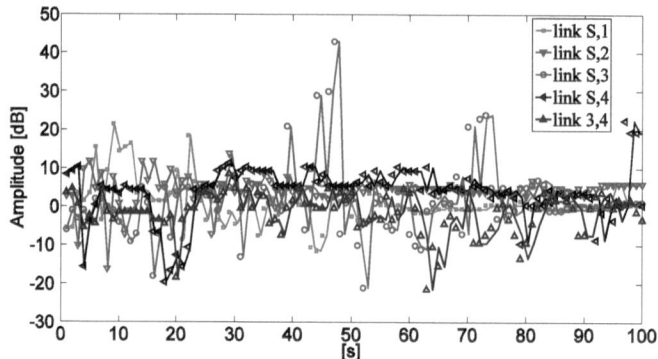

Fig. 4. Sample L_S history during the first 100 measurement seconds with sampling rate of 1 second

3.2   Network Packet Delivery Ratio (PRR) and Data Flow Rate Performances

From Table 1, the sensor 3 has M_0 of 20 and 34 dB for the SH and MH case, respectively. Moreover, σ is 8.1 and 5.0 dB for the γ_{S3} and γ_{34} cases, respectively. The probability of exceeding M_0 (or link blockage probability) is about $7 \cdot 10^{-3}$ for the SH and about $5 \cdot 10^{-12}$ for the MH case. Thus, a γ_{S3} blockage is significantly more likely than a γ_{34} link blockage. Figure 5 shows the SH PRR (primary y-axis on the right) and r (secondary y-axis on the left) for γ_{S3} with and without link blockage. The results are compared with the MH PRR and r with no link blockage on the γ_{34} link. The cases for $T_w = 93.75$ and 250 ms are considered. The PRR is > 0.9 for both SH and MH schemes with no links blockage. In case of MH network, it is shown the capability of sensor 4 to receive and route to the sink at least the data from the sensor 3 with a PRR comparable (e.g. *PRR > 0.9*) to the SH case with no blockage. In case of γ_{S3} link blockage, the SH PRR degrades of about 23% compared to the MH with no link blockage for both T_w cases, while the SH r reduction is 21% and 25% for the T_w case of 93.75 ms and 250 ms, respectively. This means that the MH topology can be used to overcome SH link blockages theoretically without PRR degradation, as the MH lower r compared to SH scheme is merely due to the synchronization basic approach discussed beforehand and it will be deepened later in this section.

As mentioned in Section 2, the PRR (and consequently r) depends directly on the waiting time (T_W) value. For this reason, both the PRR and r are preliminary studied against the T_W to maximize the data r while keeping at minimum the packet losses. Figure 6 compares the measured PRR (primary y-axis on the right) and the r (secondary y-axis on the left) against T_w for a SH and MH schemes with the link costs as defined in Table 1. The average per each sensor and the total network r are included. For $T_W \geq 93.75$ *ms*, the *PRR is ≥ 0.9* for both schemes.

Table 1. Average path loss, available margins and statistical parameters of L_S per each link of interest

Link	L_{AVG} [dB]	M_0[dB]	L_S [dB]			
			σ	Range	Min.	Max.
γ_{S1}	-44	24	7.2	53	-31.4	21.52
γ_{S2}	-62	42	6.7	43	-25.11	17.89
γ_{S3}	-75	20	8.1	66	-23.02	42.98
γ_{S4}	-54	34	7.4	44	-21.57	22.43
γ_{34}	-61	41	5.0	32	-21.33	10.67

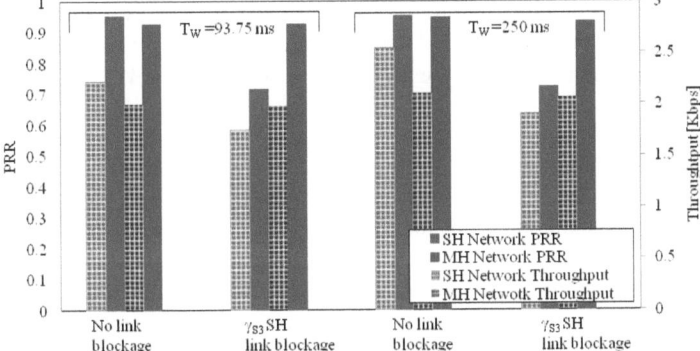

Fig. 5. Total Packet Delivery and throughput r for the SH and MH cases

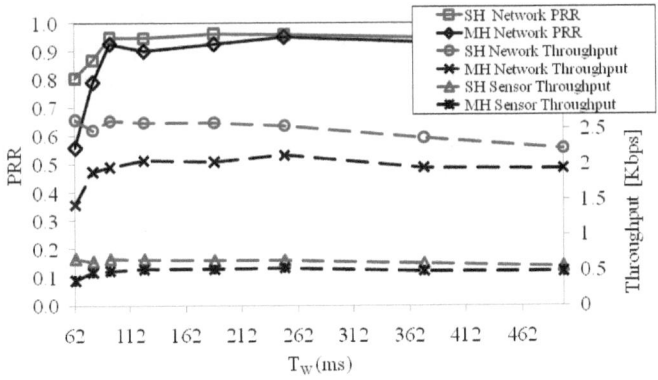

Fig. 6. PRR, total and average r against T_w for SH and MH schemes

3.3   Analytic Energy Consumption Analysis

As path loss L_S can change significantly in time even for sitting postural because of body movements, it is important to compare M against the energy consumption. The relationship between the transmit power and the sensor current consumption is not linear. The energy consumption can be estimated as a function of data packets transmitted, based on the exact circuitry being used. As a 1.8V chipset voltage is used and the defined bit rate is 250 Kbps [22], $\tilde{E}_{rx}$ is 135.4 nJ/bit, while $\tilde{E}_{tx}$ at $P_T = 0\ dBm$ is 125.28 nJ/bit. The microcontroller energy costs are not considered. From [22], the current consumption in idle and sleep modes are significantly smaller (>500μA) compared to the maximum transmit and receive currents (17.7 and 18.8mA, respectively) and they are not considered neither.

The energy consumptions estimation only represents the energy per bit dissipated in the transceiver. As the extra energy dissipated during overhead processing (data generation, data serializations, etc.) and the media access control (MAC) related (such as the waiting time T_W) are not considered, this approach provides more general results as the energy is approximate using only the network topology, the transmitted power, the chipset implementation, the bitrates and the target reliability. The energy consumption at sensor 4 is estimated using formula (7) and with $n=1$. In MH case, the sensor 4 receives and retransmits the 75 bytes sent from sensor 3.

4   Conclusions

In this paper the potential benefits and limitations of cooperative networks as a means of augment the reliability in body-wearable sensor are studied. These trade-offs have been quantified for a sensor network prototyping a real-world platform for continuous ECG healthcare monitoring. For a packet delivery ratio >0.9, the MH scheme can provide the network with a margin gain up to 14 dB traded off with an energy demand up to 30.7% higher and an average sensors r 20% lower than a SH scheme. The network lifetime of the MH scheme ranges from the 27% to 45% of the SH lifetime in cases of 0 dB and 20 dB margins, respectively. This work is a first exercise step in assessing reliability and life time trade off with real-world platforms for body area sensor networks. Follow-up studies will address wireless ECG emulators with higher number of sensors (e.g. up to 10 for a typical 12-leads ECG system) employing ultra-low power chipsets in different specific health monitoring environments, such as critical care in hospitals, aged care or athlete monitoring.

References

1. IEEE std. 802.15.4 - 2003: Wireless Medium Access Control (MAC) and Physical Layer (PHY)
2. Otto, C., Milenkovic, A., Sanders, C., Jovanov, E.: System Architecture of a Wireless Body Area Sensor Network for Ubiquitous Health Monitoring. Journal of Mobile Multimedia 1(4), 307–326 (2006)
3. Jovanov, E., Milenkovic, A., Otto, C., De Groen, P.C.: A wireless body area network of intelligent motion sensors for computer assisted physical rehabilitation. Journal of NeuroEngineering and Rehabilitation 2, 6 (2005)
4. Yazdandoost, K.Y., et al.: Channel models for body area network, IEEE P802.15-08-0780-08-0006 (April 2009)

5. Strömmer, E., Hillukkala, M., Ylisaukkooja, A.: Ultra-low Power Sensors with Near Field Communication for Mobile Applications. Presented at 2007, Int. Conf. on Wireless Network, Las Vegas, Nevada (2007)
6. Sagan, D.: RF Integrated Circuits for Medical Applications: Meeting the Challenge of Ultra Low Power Communication. In: Ultra-Low-Power Communications Division, Zarlink Semiconductor, San Diego, CA (2005)
7. Falck, T., Baldus, H., Espina, J., Klabunde, K.: Plug 'n play simplicity for wireless medical body sensors. Mobile Networks and Applications 12(2-3), 143–153 (2007)
8. Mikami, S., Matsuno, T., Miyama, M., Yoshimoto, M., Ono, H.: A Wireless-Interface SoC Powered by Energy Harvesting for short range data communication, for Short range Data Communication. In: Proceedings of the 2005 IEEE Asian Solid-State Circuits Conference, Hsinchu, Taiwan, pp. 241–244 (2005)
9. Moerman, I., Blondia, C., Reusens, E., Joseph, W., Martens, L., Demeester, P.: The Need for Cooperation and Relaying in Short-Range High Path Loss Sensor Networks. In: Proc. of the 2007 IEEE Int. Conf. on Sensor Technologies and Applications, Washington, DC, pp. 566–571 (2007)
10. Chen, Y., Teo, J., Lai, J.C.Y., Gunawan, E., Low, K.S., Soh, C.B., Rapajic, P.B.: Cooperative communications in ultra-wideband wireless body area networks: channel modelling and system diversity analysis. IEEE J. Sel. Areas Commun. 27(1), 5–16 (2009)
11. Latre, B., Braem, B., Moerman, I., Blondia, C., Reusens, E., Joseph, W., Demeester, P.: A low-delay protocol for multihop wireless body area networks. In: Proc.of 4th Int. Conf., MobiQuitous, pp. 1–8 (2007)
12. Braem, B., Latré, B., Benoît, M., Blondia, C., Demeester, P.: The wireless autonomous spanning tree protocol for multi-hop wireless body area networks. Presented at 2006, 3rd Annual International Conference on Mobile and Ubiquitous Systems, San Jose, CA (2006)
13. Su-Ho, S., Gopalan, S.A., Seung-Man, C., Ki-Jung, S., Jae-Wook, N., Jong-Tae Park, P.: An energy-efficient configuration management for multi-hop wireless body area networks. In: 3rd IEEE Int. Conf. on Broadband Network and Multimedia Technology, pp. 1235–1239 (2010)
14. Djenouri, D., Balasingham, I.: New QoS and Geographical Routing in Wireless Biomedical Sensor Networks. In: Proc. of the 6th Int. Conf. on Broadband Communications, Networks, and Systems, Madrid, Spain, pp. 1–8 (2009)
15. Felemban, E., Lee, C.-G., Ekici, E.: MMSPEED: Multipath multi-speed protocol for QoS guarantee of reliability and timeliness in wireless sensor networks. IEEE Transaction on Mobile Computing 5(6), 738–754 (2006)
16. Razzaque, A., Alam, M.M., Or-Rashid, M., Hong, C.S.: Multi-constrained QoS geographic routing for heterogeneous traffic in sensor networks. IEICE Trans. on Communications 91B(8), 2589–2601 (2008)
17. Chipara, O., He, Z., Xing, G., Chen, Q., Wang, X., Lu, C., Stankovic, J., Abdelzaher, T.: Real-time power aware routing in sensor networks. In: Proc. of the IEEE 14th International Workshop on Quality of Service, pp. 83–92 (2006)
18. Sapio, A., Tsouri, G.R.: Low-Power Body Sensor Network for Wireless ECG Based on Relaying of Creeping Waves at 2.4GHz. In: International Workshop on Wearable and Implantable Body Sensor Networks, pp. 167–173 (2010)
19. Heinzelman, W.R., Chandrakasan, A., Balakrishnan, H.: Energy-efficient communication protocol for wireless microsensor networks. In: Proc. of the 33rd Annual Hawaii Int. Conf. on System Sciences, January 4-7, vol. 2, p. 10 (2000)

20. Xigang, H., Hangguan, S., Xuemin, S.: On energy efficiency of cooperative communications in wireless body area network. Presented at 2011 IEEE Wireless Communications and Networking Conference, pp.1097–1101 (March 2011)
21. ZigBee RF transceiver datasheet, http://www.ti.com/lit/ds/symlink/cc2420.pdf
22. Sentilla webpage, http://www.sentilla.com/blogs/2008/05/sentilla-announces-worlds-smal.php
23. Fan, Y., Songwu, L., Lixia, Z.: A Scalable Solution to Minimum Cost Forwarding in Large Sensor Networks. In: Proc. of 10th Int. Conf. Comp. Communications and Networks, pp. 304–309 (2001)
24. Holland, M.M., Aures, R.G., Heinzelman, W.B.: Experimental investigation of radio performance in wireless sensor networks, Presented at 2nd IEEE Workshop on Wireless Mesh Networks, pp.140–150 (2006)
25. Madan, R., Lall, S.: Distributed algorithms for maximum lifetime routing in wireless sensor networks. IEEE Transactions on Wireless Communications 5(8), 2185–2193 (2006)
26. Bradie, B.: Wavelet packet-based compression of single lead ECG. IEEE Trans. Biomed. Eng. 43(5), 493–501 (1996)
27. Sha, K., Shi, W.: Modeling the lifetime of wireless sensor networks. Sensor Letters 3, 1–10 (2005)
28. Barsocchi, P., Oligeri, G., Potortì, F.: Measurement-based frame error model for simulating outdoor Wi-Fi networks. IEEE Transactions on Wireless Communications 8(3), 1154–1158 (2009)

Device-Free Indoor Localization
for AAL Applications

Paolo Barsocchi[1], Francesco Potortì[1], and Paolo Nepa[2,*]

[1] ISTI-CNR, Pisa Research Area, Via G.Moruzzi 1, 56124, Pisa, Italy
{paolo.barsocchi,Potorti}@isti.cnr.it,
[2] Department of Information Engineering, University of Pisa,
Via Caruso 16, 56122, Pisa, Italy
paolo.nepa@iet.unipi.it

Abstract. We present a device-free localization method oriented to Ambient Assisted Living applications. The system exploits the received signal strength (RSS) measured by fixed wireless communications devices, whose position is known a priori, in order to localize a person in the transmission coverage area. The proposed localization system is passive, by not requiring the user to wear anything, and is able to trade complexity for accuracy by simply changing the number of deployed devices. The presentation is validated by an indoor experimental study.

Keywords: RSS-based localization, AAL, tracking.

1 Introduction

Localization and tracking of mobile users in indoor environments is one of the main components (often an enabling one) in Ambient Assisted Living (AAL) [1] applications. AAL aims at improving the quality of life of elderly or disabled people, by assisting them in their daily life, in order to preserve their autonomy and by making them feeling included, protected and secure in the places where they live or work (typically their home, their office, the hospital and any other place where they may spend a significant part of their time). These objectives can be granted only if the appropriate services are delivered to the users in the right place at the right time. Localization and tracking of objects can be achieved by means of a large number of different technologies, however only few of them are suitable for AAL applications, since they should be non-invasive on the users, they must be suited to the deployment in the user houses at a reasonable cost, and they should be accepted by the users themselves. Accuracy in the position estimation is less critical than in other applications (accuracies in the order of the centimeter or below are typically not required). As an example, the EvAAL (Evaluating AAL system through benchmark [1,2]) competition compares indoor localization systems for AAL applications by taking into account metrics

* This work was supported by the European Commission under the UNIVERsal open platform and reference Specification for Ambient Assisted Living IP (universAAL, FP7-247950) within the 7th Research Framework Programme.

B. Godara and K.S. Nikita (Eds.): MobiHealth 2012, LNICST 61, pp. 361–368, 2013.

like user acceptance, availability, interoperability, and installation complexity, in addition to accuracy. For AAL applications, the required accuracy depends on the specific application that uses the localization component. For example, if the application needs to know if the person goes to the living room to switch on the TV, the requested accuracy is in the order of meters. On the other hand, if the application controls the cookware, a more precise indoor localization system is required. In other words, a localization system that changes its accuracy in accordance with the application needs is desirable. The localization solutions proposed in the literature are mainly focused on achieving as good an accuracy as possible, without adapting to the different requirements depending on the environment, and do not generally provide a way to estimate the attainable accuracy in advance. All in all, the literature is lacking solutions attractive for AAL spaces, which localize a person with an accuracy performance defined in advance in accordance with the requirements of the applications.

Considering all the above constraints, a promising technology for these services is based on Wireless Sensor Networks (WSN) [3], due to their advantages in terms of costs and time for effective deployment. Within such WSNs, it is possible to estimate the location of a user by exploiting the Received Signal Strength (RSS) information, which is a measure of the power of a received radio signal that can be obtained from almost any wireless device. The RSS measured among fixed devices (whose position is known) and mobile devices (carried by the user) is leveraged by algorithms that estimate the coordinates of the user positions. In a smart environment, where the ambience is instrumented with sensors and wireless communication devices, the marginal cost of implementing an RSS-based localisation system can be very low, as it can leverage the existing installed hardware.

Device-free localization techniques are a subset of the above ones: they do not need a mobile device worn by the person to be localized [4,5]. These systems are based on large set of small wireless devices spread over the area of interest in order to create a dense mesh, and exploit the RSS observed by each device on the links connecting it to other devices. A user moving within the area modifies the RSS pattern in a way that depends on his location; radio imaging therefore exploits the RSS measurements observed along the inter-device links to obtain a reconstruction of the object trajectory. The two main drawbacks of these methods are the large number of devices that must be deployed in the environment and the incapability of discriminating among users. Association with a sufficiently smart tracking system may help with the latter problem, while a complete solution is only possible in association with other techniques (usually non device-free, like RFID). The achieved accuracy is usually around a dozen centimeters, which is more than enough for AAL applications, where 50 cm can be considered acceptable [1,2].

In this paper we propose an indoor localization system that is able to estimate in advance the maximum error, thus matching the AAL application needs, and is particularly indicated for AAL environment where good user acceptance is essential. The proposed system works even with a small number of installed devices, thus eliminationg the first of the mentioned drawbacks of device-free localization techniques.

2   Our Solution in a Nutshell

The proposed localization system works by placing a number of sensors (hereafter called anchors) around the area of interest. Each device is capable of transmitting and receiving wireless thus creating a network of radio links that encompasses the whole area (figure 1). A user crossing the Line-of-Sight (LOS) link between two anchors causes signal fading through the link. Identifying power reduction on a given radio link can be exploited to know the area where the user is going into. As shown in figure 1, if the user enters the room and the detection algorithm detects that the LOS link between anchors 1 and 2 is affected, the localization system infers that the user is entering the subarea A_1, and will indicate the coordinates of the centroid of that subarea. The proposed localization system is strongly influenced by the detection algorithm, which will be described and evaluated in section 3.3.

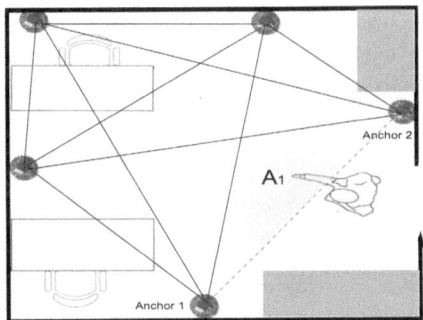

Fig. 1. The proposed AAL compliant device-free localization system

The proposed localization system is able to:

- make a priori estimation of the maximum error by evaluating the maximum distance between the centroid and the farthest point of each subarea;
- adapt the required accuracy to the application needs at installation time. If the application needs a higher location accuracy in a given area, the anchors can be deployed in order to create smaller subareas—on the contrary, if the application needs a lower accuracy, larger subareas can be planned.

According to the metric proposed in [1,2], the proposed system is particularly suitable for AAL applications, since:

- the installation complexity can be made low by simulating the anchor deployment before deployment;
- user acceptance benefits from the users not having to carry anything on them.

3   Experimental Evaluation

In this section we describe the environment setup of the measurement campaign conducted at the first floor of CNR-ISTI, the detection algorithm and its performance, and comment on the proposed localization algorithm.

3.1   Setup

We deployed a network of five IRIS wireless sensors nodes [6] in a 23 m^2 indoor laboratory, at about 120 cm above the floor. The nodes operate in the 2.4 GHz frequency band using the IEEE 802.15.4 transmission protocol. We used a modified version of the management software Spin [7], which implements a token-passing protocol to schedule node transmission. Anchors transmit a packet in broadcast, so all other anchors receive the packet and perform the RSS measurements. Packets contain the previous RSS measurements and are collected by a base station along with the node's unique ID, for storage and later processing. The data collected during the experiment consisted of more than 40000 RSS measurements for a total time of 668 s. The experimental setup is shown in Figure 2. Only the user to be localized was present in the area during the experiment.

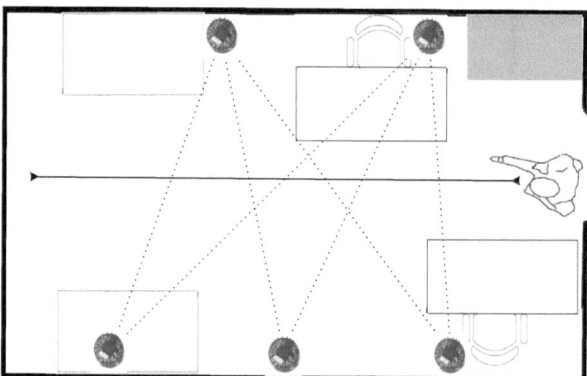

Fig. 2. Environment setup: 5 anchors placed close to the lateral walls of the room, at about 120 cm height. The straight line indicates the actual path followed during the experiment.

3.2   RSS Behaviour

In this section we show the RSS behavior during one of the data acquisition phases. Each anchor j collect the experienced RSS $r_{i,j}$ from all other anchors $i \in N_j$, where N_j is the set of neighbors of j. Figure 3 shows the RSS and the variance $\sigma_{1,4}^2$ experienced between anchors 1 and 4. When the user interferes with the LOS link between the anchors 1 and 4, the RSS value decreases; when the user passes over the 1-4 radio link, the RSS value returns to normal. Estimating $\sigma_{1,4}^2$ is a reliable way of detecting the crossing event. As illustrated in figure 3, the temporal variance of the RSS values experiences 60 peaks, as expected since during the experiment the user crossed the link 60 times.

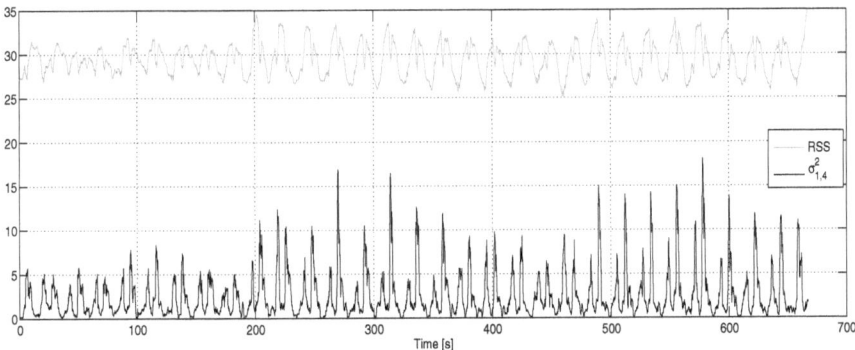

Fig. 3. RSS values and variance of the link between anchors 1 and 4

3.3   Detection Algorithm

The proposed detection algorithm is based on the observation of the RSS characteristics highlighted in previous section. As shown in related papers [8], the RSS variance is a valuable parameter to detect events in wireless systems. When the RSS variance increases it means that something happens that changes the RSS behavior for a while. In this particular case, the variance of the RSS increases when a person crosses the LOS link between a couple of anchors. When this event ends, the RSS variance goes back to its unperturbed value. Starting from such considerations we deployed an algorithm as follows:

1. given a receiver j and a transmitter $i \in N_j$ (where N_j is the set of neighbors of j) a number W of RSS measurements is collected $R_{i,j} = \{r_{i,j}^{(w)}\}_{w=1}^{w=W}$
2. the RSS variance $\sigma_{R_{i,j}}^2$ of the W measures is evaluated;
3. when $\sigma_{R_{i,j}}^2 <= \gamma$, the link between i and j is assumed to be unaffected and we go back to step 1 for the first measurement of the next window;
4. when $\sigma_{R_{i,j}}^2 > \gamma$, user crossing is detected and we go back to step 1 for the first measurement of the next window.

Performance. The detection test can be viewed as a choice between two events H_0 and H_1.

$$H_0 : \sigma_{R_{i,j}} \leq \gamma$$
$$H_1 : \sigma_{R_{i,j}} > \gamma \tag{1}$$

Since the variances $\sigma_{R_{i,j}}^2$ are random variables, their conditional density functions are denoted as $f_{\sigma_{i,j}}(\sigma|H_0)$ and $f_{\sigma_{i,j}}(\sigma|H_1)$. The performance of a detector will be given by using the probability of false alarm P_{FA} and probability of detection P_D defined, on a 1 s window time, as:

$$P_{FA} = \int_{x=\gamma}^{\infty} f_{\sigma_{i,j}}(x|H_0)\, dx$$
$$P_D = \int_{x=\gamma}^{\infty} f_{\sigma_{i,j}}(x|H_1)\, dx \tag{2}$$

The probability of missed detection P_M, is $P_M = 1 - P_D$. Since these probabilities are a function of γ, we can trade lower false alarm for missed detection. The objective of the experimental activity is to evaluate the above trade-off and show the achievable performance. To this purpose the receiver operating characteristic (ROC) curve is computed. The ROC curve is a classical method for displaying the performance of a detection algorithm by plotting the probability of false alarm P_{FA} versus probability of detection P_D (hit rate). The threshold γ is not shown explicitly, but for a particular value of γ, the detector would achieve specific $P_{FA}(\gamma)$ and $P_D(\gamma)$ values. We tested a range of γ values and plotted $P_D(\gamma)$ versus $P_{FA}(\gamma)$ in a single ROC curve.

The quality of the links is higly variable, as shown by the distance between the curves relative to the worst and the best link. Also, the performance of even the best link is not very good. It will be interesting to note that the localization performance is good even in the presence of a rather poor and highly variable ROC performance.

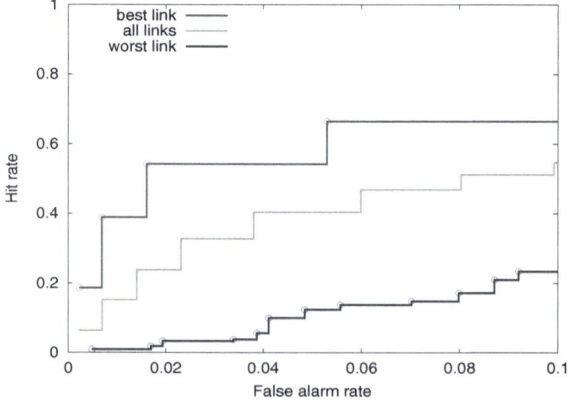

Fig. 4. ROC curve of the proposed detection algorithm. Window length is 1 s.

The values of γ relative to the points on the curve are roughly inversely proportional to the false alarm rate with a value around $range(r_{i,j})/20$ for a 10% false alarm.

3.4 Localization Error

We define the performance of the localization algorithm in terms of *error*, that is the distance between the estimated and the actual position.

It may happen that two or more events (LOS link obstruction) are detected simultaneously, either because two rays are obstructed or because of false alarms: in this cas the localization algorithm estimate is the centroid of the positions indicated by all the events. In this experiment we set the optimal detection algorithm parameters as described in section 3.3. Figure 5 shows the CDF obtained by using the proposed localization algorithm (solid line) compared to the one that the algorithm would obtain for a 100% detection probability and a null false alarm probability (dotted line). In our experiment, the localization algorithm exhibited a median error of 1 m, with an error less than 2 m in 80% of cases; the theoretical median error is about 0.4 m and in 80% of cases the error is below 1 m. Root mean square error is 1.7 m for the real case, 0.8 m for the theoretical case. We can decrease the theoretical error at will by increasing the number of deployed anchors.

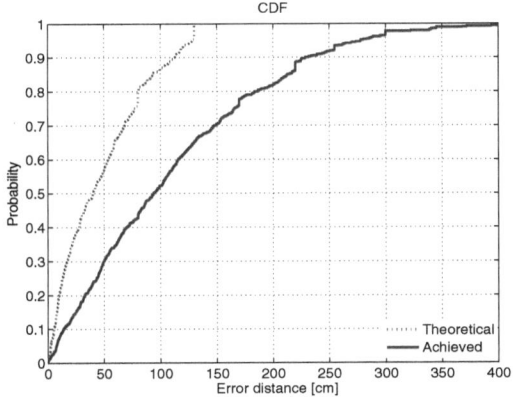

Fig. 5. Cumulative distribution function of the error measured during the experiment depicted in 3. The theoretical case assumes perfect detection.

4 Conclusion

We have experimentally observed that, with as few as 5 anchors in a room of about 23 m², our method achieves a median error of 1 m, with an RMS of 1.7 m, and an attainable median error of 0.4 m, with an RMS of 0.8 m. Work is in progress to improve the performance of the detection algorithm, to minimize the probability of false alarm and to increase the detection probability.

References

1. Barsocchi, P., Potortì, F., Furfari, F., Gil, A.M.M.: Comparing AAL indoor localization systems. In: Chessa, S., Knauth, S. (eds.) EvAAL 2011. CCIS, vol. 309, pp. 1–13. Springer, Heidelberg (2012)
2. Salvi, D., Barsocchi, P., Arredondo, M.T., Ramos, J.P.L.: EvAAL, evaluating AAL systems through competitive benchmarking, the experience of the 1st competition. In: Chessa, S., Knauth, S. (eds.) EvAAL 2011. CCIS, vol. 309, pp. 14–25. Springer, Heidelberg (2012)
3. Barsocchi, P., Lenzi, S., Chessa, S., Furfari, F.: Automatic virtual calibration of range-based indoor localization systems. Wireless Communications and Mobile Computing (2011)
4. Savazzi, S., Nicoli, M., Riva, M.: Radio imaging by cooperative wireless network: Localization algorithms and experiments. In: WCNC, pp. 2357–2361 (2012)
5. Wilson, J., Patwari, N.: Radio tomographic imaging with wireless networks. IEEE Trans. Mob. Comput. 9(5), 621–632 (2010)
6. Crossbow Technology Inc.: Iris crossbow data sheet
7. Wilson, J., Patwari, N.: Spin: A token ring protocol for RSS collection
8. Wilson, J., Patwari, N.: See-through walls: Motion tracking using variance-based radio tomography networks. IEEE Trans. Mob. Comput. 10(5), 612–621 (2011)

A Distributed Dynamic Mobility Architecture with Integral Cross-Layered and Context-Aware Interface for Reliable Provision of High Bitrate mHealth Services

András Takács[1] and László Bokor[2]

[1] Hungarian Academy of Sciences, Computer and Automation Research Institute,
Kende u. 13-17, H-1111, Budapest, Hungary
andras.takacs@sztaki.hu
[2] Budapest University of Technology and Economics, Department of Telecommunications,
Magyar Tudósok krt. 2, H-1117, Budapest Hungary
bokorl@hit.bme.hu

Abstract. Mobile health (mHealth) has been receiving more and more attention recently as an emerging paradigm that brings together the evolution of advanced mobile and wireless communication technologies with the vision of "connected health" aiming to deliver the right care in the right place at the right time. However, there are several cardinal problems hampering the successful and widespread deployment of mHealth services from the mobile networking perspective. On one hand, issues of continuous wireless connectivity and mobility management must be solved in future heterogeneous mobile Internet architectures with ever growing traffic demands. On the other hand, Quality of Service (QoS) and Quality of Experience (QoE) must be guaranteed in a reliable, robust and diagnostically acceptable way. In this paper we propose a context- and content-aware, jointly optimized, distributed dynamic mobility management architecture to cope with the future traffic explosion and meet the medical QoS/QoE requirements in varying environments.

Keywords: eHealth, mHealth, reliable and scalable mHealth service provision, DMM (Distributed and Dynamic Mobility Management), cross-layer (X-layer) design, context-awareness, content-awareness mobile IPv6 protocol family.

1 Introduction

Being part of modern telemedicine – which generally offers higher diagnosis and treatment quality standards, reduces medical costs, and provides possibilities to handle problems of the aging human society [1] – mHealth rises in parallel with the rapid adoption of mobile communications, computing, and advanced wireless technologies into our daily life. New, immersive, multimedia-driven, pervasive and interactive mHealth services (like self-diagnosis and preventive care [2], mobile-assisted telerehabilitation and therapy [3], medical care in emergency situations [4], etc.) are rising to provide timely and prompt medical attention while also saving monetary resources. The wide variety of promising application areas together with the

B. Godara and K.S. Nikita (Eds.): MobiHealth 2012, LNICST 61, pp. 369–379, 2013.
© Institute for Computer Sciences, Social Informatics and Telecommunications Engineering 2013

continuous growth in consumer use of mobile Internet to obtain health-related services help the novel paradigm of mHealth in reshaping healthcare.

However, like other services running in mobile and wireless environments, the efficiency and usability of mHealth applications are substantially impacted by the continuously varying environmental characteristics, scarce network resources, sparse radio bands and bandwidth, fluctuating delay, jitter and other QoS parameter values. This clearly implies the need of context- and content-aware mechanisms making applications, service provision and delivery procedures adaptable to the extremely diverse mobile environments [5]. The impacts of fluctuations in context and resources are further aggravated by the current trends that prognosticate a massive traffic volume growth in mobile telecommunications during 2011-2020 [6]. To date, this traffic explosion is mostly driven by Internet applications providing interaction, information, and entertainment for human users. But with the widespread deployment of sensor technologies, another form of communications called M2M (Machine-to-Machine) is emerging which supposedly will be the leading traffic contributor for mobile Internet evolution [7] and also has the potential to become a major enabler of successful live mHealth deployments [8]. Another prominent force in mobile traffic growth is the advancement of high bitrate data-hungry multimedia applications: television/radio broadcasting and high-definition Video on Demand will increase mobile video volumes with 25-fold between 2011-2016, accounting for over 70 percent of total mobile data traffic by the middle of the decade [6]. This trend is also substantial in mHealth: the spreading of multimedia technologies and developments in mobile connectivity gives doctors and medical institutions a new set of tools for managing patient care, using high definition 2D/3D imaging for diagnostic purposes and providing new types of multimedia services, such as multi-view, stereoscopic and holographic video communications for tele-diagnosis and remote operations.

The high requirements of diagnostically useful multimedia transmission techniques and the thriving traffic demands pose serious research challenges for mobility architectures of mHealth [9] [10]. In this paper we propose a novel, jointly optimized mobility architecture for the challenges: the concept of distributed dynamic mobility management (DMM) is employed to cope with the growing traffic demands, the appropriately chosen and integrated protocol components solve various handover, security and multi-access issues, while the naturally integrated cross-layer design with high adaptivity based on context- and content-awareness helps to handle varying environmental resources and meet the medical QoS/QoE requirements.

The remainder of the paper is organized as follows. In Section 2, we introduce the related work on the existing solutions for challenges of emerging mHealth applications. Section 3 introduces our design choices and the main protocol components of the system. Section 4 in turn details our proposed integrated mobility management architecture together with the API framework created for supporting sophisticated cross-layer control and flexible adaptation. In Section 5 we conclude the paper and describe our ongoing work and future plans.

2   Related Work

To address the dynamic and fluctuating nature of mobile networks, the paradigm of context- and content-awareness started to emerge [11] [12]. The change in the context (i.e., in any information that can be used to characterize the situation of a mobile entity) or in the content (i.e., in any parameter classifying the media under transmission) would require e.g., to move specific users to alternative access networks [5] or to assign different security measures/interfaces for specific contents during mobility events [13]. However, being context- and content-aware requires an extremely flexible session and mobility management in a deeply integrated network support system. This can be achieved only with the elimination of strict boundaries between traditional layers of the communication model by introducing cross-layer design solutions that allow transport dynamic information between layers and provides jointly optimized operation for devices in wireless environments [14] [15].

The application of the above introduced advanced methods for mHealth applications has already been started. Jong-Tae Park et al. [16] presented a context-aware handover architecture for u-healthcare services in converged wireless body- and local area networks, which focuses on power efficiency. P.K. Gkonis et al. [17] designed a content-centric future Internet platform that supports added value health services (safe and accurate management of medicine prescriptions) incorporating mobility, context awareness, enhanced security and privacy. In the work of Yan Zhang et al. [18] the application of integrated WiMAX and WLAN broadband wireless access technologies for telemedicine services and the related protocol issues have been discussed together with some potential deployment scenarios. R. S. H. Istepanian et al. [19] focuses on medical QoS applied to a typical bandwidth demanding mHealth application, and proposes a novel multiobjective and adaptive rate-control mechanism for optimized delivery of diagnostically acceptable ultrasound video images over beyond 3G networks. V. Ghini, et al. introduced the m-Hippocrates software architecture [20] aiming to provide mHealth applications with constant and reliable communication using an application-level communication technology called Always Best Packet Switching (ABPS). This scheme ensures continuously available, reliable and interactive communication, but it does not consider advanced IPv6 based technologies for vertical handover support and relies on a solution, which is outside of current standardization activities.

However there are several enhancements of mobility management for mHealth applications in the literature, none of them take into account the exploding traffic demands and scalability issues of future wireless systems. Taking care of scalability problems by distributing mobile network functions and sharing the increased traffic load among the distributed elements is really a hot research topic nowadays. Several architectural improvements of existing technologies (e.g., [21]) or even green field solutions (like [22]) follow this approach, but all of them share the same issue: in such schemes it is essential to implement service continuity between the highly scattered internet points of attachment. To solve this, distributed and dynamic mobility management approaches must be envisaged [23].

In the traditional MIPv6 mobility scheme [24] all signalling and data packets are transferred via the central anchor node called Home Agent (HA).

As a first alternative for eliminating this centralized way of operation researches started to implement core-level distribution procedures: anchors are distributed but still remain in the core network. A good example to this is the Global HA to HA protocol (GHAHA) [25], which extends MIPv6 in order to remove its link layer dependencies on the Home Link and distribute the anchors at the scale of the Internet. The drawback of this design is the extreme load of the synchronization messages. The scheme of M. Fisher et al. handles this problem by distributing the Binding Cache [26], but their proposal is not implementation ready, as it does not specify mechanisms for data corruption, and HA failures.

A second alternative is when mobility functions are distributed in the backhaul and access part of the network. The multi-level system of Hierarchical Mobile IPv6 (HMIPv6) [27] and its extension proposed by Mei Song et al. [28] defines regions, in which the movement does not need binding at the Home Agent counter to the inter-region movement. It relieves the HA from the load of signalling, but it could be effective only for short-term sessions, or localized movements.

A third type of distribution scenarios is the so-called host-level (peer-to-peer) distributed mobility management where once the correspondent node is found, communicating peers can directly exchange packets. MIPv6 also uses this direction when it bypasses the HA thanks to its route optimization mechanisms [24] [29]. End-to-end mobility management protocols working in higher layers of the TCP/IP stack such as Host Identity Protocol [30] can also be efficiently employed in such schemes.

Another class of distributed mobility management is based on the capability to turn off mobility signaling when such mechanisms are not needed. The so-called dynamic mobility management schemes (like [31], [32]) dynamically execute mobility functions only for cases when Mobile Nodes (MN) are actually subjected to handover events and higher layers require address continuity. These architectures are session-based contrarily to the conventional mobility architectures, which provide the same mobility features for all of the sessions. It is not effective for long-term sessions and does not provide global reachability for Mobile Nodes, but it provides effective and on-demand resource distribution for short-term sessions.

In order to have a scalable, generic, secure, transparent and widely useable mobility architecture for mHealth services, we propose an IPv6-based, DMM- and implementation-ready solution, which focuses on the context- and content-aware operations, cross-layer optimization and integration of standard components.

3   Design Considerations

While almost all existing DMM proposals introduce new protocols and architecture, Basavaraj Patil et al. stated in their recent work [33] that *"(...) most of the needed basic protocol functionality for distributed mobility management is already there. What is missing seem to be related to general system level design and lack of mobility aware APIs for application developers"*. We share this vision with them and believe that appropriate and comprehensive integration of existing Mobile IPv6 building blocks could efficiently solve all the emerging mobility issues of current architectures. However, appropriate selection and integration of protocols is needed.

In our architecture proposal, the components were selected based on practical necessities and strictly focusing on implementability. All of them extend the original Mobile IPv6 core [24]. The most common extensions are Network Mobility (NEMO-BS) [34] which ensures the mobility of networks, and Multiple Care-of Addresses Registration (MCoA) [35] that brings the possibility of parallel usage of multiple network interfaces. Table 1 summarizes the main protocol components and their purpose, and this section details the connection of them with the DMM requirements.

The problems of low scalability and single point of failure are handled by *Hierarchical Mobile IPv6* [27] and *Global HA to HA* [25]. As we described, there are some drawbacks of them when applied alone, but their integration will result in a three level (top-level, mid-level, no mobility), distributed system with high flexibility and wide scalability options. GHAHA operates at the top-level by the global distribution of Home Agents. HMIPv6 reduces signalling overhead of the central network by defining the mid-level. Movement inside these micro-mobility regions are hidden from the central network, which could relieve the HA. However, these components do not solve the problems of non-optimal routes and high latency. That is why *Source Address Selection* [36] (SAddrSel) and *Enhanced Route Optimization* [29] (ERO) are also integrated in our scheme: these two techniques are specifically addressing routing and latency issues. ERO reduces signalling requirements of correspondent binding and makes it much faster. It could increase the efficiency of route-optimized traffic, which reduces the overhead of the central network. (Note, that for NEMO cases, on the Mobile Network Node (MNN), this API is not defined yet. A new interface will be necessary which could receive commands from the MNN, not only from the Mobile Router.) SAddrSel brings the option for the applications to optimize their sessions, and direct their traffic via the actual Access Point (AP, no mobility), the Mobility Anchor Point (micro- or mid-level mobility) or the Home Agent (macro- or top-level mobility). These options select the level of mobility and stability of the sessions according to the context of the usage in a dynamic and flexible way.

Table 1. Specifications to be employed

Name	Description	Purpose
MIPv6	Mobile IPv6 [24]	Core
NEMO	Network Mobility [34]	Core
MCoA	Multiple Care-of Addresses [35]	Core
HMIPv6	Hierarchical Mobile IPv6 [27]	Scalability, single p. of failure, distrib. op.
GHAHA	Global HA-HA [25]	Scalability, single p. of failure, distrib. op.
SAddrSel	Source Address Selection [36]	Signalling, RO, dynamic op.
RO	Enhanced Route Optimization [29]	Signalling, RO
FB	Flow Binding [37]	RO, X-layer opt., content-awareness
FMIPv6	Fast Handover for MIPv6 [38]	X-layer opt., handover speed-up
MIH	Media Independent Handover [39]	X-layer opt., handover speed-up

Two key features in our architecture further exploit the benefits of cross-layer optimization. The first one is the on-demand content-aware per-flow (per-session) route selection. It could be handled via the explicit and responsive selection of the anchor point (AP, MAP, HA) with the previously introduced SAddrSel feature. If there are multiple interfaces in the system, it could be extended with the selection from them. We should exchange the routing policies between the participants to ensure the correct routing of the backwards communication. It is solved with the help of the *Flow Binding* [37] protocol extension. Flow Binding extends the Binding Update messages to be able to synchronize the session directing rules on the MN and on the HA. The architecture should define the proper API commands to receive application interactions, and the environment should be synchronized. It does not have any effects on other components.

On the other hand, we could also optimize the (speed) of the handover processes by taking advantages of cross-layer solutions and such adapting to different network characteristics. Here we rely on handover preparation, initiation and decision schemes, like the *Media Independent Handover* (MIH) specification [39]. MIH has been designed to enable the handover of IP sessions from one Layer 2 access technology to another, to achieve mobility of end user devices. Our architecture will use MIH services and message exchange technologies to predict handover events and prepare handover executions. To be able to use the complex set of functionalities of MIH, the mobility management architecture should provide the appropriate handover execution mechanisms to make the handover faster based on the MIH operation. It could be realized by the integration of *Fast Handover* (FMIPv6) [38] protocol. Integration of FMIPv6 and HMIPv6 for appropriate mid-layer (MAP) operation has not specified yet, although there are non-standardized specifications (like [40]). Integration of MIH with the other components is handled via the FMIPv6 protocol: it lets a socket open for gathering context information to initiate handovers and the context information will be provided by MIH. The interoperability between FMIPv6 and MIH is not defined yet, but there are multiple results about this subject (i.e., [41]).

Fig. 1-A depicts the supposed interoperability between the previously listed protocols. The 'stick' sign means, that the components are compatible with each other. The interoperability process is directly or indirectly defined by RFCs. The 'warning' sign denotes questionable interoperability.

4   The Proposed Architecture and Cross-Layer API Framework

The key mobility management features of our architecture are integrated into a central module called the Mobility Management Daemon (MMD). However, some additional tasks, which are traditionally managed by other tools, are realized by external resources. The Router Advertisement Daemon handles the router advertisement tasks [42], including HA and MAP advertisements [24] [27] as well. The IKEv2 Daemon is responsible for IKEv2 key exchange [43], especially for HMIPv6 mechanisms.

MIH is not included into the core, because of logical mismatch (MMD is responsible for signalling and routing, but not for handover optimization); the API (see later) connects it to the core daemon. The MIH module is responsible for the X-layer signalling exchange between the nodes with the information about the status of the connection, gathered from different layers. The result of this message exchange is forwarded to the MMD via its API, which analyses this information, and it will initiate handover if it could make the connection faster, cheaper or more stable.

Fig. 1-B depicts the preliminary architecture of the Mobility Management Daemon. The concept is similar to the Data View Control paradigm of GUI applications [44]. The Communication part sends and receives the MIPv6 signalling messages. In addition it handles the necessary ICMPv6 messages [42] [24] too. The Data plane stores and manages the Binding Update List, Binding Cache, and other data related to binding management. The Environment is responsible for setting up the routing rules. It handles all of the management tasks, which are necessary to route the data packets to the right interface with the correct source address. The Control element manages the non-signal driven functions, for example expiration of different kind of entries. These parts don't possess direct interfaces to each other. Instead, an Internal Communication Bus (ICB) connects them. Some of the commands, which are available on the ICB, are exported for third parties through the Low-level Management Socket. An external, High-level Mobility Interface, which handles more complex operations, is also available. Additionally some key features should be integrated in separate modules. For example, movement detection is one of the most important parts, and it could be realized in many ways.

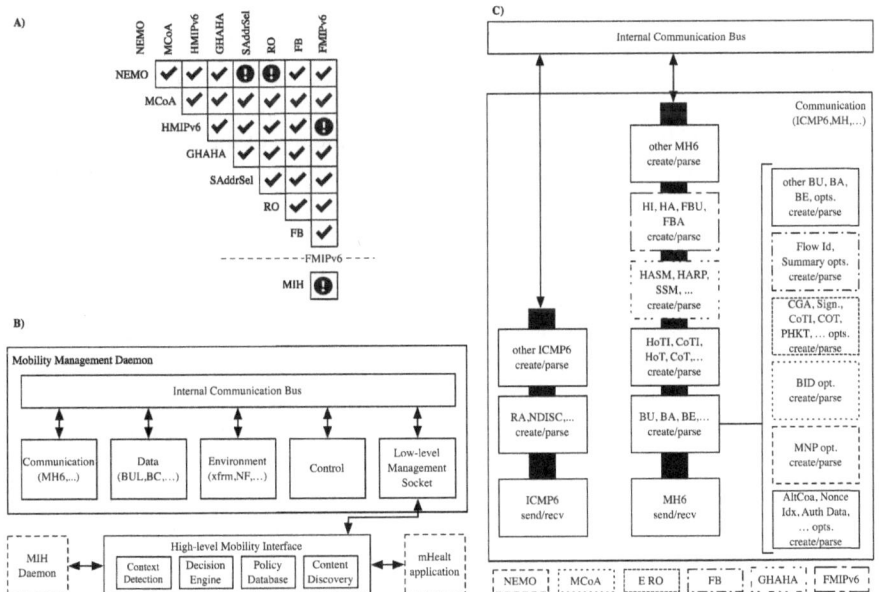

Fig. 1. A) Protocol compatibility chart; B) Proposed architecture of Mobility Management Daemon; C) Internal architecture of the Communication part

The above introduced architecture implements the core functionalities specified by [24], to which separate modules will be connected in order to integrate the wide scale of different protocol extensions to the base system. To better understand the modular architecture, we explain the details of Communication part (Fig. 1-C). While the communication core realizes the sending and receiving of ICMPv6 and MH6 messages [42] [24], the creating and parsing of different kind of messages is implemented by the modules, which belong to different protocol extensions.

Sending and receiving primitives for Mobility (MH) and ICMPv6 messages are essential for signalling functionality. The core protocol [24] defines the basic set of messages. Binding Update (BU), Binding Acknowledgement (BA) and Binding Error (BE) are indispensable for binding between the Central Network and the Mobile Nodes. Many options are defined for the Binding Update message. The most common Mobility Options are also defined in [24], but the others are specified by other protocol components like [34] [35] [37]. These options are to be inserted into the BU message by the corresponding extension modules; the core does not need to know about them. The architecture defines sockets for the modules to add further options or data to the messages before sending via handles. These should be executed at the corresponding point during the message preparation, and these could extend or re-design the messages before sending. Same as the core, all of the modules could define their own MH messages (e.g., global HA-HA's special signalling packets).

To make the MMD as powerful as it could be, it should continuously interact with the applications and other resources. A two-level API framework (Fig. 1-C) realizes this. On one hand, MMD integrates a raw interface, called Low-level Management Socket, which provides basic commands. The watchful selection of the implementation could solve the current problem between NEMO and SAddrSel (namely the lack of policy messages between the MNN and the Mobile Router). On the other hand, the High-level Mobility Interface at the top of the Management Socket realizes more complex functionalities and provides a simple API for the context- and content-aware services and specific X-layer optimization procedures.

The High-level Mobility Interface is a mid-layer between the Management Socket and the applications. It groups multiple command primitives into simple instructions, and integrates a decision engine, which provides easy to use QoS/QoE-centric control of handovers for context- and content-aware operations. This interface connects to the MIH daemon as well, and collects interface, media and other context information, which could help for the decisions. The decision engine also uses the policy database, which helps to find the best policy for the content within an actual set of environmental parameters. This application-driven, context- and content-aware API framework also brings the dynamic behaviour into our mobility management architecture: the top-level (HA) and mid-level (MAP) networks could be bypassed with on-demand binding, and the MN could perform binding only if it is necessary.

5   Conclusions

The proliferation mobile Internet applications and services tend to radically overload the current mobile and wireless architectures deployed nowadays. This traffic explosion will make the communication slower, less reliable, and also will pose serious problems for mobility management, which is essential for modern mHealth applications. To fulfil the special reliability, QoS/QoE, and bandwidth requirements of the mHealth sector, we should distribute the mobility management, and we should optimize the flow routing between the peers. The recent mobility solutions have to apply the features defined by DMM and have to integrate various optimizations, such as cross-layer optimization, context- and content-awareness. Our proposed architecture is a promising, standard-based, implementable and integrated answer for all the issues of current Mobile IPv6 systems also within the unique context of mHealth use-cases. We are currently working on the implementation [45] of the proposed architecture, which will be followed by the functional validation and the performance evaluation of our design in real-life testbed scenarios.

Acknowledgement. The research leading to these results has received funding from the European Union's Seventh Framework Programme ([FP7/2007-2013]) under grant agreement n° 288502 (CONCERTO project) and was also supported by the grant TÁMOP - 4.2.2.B-10/1--2010-0009.

References

1. Istepanian, R., et al.: M-Health: Emerging Mobile Health Systems. Springer (2005)
2. Blumrosen, G., et al.: C-SMART: Efficient seamless cellular phone based patient monitoring system. In: IEEE International Symposium on World of Wireless, Mobile and Multimedia Networks (WoWMoM), pp. 1–6. IEEE (2011)
3. Mougiakakou, S.G., et al.: Mobile technology to empower people with Diabetes Mellitus: Design and development of a mobile application. In: 9th International Conference on Information Technology and Applications in Biomedicine, pp. 1–4 (2009)
4. Malan, D., et al.: CodeBlue: An ad hoc sensor network infrastructure for emergency medical care. In: International Workshop on Wearable and Implantable Body Sensor Networks (2004)
5. Fernandes, S., Karmouch, A.: Vertical Mobility Management Architectures in Wireless Networks: A Comprehensive Survey and Future Directions. IEEE Communications Surveys Tutorials 14, 45–63 (2012)
6. CISCO: Global mobile data traffic forecast update, 20112016 (2012)
7. Wu, G., et al.: M2M: From mobile to embedded internet. IEEE Communications Magazine 49, 36–43 (2011)
8. Fan, Z., Tan, S.: M2M communications for e-health: Standards, enabling technologies, and research challenges. In: 6th International Symposium on Medical Information and Communication Technology, pp. 1–4 (2012)
9. Istepanian, R.S.H., et al.: Guest Editorial Introduction to the Special Section on M-Health: Beyond Seamless Mobility and Global Wireless Health-Care Connectivity. IEEE Transactions on Information Technology in Biomedicine 8, 405–414 (2004)
10. Adibi, S.: Link Technologies and BlackBerry Mobile Health (mHealth) Solutions: A Review. IEEE Transactions on Information Technology in Biomedicine 16, 586–597 (2012)

11. Makris, P., et al.: A Survey on Context-Aware Mobile and Wireless Networking: On Networking and Computing Environments' Integration. IEEE Communications Surveys Tutorials, 1–25 (2012)
12. Subbiah, B., Uzmi, Z.A.: Content aware networking in the Internet: issues and challenges. In: IEEE International Conference on Communications, vol. 4, pp. 1310–1315 (2001)
13. Yin, H., et al.: CASM: a content-aware protocol for secure video multicast. IEEE Transactions on Multimedia 8, 270–277 (2006)
14. Srivastava, V., Motani, M.: Cross-layer design: a survey and the road ahead. IEEE Communications Magazine 43, 112–119 (2005)
15. Foukalas, F., et al.: Cross-layer design proposals for wireless mobile networks: a survey and taxonomy. IEEE Communications Surveys Tutorials 10, 70–85 (2008)
16. Park, J.-T., et al.: Context-Aware Handover with Power Efficiency for u-Healthcare Service in WLAN. In: Proceedings of the 2009 International Conference on New Trends in Information and Service Science, pp. 1279–1283. IEEE Computer Society, Washington, DC (2009)
17. Gkonis, P.K., et al.: A content-centric, publish-subscribe architecture delivering mobile context-aware health services. In: Future Network Mobile Summit, pp. 1–9 (2011)
18. Zhang, Y., et al.: Wireless telemedicine services over integrated IEEE 802.11/WLAN and IEEE 802.16/WiMAX networks. IEEE Wireless Communications 17, 30–36 (2010)
19. Istepanian, R.S.H., et al.: Medical QoS provision based on reinforcement learning in ultrasound streaming over 3.5G wireless systems. IEEE Journal on Selected Areas in Communications. 27, 566–574 (2009)
20. Ghini, V., et al.: M-Hippocrates: Enabling Reliable and Interactive Mobile Health Services. IT Professional 14, 29–35 (2012)
21. 3GPP: Local IP Access and Selected IP Traffic Offload (2007)
22. Faigl, Z., et al.: Evaluation of two integrated signalling schemes for the Ultra Flat Architecture using SIP, IEEE 802.21, and HIP/PMIP protocols. Comput. Netw. 55, 1560–1575 (2011)
23. Chan, H.A., et al.: Distributed and Dynamic Mobility Management in Mobile Internet: Current Approaches and Issues. Journal of Communications 6 (2011)
24. Perkins, C., et al.: Mobility Support in IPv6. IETF RFC 6275 (2011)
25. Wakikawa, R., et al.: Global HA to HA Protocol Specification. IETF Draft draft-wakikawa-mext-global-haha-spec-02 (2011)
26. Fischer, M., et al.: A Distributed IP Mobility Approach for 3G SAE. In: IEEE 19th International Symposium on Personal, Indoor and Mobile Radio Communications, pp. 1–6 (2008)
27. Soliman, H., et al.: Hierarchical Mobile IPv6 (HMIPv6) Mobility Management. IETF RFC 5380 (2008)
28. Song, M., et al.: A Distributed Dynamic Mobility Management Strategy for Mobile IP Networks. In: Proceedings of the 6th International Conference on ITS Telecommunications, pp. 1045–1048 (2006)
29. Arkko, J., et al.: Enhanced Route Optimization for Mobile IPv6. IETF RFC 4866 (2007)
30. Moskowitz, R., et al.: Host Identity Protocol. IETF RFC 5210 (2008)
31. Giust, F., et al.: Flat access and mobility architecture: An IPv6 distributed client mobility management solution. In: IEEE Conference on Computer Communications Workshops, pp. 361–366 (2011)
32. Bertin, P., et al.: A Distributed Dynamic Mobility Management Scheme Designed for Flat IP Architectures. In: New Technologies, Mobility and Security, NTMS 2008, pp. 1–5 (2008)

33. Patil, B., et al.: Approaches to Distributed mobility management using Mobile IPv6 and its extensions. IETF Dratf draft-patil-mext-dmm-approaches-02 (2011)
34. Devarapalli, V., et al.: Network Mobility (NEMO) Basic Support Protocol. IETF RFC 3963 (2005)
35. Wakikawa, R., et al.: Multiple Care-of Addresses Registration. IETF RFC 5648 (2009)
36. Nordmark, E., et al.: IPv6 Socket API for Source Address Selection. IETF RFC 5014 (2007)
37. Tsirtsis, G., et al.: Flow Bindings in Mobile IPv6 and Network Mobility (NEMO) Basic Support. IETF RFC 6089 (2011)
38. Koodli, R.: Fast Handovers for Mobile IPv6. IETF RFC 4068 (2005)
39. IEEE: IEEE Standard for Local and metropolitan area networks- Part 21: Media Independent Handover (2009)
40. Lee, J., Ahn, S.: I-FHMIPv6: A Novel FMIPv6 and HMIPv6 Integration Mechanism. IETF Draft draft-jaehwoon-mipshop-ifhmipv6-01 (2006)
41. Boutabia, M., Afifi, H.: MIH-based FMIPv6 optimization for fast-moving mobiles. In: Third International Conference on Pervasive Computing and Applications, pp. 616–620 (2008)
42. Narten, T., et al.: Neighbor Discovery for IP version 6 (IPv6). IETF RFC 4861 (2007)
43. Kaufman, C., et al.: Internet Key Exchange Protocol Version 2 (IKEv2). IETF RFC 5996 (2010)
44. Buschmann, F.: Pattern-Oriented Software Architecture: A System of Patterns. Wiley (1996)
45. FP7-ICT CONCERTO project and MIP6D-NG official websites:
    http://ict-concerto.eu, http://www.mip6d-ng.net

Bridging Social Media Technologies and Scientific Research: A Twitter-Enabled Platform for VPH Modeling

Vangelis Sakkalis, Stelios Sfakianakis, and Kostas Marias

Computational Medicine Laboratory, Institute of Computer Science,
FORTH, Heraklion, Greece
{sakkalis,ssfak,kmarias}@ics.forth.gr
http://www.ics.forth.gr/cml/

Abstract. Social media and the Web2.0 technologies are ubiquitous and due to the advances in mobile communication protocols, operating systems, and internet standards they are now supported even in cell phones and tablets. We are not yet at the point where a cell phone can be used as a medical device but such small and omnipresent instruments can be used in a way that promotes research in the clinical and biomedical domain. In this paper we describe a collaborative platform for designing composite simulations for the Virtual Physiological Human (VPH) community needs. We investigate the use of pervasive mobile technologies so that scientists and researchers can easily design, share, and execute simulations. The proposed platform supports real time notification and sharing of the results, and share the results and related artifacts with their work group and colleagues.

Keywords: Social Networks, inSilico Oncology, Scientific Workflows.

1 Introduction

The focus of this paper falls in healthcare and more specifically in the research VPH community [1] [2] . Social web 2.0 and especially Medicine 2.0 refer to the generation of content by users, the power of networks, personalized health care, and the focus on collaboration across all stakeholders [3].

Starting back at the late 90's there have been a strong initiative to effectively apply Social Media tools to improve Heath care by actively engaging apart from patients themselves, researchers, practitioners and whole hospitals with the mission to promote health and fight disease. On one hand it is difficult enough to engage a busy physician and even more, specialized staff of hospitals and research centers. Fortunately, on the other hand, social media is the vehicle to decrease diffusion time for cancer research and innovations. Both patients [4] and researchers can benefit from such an empower network in very specific ways. Patients, in sites like PatientsLikeMe[1], may share intimate details of their

---

[1] http://www.patientslikeme.com

B. Godara and K.S. Nikita (Eds.): MobiHealth 2012, LNICST 61, pp. 380–387, 2013.
© Institute for Computer Sciences, Social Informatics and Telecommunications Engineering 2013

symptoms, diagnosis and treatment as well as discuss in respective groups about their condition [5]. This becomes even more crucial in diseases like cancer where treatment is merely personalized [6] and can be a controversial subject. In parallel, the research community may advocate for and against certain therapeutical schemes and computational "inSilico" models [7] [2] by rating and sharing their views on published models. Of course such online exchanges might not be ideally documented, but since they engage only experts in the field of computational oncology it is expected to disseminate accurate and noteworthy information that could pave the way towards new effective therapies.

In this paper we argue that the scientific community can gain a lot by the adoption of the social media tools and practices. As a show case we focus on the integration of a web application for the construction of scientific workflows with the micro-blogging service Twitter. In the following sections we present our application and the relevant scientific domain of interest. Then we describe the Twitter platform and we use its social networking infrastructure for the VPH modeling needs. In conclusion we present the challenges, the benefits of the approach, and future enhancements.

2   The Social Web

In spite of its success and popularity the early version of the World Wide Web lacked in many respects, ranging from user accessibility and user interface design, to the ability to repurpose and remix existing Web-based data in not pre-established ways. Most of these concerns have been addressed by advanced technologies for searching (Search engines), syndicating (RSS feeds), visualization and presentation mechanisms (CSS, SVG), etc. An additional limitation of this environment is that the people are not part of the equation. Users are expected to be the actors triggering the web interactions but content delivered should be personalized, relevant to the users context and needs, and users communication and collaboration should be promoted.

These and other requirements are the ones that the Social Web tries to tackle. Social Web does not represent a shift or radical change in technology per se but it represents rather a shift on the perception of the human – machine interaction by placing the users in the centre of the system and in control of these interactions. The requirements for implementing Social Web led to the emergence of a new breed of web applications and sites, collectively identified as "Web 2.0" by Tim O' Reilly [8], whose major design principle is to "harness network effects to get better the more people use them". The value of "Web 2.0" sites and applications therefore comes to a large extent by the number of users participating and actively communicating and sharing through them so the term "Social Web" is actually a synonym. The social nature of this Web is evident when the collaboration of people and their active contribution is considered.

Social Websites require a Social Network Infrastructure enabling of building social relations among individual researchers. Such a infrastructure provides services to represent a user by a personal profile, to develop social networks with other actors, and to generate, collect and aggregate social activity in an activity stream. The main function is to create and update User Description profiles, to develop *follower networks*, to interact in the social environment, and to build and access activity streams. Users store personal data in user profiles and publish the data in their social network. In their follower networks, users can follow the activity of other users, activity in groups and communities, or on "tags". In the next paragraph we describe Twitter, one such social network infrastructure, that we integrate with.

2.1 Twitter

Twitter is a form of free micro-blogging which allows users to send and receive short public messages called "tweets". Tweets are limited to no more than 140 characters, and can include links to blogs, web pages, images, videos and all other material online. By following other people and sources, users are able to build up an instant, personalized Twitter feed that meets their full range of interests, both academic and personal.

More than 200 million are the daily Twitter users worldwide including thousands of academics and researchers at all levels of experience and different disciplines. The hard limit of 140 characters for the tweets provides the benefit of more instant updates and better "throughput" in terms of the number of messages a user is expected to read. Especially in the research community social media seems to surpass traditional publication media: Papers are increasingly being taken apart in blogs, on Twitter and on other social media within hours rather than years, and in public, rather than at small conferences or in private conversation [9] . Twitter forms social (sub)networks of people with common intentions and interests. Such networks were found to have a high degree correlation and reciprocity, indicating close mutual acquaintances among users [10].

A Glossary of Frequently Used Twitter Terms

Tweet (noun). A message posted via Twitter containing 140 characters or fewer.

Follow. To follow someone on Twitter is to subscribe to their Tweets or updates on the site. Following another user means that all their tweets will appear in your feed.

Follower. A follower is another Twitter user who has followed you.

Hashtag. The # symbol is used to mark keywords or topics in a Tweet.

Direct Message. A tweet that is private between the sender and recipient.

Mention. Mentioning another user in your Tweet by including the @ sign followed directly by their username is called a "mention"

Retweet (noun). A tweet by another user, forwarded to you by someone you follow. Often used to spread news or share valuable findings on Twitter.

3   A Web Based Platform for Scientific Workflow Design

A *workflow management system* is a computer system that manages and defines a series of tasks within an organization to produce a final outcome. In essence, a workow can be abstracted as a composite service, i.e. a service that is composed by other services that are orchestrated in order to perform some higher level functionality. In the recent years, Scientific workflow systems have emerged as the enabling technology for e-Science. Scientists collaborate on large scale scientific experiments and knowledge discovery applications using distributed systems of computing resources, data sets, and devices [11],[12].

The Thespis Workflow system is a web based graphical workflow designer focusing on the construction of VPH "hypermodels" by connecting "simpler" (atomic) models. The objective of this tool is to provide an intuitive environment for biomedical researchers and computational biologists where simulation models retrieved from different model repositories [13], can be combined to form higher level experiments implemented and managed as "workflows". Hence, Thespis is a useful platform for linking different models reflecting multiple biocomplexity levels in order to simulate complex processes (e.g. "microscopic" for genes and enzymes, to "macroscopic" scales at the tissue level) [14]. Figure 1 illustrates a typical workflow where different simulation models and are linked together. Through the exchange of data via the connections between their inputs and outputs perform a complex high level task. Such workflows can be the tools for the implementation of multi-scale biological modeling [7].

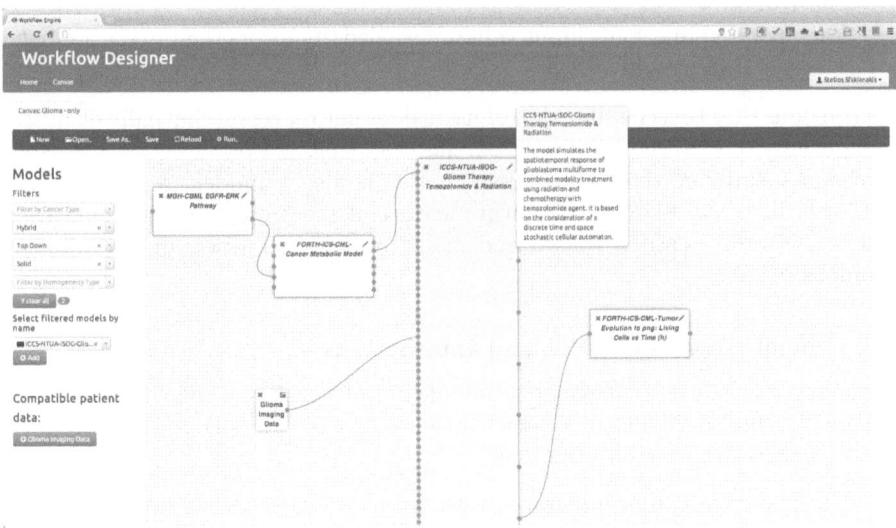

Fig. 1. A screenshot of the workflow designer

The Thespis workflow environment consists of two main components:

- The **workflow editor** (or designer) is a web application, accessible through the users' web browser. This is the graphical front-end for the editing of the workflows, the invocation of their execution, and the visualization of the results.
- The **workflow engine** is the server side, which is responsible for the management and the execution of the workflows, the communication with the model repositories, etc.

From the user point of view each user is required to register with the application and provide some information about himself, like the organization he works with, a description of his research and other interests, etc. The user authentication is supported either in a "traditional" way through some user name and password, or by linking their account with the account they maintain in some social networking site like Twitter, Facebook, or Google. In the latter case the authentication is taking place in the social networking site and the workflow application is granted authorization using the open standard oAuth [15]

In this application one can generally recognize three different types of users:

- The Model Creator (MC), who is the VPH researcher that builds new models and make them available, by publishing them in some model repository [13].
- The Workflow Creator (WC), who is the researcher that designs a new workflow by selecting existing models and tools, coupling them together based on their inputs and outputs, and possibly providing fixed parameter values for some of them.
- The Workflow User (WU), who is the user running ("enacts") existing workflows by providing some input values if needed, monitors their execution, and retrieves their results.

It is obvious that this classification of users does not represent mutually exclusive user groups. For example, it can be the case that a workflow user is also a workflow creator or that a workflow creator is also a model creator. In fact, the latter case corresponds to a future feature of the presented web application where a workflow can be reused and made available as a new model, albeit a "composite" one.

3.1   Social Based Facilities and Interactions

In the core of the user management module of the workflow application there are a number of Social Web inspired mechanisms that aim to enable the collaboration and communication among the users:

- The workflows can be annotated with "tags", i.e. free text keywords supplied by the users. These keywords can be used for the searching and classifying the workflows. By default the user submitted tags are public, which means that they are visible and can be used as filters in other users' searches, but if desired the user can make them private. Additionally private and public tags can be intermixed in the annotation of a single workflow.

- The users can have "favorite" workflows. This is useful to the workflow users so that they can better classify the most valuable workflows for their research. It is also useful to the workflow creator in order to get some feedback about the use of his/her workflows and possibly increase their "reputation" points.
- The platform keeps also statistics about the use of the workflows and the models in order to be able to answer questions like what is the most frequently used model or the workflow that has been enacted the most times.

However, to further leverage the potential of the social networks and especially Twitter we have defined a number of scenarios that reuse existing social networks and the online activity of the users. The objective of this work is to bring researchers together and to provide facilities for improving and advancing their work. To this end we have identified the following use cases where integration with a social platform like Twitter can help:

- Workflow creators and users want to know about the usage and the rating of their workflows and models, respectively.
- Workflow users want to notified when a new version of their favorite workflow is available.
- Workflow creators want to be notified when a new version of a model participating in their workflows is released.
- All users may be interested for new models become available.

For these and other scenarios the Twitter infrastructure is used to provide status updates for the interested users. First of all the workflow application maintains a twitter account (@thespisapp) as a "broadcast" account for news, notifications, etc. The users are encouraged to follow this user in order to get updates for new features of the application, general news, etc., but also for being able to receive personalized "direct messages" from the application. Furthermore, Thespis is using tweets for information that is potentially interesting to all its followers and direct messages if the information is considered more personal or of limited scope. Additionally it uses "hash tags" to annotate the messages with keywords that can be used for filtering and defining a personalized direct messaging functionality of Twitter. Examples of how this functionality is implemented through Twitter follows:

- When a new model is registered @thespisapp *tweets* about it *mentioning* the twitter user who created the model.
- When a new workflow is created @thespisapp *tweets* about it *mentioning* the twitter user who created the workflow and additionally sends *direct messages* to the creators of the models participating in this workflow.
- When a workflow is altered, the users who have annotated it as "favorite" receive *direct messages*.
- When a workflow becomes "favorite", its creator is notified with a *direct message mentioning* the twitter account of the user who liked it.

In general the methodology is to keep the status updates of the broadcast account of the application "noise-free" and prefer the use of direct messages to transmit information to the interested users. The reason for this is that `@thespisapp` can be followed by non registered users or people that are interested in the specific application domain but have not yet sign up. Another design principle is that tweets or direct messages mention related users. The rationale is that we try to connect the users and build a user research community around this workflow application.

4   Conclusions

The proposed twitter-enabled workflow creation environment is expected to provide VPH community with a social media enabled environment that facilitates knowledge management and transfer for the VPH community to benefit. Thespis concept allows researchers to design and share custom workflows but also alert users and colleagues of potential new models and workflows of interest. Ratings and usage statistics of existing models or workflows raise community awareness and builds virtual research communities where experts speak with each other and have advise to share. Such tools made available in the open source community are expected to engage more newcomers to the VPH community.

The social networking features of the workflow application presented here are currently available in a prototype version. The application will be evaluated in the context of the "YPERTHEN"[2] and there are still some ideas for future work focusing on providing more personalized information to the users. For example, the application could recommend existing models based on their rating to new workflow users [16] and notify existing modelers about newly inserted models capable of being coupled with existing ones.

There are a number of challenges though. Twitter has recently changed the rules of their API and the new rules restrict the number of tweets or direct messages made per account. This will have an impact to the workflow application when a large number of users need to be notified with direct messages. Another possible limitation is that the content in Twitter is public by default and as is the case with any Web/Cloud based platform the user can not always be pretty sure that his/her data are kept private and used for the intended purpose only. Nevertheless, for this application the data exchange are minimal and only references (through hyperlinks or tags) to the possibly intellectually protected information are shared. In any case, what worries more the expert community is finding ways to ensure that accurate information and validated models are only published online, but nevertheless countering bias and misinformation has been a long lasting concern especially during election periods!

Acknowledgements. This work was supported by the community initiative Program INTERREG III, Project "YPERTHEN", financed by the European Commission through the European Regional Development Fund and by National Funds of Greece and Cyprus, and also the TUMOR (FP7-ICT-2009.5.4-247754) project.

---

[2] `http://www.yperthen.gr`

References

1. Clapworthy, G., Kohl, P., Gregerson, H., Thomas, S., et al.: Digital human modelling: a global vision and a european perspective. Digital Human Modeling, 549–558 (2007)
2. Marias, K., Dionysiou, D., Sakkalis, V., Graf, N., et al.: Clinically driven design of multi-scale cancer models: the ContraCancrum project paradigm. Interface Focus 1, 450–461 (2011)
3. Hughes, B., Joshi, I., Wareham, J.: Health 2.0 and medicine 2.0: tensions and controversies in the field. Journal of Medical Internet Research 10 (2008)
4. Basdekis, I., Sakkalis, V., Stephanidis, C.: Towards an accessible personal health record. In: Nikita, K.S., Lin, J.C., Fotiadis, D.I., Arredondo Waldmeyer, M.-T. (eds.) MobiHealth 2011. LNICST, vol. 83, pp. 61–68. Springer, Heidelberg (2012)
5. Brownstein, C., Brownstein, J., Williams, D., Wicks, P., Heywood, J.: The power of social networking in medicine. Nature Biotechnology 27, 888–890 (2009)
6. Roniotis, A., Marias, K., Sakkalis, V., Manikis, G.C., Zervakis, M.: Simulating Radiotherapy Effect in High-Grade Glioma by Using Diffusive Modeling and Brain Atlases. Journal of Biomedicine and Biotechnology 2012, 9 (2012)
7. Sakkalis, V., Sfakianakis, S., Marias, K., Stamatakos, G., et al.: The TUMOR Project: Integrating cancer model repositories for supporting predictive oncology. In: 2nd Virtual Physiological Human Conference, VPH 2012 (2012)
8. OReilly, T.: What is web 2.0: Design patterns and business models for the next generation of software. Communications & strategies, 17 (2007)
9. Mandavilli, A.: Peer review: Trial by twitter. Nature 469, 286–287 (2011)
10. Java, A., Song, X., Finin, T., Tseng, B.: Why we twitter: understanding microblogging usage and communities. In: Proceedings of the 9th WebKDD and 1st SNA-KDD 2007 Workshop on Web Mining and Social Network Analysis, pp. 56–65. ACM (2007)
11. Barker, A., van Hemert, J.: Scientific Workflow: A Survey and Research Directions. In: Wyrzykowski, R., Dongarra, J., Karczewski, K., Wasniewski, J. (eds.) PPAM 2007. LNCS, vol. 4967, pp. 746–753. Springer, Heidelberg (2008)
12. Curcin, V., Ghanem, M.: Scientific workflow systems-can one size fit all? In: Cairo International Biomedical Engineering Conference, pp. 1–9. IEEE (2008)
13. Sfakianakis, S., Sakkalis, V., Marias, K., Stamatakos, G., McKeever, S., Deisboeck, T., Graf, N.: An architecture for integrating cancer model repositories. In: Conf. Proc. IEEE Eng. Med. Biol. Soc., pp. 6828–6831. IEEE (2012)
14. Southern, J., Pitt-Francis, J., Whiteley, J., Stokeley, D., Kobashi, H., Nobes, R., Kadooka, Y., Gavaghan, D., et al.: Multi-scale computational modelling in biology and physiology. Progress in Biophysics and Molecular Biology 96, 60 (2008)
15. Leiba, B.: Oauth web authorization protocol. IEEE Internet Computing 16, 74–77 (2012)
16. Lakiotaki, K., Delias, P., Sakkalis, V., Matsatsinis, N.: User profiling based on multi-criteria analysis: the role of utility functions. Operational Research 9, 3–16 (2009)

Depression Diagnostic and Screening Tools Using Android OS Platform

Muhammad Hafeez Shamsul Bahri, Hasmila A. Omar, Norliza Zaini,
Haryanti Norhazman, Lucyantie Mazalan, Mohd Fuad Latip,
Mohd Nasir Taib, and Saharin Ghazali

MARA University of Technology, UiTM Shah Alam, 40450 Selangor, Malaysia
{hasmila,lucyantie,drnorliza}@salam.uitm.edu.my,
{muhdhafeez.sb,haryanti7076,fuadlatip}@gmail.com,
drnasir@ieee.org, saharin.ghazali@yahoo.com

Abstract. Depression affects all walks of life and is a common form of mental health illness. Some of the common methods to diagnose depression are usually through a session with certified psychiatrist or with the aid of depression rating scales. This paper seeks to provide both clinicians and patients with an Android based mobile application that may store and calculate results based on depression rating scales i.e. DASS and MINI. A novel approach of combining both questionnaire statistics is proposed in one solution. As such, a tablet friendly application that uses a scoring algorithm and a series of psychiatric questionnaires as an indicator to a person's mental state or depression level is developed by means of an android platform.

Keywords: Mental depression level, Android application, Mobile depression questionnaire, Depression Rating Scale, DASS, MINI.

1 Introduction

Technology is aimed at making our lives easier. This in turn enables us to accomplish many things at once for multitasking purposes. Looking at the electronic gadgets for example, where the sizes are getting smaller, lighter and the processor's speed is faster. There are laptops, smartphones and the latest trend is tablets where miniaturizations take place. The electronics industry now is at its most competitive state, where a lot of companies are introducing their products into the market ever more quickly in order to get ahead in the industry. This scenario in turn makes other industries to adapt quickly to these latest of technology aiming to make our jobs easier and runs more efficiently.

The brain is one of the most hardworking organs we have. Our work efficiency is very much dictated by the state our mind, therefore it is monumental that the mind stays healthy. One of the common mental illnesses is depression, which can affect all walks of life. It can affect a person's ability to work, form relationships and destroy their quality of life. At its most severe state, depression can lead to suicide and is

B. Godara and K.S. Nikita (Eds.): MobiHealth 2012, LNICST 61, pp. 388–397, 2013.

responsible for 850,000 deaths every year. New research published in BioMed Central's open access journal BMC Medicine compares social conditions with depression in 18 countries across the world [1]. There are many levels of depression and each has its own treatment; to name a few: Major Depressive, recurrent Major Depressive, and Major depressive with Melancholic features.

At present, depression is formally diagnosed by clinicians during therapy sessions and can also be aided by the use of depression rating scales. A depression rating scale consists of a series of psychiatric questionnaires with unique scoring algorithm, which indicates the severity of the depression symptoms. There are several depression rating scales available. In this paper, a hybrid approach of combining two types of depression rating scales i.e. Depression Anxiety Stress Scales (DASS) and Mini-international neuropsychiatric interview (MINI) is proposed. Although these rating scales are commonly used by clinician to indicate the severity of depression symptoms, however there are no tablet-friendly applications that will ease the process.

The tablet usage is growing rapidly over the past few years. The APPLE iPad had started off to rave reviews, and is expected to increase its volumes and further surpasses its competition. However other tablet computers, in particular those based on Google's Android operating system, are expected to erode its share of a fast-growing market [2]. Tablets are indeed a very versatile electronic device; it is light enough to be carried by hand in extensive periods, and large enough to be used as a display for daily use or even professional use. Hence it is practical to use the tablet as a platform to house the application. The application runs on Google Android, which is the first complete, open, and free mobile platform developed by Open Handset Alliance™ (OHA) [3].

The finished application prototype has achieved these three primary goals:

1. A working algorithm which calculate the results for DASS and MINI questionnaire
2. A database which housed psychiatrist and patient's profiles and questionnaires.
3. A successfully developed application using JAVA programming language with a user interface on Android platform for displaying user profiles and results history.

2   Related Work

Depression is regarded as a mental state or chronic mental disorder characterized by feelings of sadness, loneliness, despair, low self-esteem, and self-reproach; accompanying signs that include psychomotor retardation (or less frequently agitation), withdrawal from social contact, and vegetative states such as loss of appetite and insomnia. There have been a number of research studies addressing depression that includes depression screening and detection, data analysis and classification approach [4, 5] as well as study on the effects of depression [6].

Previous works that relate to depression screening system and detection however varies ranging from software-based to hardware-based, mostly integrating not only questionnaires response and text as a subject's input to the system but also images and voice as well. Similar research was conducted by Akan et. al. by having a pilot study that screens for depressed patients using a web based application called the eScreening tool. This tool provides a graphical user interface, audio output and a database presenting the PHQ-9 and CAGE screening tests [7]. Arianti et. al. has developed a depression inventory system called the Beck Depression Inventory II Test that works as an assessment tool for the healthcare professional to diagnose depression level of a patient [8]. A different type of depression acquisition was reported by Moore et. al. using the self-rated mood data to forecast future depression ratings. The data used in the study have been collected using SMS text messaging and comprises one time series of approximately weekly mood ratings for each patient analyzed using forecasting method [9]. Some other related applications were proposed by Bevilacqua et. al [10] and Kipli et. al. [11] that presents depression detection tools using image and facial expression while Cohn et. al. [12] integrated both facial and vocal prosody in recognizing patient with depression. Another depression detection system focusing on hardware was also introduced by Leon et. al.[13] called the smart home-based detection for depressive disorder. Despite all the research works mentioned, there is no tablet-friendly application which integrates both MINI and DASS questionnaires for depression detection purposes.

3   Android Operating System

Android Operating System is a software stack for mobile devices based on Linux with a Java programming interface. The Android SDK provides the tools, e.g. a compiler, debugger and a device emulator as well as its own Java Virtual machine (Dalvik Virtual Machine - DVM). Android OS supports 2-D and 3-D graphics using the OpenGL libraries and supports data storage in a SQLite database.

A smartphone pre-installed with Google Android SDK v2.3.6 (Gingerbread) is used to showcase this application prototype. Android applications are generally forward-compatible with new versions of the Android platform and higher Application Programming Interface (API) levels [14]. The application should be able to run on all later versions of the Android platform. Android operating system uses its own Virtual Machine called Dalvik Virtual Machine (DVM), which interprets and executes portable Java-style byte code after transforming it, which is optimized to operate on the mobile platform [15]. Android phones ship with a rich array of built-in activities (services), including email, a Web browser, and a map application [16].The platform embraces a replace-and-reuse philosophy, which lets users customize the phone [17].

3.1   Android Development Tools (ADT) for Eclipse Indigo IDE

Eclipse is an integrated development environment (IDE) for Java and its SDK is free and open source software [18]. Google provides the Android Development Tools (ADT) to develop Android applications with Eclipse. ADT extends the capabilities of Eclipse by enabling quick set up of new Android projects, creating application UI, adding packages based on Android Framework API, debugging applications using the Android SDK tools, and even export signed (or unsigned) ".apk" files in order to distribute the application [19]. ADT also provides an Android device emulator (Android Virtual Device), so that Android applications can be tested without a real Android phone. The application is developed using Eclipse with ADT.

4   DASS Questionnaire

Depression Anxiety Stress Scale (DASS) is an example of a self-report instrument. Depression can be diagnosed through several methods. Traditionally, a qualified person in the psychiatric field may evaluate patient's mental state by having a one-to-one interview session. This is the commonly used method, however it is time consuming and not easily accessible by the medical practitioner since the patient's records are kept individually.

Another method in determining depression level of a person is through the use of psychiatric questionnaires. Although it is not used to ultimately decide whether a person is depressed, it is used to give advices to the patient to seek further help if needed. DASS scale is a set of three self-report scales designed to measure the negative emotional states of depression, anxiety and stress [20]. Table 1 depicts an example of DASS scoring which is used for this application.

5   M.I.N.I Questionnaire

The Mini-International Neuropsychiatric Interview (M.I.N.I.) is used during diagnostic interview. It was developed for DSM-IV and ICD-10 psychiatric disorders [21].Unlike DASS, MINI may be considered as a diagnostic tool for depressive disorders. The method of scoring and implying the questionnaire is also different to DASS which is a self-report instrument. MINI on the other hand, requires a licensed clinician to review and evaluate the patients. In order to calculate the scoring in the application, a slightly complex algorithm is required. All questions in the questionnaire must be rated by clinician who requires clinical judgment by the rater in coding the responses of either a Yes or No [21].

6   Methodology

6.1   Application Block Diagram

Fig.1 shows the general block diagram of the application. It shall have users profile and response from the questionnaire as an input. Users will be able to enter their profile information via a user's interface (UI). The output of the application is the results of the questionnaires taken and the scoring history for both depression rating scale i.e. DASS and MINI. The score history is managed by SQLite.

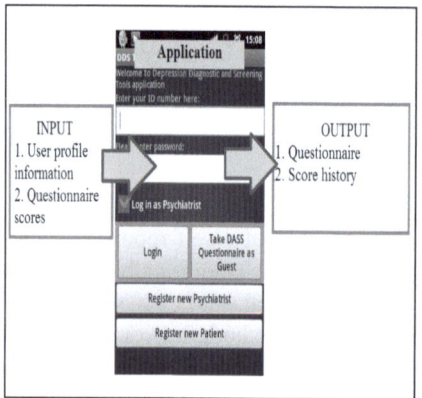
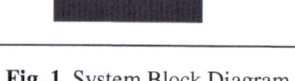
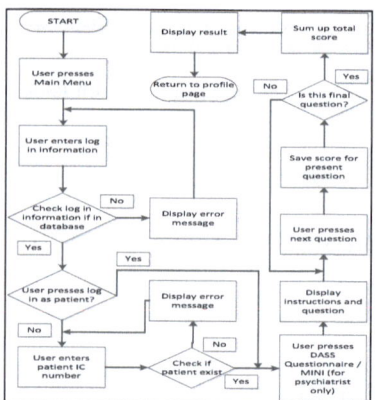

Fig. 1. System Block Diagram   **Fig. 2.** Questionnaire flowchart

6.2   User Interface

There are two types of users i.e. patient or clinician. Both have different access level and user interface due to their different roles in applying the depression rating scales. DASS is a self-report instrument meanwhile MINI can only be administered by clinicians. Therefore, a patient type user will be able to take DASS questionnaire and view previous historical scores. Meanwhile, a clinician type user will have access to patient's historical records for e.g. DASS and MINI scoring history. Clinician type user will also be able to administer MINI for registered patients.

   1) **Login Interface:** Prior to using the application, users are required to login at the register page which contains text fields for users to enter information such as user name and password. Fig. 3(a) illustrates the login interface.
   2) **Questionnaire Interface:** This mobile application contains two types of depression rating scales i.e. DASS and MINI questionnaires. The style of presentation of the questions and its answer options for both rating scales are imperative due to the nature of Android devices, which are in the form of handheld devices. These handheld devices mostly have screens smaller than 10 inches diagonally. Thus, the interface should not be too cumbersome to navigate between questions and selecting answer options. Fig. 2 shows the designed flowchart for the graphical interface on the screen which shows one question at a time. The same interface will be reused for the next question and only the question element will change at the press of either next or previous question. This way, the screen is kept clean and simple. There are not too much activity going on the screen and therefore it is easy to navigate between questions. Score options uses radio type button in which only one can be selected at any time. This prevents multiple answers for any single question. The element for this interface is set to scrolling type, so that the questions may be viewed comfortably in horizontal view. Fig. 3(b) illustrates an example of questionnaire interface.

3) Profile Interface: Fig. 3(c) illustrates a sample of profile page interface for patient type user. It displays profile of the patient, the patient's DASS and MINI result history as well as questionnaires button. The view for patient's result history is toggled between DASS and MINI due to space limitations.

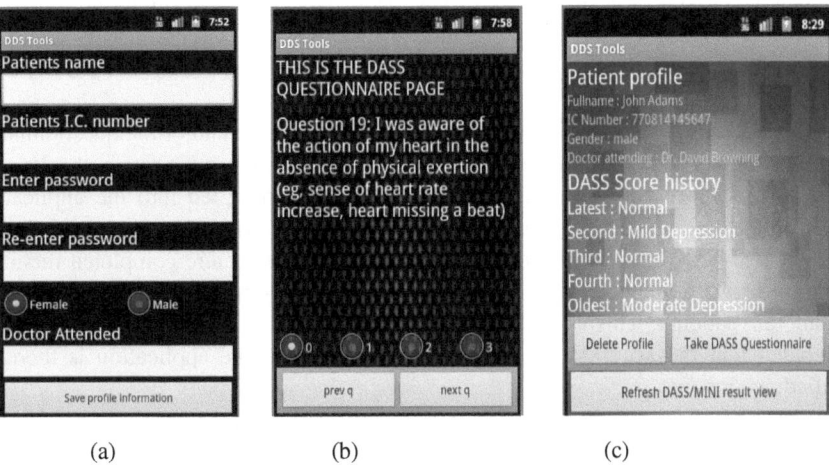

(a)   (b)   (c)

Fig. 3.

6.3   Scoring Algorithm

1) **DASS questionnaire scoring:** DASS questionnaire requires the patients to rate themselves a rating between 0-3. The number basically represents the score for each question. The scoring is done by summing up the total score and the corresponding depression classification based on the score as shown in Table 1.

2) **MINI questionnaire scoring:**   Scoring for MINI questionnaire is more complex compared to the DASS scoring system. In MINI questionnaire, patient is given two answers to choose from: Yes or No. The MINI questionnaire has a total of 16 modules, but only relevant module i.e. Module A - Depression Rating Module is selected. In Module A, there are a total of 17 questions. The session may end at any point and not necessarily for all 17 questions to be answered if certain questions are answered "No". For instance, at question 2, if the patient answered question 1 and 2 with "No", the session shall end with the result being "No Major Depressive Episode". A rule-based approach is employed for the scoring algorithm.

Table 1. DASS scoring system

	Depression(D)	Anxiety(A)	Stress(SS)
Normal	0 – 9	0 – 7	0 – 14
Mild	10 - 13	8 – 9	15-18
Moderate	14 – 20	10 – 14	19 – 25
Severe	21 – 27	15 – 19	26 – 33
Extremely Severe	28+	20+	34+

7   Results

The scoring algorithm of the application is tested by conducting experiments to verify and validate its accuracy via functionality testing. Additionally, usability testing is conducted on eighteen users to analyze user's experience via an evaluation survey.

7.1   Functionality Test

The questionnaires were administered to ten subjects. At the end of the questionnaires, the total score is summed up and compared to the scale to determine the level of depression it represents. The subject's responses were then fed into the application. The results for both types of manual and application scorings are compared against each other. It was found that the scores for DASS questionnaire completed manually using forms were identical to the scores for DASS questionnaire fed to the application for all ten patients. This is true for MINI questionnaire as well. Hence it can be concluded that the accuracy of the scoring algorithm of the application is therefore verified.

7.2   Usability Test Evaluation

A usability evaluation is administered to eighteen users. It was found that 81% of the users found that the application is nicely designed. More than 93% agreed that it was easy to navigate between pages, which is quite important since navigating between questions is the core feature of the application. The placement of the texts, buttons and boxes also plays a role in ensuring that the user experience is pleasant by making it easier for user selections and user inputs. The theme of colour used in the application is deemed suitable and appropriate by 93% of the respondent. The right choice of colour is important as it could affect the mood of the user and may have an impact on users' experience. It seems that 87.5% of users agreed that the questions were appropriately presented in such a way that it is easy to read through. The choice of font type and size for the questions also plays a role. The questions are fairly easy to understand as 77% users agreed to it. Almost 94% of the users felt the scoring method used in the application is convenient. More than 75% user prefers to take the questionnaire electronically as compared to the conventional way of using pen and paper. In conclusion, users agree that the application were easy to use. This was reflected by the fact that more than 88% of users are satisfied with the overall experience in using the application as illustrated by Fig. 4. Meanwhile, Fig. 5 shows a comparison of user's self-rating prior to using the application and user's depression level analysed by the application. The result compares well which shows that the application serves its purpose in detecting depression levels.

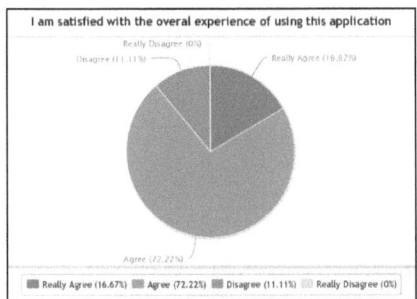
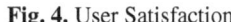

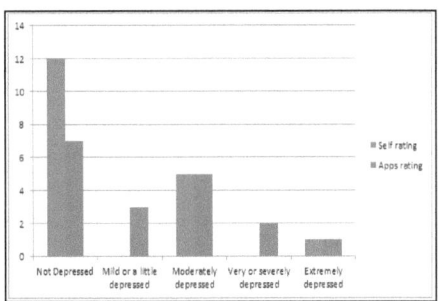

Fig. 4. User Satisfaction   **Fig. 5.** Apps v/s Self Rating Comparison

8   Conclusion

The depression diagnostic and screening tool application has been successfully developed. The Android application were created using JAVA Eclipse IDE with Android ADT plugin. It has a user-friendly graphical interface for registering profiles, answering DASS or MINI questionnaires, and viewing score history. This application has the ability to store user profile information for both patients and psychiatrist. This is done through creating and managing databases using the SQLite library. The database is stored locally on the device where the information is secured.

The application successfully replicates both DASS and MINI scoring schemes. The scoring algorithm developed based on DASS and MINI questionnaire is able to correctly classify the level of depressions. Additionally, MINI questionnaire scoring algorithm provides an extra assistance during the interview session as it automatically navigates through the questionnaire as it progresses. There are some questions that can be skipped after a certain condition is met hence cutting down processing time to administer the MINI depression rating scales significantly. This certainly eases the whole interview process. Moreover, an automated system using the Android application reduces the chances of human error while computing the results. Most importantly, the application may also serve as a mobile patient management and monitoring system as it helps clinicians to monitor patients' depression level effectively over time. The mobile application is also robust enough to be upgraded with additional features for future reference. Usability testing on real-life user shows that majority of the user is satisfied with the overall experience while using the application.

Future work calls for further development to upgrade the stand alone application to a server based application. As such, an online mobile patient monitoring and management system with extended features is to be developed. This requires online connections to the server. Clinicians shall have access to patient's records in the database anywhere and everywhere internet is available.

In conclusion, throughout the paper it is shown that a mobile device may assist in diagnosing and screening depressive disorder. It is hoped that this prototyped mobile application shall further assist the clinicians in the field of mental health for depression diagnostic and screening tool that can be used on a more widely available platform.

Acknowledgment. This research is funded by the Fundamental & Exploratory Research Grants Scheme Research, Ministry of Higher Education Malaysia.

References

1. Glover, D.H.: Scientific Press Officer, BioMed. Central
2. Kenney, M., Pon, B.: Structuring the Smartphone Industry: Is the Mobile Internet OS Platform the Key? Journal of Industrial Compet. Trade 11, 230–261 (2011)
3. Home(n.d), http://www.openhandsetalliance.com/index.html
4. Zhang, Z.-X., Tian, X.-W., Lim, J.S.: New Algorithm for the Depression Diagnosis using HRV: A Neuro-Fuzzy Approach. In: Proceedings of the International Symposium on Digital Object Identifier and Bioinformatics, pp. 283–286 (2011)
5. Li, Y., Li, Y., Tong, S., Tang, Y., Zhu, Y.: More Normal EEGs of Depression Patients during Mental Arithmetic than Rest. In: Proceedings of the International Conference on Functional Biomedical Imaging, pp. 165–168 (2007)
6. Yukimasa, T., Yoshimura, R., Nakamura, J.: Effects of High-Frequency Repetitive Transracial Magnetic Stimulation on the Treatment-Resistant Depression and Its Mechanism. In: Proceedings of 3rd International Conference on Innovative Computing Information and Control, p. 336 (2008)
7. Akan, K.D., Farrell, S.P., Zerull, L.M., Mahone, I.H., Guerlain, S.: eScreening: Developing an Electronic Screening Tool for Rural Primary Care. In: Proceedings of the Systems and Information Engineering Design Symposium, pp. 212–215 (2006)
8. Ariyanti, R.D., Kusumadewi, S., Paputungan, I.V.: Beck Depression Inventory Test Assessment Using Fuzzy Inference System. In: Proceedings of the International Conference on Intelligent Systems, Modelling and Simulation, pp. 6–9 (2010)
9. Moore, P.J., Little, M.A., McSharry, P.E., Geddes, J.R., Goodwin, G.M.: Forecasting Depression in Bipolar Disorder. In: Proceedings of the IEEE Transaction on Biomedical Engineering, pp. 2801–2807 (2012)
10. Bevilacqua, V., D'Ambruoso, D., Mandolino, G., Suma, M.: A New Tool to Support Diagnosis of Neurological Disorders by Means of Facial Expressions. In: Proceedings of the IEEE International Workshop on Medical Measurements and Applications, pp. 544–549 (2011)
11. Kipli, K., Kouzani, A.Z., Joordens, M.: Computer-Aided Detection of Depression from Magnetic Resonance Images. In: Proceedings of the International Conference on Complex Medical Engineering, pp. 500–505 (2012)
12. Cohn, J.F., Kruez, T.S., Matthews, I., Yang, Y., Nguyen, M.H., Padilla, M.T., Zhou, F., De la Torre, F.: Detecting Depression from Facial Actions and Vocal Prosody. In: Proceedings of the 3rd International Conference on Affective Computing and Intelligent Interaction and Workshops, pp. 1–7 (2009)
13. Leon, E., Montejo, M., Dorronsoro, I.: Prospect of Smart Home-Based Detection of Subclinical Depressive Disorders. In: Proceedings of the International Conference on Pervasive Computing Technologies for Healthcare (PervasiveHealth), pp. 452–457 (2011)
14. Android API Levels | Android Developers. (n.d), http://developer.android.com/guide/appendix/api-levels.html
15. Java SE Overview- at a Glance(n.d), http://www.oracle.com/technetwork/java/javase/overview/index.html
16. Gandhewar, N., Sheikh, R.: Google Android: An Emerging Software Platform For Mobile Devices (2010)

17. Butler, M.: Android: Changing the Mobile Landscape. IEEE Pervasive Computing 10, 4–7 (2011)
18. Vogel, L.: Android Development Tutorial (March 6, 2012),
    `http://www.vogella.com/articles/Android/article.html`
19. Google.Inc, ADT Plugin for Eclipse (May 30, 2012),
    `http://developer.android.com/sdk/eclipse-adt.html`
20. Lovibond, P., Lovibond, S.H.: The Structure of Negative Emotional States: Comparison of the Depression Anxiety Stress Scale (DASS) with the Beck Depression and Anxiety Inventories. Elsevier Science Ltd. (1995)
21. Sheehan, D.V., Lecrubier, Y.: MINI 5.0

Empowering Patients through a Patient Portal for an Improved Diabetes Management

Ioannis Karatzanis[1], Vasilis Kontogiannis[1], Emmanouil G. Spanakis[1],
Franco Chiarugi[1], Joanna Fursse[2], and Russell W. Jones[2]

[1] Computational Medicine Laboratory, Institute of Computer Science,
Foundation for Research and Technology - Hellas, Heraklion, Crete, Greece
`{karatzan,vasilisk,spanakis,chiarugi}@ics.forth.gr`
[2] Chorleywood Health Centre, Chorleywood, Hertfordshire, United Kingdom
`j.fursse@gmail.com, russellwjones@live.com`

Abstract. Type 2 diabetes is increasing worldwide. When compared with other chronic diseases, deaths due directly to type 2 diabetes are less. The problem though, is the mortality rates caused by the consequences of type 2 diabetes; complications that represent a major health burden which may destabilise health economies. Recognised complications are: cardiovascular disease, peripheral vascular disease, renal failure, retinal eye disease, and neuropathy leading to high levels of morbidity and mortality from heart attack, foot ulceration and leg amputation, stroke, renal failure, and blindness. Better care of type 2 diabetes and early recognition and treatment of its complications reduce levels of morbidity and mortality. There is a need to support the diabetic patient in achieving effective glucose control and life-style changes leading to improved nutrition and healthy levels of physical activity, and to early recognize and treat complications. To make this possible and efficient, a patient portal has been developed, as part of the REACTION platform, which supports interactions between the diabetic patient and both their professional and non-professional carers. Introducing the patient portal and the REACTION platform to real-life healthcare systems will empower patients more by increasing their ability to self-manage, improve the quality of their life and the overall management of their diabetes, reduce the risk of developing complications and lessen their use of health services.

Keywords: Patient empowerment, Patient portal, Diabetes management, Blood glucose measurement, Insulin delivery, Closed-loop control.

1   Introduction

Diabetes mellitus is a state of high blood glucose concentration (hyperglycaemia). It is caused by impaired secretion and/or effectiveness of insulin. There are a number of causes of diabetes mellitus and many diseases that develop because of it; it is difficult to determine a single and simple definition of diabetes mellitus. In essence, without insulin, cells cannot use glucose effectively. This metabolic fault varies in its impact

B. Godara and K.S. Nikita (Eds.): MobiHealth 2012, LNICST 61, pp. 398–405, 2013.

from an acute life-threatening illness to impaired glucose tolerance that is without apparent clinical effect.

There are two forms of diabetes. The auto-immune destruction of β-cells of the Islets of Langerhans in the pancreas causes type 1 diabetes. This occurs in children and young adults. People with type 2 diabetes, usually over 50 years old with additional health problems, exhibit reduced insulin production and resistance or reduced sensitivity to insulin [1]. There are young people now presenting with type 2 diabetes in whom there is an abnormality of the glucokinase gene and others who secrete less potent insulin because of a genetic error. There is a further group of people who become type 2 diabetics because of the impact of impaired placental function and maternal malnutrition on the development of their β-cells. Type 2 diabetes is increasing markedly and has a number of causes.

Life-style change in the last century has led to an increase of almost epidemic proportions in the incidence of diabetes worldwide. This is mainly related to type 2 diabetes. Together with genetic susceptibility in certain ethnic groups, type 2 diabetes is brought on by environmental, social and behavioural factors such as bad life-style, physical inactivity, overly rich nutrition and obesity [2]. The increased incidence and the population growth and ageing have raised the number of people with diabetes worldwide [3]. In 2010 the world prevalence of diabetes among adults (aged 20–79 years) was 6.4%, affecting 285 million adults. An increase to 7.7% and 439 million adults by 2030 can be expected. Between 2010 and 2030, there will be a 69% increase in numbers of adults with diabetes in developing countries and a 20% increase in developed countries [4]. The global health expenditure on diabetes was about $376 billion in 2010 and it is estimated to be $490 billion in 2030. Globally, 12% of the health expenditures and $1330 per person have been spent on diabetes in 2010 [5]. The human and economic burden is considerable now and is destined to grow. Diabetes complications make managing diabetes more difficult and have a profound impact on levels of morbidity and mortality.

The effective care of type 1 diabetes is achieved by reducing the likelihood of both hyperglycaemic and hypoglycaemic levels of glucose by administrating basal and bolus insulin and adjusting the dosage by continuous blood glucose monitoring. Management of type 2 diabetes consists in the control of a healthy blood glucose level through oral anti-diabetic drugs (OADs) and, when necessary, insulin. Best care also involves monitoring and advising on levels of physical activity, nutrition and maintaining optimal body weight. This helps reduce the risk of complications - particularly cardiovascular diseases. In both types, people with diabetes should receive education by a specialized team skilled in the self-management of diabetes.

Patient empowerment is a new approach in health care with the point of view of having patients as active participants in the health care process for the attainment of optimal outcomes [6]. The active participation implies a higher involvement in the decision making process. An appropriate decision making can be performed only if a proper communication between patient and clinicians is assured and the patient is provided with appropriate education material and supported with the necessary information resources. An appropriate use of healthcare best practice supported by electronic processes and communication (eHealth) may enable the patient empowerment, especially in case of patients with chronic diseases [7], where a life-long daily disease management is required.

Patient empowerment is a necessary pre-requisite of effective disease self-management. At the first European conference on patient empowerment, it was agreed that Europe cannot afford not to self-empower in case of chronic disease management, since cardiovascular diseases, cancer, diabetes, obesity, and chronic respiratory diseases cause an estimated 77% of the disease burden in Europe [8]. Although self-management cannot substitute the acute care provided by professionals, it can help people with chronic diseases stay in the workforce and remain integral and active members of their community. Programmes on chronic disease self-management teach and support patients to identify warning symptoms, measure and evaluate vital signs, decide the most suitable treatment for them, and take medications.

In the specific case of diabetes more attention has to be paid to the emotional charge related to diabetes. The stress of supervising constantly their activity, diet and medication implies an emotional involvement of patients with their disease. Depression is common in diabetes and worsens levels of morbidity and mortality. Emotional distress results in poor motivation for self-management and inadequate adherence to the treatment. Thus, monitoring of depression and patient motivation are other major tasks for general practitioners in the primary care environment [9].

eHealth technological platforms can support both clinicians and patients in the short and long term management of diabetes. A key component, specifically focused on supporting patient empowerment and self-management, of such solutions is the patient (web) portal because it can provide at any time and in any place the relevant information to patients, improve their interaction with the clinicians, support education and motivation, and provide information about life-style, behaviour and emotional status. Patient portals integrate the electronic health record and the patient health record since patients themselves contribute to the maintenance of their health care information. Patient portals are more and more used in chronic disease management, but in diabetes management they have an even more fertile ground.

A recent review about patient portals for people with diabetes showed that such systems enhance interactions between patients and clinicians, increase patient overall satisfaction with care, provide better, more prompt and ubiquitous access to health information, and improve diabetes management and patient outcomes. Key points in the delivery of patient portals to patients are good usability, reliability and availability of user choices for patients, while providers should apply more extensive training and assistance when the portal addresses elderly and not highly computer-literate populations [10]. In fact, although diabetes is today quite common even to young adults, it is mainly prevalent among adults aged 65 and older. Thus, the interface design should be made trying to avoid potential design problems for this specific target group.

Another recent study [11] proved that patient portals have the ability to provide patients with the opportunity to be increasingly involved in their own care (thus increasing self-management capability) and to reduce inequity in the access to care.

Patient portals can help in increasing the health literacy and the capability for self-management of diabetes if designed with high usability criteria for not highly computer-literate populations, otherwise the health literacy barrier will not be removed [12].

2   Methods

The REACTION project [13] aims to support management of diabetes in different clinical settings through a platform that will offer professional management and therapy services to diabetes patients [14]. This platform provides healthcare services to diabetes patients and caregivers such as blood glucose monitoring, monitoring of other relevant parameters (e.g. complication indicators, activity, and food and medication intake), decision support systems, therapy management, support of life-style changes, and crisis detection and management.

When at home, the diabetic patient is managed through the platform and the services provided by the primary health care centre. Main components of the system from the stakeholders' point of view are: a) the home or mobile platform composed of medical and environmental devices and a home or mobile gateway for the secure connection with the back-end servers; b) the health professional (clinician) portal; c) the patient portal. All components have also the capability to interoperate with each other and at least weakly with the electronic health record of the primary care centre.

The home or mobile platform is dedicated to the automatic collection of vital sign, environmental and context measurements with a focus on user friendliness, low costs, use of standards and use of wireless medical and other devices. The health professional portal supports the clinicians with the following main functionalities: a) system administration; b) user management; c) patient management; d) education and care plan (life-style and medication) management; e) remote monitoring scheme plan; f) daily measurement management; g) view of additional data and questionnaire responses; h) risk management; i) notification management. The patient portal supports the patients and informal carers with the following main functionalities: a) capture of life-style data (activity, diet, emotional status); b) capture of medication data (insulin, OADs); c) support of life-style and compliance questionnaires; d) view of care plan (life-style and medication); e) view of own measurements; f) view of feedbacks; g) view of notifications, alerts and reminders; h) view of material in support of education and motivation; i) manual input of measurements (as back-up solution).

All components of the overall solution have been developed in order to be simple, easily usable by elderly people (hiding technology as much as possible), with low cost and with easy procedures for installation and removal.

This paper will focus on the design, development and first usability tests of the prototype patient portal.

2.1   The REACTION Patient Portal

The REACTION patient portal is a secure multiplatform web application built on previous experiences of the Foundation for Research and Technology - Hellas (FORTH). The creation of the REACTION patient portal was based on a multi-step procedure, where every step was carefully designed and validated. The procedure started from the general requirements of the platform, created by the stakeholders, selecting the specific requirements for the patient portal including the ones specifying its interactions with the other components. All these requirements were translated into functionalities that were analysed and described in detail. The functionalities were logically grouped, optimizing the typical workflows performed by patients and, thus, organizing the patient portal into logically distinct sections. The functionalities were decoded as software modules and graphically represented in the user interface by big buttons that contain easily identifiable icons and easily readable captions. Special attention was given to the design of the user interface, having in mind accessibility, user-friendliness and usability criteria. The colour of the text, the icons, the button control sizes, the graphical unit display of the glucose and the other vital signs were carefully selected in such a way to fulfil the usability criteria specified in the requirement list (e.g. using high contrast with the background of the buttons). This, in addition to the careful design of the layout and the organization of the functionalities, contributed to the creation of a modern and friendly user environment.

The REACTION patient portal was implemented in C# using the ASP.NET v4.0 framework. The selected database engine was the Microsoft SQL Server 2008 R2. The implementation of the user interface was performed using html5 and css3 technologies. Complementary technologies to design a modern and user friendly interactive interface include the latest versions of the JavaScript libraries of jQuery and jQuery UI and an interactive JavaScript library for the chart drawing elements. The development environment used was mainly composed of an integrated development environment (Microsoft Visual Studio 2010) and an integrated environment for the database management (SQL Server Management Studio). The target environment, where the application was deployed, was a Microsoft Server 2008 R2 standard server with IIS as web server on board.

Since the patient portal has been designed as a web application, any type of device, personal computer, smart phone or tablet PC, can access it, as long as it has a web browser (that supports the present common web standards and technologies defined by the World Wide Web Consortium (W3C)) and it is connected to the Internet. The REACTION patient portal has been accurately tested to operate properly with the last versions of all the major web browsers (Internet Explorer 8+, Mozilla Firefox12+, Google Chrome15+, Opera 10+, Safari 5+ & Dolphin HD+) in the three major desktop operating systems (Windows XP+, Mac OS X 10.7+, Ubuntu Linux 10.04+) as well as in the three major mobile operating systems (iOS5, Android 3+, WP7+).

Some interactive screenshots of the patient portal on tablet PC are shown in Fig. 1.

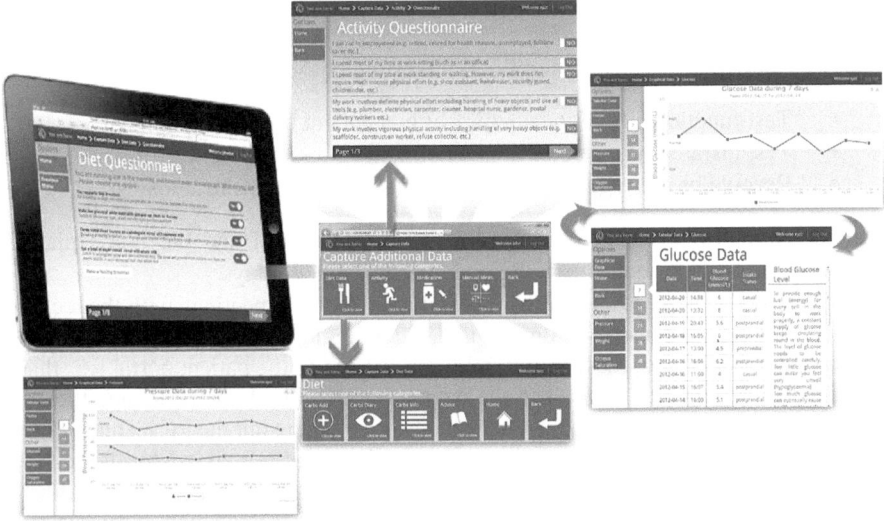

Fig. 1. Some interactive screenshots of the REACTION patient portal

Several reviews of functionalities and user interface on paper and then with mock-ups were performed with simulated end-users. The adopted design choices were verified by usability tests, performed in the sites of the clinical partners, scoring high on the "ease of interaction" and "user satisfaction". Usability tests were also performed with actual elderly users and users with little computer-literacy focused on the optimization of the user friendliness of the patient portal. Retrofits were continuously provided and modifications implemented and deployed in an iterative process, towards the attainment of a version suitable for clinical use.

3   Results

Prior to commencing the primary care field trials, a series of tests on the overall platform have been undertaken in the clinical site. The testing process has been undertaken in 2 stages, friends and family testing and field testing.

Friends and family testing involved users that were not from the target population. They included researchers, friends and neighbours of those working within the study.

The main objectives of the friends and family phase were to:

- Test reliability and robustness in a non-lab environment
- Test functionality of the equipment in a non-lab environment
- Test usability and functionality of patient and clinician portals
- Receive usability feedback

A small number of users undertook this testing for 7 days following a test script protocol. Following the friends and family testing, a number of patients with very basic computer-literacy from the target sample were approached and asked to take part in a series of field tests.

The main objectives of the pre-pilot field testing phase were to:

- Test functionality of the equipment in a patient home environment
- Test installation procedures in a home environment
- Receive usability feedback from end-users to the technical teams

Patients were trained and asked to use the patient portal and the home platform following specific protocols for a period between 7 and 28 days.

In both test phases actions were reviewed regularly via meetings with the technical partners and the technical solution was updated and improved in an iterative process.

The main outcome of these initial field tests related to the patient portal was that all patients were able to gain access to the patient portal on both the tablet and their own PC. There was one functional error reported by a patient using the PC. This was to do with the date range when entering manual readings and was fixed by the technical team updating the patient portal version.

Patients using a personal computer generally stated that the patient portal was easy to use. It was simple to log onto and was quick to navigate and complete the tasks. A minor usability raised by the patients was solved by changing the yes/no check box control in the questionnaires and in all parts of the portal with a different one, which, in subsequent tests, was considered very satisfactory by patients. Another minor usability issue came from a patient accessing the patient portal with an old version of web browser not matching the patient portal pre-requirements. In that case, the solution was to update the browser version.

In case of use of a tablet PC, it was verified that when there is a level of reduced mobility in hands, the use of a standard PC is preferred, thus the multi-platform design adopted for the patient portal is a clear advantage being able to address a heterogeneous set of end-users.

Finally, all patients considered the patient portal helpful in their daily self-management of diabetes.

4   Conclusion

Diabetes management is complex. The impact of physical activity, diet variation and stress on glucose levels must be assessed and taken into account. This, along with blood glucose measurements will determine the insulin dose or the appropriate use of hypoglycaemic drugs. The complexity of professional care and self-management increases with the necessary effort to achieve the best care and treatment of co-morbidities along with effective life-style changes. Daily management has to be performed appropriately by the patients themselves, and proper education, information and support have to be provided. It is also necessary to take into account the difficulties that older adults may experience due to the decline in cognition, vision, and motor skills, and for this reason, before the deployment, an evaluation and comparison of results against the Web Content Accessibility Guidelines 2.0, in order to determine the e-accessibility level of services offered, will be performed and eventual retrofits applied.

The proposed patient portal within the framework of the REACTION platform, deployed in real-life healthcare systems, is expected to greatly empower the patient, increase the self-management capacity, improve the quality of life and the overall management of diabetes, reducing the risk of developing complications in general, and the rate of hospital admissions. Results of initial tests and first experiences with real end-users are encouraging and seem to confirm these expectations.

Acknowledgments. This work was performed in the framework of the FP7 Integrated Project REACTION (Remote Accessibility to Diabetes Management and Therapy in Operational Healthcare Networks) partially funded by the European Commission under Grant Agreement 248590.

References

1. Spanakis, E.G., Chiarugi, F.: Diabetes Management: Devices, ICT Technologies and Future Perspectives. In: Nikita, K.S., Lin, J.C., Fotiadis, D.I., Arredondo Waldmeyer, M.-T. (eds.) MobiHealth 2011. LNICST, vol. 83, pp. 197–202. Springer, Heidelberg (2012)
2. Zimmet, P., Alberti, K.G., Shaw, J.: Global and societal implications of the diabetes epidemic. Nature 414(6865), 782–787 (2001)
3. Wild, S., Roglic, G., Green, A., Sicree, R., King, H.: Global prevalence of diabetes: estimates for the year 2000 and projections for 2030. Diabetes Care 27(5), 1047–1053 (2004)
4. Shaw, J.E., Sicree, R.A., Zimmet, P.Z.: Global estimates of the prevalence of diabetes for 2010 and 2030. Diabetes Res. Clin. Pract. 87(1), 4–14 (2010) (Epub November 6, 2009)
5. Zhang, P., Zhang, X., Brown, J., Vistisen, D., Sicree, R., Shaw, J., Nichols, G.: Global healthcare expenditure on diabetes for 2010 and 2030. Diabetes Res. Clin. Pract. 87(3), 293–301 (2010) (Epub February 19, 2010)
6. Brennan, P., Safran, C.: Report of conference track 3: patient empowerment. Int. J. Med. Inform. 69(2-3), 301–304 (2003)
7. Alpay, L.L., Henkemans, O.B., Otten, W., Rövekamp, T.A., Dumay, A.C.: E-health applications and services for patient empowerment: directions for best practices in The Netherlands. Telemed. J. E. Health 16(7), 787–791 (2010)
8. The Lancet. Patient empowerment - who empowers whom? Lancet 379(9827), 1677 (2012)
9. Unger, J.: Diabetes management in primary care. Lippincott Williams & Wilkins, A Wolter Kluwer business (2007)
10. Osborn, C.Y., Mayberry, L.S., Mulvaney, S.A., Hess, R.: Patient web portals to improve diabetes outcomes: a systematic review. Curr. Diab. Rep. 10(6), 422–435 (2010)
11. Shaw, R.J., Ferranti, J.: Patient-provider internet portals - patient outcomes and use. Comput. Inform. Nurs. 29(12), 714–718 (2011)
12. Sarkar, U., Karter, A.J., Liu, J.Y., Adler, N.E., Nguyen, R., Lopez, A., Schillinger, D.: The literacy divide: health literacy and the use of an internet-based patient portal in an integrated health system - results from the diabetes study of northern California (DISTANCE). J. Health Commun. 15(suppl. 2), 183–196 (2010)
13. http://www.reaction-project.eu/news.php
14. Spanakis, E.G., Chiarugi, F., Kouroubali, A., Spat, S., Beck, P., Asanin, S., Rosengren, P., Gergely, T., Thestrup, J.: Diabetes management using modern information and communication technologies and new care models. Interact J. Med. Res. 1(5), e8 (2012)

E-Procurement in Hospitals – An Integrated Supply Chain Management of Pharmaceutical and Medical Products by the Usage of Mobile Devices

Patrick Bartsch[1], Thomas Lux[2], Alexander Wagner[1], and Roland Gabriel[1]

[1] Competence Center eHealth Ruhr, chair of business informatics,
Ruhr-University Bochum, Universitätsstr. 150, 44801 Bochum
{awagner,pbartsch,rgabriel}@winf.rub.de
[2] University of Technology Chemnitz, Chair of Business Information Systems I,
Thueringer Weg 7 (#222), 09107 Chemnitz Germany
tlux@tu-chemnitz.de

Abstract. The optimization of procurement processes for medical and pharmaceutical products helps hospitals reducing costs and increasing their cost transparency, treatment quality and patient safety. However, due to the great amount of actors and interfaces taking part in procurement processes a structured methodology is required for holistic documentation and analysis. Therefore, this paper elaborates and describes the main optimization goals for procurement processes and develops methods for process analysis and the ability of a goal-targeted optimization using specialized ICT systems.

Keywords: supply chain management, hospital engineering, E-Procurement, cost transparency, patient safety, healthcare process engineering, medical ICT, eHealth.

1   Problem Statement

There are many rough economic challenges for hospitals nowadays. Especially because of the implementation of G-DRGs[1] in German hospitals there is currently a focus on the minimization of costs, so that hospitals can retain their competitiveness. With 12% of the total costs logistics is one of the key cost drivers in the hospital business. 75% of these costs are personnel costs [1]. This high percentage of personnel costs in hospital logistics is strongly correlated to unusual work of the nursing staff which takes up 28% of their regular working time [2]. But supply chain management is also seen as a chance to improve the hospital's organizational aspects [3].

The logistics of medical products and pharmaceuticals in hospitals represents a vast field of activity in which many people of various professional groups are involved [2]. It extends from the identification of needs in the functional areas and

---

[1] G-DRG: German Diagnosis Related Groups.

B. Godara and K.S. Nikita (Eds.): MobiHealth 2012, LNICST 61, pp. 406–412, 2013.
© Institute for Computer Sciences, Social Informatics and Telecommunications Engineering 2013

wards, the consumption of products up to the health care processes in internal supply departments where the used products are delivered from external suppliers. On the one hand pharmaceuticals and medical products need to be administered in accordance to medical or nursing prescriptions at the right time in the right quantity to the right patient, and on the other hand the resulting demand of these products for hospital wards and departments needs to be ensured. There are already many different isolated applications that are focusing on these logistic problems, but a solution facing the total procurement-process of medicine and medical products is missing [4]. When looking at the whole procurement-process – from the external supplier over the purchasing department and the ward to the patient – various potentials for optimization can be identified that not only decrease the costs but also raise the transparency, the patient safety and the global economic efficiency in the hospitals [5]. Most hospitals have no ICT-solutions to record patient-related consumption of products, thus comparisons of DRG revenues with the costs of the consumption of goods are not possible (cost transparency) [6].

Furthermore there are only very few inventory controlled storage facilities in hospital wards – unlike in central storages or external suppliers –as a result it is often unclear which materials are in store and in what quantity. This complicates the planning and documentation of the demand compared to automatic management by ICT, and also leads to the fact that orders need to be placed manually "on paper" and can only be done after "visual inspection" of the storage facilities. Because of these points it is not easy to plan optimized storage-balances with respect to delivery-loops. This results in uncontrollable stocking of products by the nursing staff and inefficient capital-binding. In case of a callback of problematic products the missing location information makes it necessary to get a manually overview of all storages at the site.

The urgent need of ICT solutions in the field of medicine is driven by the doctor's prescription of medication. In this regard, there are possibilities of ADE (adverse drug events) by e.g. a wrong dosing, mistakes in medication setting and mistakes in application of medicine. Studies are showing that up to 10% of the anamneses in hospitals are flawed and thereof 60% pertaining to medication [7]. The implementation of specialized ICT systems aims to prevent these ADEs. Additional special measures and technical equipment (e.g. patient bracelets with barcodes) help to get the right medication to the right patient in the right time [8].

2   Project Goals

The project "e-med PPP – patient safety and procurement-processes" [2] is endorsed by the German State of North Rhine-Westphalia and the European Union and develops integrated strategies and solutions to optimize the logistic processes of pharmaceuticals and medical products in hospitals on the base of the problems mentioned above. The complete ecosystem of the procurement in a hospital is reflected by the partners in the project. There are for example two reference hospitals,

---

[2] http://www.e-medppp.de

several partners from all steps of the value-added chain like business and industry partners as suppliers, and the patient as customer. One of the project's targets is to find strategies to solve existing problems and as well concrete recommendations for the implementation of ICT solutions. The project goals can be divided in two distinct areas. Firstly, overall-goals concerning all activities and departments, and secondly, direct goals facing the above mentioned problems to optimize single processes in the hospital with potentially structural changes.

One specific objective is the evaluation of technical methods for accurate tracking of each patient's consumption of pharmaceuticals and medical products. In addition to an automated documentation it should be possible to identify every single patient as a single cost unit. In this connection the project aims to identify patients and products by auto-ident-technologies such as barcodes, data matrices or RFID chips. With these, it is possible to integrate these data into heterogeneous hospital ICT systems (e.g. hospital information systems (HIS), stock management). The respective concept that will be developed to fulfill these specs, should integrate Computerized Physician Order Entry (CPOE) Systems. Like mentioned above, for this concrete use case it is also necessary to develop concepts for the efficient integration in the heterogeneous ICT systems in hospitals (e.g. HIS, LIS, stock management).

Another goal in this project is to work out a foundation of conditions and methods to implement inventory controlled ward-storages. This process has to be integrated with other goals like patient as cost unit, automated documentation and CPOE-Systems. Finally, it is important to create the possibility of automated and electronic supply-processes of pharmaceuticals and medical products between all players. This includes, on the one hand, business connections between the hospital and the external supplier, and, on the other hand, the transactions between wards and departments and the central warehouse and pharmacy in the hospital. For each use case electronic order platforms need to be developed that enable integration with the remaining ICT systems, so that orders are integrated efficiently in the process of ordering and purchasing [9].

Figure 1 shows a structural overview of the logistic process chain in a hospital and the respective actors. The ultimate purpose of the logistic process is a secure and efficient realization of a correct consumption of pharmaceuticals and medical products for the patient (process "Consumption"). To fulfill this aim, hospital wards need to report demand of these products (process "Ordering"), which at the end leads to the delivery of the ordered products (process "Supply"). Internal purchasing departments have to order their needed products themselves from suppliers (processes "Procurement" and "Delivery"). In the case of pharmaceuticals, this would be the central pharmacy, in the case of medical products this would be the purchasing department or the central storage.

One of the major goals of this project is to develop recommendations for our reference-hospitals based on scientific studies and process analyses, which lead to better process quality for all procurement processes. For achieving a better process-quality it is important to clear the personnel responsibilities, the binding character of the processes in the departments and the development of escalation scenarios for exceptional cases. With respect to lower costs, there have to be solutions to unburden the nursery staff from unconventional work (e.g. by delegating the work to other professional groups) in due consideration of process length, process frequencies and process costs.

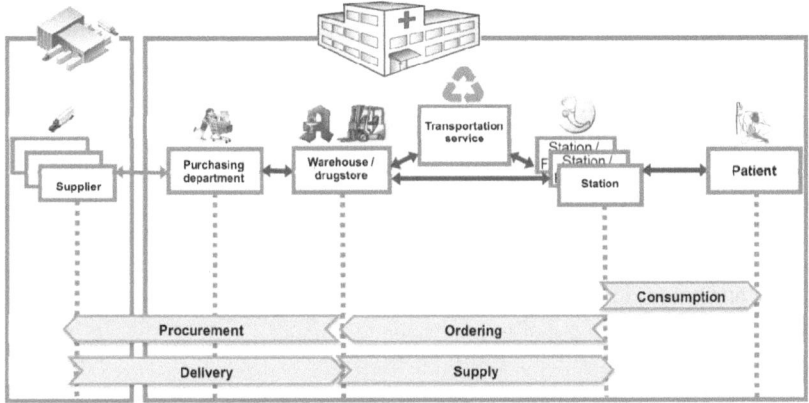

Fig. 1. procurement-process in hospital

To ensure the data safety and security in all steps of the total procurement process, measures for the implementation and integration of data security and safety must be taken and considered in the complete concept [10].

3   Method

For achieving the four objectives of the project (high process quality, economical process design, information security and relief of human resources), the knowledge of the current situation of processes was essential. The first milestone was therefore the recording and modelling of the actual processes. After an initial screening of the scope, we interviewed all process owners. In order to detect all logistic and supply processes of the relevant departments of the internal supply up to typical consuming areas, we interviewed the process owners of "standard ward", "general reception", "intensive care unit", "operating room", "warehouse" and "pharmacy". To ensure consistency, we have created a detailed questionnaire.

During the interviews the processes were documented with function templates, and image and sound recordings. The next step was the creation of process models by using ARIS software. We set up an ARIS server, so that all relevant project partners could work collaboratively. The publications of the process models within the project team were done by using the ARIS Business Publisher, a Web-based interface for accessing the model database. The relevant processes are modelled as extended event-driven process chains (eEPC). It was important to describe the processes as detailed as possible with the help of attributes to get a solid foundation for the subsequent assessment [11].

In addition to the description of functions it was also important to document the durations and execution cycles of relevant functions. Then we measured the durations of all relevant functions in the hospital with the time-measuring instruments "Timeboys" of the company Datafox. Each department or station was observed for two weeks. Finally, we evaluated and implemented the results in the analysis of the current situation.

The objectives of information security are also very important in this project. This aim requires a detailed identification, modelling and documentation of all relevant assets in this scope [10]. In addition to the usual elements of an eEPC (roles, data, application systems), we integrated additional elements, such as infrastructural components, devices or transportation elements into the eEPC-models. Furthermore, the documentation of the requirements for the security objectives, threats and vulnerabilities of each asset were necessary. This information has been documented in the object attributes [11].

4   Valuation

To analyse and valuate the current situation was the next step. The focus here was on both, the pharmaceutical processes and also on the medical-product processes. It was based on different criteria: documentation procedures, software and hardware systems, information flows, process costs, etc. The outcome of this step was a detailed overview of the identified weaknesses and potentials for improvement. As expected, numerous vulnerabilities can be uncovered in connection with hand-written documentation, which is a serious hazard in matters of the patient safety and information security. Unreadable or incorrectly written prescriptions can simultaneously affect all the security objectives, threaten the patient's health and in the worst-case even the patient's life.

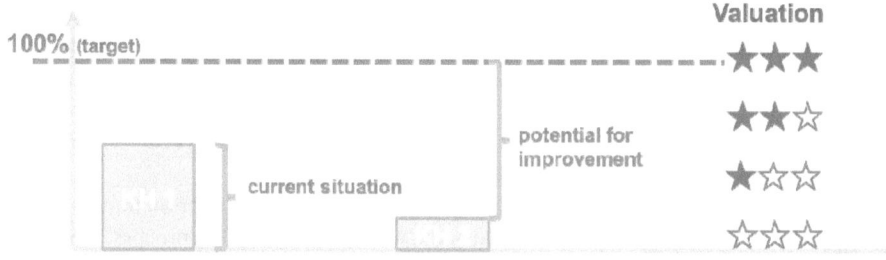

Fig. 2. Current situation

As part of the process-based cost accounting we identified specific cost drivers [11]. A comparison between the two hospitals shows that an electronic inventory of medical products in "KH1" (Figure 2) brings significant cost advantages. Figure 2 also shows the evaluation system that was developed in this project. The 100 % target line lights the best possible status with respect to the project objectives. The distance between the current situation and the 100% target line represents the achievable potential for improvements [11]. The project is currently in the conceptualization phase of target scenarios. A scientific comparison between the target and actual situation is not yet possible. However, the analysis of the current situation has shown potentials for optimization for both hospitals "KH1" and "KH2". Our next step is to provide an integrated approach along the entire supply chain with the help of a targeted use of ICT like mobile Handhelds (Figure 3) or Smartphones.

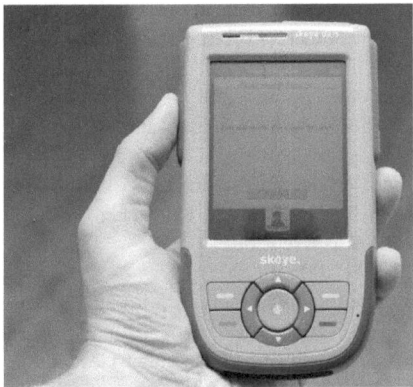
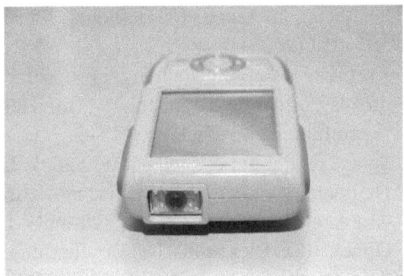

Fig. 3. Mobile Barcode Scanner

5   Target Scenarios and Outlook

On the base of the above mentioned valuation we will create concepts that bridge the gap between current and target situation in total or partially. However, our goal is not to develop a monolithic solution. We want to develop different, customizable scenarios as a modular system with various potentials to achieve the project goals. For example, the use of RFID offers enormous potential for improvement especially in the logistics of medical products [12].

The supply chain in reference to the pharmaceutical processes can be optimized by using a unit-dose system in combination with identification technologies, patient wristbands and RFIDs or data matrix. In the medicine supply a unit dose system is conceivable in conjunction with scanners and patient wristbands. This allows to record, which drug is given to which patient at which time. Alternatively, a CPOE system could already trigger a demand of pharmaceuticals as the medication is prescribed on the ward, assuming that a modern ward storage system is used. In all scenarios, the solution is connected to the existing software systems in the hospital through defined interfaces. The developed "modular solutions" will be tested and valuated regarding their potential and practicality in laboratory experiments and exemplary applications in the real environment. The outcome is a flexible solution, because at least the hospital decides about the optimal configuration for its own scenario.

References

1. Siepermann, C.: Stand und Entwicklungstendenzen der Krankenhauslogistik in Deutschland. Verlag für Wissenschaft und Forschung, Berlin (2004)
2. Blum, K.: Pflegefremde und patientenferne Tätigkeiten im Pflegedienst der Krankenhäuser. Deutsche Krankenhaus Verlagsgesellschaft mbH, Düsseldorf (2003)
3. Schneller, E.S., Smeltzer, L.R.: Strategic Management of the Health Care Supply Chain. Jossey-Bass, San Francisco (2006)
4. van de Castle, B., Szymanski, G.: Supply Chain Management on Clinical Units. In: Hübner, U., Elmhorst, M. (eds.) eBusiness in Healthcare - From eProcurement to Supply Chain Management. Springer, London (2008)
5. Holmes, S.C., Miller, R.H.: The strategic role of e-commerce in the supply chain of the healthcare industry. International Journal of Services Technology and Management 4, 507–517 (2003)
6. Kreysch, W.: Verzahnung von Pfad- und Budgetkalkulation als Basis für das prozessgesteuerte Krankenhaus. In: Hellmann, W. (ed.) Praxis Klinischer Pfade: Viele Wege führen zum Ziel, pp. 214–227. Ecomed, Landsberg (2003)
7. Sauer, F.: Patient & Medication Safety. EJHP-P 11 2005-4 (2005)
8. Hellmann, G.: Elektronische Arzneimitteltherapiesicherheitsprüfung. Deutsche Krankenhaus Verlagsgesellschaft mbH, Düsseldorf (2010)
9. Oppel, K.: Elektronische Beschaffung im Krankenhaus – Nutzung, Gestaltung und Auswirkungen von B-to-B-Marktplätzen. Deutscher Universitäts-Verlag, Wiesbaden (2003)
10. Lux, T., Wagner, A.: Informationssicherheit im Gesundheitswesen – Eine prozessorientierte Analyse. Competence Center eHealth Ruhr, Bochum (2010)
11. Junginger, S., Kabel, E.: Business Process Analysis. In: Hübner, U., Elmhorst, M. (eds.) eBusiness in Healthcare - From eProcurement to Supply Chain Management. Springer, London (2008)
12. Mohr, J., Sengupta, S., Slater, S.: Marketing of High-Technology Products and Innovations, 3rd edn. Pearson Education Inc., New Jersey (2010)

SNS as a Platform of the Activity Monitoring System for the Elderly

Ismo Alakärppä[1], Simo Hosio[2], and Elisa Jaakkola[1]

[1] University of Lapland, Yliopistonkatu 8,
FI-96101 Rovaniemi, Finland
{ismo.alakarppa,elisa.jaakkola}@ulapland.fi
[2] University of Oulu, Pentti Kaiteran katu 1,
FI-90014 Oulun yliopisto, Finland
{simo.hosio}@ee.oulu.fi

Abstract. Social networking services (SNS) offer new ways of tackling challenges related to maintaining elders' autonomy in their later life, ageing in place, loneliness and cost pressures of welfare system in ageing communities. In this paper we present a communal activity-monitoring concept that utilizes SNS and sensor technology. We propose that acceptability of the activity-monitoring system can be increased with context aware data delivery and by using social media as a platform for the monitoring system.

Keywords: Elderly, Social media, Monitoring, Context aware.

1 Introduction

Social media continues to expand popularity among all age groups. In the past two years, social media use among Internet users age 65 and older has grown 150% between April 2009 and May 2011 [1]. Besides professional help, the psychological and perceived wellbeing can be achieved through the social support given by friends and other related parties. Social support is found to have an indirect link to the subjective health experience through the psychological effects [2]. Connections and interaction with the community have increasing role of preventing loneliness, which forms an important health and safety risk for the elderly. For those older people living alone, social participation can become more difficult, and they may need encouragement, communication and participation [3]. Although high degree of acceptance of the Ambient Assisted Living (AAL) has been found and it would likely make seniors feel safer and more secure in their homes, the main concern is still how it will impact their daily lives. This question has been largely overlooked. Seniors have identified and valued the positive impact of AAL system on their daily life as providing possibility to age-in-place and remaining safe in their homes. On the other hand seniors were concerned of intrusiveness of the system and how AAL could affect their behavioral freedom within home space [4].

The safety systems should not replace the existing safety nets, but should rather act as complementary solutions. In particular, monitoring through technology should not

B. Godara and K.S. Nikita (Eds.): MobiHealth 2012, LNICST 61, pp. 413–420, 2013.
© Institute for Computer Sciences, Social Informatics and Telecommunications Engineering 2013

increase isolation, but should ideally lead to strengthening of social networks and increase in user independence.

In this paper we will contribute to field of Mobile Monitoring and Social Media Pervasive Technologies by presenting communal caring concept (Comcare) that is built on online communication and simple sensors. The main idea of the Comcare is to form a social aware, bi-directional and equal care-giving community to take care of a certain person. Social awareness is defined as a system that is able to distinguish and understand user's social environment, like social structures, human relationships, community and user's roles in it [5]. The Comcare is designed to keep relatives informed through SNS on everyday routines of their loved ones in a positive way. The source data may come from sensors or community members. However, all the information of the target is presented as status updates.

2   Challenges with Older Population and Technology

There is little knowledge about older adults' experiences and perceptions of social media as well as on seniors' attitudes towards communication overall [5, 6]. The lack of studies reflects clearly a brief history of social media in contemporary society. It has been noted that strong social integration and interactivity often play a beneficial role in maintaining quality of life and contributing to a better mental health of older adults [7, 8]. Elders that have weak social network are more likely suffering cognitive decline, which is a result of isolation or high stress levels caused by the loss of a spouse [9]. On the contrary, socially active seniors are physically and mentally healthier [7]. In this light, the main challenge is how to improve seniors' capability and possibilities to communicate with their friends and relatives, and how to prevent isolation. In recent years there have been many publications dealing with social media and the elderly, see e.g. [10, 11, 12, 13, 14]. It seems that social networking sites can be used to assist users in sustaining and strengthening ties with the circle of important people, but there is a risk that non-technical elders are left out within their own family [7].

2.1   Acceptance and Attitudes

Seniors' attitudes towards communication and assisted living can be shaped by how they perceive technology from the perspective of privacy, security and independence. It is suggested that relevant factors to the use of in-home technologies are perceived usefulness, key social relationships, data granularity, and sensitivity of activities, i.e. where, when and in which situations the user is monitored. Also seniors' perceptions of privacy related to these technologies are highly contextual, individualized, and influenced by psychosocial motivations [15]. Beringer et al. [4] suggest that the future research should be directed and emphasized on probing how users would feel to live with such technologies on a daily basis. The study [16] presents a practice-based approach for technology acceptance evaluation that is in line with above-mentioned suggestions. In this approach, contextual and dynamic user-product relationship is a starting point, as it is seen strongly affecting technology adoption. In this light, acceptance is seen as part of user experience and is built on the willingness of users to bring monitoring technology into their existing practices in daily lives and on the appropriateness of the technology to user practices and their social and cultural environment.

There is evidence that physical spaces and environments, as well as techno-logy itself, affect to acceptance [17, 18]. For example, the room types have found to be in relation to acceptance of the monitoring technology [17]. Several researchers have presented multiple constructs on environmental classifications covering at least three levels [19, 20, 21, 22]. In the study [18] different levels of these environments are classified, and they were used in the study on acceptance of health care applications. The classification consisted following levels: 1) private/personal level, 2) semi-public/group level, and 3) public/organization and community level. This classifica-tion can be applied with the Comcare like it was presented in research of Lindley et al. [5]. They proposed that interaction with peripheral circle of friends can be less focused and less personal, and therefore lightweight communication could be a proper tool to maintain contact with those that it might otherwise be lost.

Privacy concerns are major barrier to Internet usage, and the elderly are also more concerned about their privacy than younger generations. In the study of Maaß [23], 67% of people in age 18-24 reported concerns about privacy where as the same figure among people age 55 and more was 86%. Privacy and things what are considered to be private ultimately depend on the context. Depending on the situation, the norms as well as behavior and how they are fitted with the prevailing norms change. However, it is always a risk that a particular set of norms spread to another context in which they are interpreted incorrectly [24]. Using surveillance technology at home raises ethical questions regarding the treatment of human dignity and self-determination and good life. Due to these tensions, a need for ethical choices between safety, transpa-rency and security must be considered case by case [25].

Xie et al. [6] conclude that major barriers to older adults' adoption of social media are technological and social or cultural. It is similarly important that they feel to be in control of technology. Related results were also found in a more recent study [15], in which it was discovered that if seniors rely on others to manage the technolo-gical devices in their homes, it may place them at disadvantage and may reduce their ability to stay in control of decision-making. Therefore, the collected data should be transparent and verifiable by the senior, who should be able to easily and flexibly control when and what data is collected, and with whom it is shared.

As a summary, we conclude that the Comcare should combine contextual aware-ness, and personal communication as well as sensory data in a sensitive, ethical and privacy requirements fulfilling fashion. To achieve this general objective, the following design requirements were considered for system development;

- leave time to react before a response is expected
- provide freedom to control communication and technology
- provide multilevel interaction with different circles
- avoid high cognitive load in user interface
- consider seniors' special needs in the user interface

3   A Context Aware Monitoring Solution for the Elderly

The Comcare is built to monitor daily interaction and activity of an elderly person. It combines sensor technology and manual updates from the elderly person's peers to form a lightweight, semi-automated monitoring system. Both sensor and manual updates are relayed by Comcare server to corresponding recipients, according to predetermined rights and rules in server configuration.

The main difference of the Comcare compared to existing SNS is context sensitive data delivery, which means changing data content and representation in the followers' user interfaces. For example, certain peers can see exactly what is happening in the elderly person's environment, but other peers might only know that an activity took place, oblivious to the finer details. For this purpose, peers with different permissions have dedicated user interfaces, as depicted in Figure 1.

The Comcare has three different modes for monitoring activity of an elderly person; normal, enhanced, and continuous monitoring. Normal monitoring checks and forwards updates and sensor inputs once per day, while enhanced monitoring does the same four times a day (6-hour intervals). Continuous monitoring forwards all events realtime to the followers.

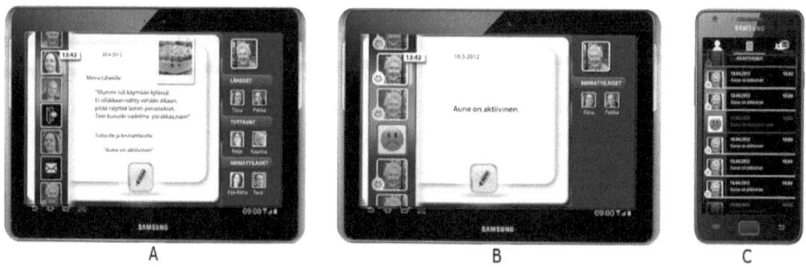

Fig. 1. Screenshots of the user interface; a) Target, b) Relatives and c) Professionals.

3.1   Target and Circles

Target refers to a person, who is the subject of monitoring (i.e. an elderly person). The target has three different circles that together are called a Comcare community. The circles have different access rights for activity updates coming from the target, relatives, professionals and sensors. The target is always aware of the sent messages through the transparent presentation of status updates, shown on the target's client software. In addition, the target is able to switch off the system at any time. Communication with the elderly (target) includes two options; 1) status updates, and 2) private messages.

Relatives circle consists of family and friends. All the updates from the target are presented authentically and appear in their original written form. *Acquaintances* circle may comprise for example of neighbors or voluntary support staff, as well as other acquaintances, with whom the target has regular contact. *Professional* are persons who are in a professional relation with the target, e.g. home or health care personnel. With these persons, the target is supposed to share activity information for professional purposes. The status updates are shown to the acquaintances and professional circle as the activity information without the original written text. However, all community members can send private messages to each other and the relatives or the acquaintances can make updates on behalf of the elderly on the basis of personal observations.

4   Implementation

In our initial Comcare concept the plan was to utilize existing online social networking platforms, such as Facebook and Google+, for realizing all the desired functionalities. However, due to several restrictions in the APIs offered by existing solutions, we ended up in implementing our own social networking application. Another reason for this was retaining full control and ownership of the system and the possibly sensitive data that it handles daily. Technically the Comcare system is loosely based on client-server model, but with communication functionality relying on a third party publish/subscribe mechanism instead of direct point-to-point communications. An overview of the technical functionality is depicted in Figure 2.

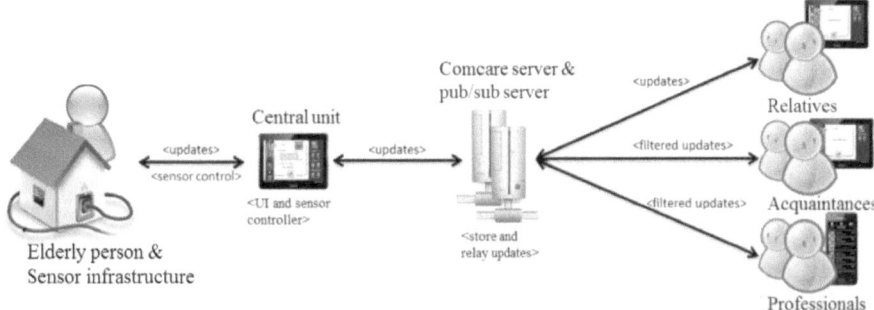

Fig. 2. The Comcare system overview: elderly person controls the sensors via a central unit, which delivers all updates to the Comcare server. Server relays filtered messages to and receives messages from all the three circles.

4.1   Server

The Comcare server was implemented using Java Platform, Standard Edition (Java SE) 6 and MySQL. The Comcare Server is used for configuring the Comcare environment including targets, their circles, and contact data points. The targets belonging to a Comcare environment are defined at server side in separate XML files, which can be manually modified and reprocessed by the server runtime, if requested. Secondly, the server is responsible for logging all messages in the Comcare for analysis purposes. Thus, all messages are relayed also to the server and stored in a local MySQL database, which is mirrored to a backup server once per day to prevent data loss in case of hardware failures. Finally, the server provides the clients their message history and other information about the Comcare environment in runtime.

4.2   Clients

The Comcare client software was developed for tablet PCs and mobile phones using Android OS (version 3.2 or higher), and it primarily serves as the user interface for making and receiving updates. Upon first startup, administrators of the Comcare are required to define the unique user ID of the client, matching one of the user IDs defined in the configuration of the Comcare environment at server side. Using this ID, the client is able to request information from the server and auto-configure itself and the user interface to match the corresponding Comcare environment and the role of the defined user. The client of the elderly person, i.e. of the target, has a secondary role as well: it serves as the connecting computational resource for sensors at the target's home. The sensors are attached directly to the client tablet via USB connection, and the raw sensor data is abstracted to high level, human readable sensor events at client side to be dispatched to the server.

4.3   Sensors

Sensors are realized using a do-it-yourself sensor kit called Phidgets (http://www.phidgets.com/). The sensors connect to the client tablet, and provide automated activity updates by monitoring the elderly person's environment. The sensors to be used are as follows; 1) *the front door*, detect tenant's movement: magnetic switch and motion sensor, 2) *the mailbox*, detect mail pick-up: pressure sensor, 3) *the fridge door*, detect door opening: magnetic switch and 4) *the central unit*, control the other sensors: hub with an on-off switch.

4.4   Communication

The Comcare is designed for large-scale deployments. Its environment is anticipated to be fragmented with problems in connectivity and serendipitous data events from tens of sensors in geographically varying locations. For stability reasons, we chose to utilize a third party lightweight publish/subscribe system, Message Queue Telemetry Transport (MQTT) from IBM (http://mqtt.org/). MQTT is an "Internet of Things" connectivity protocol, designed for such environments as ours and for high volume sensor data with very low overhead. Clients subscribe to events belonging to them, and all sensor messages and updates from clients are relayed directly peer-to-peer using MQTT. Simultaneously, copies of messages are dispatched to the server for logging. Thus, clients never have to directly connect to the server, and the environment can operate in "Comcare namespaces", instead of e.g. handling IP addresses.

5   Discussion

We have presented a new concept for communal activity-monitoring service that utilizes SNS. We believe that social media applications combined with context sensitive data delivery could increase acceptance of monitoring systems and engage young generations to take care of their older relatives. The Comcare is directed to independently living elders and their close ones, providing a new way to take care of relatives living far away and strengthen ties in the community. The main difference of the Comcare compared to existing SNS services is context sensitive data delivery, members' ability to make updates on behalf of the elderly and transparent monitoring messages shown on the target's Comcare client software. Our starting point is to empower older people to decide who gets their monitoring data and who do not. Thus, the target has to be able to switch off the system at any time and also decide who are included in the Comcare community. We see that security systems should provide equal communication ability between the elderly and relatives. In other words, activity monitoring should combine contextual awareness and personal communication as well as the sensory data in a sensitive, ethical and privacy requirements fulfilling fashion.

While we have chosen to construct a standalone social networking system, we acknowledge the potential of integrating existing online social networking solutions. Even though the limitations of their current APIs prohibit relying solely on them, their features such as getting profile pictures and other details of contacts could be leveraged especially in the setup phase of a Comcare deployment. Further, users in any of the three circles might prefer to receive non-sensitive activity information as private or chat messages in Facebook, instead of using the dedicated Comcare client.

In the next step, we will setup the system and start preparations for a longitudinal field study in authentic settings, where the system will be used for 3 months. Data from the pilot will be collected through observations and extensive follow-up surveys.

References

1. Pew Research Center, http://pewinternet.org/Reports/2011/Social-Networking-Sites.aspx
2. Guindon, S., Cappeliez, P.: Contributions of Psychological Well-Being and Social Support to an Integrative Model of Subjective Health in Later Adulthood. Ageing International 35, 38–60 (2010)
3. Mankkinen, T.: Turvallinen elämä ikääntyneille, Toimintaohjelma ikääntyneiden turvallisuuden parantamiseksi, Sisäministeriön julkaisuja19/2011, Helsinki (2011) (in Finnish)
4. Beringer, R., Sixsmith, A., Campo, M., Brown, J., McCloskey, R.: The "Acceptance" of ambient assisted living: Developing an alternate methodology to this limited research lens. In: Abdulrazak, B., Giroux, S., Bouchard, B., Pigot, H., Mokhtari, M. (eds.) ICOST 2011. LNCS, vol. 6719, pp. 161–167. Springer, Heidelberg (2011)
5. Lindley, S.E., Harper, R., Sellen, A.: Desiring to be in touch in a changing communications landscape: Attitudes of older adults. In: Proceedings of the 2009 SIGCHI Conference on Human Factors in Computing Systems, ACM, New York (2009)
6. Xie, B., Huang, M., Watkins, I.: Technology and retirement life: A systematic review of the literature on older adults and social media. In: Wang, M. (ed.) The Oxford Handbook of Retirement, Oxford University Press, New York (2012)
7. Cornejo, R., Favela, J., Tentori, M.: Ambient Displays for Integrating Older Adults into Social Networking Sites. In: Kolfschoten, G., Herrmann, T., Lukosch, S. (eds.) CRIWG 2010. LNCS, vol. 6257, pp. 321–336. Springer, Heidelberg (2010)

8. Perakis, K., Tsakou, G., Kavvadias, C., Giannakoulias, A.: HOMEdotOLD, HOME Services aDvancing the sOcial inTeractiOn of eLDerly People. In: Bravo, J., Hervás, R., Villarreal, V. (eds.) IWAAL 2011. LNCS, vol. 6693, pp. 180–186. Springer, Heidelberg (2011)

9. Seeman, T.E.: Social ties and health: the benefits of social integration. Ann. Epidemiol. 6, 442–451 (1996)

10. Takahashi, H., Yamanaka, K., Izumi, S., Tokairin, Y., Suganuma, T., Shiratori, N.: Gentle supervisory system based on integration of environmental information and social knowledge. International Journal of Pervasive Computing and Communications 6, 229–247 (2010)

11. Lindley, S.E.: Shades of lightweight: Supporting cross- generational communication through home messaging, http://research.microsoft.com/pubs/121333/CrossGenerationalCommunication_Lindley.pdf

12. The Shoutwark Circle, http://www.southwarkcircle.org.uk/index.php

13. López-de-Ipiña, D., Blanco, S., Laiseca, X., Díaz-de-Sarralde, I.: ElderCare: An Interactive TV-based Ambient Assisted Living Platform. In: Liming, C., Nugent, C.D., Biswas, J., Hoey, J. (eds.) AAPI, vol. 4, pp. 111–125. Atlantis Press (2011)

14. Bothorel, C., Lohr, C., Thépaut, A., Bonnaud, F., Cabasse, G.: From Individual Communication to Social Networks: Evolution of a Technical Platform for the Elderly. In: Abdulrazak, B., Giroux, S., Bouchard, B., Pigot, H., Mokhtari, M. (eds.) ICOST 2011. LNCS, vol. 6719, pp. 145–152. Springer, Heidelberg (2011)

15. Lorenzen-Huber, L., Boutain, M., Camp, L.J., Kalpana, S., Connelly, K.H.: Privacy, Technology, and Aging: A Proposed Framework. Ageing International 36, 232–252 (2011)

16. Alakärppä, I., Valtonen, A.: Practice-Based Perspective on Technology Acceptance: Analyzing Bioactive Point of Care Testing. International Journal of Marketing Studies 3, 13–29 (2011)

17. Ziefle, M., Himmel, S., Wilkowska, W.: When your living space knows what you do: Acceptance of medical home monitoring by different technologies. In: Holzinger, A., Simonic, K.-M. (eds.) USAB 2011. LNCS, vol. 7058, pp. 607–624. Springer, Heidelberg (2011)

18. Alakärppä, I., Riekki, J., Koukkula, R.: Pervasive pain monitoring system: User experiences and adoption requirements in the hospital and home environments. In: Proceedings of the 3rd International ICST Conference on Pervasive Computing Technologies for Healthcare (2009) ISBN: 978-963-9799-42-4

19. Altman, I.: The environment and social behavior, privacy, personal space, territory, crowding. Brooks/Cole, California (1975)

20. Forlizzi, J., DiSalvo, C., Cemperle, F.: Assistive robotics and an ecology of elders living independently in their homes. Human- Computer Interaction 19, 25–59 (2004)

21. Bronfenbrenner, U.: The ecology of human development. Harvard University Press, Cambridge (1979)

22. Lawton, M.P., Nahemow, L.: Ecology and the aging process. In: Eisdorfer, C., Lawton, M.P. (eds.) The Psychology of Adult Development and Aging, pp. 619–674. American Psychological Association, Washington (1973)

23. Maaß, W.: The Elderly and the Internet: How Senior Citizens Deal with Online Privacy. In: Trepte, S., Reinecke, L. (eds.) Privacy Online: Perspectives on Privacy and Self-disclosure in the Social Web, pp. 235–249. Springer, Heidelberg (2011)

24. Hull, G., Lipford, H.R., Latulipe, C.: Contextual gaps: privacy issues on Facebook. Ethics and Information Technology 13, 289–302 (2011)

25. Ganascia, J.-G.: The new ethical trilemma: Security, privacy and transparency. Comptes Rendus Physique 12, 684–692 (2011)

SIXTH: A Middleware for Supporting Ubiquitous Sensing in Personal Health Monitoring

Dominic Carr, Michael J. O'Grady, Gregory M.P. O'Hare, and Rem Collier

Clarity: Centre for Sensor Web Technologies
School of Computer Science & Informatics
University College Dublin (UCD)
Belfield, Dublin 4, Ireland
dominic.carr@ucdconnect.ie,
{michael.j.ogrady,gregory.ohare,rem.collier}@ucd.ie
http://www.ucd.ie

Abstract. For an arbitrary event, a lack of the prevailing context compromises understanding. In health monitoring services, this may have serious repercussions. Yet many biomedical devices tend to exhibit a lack of openness and interoperability that reduces their potential as active nodes in broader healthcare information systems. One approach to addressing this deficiency rests in the realization of a middleware solution that is heterogeneous in a multiplicity of dimensions, whilst supporting dynamic reprogramming as the needs of patients change. This paper demonstrates how such functionality may be interwoven into a middleware solution, both from a design and implementation perspective.

Keywords: Middleware, Ambient Assisted Living, WSN.

1 Introduction

Two key perspectives characterize pervasive healthcare. The first concerns the application of mobile computing and sensing technologies to the provision of remote healthcare services, frequently using a variety of wearable biomedical sensor devices. The second concerns the objective of making healthcare truly pervasive both in the spatial and temporal dimensions [3]. A key motivation for pervasive healthcare is its potential as an enabler of preventative medicine. One popular interpretation of pervasive healthcare is that of Ambient Assisted Living (AAL). AAL envisages a home environment capable of monitoring and appropriately supporting the resident. The raison d'être of AAL is to enable older adults to live in their preferred home environment for longer than would normally be the case with all the personal, health, societal and financial benefits that accrue from this. AAL envisages embedded sensors dispersed throughout the home that continuously monitor inhabitant behavior and evolve as the circumstances of the inhabitant change, possibly due to increasing infirmary for example [7].

B. Godara and K.S. Nikita (Eds.): MobiHealth 2012, LNICST 61, pp. 421–428, 2013.

A cursory analysis of the literature will indicate that significant research is taking place in wearable Body Area Networks (BANs) as well as embedded sensor networks for AAL. Much of this is progressing in parallel but independently, with little cross over. It is conjectured that harnessing both research streams could lead to better and more robust outcomes. In particular, the potential of harnessing AAL technologies as a basis for determining prevailing contexts would be particularly beneficial. For example, if a wearable sensor should detect an increased heart rate, it can only report this in the usual way. There may well be an organic reason for this, and one that requires urgent medical intervention. However, it could just be the case that some extra physical exertion is taking place. AAL configurations offer significant potential for determining prevailing contexts at arbitrary moments in time. This paper illustrates how a generic middleware architecture offers potential for fusing these disparate information sources, leading to more informed decision making on the part of the health professional.

The remainder of the paper is structured as follows: Section 2 provides a breakdown of relevant related work. Section 3 discusses the design of our system for combining sensed data streams. Section 4 showcases by way of example code how the design is built and how similar systems could be built within a generic framework. Section 5 identifies prudent future work and concluding remarks are provided in Section 6.

2   Related Work

Within this Section a breakdown of some related work is enumerated, in particular a discussion of AAL and BAN/Wearable Sensing Middleware is given.

Examples of middleware developed for AAL include SAM [10], OASIS [1], GAL [2] and openAAL [12]. openAAL is a flexible component based middleware showcasing variant behavior based upon installed bundles. The openAAL workflow moves from event detection to an invocation of a service controlling actuation in response to an identified situation. GAL is a service-oriented middleware which integrates BAN sensors with environmental sensors and combines the information from these sources to provide context to identified events. The SOPRANO Ambient Middleware (SAM) shares a common goal of providing a loop from sensory input to actuation. The OASIS project is an agent based offering attempting to facilitate the sharing of content between services in domains relevant to elderly patient care.

Middleware architectures are also an important consideration for a BAN; we look at two such relevant examples: Personal Wireless Body Area Network (PW-BAN) [11] and Self-Managed Cell (SMC) [4]. The PWBAN offering is designed to acquire sensed data and deliver to user level applications. Elements of security, node (re)tasking, and resource detection are supported. SMC describes an architecture akin to a software agent in which each SMC is autonomous and is reactive to current user activity. A discovery module maintains contact between neighboring SMC's. A policy service governs the SMC reaction to identified events.

Through this spectrum of related work the need for the continued development of platforms supporting heterogeneous sensor devices in such a way that new devices can be easily incorporated (as within GAL) is evident. Through support for heterogeneous devices we can bridge the divide between a typical AAL home scenario and a BAN within a single system to empower applications to reason about this unified data set. There must be movement towards dynamic configurability of sensor resources, as is supported within PWBAN notably. The modularity of openAAL is attractive and such capability to inject services into the system is key when system uptime is crucial as in patient monitoring systems.

3 An Integrated Middleware Approach

SIXTH [8] is a modular, extensible and scalable sensor middleware which has been developed within the CLARITY research centre in University College Dublin. SIXTH is built on the Open Services Gateway initiative framework (OSGi) [1]. SIXTH aims to provide uniform access to sensing resources by abstracting the details of connection to the sensing apparatus. Extensibility is a core tenet of the SIXTH philosophy and is supported by its OSGi basis thus accommodating the dynamic addition of new functionality at runtime. The connection mechanisms to sensor networks are implemented as plug and play components termed *Sensor Adaptors*. A simplified description of the SIXTH system architecture is shown in Figure 1, this shows how adaptors connect to the SIXTH core, the architecture is described in detail in [8].

SIXTH is open, allowing for the replacement of functional components, such as the data dissemination policy, with a more tailored solution to suit application requirements. Support for heterogeneity of data source is key to a successful middleware solution; this is why SIXTH has been designed to provision support for any data provider through the introduction of a new adaptor. Adaptors have been developed for Tyndall iWSN nodes, TinyOS nodes, Oracle SunSpots, Shimmers, Arduinos and a multitude of web-based sources such as Twitter, Cosm and Foursquare.

To be reactive to the shifting demands of user applications, such as the applications monitoring the home environment and wearable sensors, there is necessity for dynamic sensor reprogramming e.g. to sample for light when no movement has been detected. SIXTH supports dynamic reprogramming; this is handled through the *RetaskingMessage* class and the passing of these messages to the nodes is handled by their *Sensor Adaptor*.

For our purpose herein we utilise Shimmer sensors as wearable sensors and Tyndall iWSN [6] nodes as those located within the home environment. These sensors are shown in Figures 5 and 6 respectively.

---

[1] OSGi: `http://www.osgi.org/Main/HomePage`

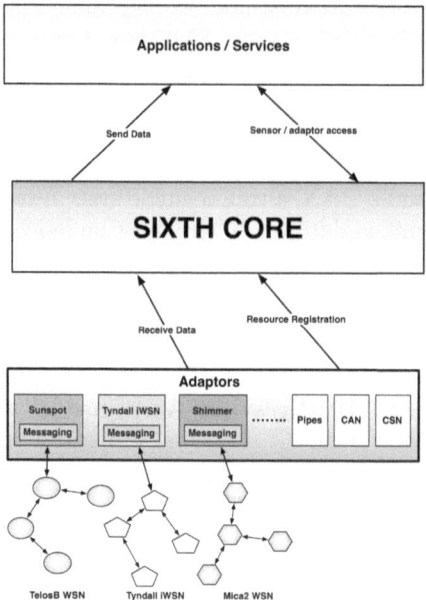

Fig. 1. The SIXTH Architecture

4   Adaptors for Heterogeneous Sensing

In this Section we discuss the implementation of SIXTH adaptors making reference to the implementation issues of the Tyndall iWSN and Shimmer adaptors. We convey our intention that heterogeneous sensor resources appear as like entities to the user application after SIXTH has isolated the heterogeneity of interaction within the adaptor layer. A showcase is provided of the data handling element of the middleware wherein we show how any component can be set up to receive data.

4.1   Creating An Adaptor

A Sensing Adaptor is created by implementing the *ISensorAdaptor* interface and enacting the required methods. As a means of relieving the burden of programming the *AbstractSensingAdaptor* has been defined with default functionality for handling component registration and data dissemination. Each adaptor is responsible for the connection to its external source(s) e.g. via USB to a WSN base station, when data is received from a source it must be translated to the *ISensorData* standard and the *send(ISensorData)* method invoked to disseminate the data to the registered listeners. Figure 3 shows the creation of a skeleton Adaptor extending *AbstractSensingAdaptor*. The *AbstractSensingAdaptor* is utilised as a common basis for both the Tyndall iWSN and Shimmer adaptors. The connection mechanism of each is different; the Shimmer adaptor is coupled with

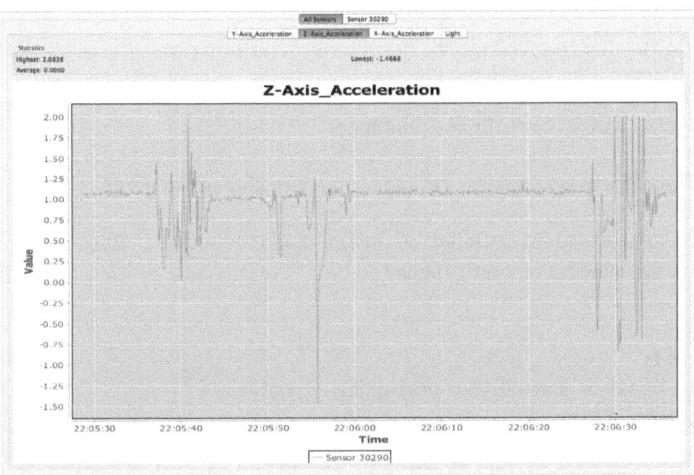

Fig. 2. Accelerometer values from a Tyndall iWSN sensor

a Bluetooth bundle for communication, whereas communication to the Tyndall motes is done via a USB connected base station. In both cases message translation must be performed to achieve a unified end result. Both adaptors support translation of *RetaskingMessage* instances to device messages for runtime device (re)tasking, this system is flexible allowing an adaptor to reject an invalid request i.e. for too high a frequency, or for an unsupported modality.

4.2 Receiving Data

The simplest method of receiving data is to implement the *IDataReceiver* interface and register the class as such on the OSGi service registry, this class will then be notified of all data which is produced by sensing entities. Figure 4 illustrates an example of a simple *IDataReceiver* implementation

To receive a filtered data stream an *INotifiier* implementation can be utilised typically with some set Query which specifies rules for the set of Sensor Data which is passed on to its associated *INotifiable* e.g. the application. Figure 2 shows a visualisation of accelerometer data from a Tyndall iWSN node. The code driving this is implemented as an *IDataReceiver* which creates a visualisation element for each numerical piece of sensed data for each newly identified sensor node.

4.3 The Wider AAL Context

SIXTH empowers connection to heterogeneous sources allowing their data to be easily combined in a single system. By utilizing Tyndall motes as door contact sensors we can reason as to where the patient is when unusual acceleration values are detected from the wearable sensor, giving inference as to an activity that might be taking place. Utilizing a wider toolkit of internal room sensors we could, for instance, discern if a patient was sitting from pressure mat data.

```
package ie.ucd.sixth.core.adaptor;

import org.osgi.framework.BundleContext;
import ie.ucd.sixth.core.RetaskingMsg;

public class ExampleAdaptor extends AbstractSensorAdaptor {

    public ExampleAdaptor(BundleContext bundleContext, String type) {
        super(bundleContext, type);
    }

    @Override
    public boolean retask(RetaskingMsg message) {
        return false;
    }

    @Override
    public String getSpecification() {
        return null;
    }

}
```

Fig. 3. Example of A sketeton Sensor Adaptor

```
package ie.ucd.sixth.core;

import ie.ucd.sixth.core.receiver.IDataReceiver;
import ie.ucd.sixth.core.sensor.data.ISensorData;

public class DataReceiverExample implements IDataReceiver {

    public DataReceiverExample(){
        Activator.getContext().registerService(IDataReceiver.class, this, null);
    }

    @Override
    public void receive(ISensorData data) {
        // perform operation on data
    }

}
```

Fig. 4. IDataReceiver implementation example

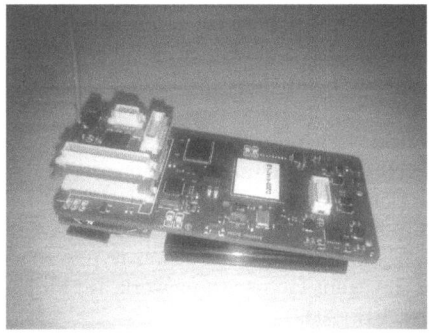

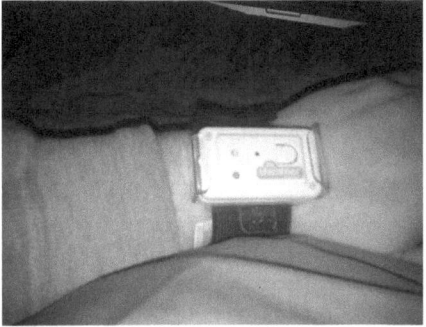

Fig. 5. Tyndall iWSN Sensor Node   **Fig. 6.** Shimmer as a wearable sensor

5   Future Work

In future, to provide a means for automatic event detection, while taking into account all contextual information, an agent driven solution will be utilized. This would be realised via a deep integration with the agent programming framework Agent Factory [5], and, in certain cases, adopting agile agents [9]. To further illustrate this solution, we plan to instrument a home environment and perform a large battery of tests with many sensors. We also plan to develop SIXTH adaptors for a range of smart clothing products, for example, the StatSports vest [2], so as to provide more fine grained information on patient health.

6   Conclusion

We have motivated the development of SIXTH, looking at the importance of context identification in an AAL configuration and how this can be best achieved through the convergence of multiple heterogeneous data sources. We provided a overview of the state of other initiatives and how these important issues are dealt with. SIXTH was showcased as an open, extensible middleware offering the integration of typical AAL configurations and wearable sensing devices.

Acknowledgements. This work is supported by Science Foundation Ireland (SFI) under grant 07/CE/I1147.

References

1. Bekiaris, E., Bonfiglio, S.: The OASIS concept. In: Universal Access in Human-Computer Interaction, pp. 202–209. Addressing Diversity (2009)
2. Büsching, F., Bottazzi, M., Wolf, L.: The GAL monitoring concept for distributed AAL platforms. In: 2012 IEEE 14th International Conference on e-Health Networking, Applications and Services (Healthcom) (IEEE Healthcom 2012), Beijing, P.R. China (2012)

---

[2] Stat Sports: http://www.statsports.ie/

3. Istepanian, R., Jovanov, E., Zhang, Y.: Guest editorial introduction to the special section on m-health: Beyond seamless mobility and global wireless health-care connectivity. IEEE Transactions on Information Technology in Biomedicine 8(4), 405–414 (2004)
4. Keoh, S., Dulay, N., Lupu, E., Twidle, K., Schaeffer-Filho, A., Sloman, M., Heeps, S., Strowes, S., Sventek, J.: Self-managed cell: A middleware for managing body-sensor networks. In: Fourth International Conference on Mobile and Ubiquitous Systems: Networking & Services (MobiQuitous 2007), pp. 1–5. IEEE (2007)
5. Muldoon, C., O'Hare, G.M.P., Collier, R.W., O'Grady, M.J.: Towards pervasive intelligence: Reflections on the evolution of the agent factory framework. In: Multi-Agent Programming, pp. 187–212. Springer, US (2009)
6. O'Grady, M.J., Angove, P., Magnin, W., O'Hare, G.M.P., O'Flynn, B., Barton, J., O'Mathuna, C.: Enabling intelligence on a wireless sensor network platform. In: Pérez, J.B., Sánchez, M.A., Mathieu, P., Rodríguez, J.M.C., Adam, E., Ortega, A., Moreno, M.N., Navarro, E., Hirsch, B., Lopes-Cardoso, H., Julián, V. (eds.) Highlights on PAAMS. AISC, vol. 156, pp. 299–306. Springer, Heidelberg (2012)
7. O'Grady, M.J., Muldoon, C., Dragone, M., Tynan, R., O'Hare, G.M.P.: Towards evolutionary ambient assisted living systems. Journal of Ambient Intelligence and Humanized Computing 1, 15–29 (2010), 10.1007/s12652-009-0003-5
8. O'Hare, G.M.P., Muldoon, C., O'Grady, M.J., Collier, R.W., Murdoch, O., Carr, D.: Sensor Web Interaction. Int. Journal on Artificial Intelligence Tools, 21(2) (2012)
9. O'Hare, G.M.P., O'Grady, M.J., Keegan, S., O'Kane, D., Tynan, R., Marsh, D.: Intelligent agile agents: Active enablers for ambient intelligence. In: ACM's Special Interest Group on Computer-Human Interaction (SIGCHI), Ambient Intelligence for Scientific Discovery (AISD) Workshop, Vienna, Austria, April 25 (2004)
10. Sixsmith, A., Meuller, S., Lull, F., Klein, M., Bierhoff, I., Delaney, S., Savage, R.: Soprano–an ambient assisted living system for supporting older people at home. In: Ambient Assistive Health and Wellness Management in the Heart of the City, pp. 233–236 (2009)
11. Waluyo, A., Pek, I., Chen, X., Yeoh, W.: Design and evaluation of lightweight middleware for personal wireless body area network. Personal and Ubiquitous Computing 13(7), 509–525 (2009)
12. Wolf, P., Schmidt, A., Otte, J., Klein, M., Rollwage, S., König-Ries, B., Dettborn, T., Gabdulkhakova, A.: openAAL - the open source middleware for ambient-assisted living (AAL). In: AALIANCE Conference, Malaga, Spain (2010)

Evaluating Energy Profiles as Resource of Context and as Added Value in Integrated and Pervasive Socio-Medical Technologies using LinkSmart Middleware

Stefan Asanin, Peter Rosengren, and Tobias Brodén

CNet Svenska AB,
Svärdvägen 3b, 18233 Danderyd, Sweden
{stefan.asanin,peter.rosengren,tobias.broden}@cnet.se

Abstract. The EU funded project inCASA has brought new insights in the field of socio-medical technology using the context-aware LinkSmart middleware. One of the main concerns that were experienced was whether separate medical devices could aggregate contextual information given by multiple environmental sensors within social care. Energy profiles were hypothesised to be able to substitute many of these in exchange for context information about a patient's behaviour. A small study was conducted to review the energy profiles given by medical devices at dispose. Unluckily, the results showed that the medical devices do not expose relevant information in order to construct such profiles.

Keywords: Energy ontology, Context, Remote Patient Monitoring, AAL, HL7.

1 Introduction

In our everyday lives and environments any computational device that is able to be interwoven or perceptually hidden from us is usually referred to as artefact targeted by pervasive computing. This term is often used in wireless networks, real-time multimedia transmissions over mobile communication protocols, and when working with ubiquitous embedded devices, sensors and actuators. Pervasive computing is prone to get more involved in areas of mHealth and Assisted Ambient Living (AAL) and improve the way healthcare is delivered [1]. Besides changing the way of healthcare delivery, pervasive data gathering opens up for new and more profound approach to how context data can be interpreted.

Solutions that cover eHealth or mHealth alone are generally more directed to raise context-awareness about physiological measurement values and semantics for understanding patient-related information [2][3]. On the other hand, social and elderly care solutions such as what can be found within most European AAL projects [4][5][6] and socio-medical research [7][3] point at the need to contextualise more of the environmental and situational events in order to better understand and anticipate emergencies and social efforts. AAL consequently leads to some kind of Smart Home deployment using sensors and actuators to gather information about and control the environment. The field of Smart Homes is broad and commercially more adopted

B. Godara and K.S. Nikita (Eds.): MobiHealth 2012, LNICST 61, pp. 429–436, 2013.

bringing forth AAL as side-effect. Here, devices and appliances are often able to fall into the term of energy efficiency and remote control by exposing relevant information referred to energy profiles. The use of these profiles enables the extraction of valuable contextual information that can be utilized to identify user behaviour and expectancy of energy consumption and cost [8][9].

The fundamental principles behind pervasive computing environment design evolved with distributed systems, wireless networks, LAN, WAN, middleware technologies, and the WWW. The LinkSmart middleware [16] fulfils some key requirements of mobile and pervasive computing by enabling access to critical services and data at any point in time and location by using wireless networking and infrastructure network support. LinkSmart is a successful technology adopted in multiple EU funded projects where energy and control of the environment are essential areas and where context-awareness has a major impact on operating ranges. But it is also used in a socio-medical project addressing AAL [10][11] and this is where this paper has been elaborated to give more knowledge whether medical devices may provide the same type of information on energy profiles leading later to an enhancement of the contextual representation.

2   Energy Semantics and Context-Aware Middleware

While the inCASA project has the mission to help elderly people to handle ageing by using an age calibrated integrated solution that enrols ICT and social and health care resources, LinkSmart, due to its flexible ontology support, has gained wide popularity by the public and at least three EU funded projects to refer to. The SEEMPubS project is about smart energy efficiency for public spaces and uses LinkSmart to develop an intelligent Context Energy Awareness Service Framework capable of managing sensor data and events across different contexts and situations [12]. The Me3Gas project [13] uses almost the same approach to reach its goal of placing the consumers in control of their energy efficiency and appliances at home while the SEAM4US project adopts a isolated solution where models for agent-based distributed and coordinated context-aware and energy resource constrained multi-project scheduling of the different subsystems in the Barcelona subway network [14]. Regardless, the point is that LinkSmart per se offers a stable ground for creating and energy awareness framework that will be reusable in future Smart Home and M2M solutions.

2.1   2.1 Developing with SOA and MDA Middleware

The LinkSmart Middleware was an EU co-funded four years Integrated Project that developed a middleware for Networked Embedded Systems. It ended on 31st December 2010 and due to property rights to its original name "Hydra" the project decided to change it to LinkSmart Middleware and to release it as Open Source reference implementation [15]. By offering a design of a generic semantic model-based architecture that supports model-driven development of applications [16], the middleware allows its developers to easy and quickly incorporate heterogeneous physical devices by using Web Service interfaces for controlling them irrespective underlying communication technology and still present them as semantic entities irrespective network setup.

By describing device related information the LinkSmart device ontology is able to present some basic high level concepts usable during development as well as in run-time processes. A developer is able to use the device ontology to create new instances and detailed data for any device type whereas each of these instances then represents the specific device model. This approach allows the model to be used as the template for the run-time instances so that real devices connected to the middleware can be exposed as virtual devices and accessed on remote.

2.2   Ontology Structure and Modules

The LinkSmart Ontology structure was designed to support and maintain its current setup of ontologies and ensure that future extensions of used concepts could with favour be adopted. Using the OWL language, the LinkSmart developing team differentiated between parts of the device model into separate ontology files from where these can be imported. In LinkSmart the core of device ontology relies on the access to basic device information and as concept the IoTDevice is sub classed by the taxonomy of all device types. This means that it serves as the root ontology concept from which one important property is the deviceId. This represents the unique device URI that is the identifier of the device template assigned to specific run-time instance of that particular device [17].

The semantic device description and structure is divided into three modules 1) device malfunctions, 2) device capabilities, and 3) device services. These are all connected to the core ontology concept from which the initial device ontology structure has been extended (FIPA device ontology specification and AMIGO project vocabularies for device descriptions) and is now covered by the basic device taxonomy and information in the ontology Device.owl that imports all other model parts [16][17].

Basing the semantic service specification on OWL-S standard the LinkSmart service model is able to enable the interoperability between devices and services by exposing the device service capabilities (e.g. device or service states and transitions) as well as tell the developer/end user what the input and output parameters are. As such, the device service ontology component will always present the device's services on a higher and a technically independent level maintaining the service concept. Having the service concept allows each service to be represented whereby the service concept will act as the root concept for all sub classes creating their service taxonomy. On the other hand, a service can respond to several service taxonomies and therefore each taxonomy represents a certain type of categorisation where the ins instance of specific service may be of more rdf:types representing several categories (see below for energy example) [17].

```
<rdf:RDF
    xmlns:rdf="http://www.w3.org/1999/02/22-rdf-syntax-
ns#"
xmlns:property="http://localhost/ontologies/StaticPrope
rtyModel.owl#"
    xmlns:owl="http://www.w3.org/2002/07/owl#"
    xmlns:xsd="http://www.w3.org/2001/XMLSchema#"
    xmlns:unit="http://localhost/ontologies/Unit.owl#"
    xmlns="http://localhost/ontologies/Energy.owl#"
    xmlns:rdfs="http://www.w3.org/2000/01/rdf-schema#"
  xml:base="http://localhost/ontologies/Energy.owl">
</rdf:RDF>
```

The categorisations are implemented as WSDL operations where each service is represented while the property of serviceOperation in the service concept contains the WSDL operation name and works as the service identifier during run-time execution. There is no limit on IoTDevice concept services and this makes the LinkSmart device ontology one of the key components in the middleware being able to store information and knowledge about different devices and device types.

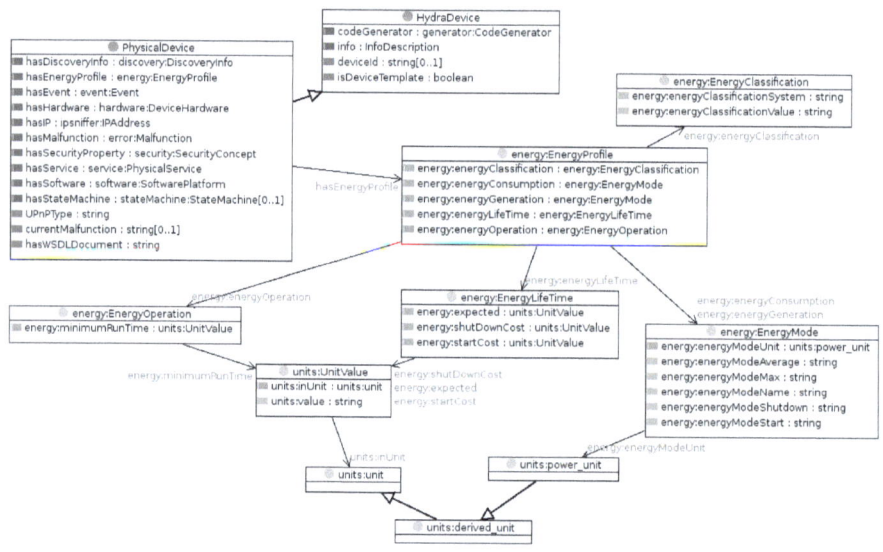

Fig. 1. Model of LinkSmart energy profile ontology

All devices enabled in LinkSmart have automatically attached the model representing their energy profile (Figure 1). This means that every device although not inherently providing the functionality for it will contain the static information related to their device's energy consumption or generation modes; basic energy classification, life-time and operation information. In sum, all ontology properties in LinkSmart that are related to the energy units defining the amount of energy spent, generated, remaining, average, etc. are tied to the power unit instances in LinkSmart QoS ontology [15].

2.3   Context in Socio-Medical Environments

There are two resources for context in the environment where patients and elderly move. One is adopted by the social care and one by the healthcare division. The LinkSmart uses [11] the Continua Guidelines [18] and the HL7 standards [19] as framework for medical data exchange and semantic integration of health services. Most AAL, i.e. Smart Home devices and appliances follow the XML text format for Web-based data exchange [20].

While context for the social care [21][22] will require specific sensors in order to extract enough data to estimate behavioural and social patterns, the medical side and device context is, as stated, rather narrowed down to only include information about physiological and measurement information or the context of medical records, history logs and rules [23][24]. Both have great value to better understand how treatment vs. care is accomplished but few note the fact that a synergy in between would possibly give even greater value in remote monitoring. As medical devices usually do not broadcast environmental data in the way that sensors for assisted living do we need to understand what features are exploitable and what parameters should be accounted for future medical devices.

3   Evaluation Study of Potential Device Energy Services

A first step in evaluating the possibilities to incorporate medical devices as contextual from other perspectives other than what they are originally designed for, i.e. to be used in socio-medical environments, is to eliminate the need to add environmental sensors as IR presence, activity sensor, etc. in order to facilitate recognition of user behaviour parameters for a certain situation. Context information about energy consumption could with ease be translated into activity context and hence behavioural data. An energy profile are therefore hypothesised to be able to substitute plenty of environmental sensors for exchange to context information about a patient's behaviour, e.g. how often is the device used, is the device used, how many times per day does the patient take measurements contra what is actually received at server side.

We have conducted a small study evaluating what energy profiles are available for each field. The idea was to use the experience and knowledge we have using Smart Home devices and appliances and to highlight what features and thereby parameters would be relevant to find in the medical devices. For Smart Home appliances and energy efficiency solutions we mainly use the Plugwise home basic kit and plugs named circles [25] and expose them as Web Services over a P2P network to be monitored and controlled by some end-user. The Plugwise covers many AAL related appliances and is therefore a good example for this comparing study trial.

Table 1. Evaluation of *Smart Home/AAL* IoT device energy service features in LinkSmart using common PlugWise devices. 'A' means that the service is available in LinkSmart while 'C' means that the service is compatible once mapped at application level.

Device description	AVG effect	Current usage	Device energy policy	Energy class	Energy mode	Energy policy status	Energy profile	Max effect	Min effect	RMNG life time	Total usage
PlugWise:: Refrigerator	C	A		C				A	A		A
PlugWise:: Light	C	A						A	A		A
PlugWise:: Microwave	C	A		C				A	A		A
PlugWise:: SmartTV	C	A		C	C	C		A	A		A
PlugWise:: Coffeemaker	C	A						A	A		A
PlugWise:: Cooling fan	C	A						A	A		A

Table 1 shows the study review of some usual LinkSmart enabled devices. We then continued to review the medical devices (Table 2) we have purchased to see if we could find any embedded services within the devices themselves that could be either exploited and defined on application level through coding or directly consumed by the LinkSmart Energy Profile Ontology.

Table 2. Evaluation of *medical* IoT device energy service features in LinkSmart in conjunction with the LinkSmart enabled medical devices at dispose. 'A' means that the service is available in LinkSmart while 'C' means that the service is compatible once mapped at application level.

Device description	AVG effect	Current usage	Device energy policy	Energy class	Energy mode	Energy policy status	Energy profile	Max effect	Min effect	RMNG life time	Total usage
A&D BPM UA-767PBT-C.					C						
A&D WS UC-321PBT-C.					C						
Nonin Pulse Oximeter 9560.					C						C
Pivotell Pill Dispenser GSM.					C						C
Bayer USB Contour.					C						
Ambulatory Inc. Actigraph.					C						

4   Results and Discussion

Context for social care and context for healthcare does not immediately mean that the two concepts fall under the same area of use. Still, what we now know is that context as resource for added value or additional information about a patient's well-being is subdivided and handled separately for healthcare and social services. Projects such as the inCASA and alike that adopt a socio-medical approach in the remote monitoring of patients are likely to have a consolidation of the two resources and hence realise sustainable solutions for joint social and healthcare delivery. On the other hand, the study showed that our medical devices in general do not possess the ability in expose energy profiles or services and what can be concluded is that they, in their current model versions, will not be able to provide added contextual value as anticipated. We encourage pursuing the topic as it could have great relevance in the forward planning of Internet of Things and socio-medical technologies.

Acknowledgments. This work was performed in the framework of CIP-ICT-PSP Project inCASA (Integrated Network for Completely Assisted Senior citizen's Autonomy) partially funded by the European Commission. The authors wish to express their gratitude to the other members of the inCASA Consortium for valuable discussions on the topic of context and how to express such information throughout our common platform.

References

1. Orwat, C., Graefe, A., Faulwasser, T.: Towards pervasive computing in health care – A literature review. In: BMC Medical Informatics & Decision Making 8, 26 (2008)
2. Ganguly, S., Kataria, P., Juric, R., Ertas, A., Tanik, M.: Sharing information and data across heterogeneous e-health systems. Telemedicine Journal and e-Health 15(5), 454–464 (2009)
3. Bricon-Souf, N., Newman, C.: Context awareness in health care: a review. International Journal of Medical Informatics 76(1), 2–12 (2007)
4. Care project, http://care-aal.eu/
5. ExCITE project, http://www.oru.se/excite
6. WayFIS project, http://www.wayfis.eu/
7. Hagler, S., Austin, D., Hayes, T., Kaye, J., Pavel, M.: Unobtrusive and Ubiquitous In-Home Monitoring: A Methodology for Continuous Assessment of Gait Velocity in Elders. IEEE Transactions on Biomedical Engineering 57(4), 813–820 (2010)
8. Rahmati, A., Zhong, L.: Context-Based Network Estimation for Energy-Efficient Ubiquitous Wireless Connectivity. IEEE Transactions on Mobile Computing 10(1), 54–66 (2011)
9. Inca Project, http://www.oulu.fi/cse/node/8003
10. InCASA project, http://incasa-project.eu/

11. Lamprinakos, G., Asanin, S., Rosengren, P., Kaklamani, D.I., Venieris, I.S.: Using SOA for a Combined Telecare and Telehealth Platform for Monitoring of Elderly People. In: Nikita, K.S., Lin, J.C., Fotiadis, D.I., Arredondo Waldmeyer, M.-T. (eds.) MobiHealth 2011. LNICST, vol. 83, pp. 233–239. Springer, Heidelberg (2012)

12. SEEMPubS project, http://seempubs.polito.it/

13. Me3Gas project, http://www.me3gas.eu/

14. SEAM4US project, http://seam4us.eu/

15. Hydra Project, http://www.hydramiddleware.eu/

16. Kostelnik, P., Sarnovsky, M., Hreno, J.: Ontologies in Hydra – Middleware for Ambient Intelligent Devices. In: Cech, P., et al. (eds.) Ambient Intelligence Perspectives II. IOS Press, Amsterdam (2009)

17. Kostelnik, P., Ahlsén, M., Rosengren, P.: Ontologies Prototype, Technical Report D6.4, Hydra Consortium, IST-2005-034891 (2009)

18. Continua Health Alliance, http://www.continuaalliance.org/index.html

19. HL7, http://www.hl7.org/

20. W3C Ubiquitous Web Domain, http://www.w3.org/XML/

21. Jih, W., Yung-jen, J., Tsai, T.M.: Context-Aware Service Integration for Elderly Care in a Smart Environment. In: AAAI 2006 Workshop: Modeling and Retrieval of Context Retrieval of Context, Boston, Massachusetts, USA, pp. 44–48 (2006)

22. Kim Zapf, M.: Social Work and the Environment: Understanding People and Place. Critical Social Work 11(3), 30–46 (2010)

23. Jih, W., Cheng, S., Yung-jen Hsu, J.: Context-aware Access Control on Pervasive Healthcare. In: EEE 2005 Workshop: Mobility, Agents, and Mobile Services (MAM), Hong Kong, pp. 21–28 (2005)

24. Devlin, A.S., Arneill, A.B.: Health Care Environments and Patient Outcomes - A Review of the Literature. Environment and Behavior 35(5), 665–694 (2003)

25. Plugwise, http://www.plugwise.com/idplugtype-f/home/home-basic

Adopting Rule-Based Executions in SOA-Oriented Remote Patient Monitoring Platform with an Alarm and Alert Subsystem

Stefan Asanin[1], Peter Rosengren[1], Tobias Brodén[1], Ivo Ramos Maia Martins[2], Carlos Cavero Barca[2], Manuel Marcelino Pérez Pérez[2], Lydia Montandon[2], Manolis Stratakis[3], and Stelios Louloudakis[3]

[1] CNet Svenska AB, Svärdvägen 3b, 18233 Danderyd, Sweden
{stefan.asanin,peter.rosengren,tobias.broden}@cnet.se
[2] ATOS, Albarracín 25, 28037, Madrid, Spain
{ivo.ramos,carlos.cavero,manuel.perez,lydia.montandon}
@atosresearch.eu
[3] Forthnet S.A., ETEP Crete, Heraklion, Greece
{stratakis,slou}@forthnetgroup.gr

Abstract. Monitoring and event handling are important aspects in the EU funded REACTION project and its remote patient monitoring services. The REACTION platform is designed to let any application to be able to react ubiquitously to change in a patient's health state and environment and perform pre-defined activities such as alarm handling according to pre-programmed rules. This paper presents and discusses the platform's alarm and alert handling system out of technical perspectives.

Keywords: Alarm handling, Remote Patient Monitoring, Rules, XSLT, SOA.

1 Introduction

REACTION is a research and development project, partially funded by the European Commission, for devising and implementing a platform allowing the remote management of medical data related to diabetes patient's treatment and health care. The strict control of blood sugar levels is necessary for assessing precisely patients' insulin doses in every specific situation. A tight blood glucose level control requires frequents measurements and complex algorithms for assessing the insulin dose needed to adjust for short term variations in activity, diet and stress. One of the main features of REACTION is to provide a safe environment by minimizing, but still managing potentially life-threatening situations. Therefore, the platform offers closed-loop feedback to patients, carers and healthcare professionals with important information for effective control of blood glucose levels in all situations. The ultimate goal is to minimize health risks and improve the lives of patients [1]. In this paper we present and discuss the alarm and alert handling system of the REACTION platform.

B. Godara and K.S. Nikita (Eds.): MobiHealth 2012, LNICST 61, pp. 437–444, 2013.

2   REACTION Notification System

The REACTION's Notification System allows healthcare professionals to pre-define notifications and activities to be performed according to a set of pre-defined rules based on individual changes in patients' health status and/or their environment. These notifications, in turn, will facilitate the day-by-day work of healthcare professionals, as well as formal and informal carers, in addition to provide support to patients related to their individual health status. The system is based on a closed cycle that involves patients, healthcare professionals and the informal carers.

It combines the orchestration of services with an underlying efficient networked-based event management solution. The system is composed by the *Global Settings, Alarm Handling, Alarm Tray Details, Personalized Settings* and *Reports.*

The *Global Settings* contains the Rule editor and the Notification editor. The aim of the Rule editor is to set global thresholds in order to identify patients' adverse events based on the analysis of the received information. By default any new rule is defined to be applied to all the patients under the same pathological condition. It is possible to Add/Remove global rules, as well as to combine different parameters such as age, weight, blood glucose, etc. The Notification editor sets the communication channels that will be used (email, short message service or other), the level of the notification (advice, warning, critical), which is associated with different colours (green, yellow and red) depending on the severity of the event.

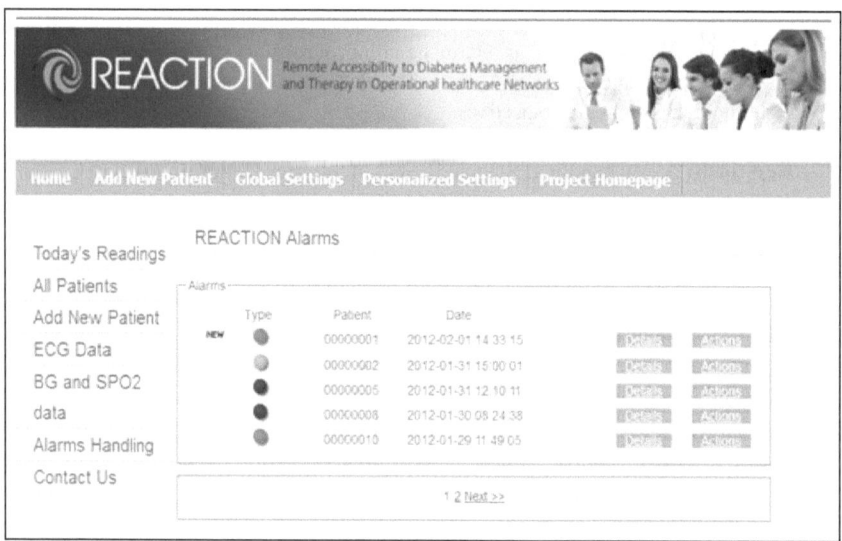

Fig. 1. Alarm Handling Graphical User Interface (GUI)

Fig 1 represents the *Alarm Handling,* where it is possible to visualize the alarms list to better follow the events in the system. The information displayed is the type of alarm, the time and status of the alarm management. It is possible to visualize the alarm details and to enter manual actions required in each specific case. The aim of the *Alarm Tray Details* is to allow the study of the reasons for the alarm, to analyse the different parameters stored in the system (Electrocardiograph (ECG), blood analysis results, etc.) and to know in details the patient status. With this functionality, clinicians will be able to introduce additional actions manually and generate reports.

The *Personalize Settings* (divided in patient selection, alerts and rule editor) module contains the global settings applied by default that can be adapted to the individualized patient's features; it is possible to filter data by status, name or NHS ID (National Health Service Identification). The thresholds can be modified if needed and different ways of communication can be configured for a particular patient. Finally in *Reports*, the clinicians can personalize the information required and add extra information in order to generate .Pdf files summarizing the status of the alarm and the actions taken. It is possible to add to the report snapshots of the parameters, annotations, tables, etc.

3   LinkSmart Web Service Exposure and Rules

The REACTION project uses the former FP6 EU funded project results of the Hydra Middleware [2] (today called LinkSmart) and its semantic model-driven architecture. By a secure Peer-to-Peer (P2P) tunnelling REACTION is able to exploit remote control of medical devices in diverse patient environments [1]. The REACTION platform is based on a Service-Oriented Architecture (SOA) model [3] that supports the collection of loosely coupled services that communicate with each other and where ensembles of them are orchestrated by a specific high-level workflow using the REACTION Service Orchestrator. The rules are executed at any new received data in both automatic and manual transparent way to the end-user facilitating usability.

3.1   Declaring Rules by XSLT

In REACTION there is a need to process incoming events, mainly observations, and for instance generate different types of alerts and or alarms. Event-driven architectures especially in combination with service-oriented approaches are a topic that has drawn much attention recently. The advantage of event driven system is that it provides a loose coupling between different subsystems which provides flexibility.

When an event occurs then a transition (change of state) take place and any alarm responses can be initiated by the occurrence and detection of events corresponding to a pre-defined scheme. In real life, events are typically combined to yield more accurate assessment of the situation (e.g. is the blood sugar level higher than 7.0 mmol/L? AND has the patient been eating within the last 20 minutes?).

The REACTION Data Fusion Engine is able to aggregate data monitoring events with the semantic annotations provided by the REACTION Context Manager. This fulfils the project's strive for the multi-parametric monitoring where methods for fast and reliable evaluation of complex conditions are implemented.

In order for clinicians to express how different events and combinations of events are to be processed we need to provide mechanisms that make it easy to configure rules. These rules are expressed using the Alarms and Alerts GUI, in a semi-natural language form. This includes setting up the rule triggering criteria as well as defining the actions to take. The rules that are entered are translated into an eXtensible Stylesheet Language Transformation (XSLT) format [4]. The use of XSLT then allows easy matching of the rules against the incoming Health Level 7^1 (HL7) message [5] in eXtensible Markup Language (XML) format.

An important aspect of the rule engine is that this approach makes it possible to individualise monitoring schemes for patients depending on the clinician's knowledge of the patient health status.

3.2   Executing Set of Rules

Monitoring and event handling are important aspects of the services and by combining the orchestration of services with an underlying efficient networked-based event management solution a set of pre-programmed rules are able to react ubiquitously to change in the patient's health state and perform some defined activities such as raising an alarm.

Since every device, application and subsystem in REACTION is available as a Web Service (WS), these components can easily be incorporated into the action part of the rules, and used when a rule is triggered. This makes the rules very powerful and the system extensible and customisable to meet different application needs. It is also possible to prioritise the rules depending on their importance in different situations. In certain situations it might be more critical if the blood glucose is out of range then if the blood pressure is, and vice versa.

4   Feedback Generating Services

The main objective of the SMS service is to provide advanced and targeted alerts and notifications to end users, with the use of an instant communication method, the Short Messaging System (SMS), which is available over Global System for Mobile Communications (GSM) networks, to mobile users.

4.1   REACTION SMS Alert and Notification system

The key issues for this service is the advanced user profiling and the cognitive techniques which should be used in order to dynamically compose and send alert and notification messages to the REACTION platform end users, depending on their personal profile and attributes (carers or patients). In general, SMSs are sent as:

- Notifications: If all the requested readings from the sensors have been successfully received, stored and properly examined by the system in the central database, a confirmation SMS is sent to the patient. The text message in this case is also predefined and the purpose of its transmission is basically to reassure the patient that all the readings have been properly received.

---

[1] Framework on related standards to exchange, integrate and share electronic health data.

- Alerts: This function is used for transmitting warning SMSs in order to alert both the carers and the patients, in case the readings received by the REACTION medical sensors used by a patient, show a recrudescence of their vital signs, or in case a serious health risk is detected by the system. These messages will be automatically triggered by the platform, in cases where the data received from the sensors is below or above individually desired levels. This kind of data examination is performed in the central REACTION database through the Rule Engine services. SMS messages may also be composed by carers, through the official REACTION carers' interface. In this case the SMSs are dynamically generated, providing the superintendent carers with the option of writing targeted SMS messages to their patients, including specific medical instructions.

Why use SMS for alerting? SMS is a globally accepted wireless service that enables the transmission of alphanumeric messages among GSM mobile subscribers. The initial version of GSM's short message service was limited to 160 characters per message. Despite that limit, the service became very popular in Europe as a mechanism to exchange text messages between various devices, such as GSM phones, laptops, tablets, Personal Digital Assistants (PDA) and others.

SMS is actually a store-and-forward service that is based on a Short Message Service Center[2] (SMSC) which operates as the store and forward system. Messages can be sent or received over both GSM and General Packet Radio Service (GPRS) channels. GSM uses a large number of logical channels which are mapped onto the physical channels in the radio path. The logical channels are divided in two categories: 1) the Traffic Channels (TCH), and 2) the control channels.

The *control channels* consist of Broadcast Control Channel (BCCH), Common Control Channel (CCCH) and the Dedicated Control Channel (DCCH). The BCCH is a one-to-many unidirectional control channel for broadcasting information from the Base Station (BS) to the mobile terminals (e.g. mobile phones). The CCCH is a point-to-multipoint bidirectional control channel primarily intended to carry signalling information, necessary for handshaking and access management. Finally, the DCCH is a point-to-point, directional control channel. SMS messages are carried from the terminal to the base station over the DCCH channel which consists of the Stand-alone Dedicated Control Channel (SDCCH) and the Slow Associated Control Channel (SACCH). The SDCCH is used before the mobile terminal is assigned a traffic control channel (TCH). It is used to provide authentication to the mobile terminal, for voice call setup and location updates, as well as assignments of TCHs. It is also used for system signalling during idle periods. A slow associated control channel (SACCH) can be linked to either a TCH or a SDCCH. This is continuous data channel carrying information from the mobile, like, for example, measurement reports of received signal strength.

SMS messages are carried on either SDCCH or SACCH depending on the use of the TCH. When the TCH is not available, for example, when there is no voice call or data transfer in progress, SMS messages are delivered over the SDCCH. If a TCH is allocated before a SMS message transfer initiates, the short message uses the SACCH which is associated with that particular TCH. If a TCH is allocated during a short message delivery over a SDCCH (i.e., a voice call or data transfer starts during short

---

[2] An element in the mobile telephone network that handles SMS operations.

message transfer), the short message transaction stops and continues on the SACCH associated with the TCH. If the voice call or data transfer ends, during short message transfer, the short message may either continue on the SACCH associated with the TCH or it may stop and continue delivery using a SDCCH. The sequence of the exchanged messages is similar to that of the voice call setup, with the difference that in the case of SMS message transfer when a traffic channel is not allocated, the SDCCH is not released after authentication, cipher and routing but it is retained, in order to deliver the short message [6].

The fact that SMS messages are being transmitted over data channels means that an active SMS enabled mobile terminal is able to send or receive a short message at any time, independent of whether or not a voice or data call is in progress, while it is possible to deliver a short message even if, due to overloaded network, it is impossible to allocate a voice channel. SMS also guarantees delivery of the message by the network. If the recipient's device is out of range or turned off, or in case that any other failures are identified, the message is stored at the SMSC, until recipient's headset becomes available.

The alert notification system was developed to offer sophisticated end-user services and a medium of immediate feedback to patients and clinicians. The SMS gateway, developed for the REACTION notification system, is a middleware application that accepts requests on a Transmission Control Protocol (TCP) port. The gateway was developed as an external module to REACTION's middleware with the intention to disengage the two and run them on separate boxes, if so required. To this end, the module accepts XML-based requests from the rule engine, instead of using a language specific Application Programming Interface (API).

The SMS routing gateway is a multi-threaded server. The XML-based protocol that was adopted for communication allows any number of clients to interact with the gateway. Each client is responsible for obtaining credits for the gateway, which define the amount of SMS messages the client may send. As stated above, the main communication medium will be text mobile messaging service delivered to personal mobile phones in order also to address the patient confidentiality matters.

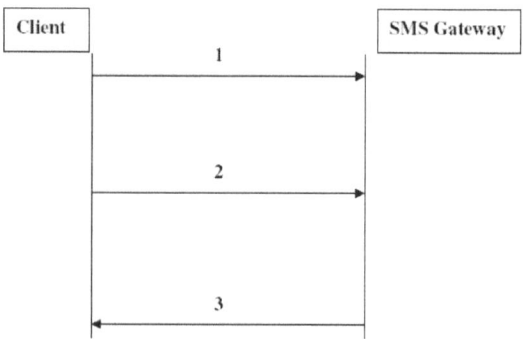

Fig. 2. Client/Server communication on SMS Gateway

Fig 2 illustrates the interaction between the gateway server and a client as a 3-stage process: 1) the client opens a TCP/IP socket connection with the gateway, 2) the client sends through the socket, a request in XML format, and 3) the gateway sends and XML-based response to the client.

4.2   Reading Action XML and Sending Sms

Exactly one message text can be delivered to an arbitrary number of GSM recipients per Hypertext Transfer Protocol (HTTP) request. Elements XML, REQUEST and REACTIONUSER are mandatory in every request. The [request-body] depends on the value of element REQUEST. In order for the SMS gateway to process a request it must first authenticate the client that submits it. The credentials of the client consist of a *username* and a *password* that are issued for every valid client of the gateway. The credentials are part of the REACTION request, enclosed element REACTIONUSER, in child-elements USERNAME and PASSWORD. The *XML elements* to be used are:

- **XML** (mandatory; XML Document Root)
- **REQUEST** (mandatory; transaction type)
- **REACTIONUSER**
    - o **USERNAME** (mandatory; username of REACTION account)
    - o **PASSWORD** (mandatory; password of REACTION account)
- **SUBJECT** (optional; desired originator text "REACTION")
- **RECIPIENTS** (mandatory; list of one or several REACTIONUSERS phone number to receive the SMS message)
- **PHONE** (recipient phone number)
- **MESSAGE** (mandatory)
    - o **TEXT** (mandatory; message text, 1-160 characters in length)
- **MESSAGEID** (optional; message ID number to check status)

The request that the REACTION rule engine submits to the SMS gateway has the syntax displayed above.

```
<?xml version="1.0" standalone="no"?>
<!DOCTYPE XML SYSTEM
"http://gsms.REACTION.com/sms.dtd">
<XML>
   <REQUEST>SENDMESSAGES</REQUEST>
   <REACTIONUSER>
        <USERNAME>user</USERNAME>
        <PASSWORD>pass</PASSWORD>
   </REACTIONUSER>
   <SUBJECT>REACTION</SUBJECT> — [request-body]
   <RECIPIENTS>
        <PHONE>4469XX123456</PHONE>
        <PHONE>3069YY654321</PHONE>
   </RECIPIENTS>
   <MESSAGE>
        <TEXT> Demo REACTION readings-</TEXT>
   </MESSAGE>
</XML>
```

Fig. 3. REACTION request as XML based SMS message

Fig 3 describes the following: the requirements of the project has specified the need for two types of server requests, one for dispatching an SMS and one for retrieving the number of available credits for the REACTION account (latter not depicted in figure). The value of element REQUEST defines the type of instruction submitted to the gateway. The types of requests and a short description for each one are: a) SENDMESSAGES sending the message specified in the request body to a list of recipients, and b) GETCREDITS which returns the number of available credits for the REACTION account.

5   Discussion

The REACTION Alarm and Alert handling system using XSLT as rule format for configuring thresholds and actions to be taken for patients on remote monitoring programme is an efficient and constructive way to demonstrate how the rule engine is able to individualise monitoring schemes for patients.

Consequently, the Alarm notification system is, on a high level, able to react ubiquitously to change in a patient's health state and environment and invoke pre-defined activities according to some pre-programmed rules. These rules may include more complex expressions. The REACTION SMS service is a reliable way to ensure that correct receiver is notified once alarm or alerts are triggered. We suggest XSLT as basis for declarations for rule-oriented electronic health solutions where "smart spaces", interoperability and sensor data are seen as heterogeneously processed [7] or simply where adjacent notifying or actuating subsystems impose XML dependence.

Acknowledgments. This work was performed in the framework of FP7 Integrated Project REACTION (Remote Accessibility to Diabetes Management and Therapy in Operational Healthcare Networks) partially funded by the European Commission. The authors wish to express their gratitude to the members of the REACTION consortium for valuable discussions.

References

1. REACTION project, http://www.REACTION-project.eu
2. Hydra project, http://www.hydramiddleware.eu
3. Ahlsén, M., Asanin, S., Kool, P., Rosengren, P., Thestrup, J.: Service-oriented middleware architecture for mobile personal health monitoring. In: Nikita, K.S., Lin, J.C., Fotiadis, D.I., Arredondo Waldmeyer, M.-T. (eds.) MobiHealth 2011. LNICST, vol. 83, pp. 305–312. Springer, Heidelberg (2012)
4. W3C XSLT, http://www.w3.org/TR/xslt
5. HL7, http://www.hl7.org/
6. Agarwal, N., Chandran-Wadia, L., Apte, V.: Capacity analysis of the GSM short message service. In: National Conference on Communications, Bangalore, India (February 2004)
7. Vergari, F., et al.: An Integrated Framework to Achieve Interoperability in Person-Centric Health Management. Int. J. Telemed. Appl. (2011), doi: 10.1155/2011/549282

Usability Evaluation Plan for Advanced Technology Services for Prevention and Management of Chronic Conditions for the Elderly

Angelina Kouroubali, Ilia Adami, Michalis Foukarakis,
Margherita Antona, and Constantine Stephanidis

Institute of Computer Science, Foundation for Research & Technology-Hellas
100 N. Plastira St, Heraklion, 70013, Crete, Greece
{kouroub,iadami,foukas,antona,cs}@ics.forth.gr

Abstract. This paper analyzes the methodology and preliminary results of the usability evaluation of large scale technology services for the prevention and management of chronic conditions of elderly people. REMOTE, a three years European project in the Ambient Assisted Living domain, aims to define and establish a multidisciplinary and integrated approach to research and development of advanced technology services for addressing real needs of elderly people. The target population included citizens at risk due to geographic and social isolation in combination with specific chronic conditions and the coexistence of lifestyle risk factors, such as obesity, blood pressure, poor eating/drinking habits, stress and others. Technology services provided by the project include wearables and sensors for detecting body temperature, heart rate, human posture, as well as sensors and actuators to be installed in premises for providing context information, such as air temperature, human location and motion. The article presents the usability evaluation plan that was developed for the purposes of the project, as well as some preliminary results from the usability evaluation.

Keywords: Usability evaluation, ambient assisted living, sensors & wearables.

1 Introduction

The elderly population is rising throughout Europe and it has been estimated that between 2010 and 2030 the number of people aged from 65 to 80 will rise by nearly 40%, posing enormous challenges to Europe's society and economy [1]. Policies which address the ageing of the population and the work force focus on enabling older workers to remain active and productive for a longer proportion of their life span [2]. Advanced information and communication technologies (ICT) have the capacity to assist in this issue [3]. For example, using telemonitoring for disease management of heart conditions reduces mortality rates by an estimated 20%. It has also been demonstrated that telemedicine influences the attitudes and behaviour of patients, resulting in better clinical outcomes. In addition, ICTs can assist elderly people, especially individuals with chronic conditions and/or at risk of exclusion, in

B. Godara and K.S. Nikita (Eds.): MobiHealth 2012, LNICST 61, pp. 445–454, 2013.

increasing their self-management capacity [4]. ICTs are particularly useful in establishing a feeling of security and command for aged people in the European countryside [5], strengthening people confidence in leading an independent life at home and delaying, or even fully avoiding, institutionalisation.

The REMOTE project, recognising that isolation of the elderly- both geographical and social- is often a common multiplying risk factor, developed and tested ICT applications and services for health care and management [6]. A user-centred design approach was adopted from planning to execution of the project, with continuous involvement of users to ensure that all relevant facets of subjective quality were successfully delivered, ranging from ethical aspects to accessibility, usability, safety, security, and "customer relationship". The REMOTE technological platform includes

Table 1. The REMOTE platform applications

Application	Explanation
Brain skills trainer	Activities and games for memory support and memory assessment.
Calendar	Allows the user to keep track of daily tasks, schedule appointments, and provides reminders. Medication list and schedule is also viewed in this application.
Environmental control	Allows for remote control of the environment such as lighting and heating.
Guardian Angel	Connects with the BioHarness belt sensor to monitor vital signs and detect falls. It provides alerts based on the thresholds for each user as they have been set in the Healthcare advisor application.
Nutritional Advisor	Provides the user with personalized nutritional content such as menus, nutritional tips, shopping assistance and cooking assistance.
Activity Advisor	Provides an activity plan which the user should follow, joint with advice and tips. The professional has access to questionnaires to understand user needs and design the appropriate activity plan.
Emergency Management	Visualise and manage the automatically driven and patient driven health emergency calls and alerts.
Healthcare Advisor	The physician sets the user's medication schedule. Establish thresholds for vital sign monitoring and review alerts based on these thresholds.
Medical Contact Center	Administrative tool to register new patients, assign services, connect them to health professionals and store personal data ensuring privacy and confidentiality.

mobile, desktop and web applications for remote monitoring of vital signs, and activity status, emergency alerts, organization of activities calendar, environmental control sensors and others[1]. The REMOTE platform offers integration of services to encompass all range of users including physicians, patients and carers. Table 1 presents the applications of REMOTE which were evaluated for usability.

In order to ensure the user-centred approach, the REMOTE project has developed and executed an extensive usability evaluation plan to address usability issues throughout application and system lifecycles. This paper describes the design and implementation of the usability evaluation plan and explains the advantages and disadvantages of this plan for large scale usability evaluations of ICTs. Some preliminary analysis of the evaluation results is also presented.

The evaluation plan was applied to all applications and systems in all pilot sites of the REMOTE project. The usability evaluation methodology aimed at examining what elderly patients, nurses, doctors as well as healthcare professionals and informal carers expected from the proposed technology, as well as assessing the developed applications against the four main usability principles, as outlined by Booth [7], usefulness, ease of use, learnability/memorability, and likeability or satisfaction.

2   Usability Evaluation Plan

This section describes in detail the evaluation plan that was formed for the usability testing of the applications that were developed for the REMOTE project. The evaluation plan was based on existing expert and user-based evaluation techniques and used a combination of recognized qualitative and quantitative usability analysis tools to report the findings. This plan was followed by a total of 9 pilot sites in 6 countries, Germany, Israel, Greece, Spain, Romania, Italy, and Norway, and involved the testing of 9 main applications implemented for mobile and desktop use.

Evaluating large scale systems that involve a variety of applications with integrated services that can be accessed through a unified platform is not an easy endeavour. The evaluation plan needs to follow a solid methodology that can be carried out easily by all parties involved, as well as to produce findings that can be presented in a consistent and homogeneous manner. There are many recognized usability methods available to choose from and many usability metric tools respectively. Jakob Nielsen recommends using more than one method of evaluation, if possible, because one method may uncover issues that the other one missed   [8]. Based on this premise, an evaluation plan was designed for the REMOTE project which consisted of a combination of expert-based, user-based, and home-based evaluation tools. Also, the evaluation plan included qualitative analysis components such as user personal comments and expert observations, as well as quantitative analysis components such as metric usability questionnaires (System User Satisfaction (SUS) questionnaire and user success rate) [9, 10]. The qualitative and quantitative components of the evaluation plan are explained in more detail further down the paper. The evaluation plan consisted of three phases: 1) Expert-based evaluation

---

[1] http://www.remote-project.eu/

phase, 2) User-based evaluation phase in a controlled environment, and 3) User-based evaluation phase at home.

Phase 1 Expert Based Evaluation: The main purpose of the first phase of the REMOTE evaluation plan was to identify and correct any major design flaws and problems before they reached production and real user testing. Expert-based evaluation is generally used to identify usability problems based on established human factors principles [11]. The experts conducting this type of evaluation can be human-computer interaction specialists, usability, and accessibility specialists, or even interface designers with experience in user-centric design principles. There are a few inspection techniques available [8], but the two that were used in the evaluation of the REMOTE applications were expert walkthroughs and heuristics analysis [11, 12]. During the expert walkthroughs, two to five evaluators performed a series of application specific user tasks on working or non-working prototypes, just like a real user would, and identified the areas that could potentially cause confusion or errors to the real users. At the same time, the experts were also asked to rate the application against Jacob Nielsen's Heuristics list of usability principles and guidelines [11]. At the end of the expert evaluation, each evaluator produced a report on the observations he or she made during the inspection and completed a Heuristic analysis questionnaire. These reports were then aggregated in a single report that included the results from all the inspections and was given to the development and design team of the evaluated application. Upon completion of the expert evaluation, the developers incorporated the most important comments into the applications/systems and released the working version of the software in order to proceed for testing with real users.

Phase 2 User Based Evaluation: Once the improved working versions of the applications were released from the developers, the actual user-based evaluation phase began. During this phase, real life usage scenarios and tasks were written for each application and actual users were invited to participate in the evaluations. The tasks had to be clear, precise, and relatively short to accomplish and the chosen evaluation participants had to fit the profile of real life users of the applications/systems as close as possible.

At the beginning of each evaluation session, the participant was introduced to the purpose and the process of the evaluation and was given a brief explanation of how the application worked by the evaluator. The participant was given a User Test Consent Form to sign that stated his or her agreement to participate. The fact that the evaluation was testing the performance of the application and not the performance of the user was also emphasized at that point. A series of representative user tasks was then given to the user to complete sequentially. The participant was requested to openly express his or her thoughts, observations, feelings, and comments to the evaluator during each task. This is known as the Think Aloud method [13], which enables the evaluator to capture the thinking process of the user. The evaluators were instructed to provide assistance only when absolutely needed and keep notes on what was happening and what was being said during each task.

The following three usability measurement tools were used during Phase 2 of the evaluation: 1) System Satisfaction Scale Questionnaire (SUS), 2) User Success Rate, and 3) User Test Analysis. The first two tools were used for the quantitative analysis and the third tool was used for the qualitative analysis of the results.

The System Satisfaction Scale Questionnaire (SUS) [9] is a measurement tool that calculates the total system satisfaction. This questionnaire is a 5 point Likert scale based questionnaire that had to be completed by each test participant right after the test when everything was still fresh in the memory. The User Success Rate is a measurement tool that calculates the overall effectiveness of the system [10]. The evaluator marked in a form if the user completed each task with success (requiring no assistance from the evaluator), with partial success (requiring some assistance), or with failure (giving up on task). The User Test Analysis form was used to gather all the important comments and observations made by each test participant during the test.

It is important to note that the measurement tools are only indicative of the overall usability of the system. There are many factors that affect the scores such as user expertise, the complexity of the user tasks that were given to the participants to complete, the performance of the system and the network where the application was tested, etc. Therefore these scores are meant to be general indicators on how the applications performed.

Phase 3 – Home-Based Evaluation: During the third phase of the evaluation plan, the home-based evaluation, selected users were given a specific REMOTE application/system to use at home for a few days on their own. These users were given a demo of how the application/system worked beforehand. Each user was instructed to complete the home-based evaluation questionnaire at the end of the evaluation period.

3   Usability Evaluation Actions

Each pilot site explored the applications as part of an integrated scenario of daily living and decided upon the user tasks to test for each application. As a result, the applications were tested from different aspects focusing on the most important functions of the application/system. Table 2 provides an example of user tasks for the Guardian Angel application in three different pilot sites. User tasks were used to establish the user success rates. The evaluator introduced each task to the user, and were given to perform these tasks, the evaluator was noting the success, partial success or failure of the user to complete these tasks, in order to calculate the User Success Rate metric.

Participants were also asked to fill out the system user satisfaction questionnaire (SUS) marking each question with 1 to 5, where 1=strongly disagree and 5= strongly agree. The SUS score reflects the overall system usability as perceived by the particular user. Sample questions included *I would use this system frequently*, *The system is unnecessarily complex, I needed to learn a lot of things before using it*.

In addition to these tools, data about the users' profile were maintained taking into consideration, gender, age, health status, education and familiarity with technology. The average primary user profile was a person of 55-77 years of age, with chronic

Table 2. User tasks for Guardian Angel

Pilot Sites	User Tasks
GREECE Pilot A	T1: Once you login to the Guardian Angel application, follow the instructions displayed on the screen. Now press the "Start" button that's located on the belt and then the "Enter" button that is on the screen of the mobile phone.
	T2: Wait for the connectivity between the belt and the phone to establish and then read the vital signs measurements taken.
	T3: When you are done reading the various measurements, exit the application from the phone and take off the belt.
GREECE Pilot B	T1: You have been asked to enter the Guardian Angel application from the main menu. Navigate to the menu and check your breathing rate.
	T2: You have been asked to enter the Guardian Angel application from the main menu. Navigate to the menu and check your heart rate.
	T3: You have been asked to enter the Guardian Angel application from the main menu. Navigate to the menu and check your activity level.
	T4: You have been asked to enter the Guardian Angel application from the main menu. Navigate to the menu and check your posture.
SPAIN Pilot A	T1: Log in to REMOTE on mobile, choose health monitoring option and then Guardian Option
	T2: Place belt around chest, turn the system on; perform tasks for 10 minutes (sitting, sitting and reading; walking)
	T3: Turn off the recording on the mobile and turn off Guadian Angel; remove belt from chest
	T4: Using Health Advisor, check the data recorded

diseases and a slight familiarity with technologies such as personal computers and smart phones.

When dealing with the evaluation of large-scale systems with many sub-components and applications, as much emphasis must be given on how to aggregate and report the results of the evaluations, as on selecting the appropriate usability tools and methods to use. One of the main challenges in applying a common methodological evaluation approach to multiple sites is the accuracy and consistency of reporting the results. To overcome this challenge in REMOTE, special templates were developed to report the results in an aggregate format and were sent to each pilot site along with clear instructions on how to use them. These templates helped towards a uniform reporting of results that allowed a common analysis despite the fact that each pilot site tested different applications. So, at the end of the evaluations, each pilot site was responsible for sending the appropriate filled-out templates and reports with the results, to one central person who then processed them to produce the final results per application accordingly.

The evaluation plan that was used for REMOTE's purposes proved to be efficient and effective in drawing a comprehensive picture of the usability of the entire platform. Its success was not only based on the fact that it incorporated expert-based and user-based evaluation techniques in addition to home-based user trials, but it was also based on the fact that it provided the pilot sites with the necessary reporting tools to aggregate and send-in their results in a homogeneous format saving a great amount of time and effort in their further analysis.

3.1   Analysis and Preliminary Results

The analysis of all user responses across pilot sites per application based on the SUS scores and the User Success Rates scores indicates that the mobile applications received higher SUS scores and user success rates than the desktop ones, as it can be seen in Figure 1 and 2. However, it was concluded that this difference does not mean that one platform was more usable than the other because there are many factors that could have contributed to this difference. For example, the desktop applications offered richer functionality than their mobile counterparts and therefore the tasks used during the evaluation of the desktop applications were more complex in nature than the ones used in the evaluation of the mobile ones. It is very possible that the higher complexity of tasks used in the desktop applications could have caused the lower user success rates and SUS scores. Regardless of this differentiation, it is safe to conclude that both platforms performed above average in the scores, which means that the users perceived them to be easy to use, easy to learn, and useful.

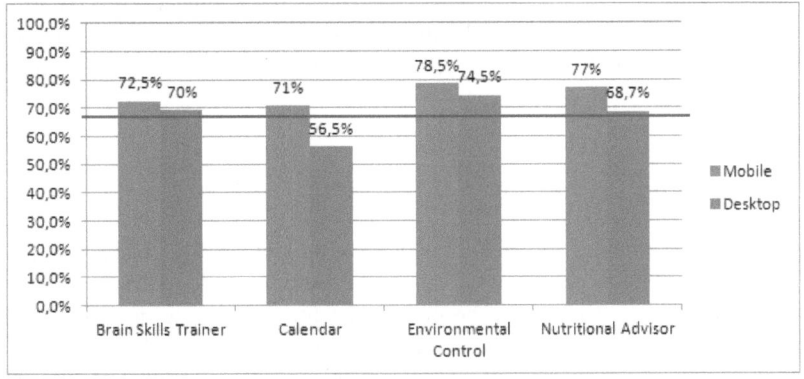

Fig. 1. Total SUS Scores Mobile vs Desktop Applications

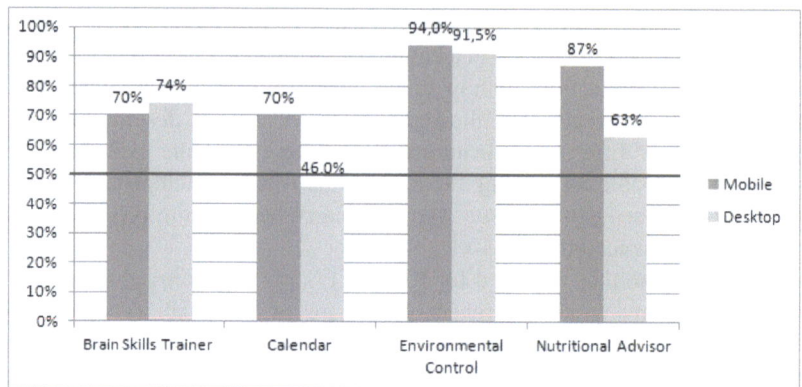

Fig. 2. Total User Success Rates Mobile vs Desktop

Looking at the user comments as they have been captured during the Thinking Aloud process, specific usability issues were identified. Overall, the users were satisfied with the concept of the interoperability of REMOTE's applications. However, difficulties were observed with using some of the application mainly due to the users' lack of experience and familiarity with the technologies involved. The touch screen functionality of the Smart Phones in combination with the small screen of these phones caused challenges in the users with chronic conditions such as Parkinson's, while the use of the keyboard and the mouse in the desktop application was also challenging for a lot of users, who had never used PCs before. Despite these barriers, the users were able to use the applications and complete the majority of the tasks given to them during the evaluations.

The home-based trials were carried out in 4 pilot sites and involved a total of 20 users who were given the Zephyr bio harness and the Nokia Smartphone to use along with the Guardian Angel and the health monitoring applications. The results aggregated from these trials further reinforced the conclusion that the users found the REMOTE platform a useful and usable tool for elderly people that can help in the monitoring of their health on an everyday basis. The platform received high marks for its ability to communicate the users' vital signs measurements directly to their assigned physicians through the mobile phone. The users appreciated the concept and thought that such health-monitoring tools can be very valuable for elderly people to have in their homes.

4   Discussion

Information and communication technologies have the potential to change health care as well as life style for people with chronic conditions [14]. These changes are occurring concurrently and need to be considered for appropriate design of sensor-enhanced health information systems. Basic functionalities of technology services include emergency detection and alarm, disease management, health status feedback and advice [14] as well as social and psychological support. These functionalities are combined differently based on individual conditions as well as individual needs of chronic patients and their informal carers.

A unified usability methodology over pilot sites distributed across Europe is an essential tool for identifying application/system design and functionality issues that go beyond cultural or user profile differences. However, it is important to offer individual evaluation moderators instructions and training not only for conducting the evaluations, but also for reporting of the results. A unified methodological approach can only express its fullest potential if data capture and data reporting is also unified. This aspect can be a great challenge for large implementation projects involving different partners from different countries.

Despite the differentiation of data reporting across sites, the data that was reported offers a valuable basis for improving the design and implementation of the REMOTE applications. Preliminary analysis of the results has shown that elderly users are open to using mobile and desktop applications that may improve their daily life and support their activities. Participants in general welcomed the technology services offered, and thought it would improve their quality of life, resulting in fewer complications. These findings are in accordance with those of other studies about technology management of chronic conditions [15, 16]. The introduction of new technologies for supporting independent living would need to involve appropriate education and adjustment periods to ensure the motivational and psychological support of users. These practices are fundamental in enhancing use of technology services.

5   Conclusions

This paper has presented the methodology and preliminary results of large scale usability evaluation conducted in pilot sites in different European countries.

Participants followed an extensive usability methodology involving heuristic analysis, user-based evaluations, and home trials. It made use of a variety of qualitative and quantitative tools in order to examine the overall usability of the system. In addition, the methodology paid extra attention in the gathering of the results and provided the pilot sites involved with clear instructions and templates to use for reporting purposes. Preliminary results indicate that this is a suitable evaluation plan for large-scale systems and provide the necessary structure to gather data for applications/systems implemented in different settings. However, the interpretation of the results should be handled with care as there are several factors at play which cannot be measured such as cultural issues, background knowledge, etc.

Further work is needed to investigate whether implementation of changes to application and systems based on user comments will improve the opinion of users and their user success rates and user satisfaction scores.

Acknowledgment. This work was performed in the context of the project "ICT based solutions for Prevention and Management of Chronic Conditions of Elderly People" (REMOTE, AAL-2008-1-147) funded but the Ambient Assisted Living (AAL) Joint Programme.

References

1. Giannakouris, K.: Ageing characterises the demographic perspectives of the European societies. In: Population and Social Conditions, Eurostat Statistics in Focus (2008)
2. Eurostat, Demography report 2012: Older, more numberous and diverse Europeans, European Commission (2011)
3. Camarinha-Matos, L.M., Afsarmanesh, H.: Active Ageing Roadmap – A Collaborative Networks Contribution to Demographic Sustainability. In: Camarinha-Matos, L.M., Boucher, X., Afsarmanesh, H. (eds.) PRO-VE 2010. IFIP AICT, vol. 336, pp. 46–59. Springer, Heidelberg (2010)
4. MacAdam, M.: Frameworks of integrated care for the elderly: a systematic review. Canadian Policy Research Networks= Réseaux Canadiens de Recherche en Politiques Publiques (2008)
5. Heenan, D.: How local interventions can build capacity to address social isolation in dispersed rural communities: a case study from Northern Ireland. Ageing International 36(4), 475–491 (2011)
6. Bekiaris, A., Mourouzis, A., Maglaveras, N.: The REMOTE AAL Project: Remote Health and Social Care for Independent Living of Isolated Elderly with Chronic Conditions. In: Stephanidis, C. (ed.) Universal Access in HCI, Part III, HCII 2011. LNCS, vol. 6767, pp. 131–140. Springer, Heidelberg (2011)
7. Booth, P.: An introduction to human-computer interaction. Psychology Press (1989)
8. Nielsen, J.: Heuristic Evaluation. In: Nielsen, J., Mack, R.L. (eds.) Usability Inspection Methods, pp. 25–62. John Wiley and Sons, Inc., USA (1994)
9. Brooke, J.: SUS-A quick and dirty usability scale. In: Usability Evaluation in Industry, vol. 189, p. 194 (1996)
10. Nielsen, J.: Success rate: the simplest usability metric. Jakob Nielsen's Alertbox (2001)
11. Wharton, C., et al.: The cognitive walkthrough method: A practitioner's guide. In: Usability Inspection Methods, pp. 105–140 (1994)
12. Nielsen, J., Molich, R.: Heuristic evaluation of user interfaces. In: Proceedings of the SIGCHI Conference on Human Factors in Computing Systems: Empowering People. ACM (1990)
13. Lewis, C., Rieman, J.: Task-centered user interface design. A Practical Introductio (1993)
14. Haux, R., et al.: Health-enabling technologies for pervasive health care: on services and ICT architecture paradigms. Informatics for Health and Social Care 33(2), 77–89 (2008)
15. Bostock, Y., et al.: The acceptability to patients and professionals of remote blood pressure monitoring using mobile phones. Primary Health Care Research & Development 10(4), 299 (2009)
16. Verhoeven, F., et al.: The contribution of teleconsultation and videoconferencing to diabetes care: a systematic literature review. Journal of Medical Internet Research 9(5) (2007)

Author Index